W= R. Deon
2000

Lameness
in Cattle

Editor

PAUL R. GREENOUGH

FRCVS
Professor Emeritus of Veterinary Surgery
Western College of Veterinary Medicine
University of Saskatchewan
Saskatoon, Saskatchewan, Canada

Associate Editor

A. DAVID WEAVER

BSc, Dr med vet, PhD, FRCVS
Professor Emeritus, University of Missouri–Columbia
Specialist in Cattle Health and Production (Surgery)
Bearsden, Glasgow, Scotland, United Kingdom

Lameness in Cattle

THIRD EDITION

W.B. SAUNDERS COMPANY
A Division of Harcourt Brace & Company

Philadelphia London Toronto Montreal Sydney Tokyo

W.B. SAUNDERS COMPANY
A Division of Harcourt Brace & Company

The Curtis Center
Independence Square West
Philadelphia, Pennsylvania 19106

Library of Congress Cataloging-in-Publication Data

Lameness in cattle / editor, Paul R. Greenough; associate editor, A. David
Weaver.—3rd ed.

p. cm.

Rev. ed. of: Lameness in cattle / Paul R. Greenough, Finlay J. MacCallum, A. David
Weaver. 2nd ed. 1981.

ISBN 0–7216–5205–0

1. Lameness in cattle.   I. Greenough, Paul R.   II. Weaver, A. David
  (Anthony David)   III. Greenough, Paul R.   Lameness in cattle.

SF967.L3L35   1997

636.1′089758—dc20   96-28602

LAMENESS IN CATTLE, 3rd edition   ISBN 0–7216–5205–0

Printed in the United States of America.

Last digit is the print number: 9   8   7   6   5   4   3   2   1

Contributors

Jeremy Bailey, BVSc (Pretoris), MVetSc (Sask), DACVS

Professor, Large Animal Surgery, Western College of Veterinary Medicine, University of Saskatchewan, Saskatoon, Saskatchewan, Canada

Wounds

Uri Bargai, AB (Zool), VMD, DVSc

Head of Large Animals Clinic and Radiology Department, Koret School of Veterinary Medicine, The Hebrew University of Jerusalem, Rehovot, Israel

Radiology

Christer Bergsten, DVM, PhD

Director of Research, Swedish University of Agricultural Sciences Veterinary Faculty, Experimental Station, Skara, Sweden

Infectious Diseases of the Digits

William G. Bickert, PhD, MS

Professor, Agricultural Engineering Department, Michigan State University, East Lansing, Michigan

Housing Considerations Relevant to the Lameness of Dairy Cows

Donald M. Broom, PhD, MA

Professor of Animal Welfare, Department of Clinical Veterinary Medicine, University of Cambridge, Cambridge, United Kingdom

Basic Concepts of Bovine Lameness; Behavior

Jan Cermak, BSc, PhD

ADAS Guildford, Guildford, United Kingdom

Housing Considerations Relevant to the Lameness of Dairy Cows

Donald W. Collick, BVSc, DBR, MRCVS

Private Practice, Delaware Veterinary Group, Castle Cary, Somerset, United Kingdom

Pododermatitis Circumscripta (Sole Ulcer), White Line Disease at the Heel, Traumatic Injuries to the Sole, Heel Horn Erosion, Interdigital Hyperplasia

Nadia F. Cymbaluk, DVM, MSc

Professional Research Associate, Department of Animal and Poultry Science, University of Saskatchewan, Saskatoon, Saskatchewan, Canada

Role of Nutritional Supplements in Bovine Lameness—Review of Nutritional Toxicities

Richard J. Esslemont, BSc, PhD

Senior Lecturer, Department of Agriculture, University of Reading, Reading, Berkshire, United Kingdom

Basic Concepts of Bovine Lameness

James G. Ferguson, DVM, Dr med vet, MSc

Professor, Large Animal Surgery, Western College of Veterinary Medicine, University of Saskatchewan, Saskatoon, Saskatchewan, Canada

The Physis; Principles of Bovine Orthopedics; Surgery of the Distal Limb; Surgical Conditions of the Proximal Limb

Francisco A. Galindo, PhD, MVZ

Professor and Head of the Department of Ethology, Facultad de Medicina Veterinaria y Zootecnia, Universidad Nacional Autonóma de México, Coyoacán D.F, México

Basic Concepts of Bovine Lameness; Behavior

Paul R. Greenough, FRCVS

Professor Emeritus of Veterinary Surgery, Western College of Veterinary Medicine, University of Saskatchewan, Saskatoon, Saskatchewan, Canada

Basic Concepts of Bovine Lameness; Conformation, Growth; White Line Disease at the Toe (Toe Ulcer), Vertical Fissure (Sand Crack), Horizontal Grooves and Fissures, Traumatic Exungulation; Methyl Methacrylate and Claw Prosthetics; Applied Anatomy; Laminitis: Grass Founder; Management and Control of Claw Lameness—An Overview

Pieter Kloosterman, Ing

Head of Hoofcare Division and Course Coordinator of Hoofcare, I.P.C. Livestock/Dairy Training Centre, Friesland, Oenkerk, The Netherlands

Claw Care

Jeff C. H. Ko, DVM, MS, Diplomate ACVA

Assistant Professor of Anesthesiology, Department of Large Animal Clinical Sciences, College of Veterinary Medicine, University of Florida, Gainesville, Florida

Anesthesia and Chemical Restraint

Horst W. Leipold, Dr med vet, PhD (Deceased)

Professor, Department of Veterinary Pathology, University of Kansas, Manhattan, Kansas

Congenital Defects of the Musculoskeletal System

Ben T. McDaniel, PhD, MS

Professor, Animal Science and Genetics, North Carolina State University, Raleigh, North Carolina

Genetics of Conformation

Peter Ossent, Dr med vet

Lecturer, Faculty of Veterinary Medicine, University of Zurich, Zurich, Switzerland

Laminitis

John W. Pharr, DVM, MS, Diplomate ACVR

Professor, Veterinary Radiology, Western College of Veterinary Medicine, University of Saskatchewan, Saskatoon, Saskatchewan, Canada

Radiology

Kimberly A. Redic-Kill, Pharm D, BCPS

Director of Pharmacy, Veterinary Teaching Hospitals, College of Veterinary Medicine, University of Minnesota, St. Paul; Clinical Assistant Professor, College of Pharmacy, University of Minnesota, Minneapolis, Minnesota

Clinical Pharmacology

Randy D. Shaver, PhD, MS

Extension Dairy Nutritionist, Department of Dairy Science, University of Wisconsin, Madison, Wisconsin

Nutrition

Marion Smart, DVM, PhD

Professor, Department of Internal Medicine, Western College of Veterinary Medicine, University of Saskatchewan, Saskatoon, Saskatchewan, Canada

Role of Nutritional Supplements in Bovine Lameness—Review of Nutritional Toxicities

Laura Smith-Maxie, DVM, MSc

Associate Professor, Department of Clinical Studies, Ontario Veterinary College, University of Guelph, Guelph, Ontario, Canada

Diseases of the Nervous System

Christian Stanek, Dr med vet, Dr habil

Professor, Klinik Für Orthopädie Bei Huf-und Klauenteieren, Veterinarmediziniche Universitat, Vienna, Austria

Examination of the Locomotor System; Tendons and Tendon Sheaths

John C. Thurmon, DVM, MS, Diplomate ACVA

Professor of Veterinary Clinical Medicine and Head of Anesthesiology, Department of Veterinary Clinical Medicine, College of Veterinary Medicine, University of Illinois, Urbana, Illinois

Anesthesia and Chemical Restraint

Ava M. Trent, DVM, MVSc, Diplomate ACVS

Associate Professor, Large Animal Surgery and Associate Dean, Academic and Student Affairs, Department of Veterinary Clinical Studies, College of Veterinary Medicine, University of Minnesota, St. Paul, Minnesota

Clinical Pharmacology

Jos J. Vermunt, DVM, MSc, MACVSc

Southern Rangitikei Veterinary Services, Bulls, New Zealand

Laminitis; Management and Control of Claw Lameness—An Overview

A. David Weaver, BSc, Dr med vet, PhD, FRCVS

Professor Emeritus, University of Missouri–Columbia, Columbia, Missouri; Specialist in Cattle Health and Production (Surgery), Bearsden, Glasgow, Scotland, United Kingdom

Basic Concepts of Bovine Lameness; Traumatic Injuries to the Interdigital Space; Joint Conditions; Muscles and Neoplasms; Spastic Paresis (Elso Heel); Downer Cow Syndrome

Preface

Over 20 years ago the problem of bovine lameness justified publication of the first edition of *Lameness in Cattle*. The second edition, in 1981, emphasized lameness problems arising in large intensive dairy and beef units. Increased awareness of the economic importance and animal welfare issues associated with lameness resulted in increased research and the development of a very active international forum for workers interested in bovine digital disorders. A third edition was needed to reflect these changes.

The significant advance of the past decade has been to consider lameness as a herd problem rather than one that affects the individual animal. The adoption of herd health programs has led to the maintenance of better records and the emergence of hard facts concerning lameness. There is a widespread and better appreciation of the economic losses.

Numerous risk factors are involved in the etiology of lesions that cause lameness. The complicated meshwork of these factors has resulted in a need for a multiauthor format to cover the numerous disciplines and specialties. The combination of contributions from nonveterinarians (nutritionists, animal behaviorists, animal scientists) and veterinary scientists (anesthetists, radiologists, surgeons, clinicians) is our attempt to present recent research and contemporary views rather than anecdotal concepts.

Every effort has been made to retain the basic information needed to manage lameness in the "on farm" situation. As in previous editions, we write for the applied scientist in the broadest sense—the practicing veterinarian, the progressive farmer, and the range of professional agricultural advisors—as well as for undergraduate veterinary and agricultural students. Our aim also has been to establish an internationally acceptable basis for applied research that will be conducted under varying conditions around the world. This effort will prove worthwhile if there is an increased perception of the suffering caused by lameness and an appreciation of the scientific measures that can be adopted to ameliorate the problem.

We wish to express our appreciation to our contributors. They have all accepted our editorialization with good grace. Creating uniformity without duplication or overkill has imposed constraints on some. Their generosity to the cause is appreciated. We wish to pay tribute to our late colleague, Finlay MacCallum, who made great contributions to the first two editions. We also wish to acknowledge contributions by the late Horst W. Leipold. Finally, we wish to thank the staff of W.B. Saunders for their help, patience, and exertive encouragement.

PAUL R. GREENOUGH
A. DAVID WEAVER

NOTICE

Food animal medicine is an ever-changing field. Standard safety precautions must be followed, but as new research and clinical experience grow, changes in treatment and drug therapy become necessary or appropriate. The authors and editors of this work have carefully checked the generic and trade drug names and verified drug dosages to assure that dosage information is precise and in accord with standards accepted at the time of publication. Readers are advised, however, to check the product information currently provided by the manufacturer of each drug to be administered to be certain that changes have not been made in the recommended dose or in the contraindications for administration. This is of particular importance in regard to new or infrequently used drugs. Recommended dosages for animals are sometimes based on adjustments in the dosage that would be suitable for humans. Some of the drugs mentioned here have been given experimentally by the authors. Others have been used in dosages greater than those recommended by the manufacturer. In these kinds of cases, the authors have reported on their own considerable experience. It is the responsibility of those administering a drug, relying on their professional skill and experience, to determine the dosages, the best treatment for the patient, and whether the benefits of giving a drug justify the attendant risk. The editors cannot be responsible for misuse or misapplication of the material in this work.

THE PUBLISHER

Contents

General Considerations

Paul R. Greenough   *Canada*

A. David Weaver   *United Kingdom*
Donald M. Broom
Richard J. Esslemont

Francisco A. Galindo   *Mexico*

1

Basic Concepts of Bovine Lameness

ANIMAL WELFARE

Interest in animal welfare has increased spectacularly in recent years, and the Animal Welfare Foundation of the British Veterinary Association annual review 1993–1994 "identified lameness in farm animals as a welfare issue of particular concern and lists research on lameness as a priority for the future." The same review points out that "if it were possible to reduce substantially the incidence of lameness (in all farm species [including poultry]), this single initiative, more than any other would benefit more animals than any others."[1]

How serious is lameness for an individual animal? In what ways does it affect the welfare of that animal? If welfare is defined as the state of the animal in terms of its attempts to cope with its environment, how is it best assessed in lame animals? The assessment of pain is far from simple because in certain situations it might be wholly disadvantageous for an animal to display signs of pain. For lame cattle, indications of pain are obvious in the changed gait of an animal, and it seems reasonable to assume that the greater the disruption of this normal movement, the more intense the pain is likely to be. The degree of pain, however, remains unknown.

Various techniques such as measuring the effects of administering analgesics or even direct recording, such as from the sensory nerves from pain receptors, might provide some information about pain level. Locomotion scoring can be a system for assessing the prevalence, severity, and duration of lameness (see Fig. 1–2). Cows do not change their pattern of locomotion to any great extent on any particular surface unless they have some pain or discomfort. Such abnormalities of walking may also have adverse consequences for muscles or bones or may increase the likelihood of injury.

Another way in which behavior measurements can give information about welfare in relation to lameness is by indicating how much an animal is prepared to work or to forgo reward to avoid discomfort. An animal may give up its social position and reduce the number of times it walks to obtain resources. In extreme circumstances, a cow may reduce its consumption of food and water to avoid painful experiences during walking.

The social structure within the group and the building design are important factors to consider when using behavioral measures to assess lameness and its effect on welfare. These factors are discussed in Chapter 19.

Farmers in the United Kingdom are forbidden to transport lame farm stock to markets or slaughterhouses. Such stock must be slaughtered on the farm. The phrase "causing unnecessary pain and suffering" is the key. Because certification as "fit to travel" may be issued by the farmer's veterinarian or by the farmer himself, the responsibility can be placed on either person. This policy of the Ministry of Agriculture, Fisheries and Food has undoubtedly contributed to the awareness of lame cattle on the farm.

The ethical responsibilities of the owner, manager, or stockperson involved with these animals should be directed toward attainment and maintenance of freedom from pain, injury, and disease; from fear and distress; and, in chronically ill animals, from prolonged discomfort.

ECOPATHOLOGY AND EPIDEMIOLOGY AS TOOLS

Lameness has a multifactorial etiology. The term *ecopathology* has been used to describe the study of the relationships between the pathology and the risk factors that may be implicated in the etiology of the disease process (Fig. 1–1).[26]

Another investigative tool in research and herd health management is epidemiological evaluation. The process, widely adopted in bovine herd lameness studies, uses ecopathologically defined parameters[13] for the purpose of

• Problem recognition

• Data collection

• Data analysis

• Prediction

- Establish farmer's confidence
- Intervention (treatment, control)

TERMINOLOGY

Terminology continues to confuse the understanding of different digital problems. New and accurate terminology has been published with appropriate descriptions, but the use of these guidelines is not universal. This observation was underlined by the need to specially train veterinarians who were cooperating in recent research projects during which they were required to correctly identify lameness-causing lesions.[8, 26, 36]

Colloquial expressions continue to be used commonly in many languages. The classical example is the North American term *footrot*, which includes interdigital necrobacillosis but, depending on the particular textbook, may include almost any bacterial infection of any part of the digit including the coronary band and heels. After meetings of a specialist group interested in bovine digital disease in Utrecht (1976) and Skara (1978), 11 terms were established. The principle was to use Latin and to describe in each term the area of the digit and characteristics of the lesion. These terms are given throughout this text (see Chapters 7 and 8). These terms have also been illustrated in a small color atlas.[14]

It is therefore recommended that scientists should whenever possible use the established terminology in the title of papers or for the first mention of a disease (with the colloquial term in parentheses).

Anatomical terminology is clarified in Chapter 14. Misuse of this terminology is exemplified by the regular appearance of the term *P3* to describe the distal phalanx, which is otherwise called the *pedal* or *coffin bone*. The term *foot* may continue in lay parlance, but in descriptive literature, *digital region* or *claw* is preferable.

SYSTEMIC DISEASE

Bovine lameness is a classical multifactorial problem (see laminitis, p. 277, and nutrition, p. 293). Lameness may be a sign of systemic disease, and it would be remiss to ignore the fact that the most infectious systemic bovine condition, foot and mouth disease (FMD), may herald its arrival in a particular region by signs of lameness in one or more stock. This was the case in the last (1981) United Kingdom outbreak of FMD on the Isle of Wight, when a farmer noticed a lame animal in a group of 19 dry cows one day and found 16 of the group to be lame, as well as showing other systemic signs, the following morning.[10] Any investigation of lame cattle should therefore rule out the possibility of FMD.

INCIDENCE AND PREVALENCE

How big a problem, in numerical terms, is bovine lameness? Clarkson[7] has pointed out the pitfalls in

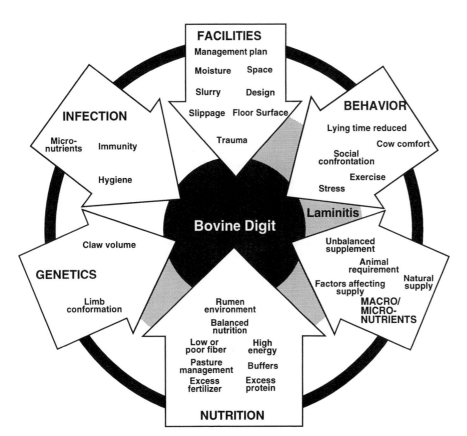

Figure 1–1. Lameness has a multifactorial etiology. Many of the "risk factors" are of concern to the ecopathologist.

various methods of data collection, with particular reference to lameness. Few countries have published any accurate data, and recording methods vary widely. Some extensive surveys (United Kingdom) have covered only veterinary visits to lame cattle, inevitably leading to a gross underestimation of total lameness because most cattle are not examined by a veterinarian or indeed even by a farmer or stockperson. Programs that have been devised for accurate recording of all lame cattle tend to be biased toward selected farms with a relatively high standard of management. Ten years ago, incidence figures in the United Kingdom were about 25% (lame dairy cows per annum). A recent extensive survey of 37 farms in England and Wales revealed that about 60% of dairy cows were lame annually,[8] whereas another source[15] recorded 36% in 63 dairy herds linked by the DAISY program of Reading University.

National data do not exist for any country except Israel,[4] where the incidence was less than 5% in the Hachaklait computer database (covering more than 95% of all dairy cattle). This 10-fold variation in incidence reflects very different husbandry conditions in areas of high-producing dairy cattle. The Israeli dairy herds, the highest producers in the world, are fed a total mixed ration in covered yards, where climate ensures a dry floor for the entire year. Data recording in the Israeli herd is veterinarian generated, and some underreporting can have artificially arisen.

In Chiba, Japan,[39] the average incidence of lameness in dairy cows is low, at 2.7%.

Caution must be exercised when interpreting reports flowing from studies of the incidence of locomotor problems. Variables include not only the region, climate, and type of husbandry (dairy, beef intensive or extensive) but also the method of data collection (farmer, veterinarian), classification (diagnosis, severity, incidence or prevalence), and statistical evaluation of the data. Hence, direct comparisons should be made with caution.

Data are essential to establish the economic significance of lameness and to evaluate the descriptive epidemiology of lameness or the major trends such as the impact of intensive management on the emergence of new problems (e.g., digital dermatitis). In 1994, digital dermatitis in dairy cows had reached nearly epidemic proportions in certain regions of some countries (e.g., California) but is almost unknown in the western Canadian plains. Vertical fissures are a plague on the Canadian prairies but of little significance elsewhere in the country. Subclinical laminitis was only recognized some 15 years ago, but by virtue of increased awareness, it appears to have a higher incidence today than it did then. The accuracy of changes in the incidence over time is uncertain because knowledge and awareness have also changed.

The frequency of the occurrence of lameness can be expressed in several different ways, including annual incidence, prevalence, and case, herd, and seasonal incidence.

ANNUAL INCIDENCE

Annual incidence measures the total quantity of lameness that veterinarians, farmers, or other persons observe in a population of cattle in 1 year. A new case of lameness is defined as the first occasion on which a lame cow was examined or when the same cow was lame in a different limb or in the same limb 28 days or more since the previous record. One United States university Holstein herd had an incidence of 35% to 56% during a 5-year period.[35] Clarkson[8] reports a mean annual incidence rate for 37 farms in England and Wales of 59.5%. This is much higher than those reported by previous workers,[2, 28, 38] whose figures range from 25% to 30%.

Other workers have reported much lower figures (7.3%, 5.5%), probably because their studies were based on records kept by veterinary surgeons and did not include cows treated by farmers.[12, 30] Whitaker and colleagues,[38] in recording an incidence of 25%, found 6.3% being treated by veterinarians and 18.7% by farmers.[38]

Beef cattle on slatted floors had a 43% incidence of septic traumatic pododermatitis after penetration of the toe region or white line, compared with 1% incidence in cattle in straw yards.[24]

Weaver[35] recorded an average of 31 days' duration for 303 digital lameness cases and 22 days for 63 non-digital lameness cases (difference not statistically significant). Tranter and Morris[33] found the average duration of lameness to be 27 ± 19 days.

PREVALENCE

No large-scale surveys of prevalence of lameness (number of cases at any given time), as opposed to incidence, have been published. It is theoretically possible to have an annual lameness incidence of 50% in a 100-cow herd yet to have, if each lame cow shows signs for 7 days and the incidents are equally spread throughout the year, a prevalence rate of 1%.

Seventeen midwestern United States herds had a prevalence of clinical lameness of 13.6% in the summer and 16.7% in winter/spring. These figures are more than twice the values estimated by the herd personnel.[37] The annual incidence was not stated in this abstract.

In a Dutch study[32] of 2121 dairy cows, only 1.2% of which were clinically lame, most cows had at least one disorder of the hind claws: interdigital dermatitis was very common (83.1% of examined cows). Digital dermatitis (17.6%), discrete (75%) or diffused (75%) lesions of pododermatitis aseptica (laminitis), solar ulceration (5.5%), white line lesions (12.1%), and sole cavitation (4.9%) were important; and only 0.4% showed phlegmona interdigitalis (interdigital necrobacillosis).

Confusion can also arise in distinguishing "lesions" from "lesions causing lameness." The Dutch study revealed that most of these Dutch cows had lesions indicative of subclinical digital disorders. Similarly, foot disorders were diagnosed in 97.8% of 759 milking cows in a Costa Rica survey.[5] The most prevalent diseases were laminitis (77%), interdigital dermatitis (52%), white line separation (66%), solar contusion (13%), and double sole (12%).

CASE INCIDENCE OF LAMENESS

The case incidence of lameness represents the number of cases (= occurrences) of lameness in a given period of time. For example, Esslemont and Spincer[15] stated that the average quantity of lameness in 63 herds involved in the DAISY scheme was 35.6 cases per 100 cows, or 20.4% of the herd affected, with each cow having an average of 1.4 incidents.

HERD INCIDENCE OF LAMENESS

The frequency distribution of cases of lameness in 63 herds studied by Esslemont and Spincer[15] showed that the best quartile (top quarter of the population) of herds, considered to be target levels, achieved as low as 6.2 cases per 100 cows and the worst quartile 74.8 cases. Arkins in Ireland[2] found that the dairy herd incidence (cases) varied from 7% to 61% whereas the animal incidence varied from 6% to 44%. In contrast, Clarkson and colleagues[8] report an annual herd animal incidence of lameness in 37 herds varying from 9.3% to 200.7%.

SEASONAL INCIDENCE OF LAMENESS

The 3-month period postpartum has the highest incidence of lameness. The seasonal incidence of lameness in dairy cows[12, 28, 30] may be skewed by the calving season. Wells and colleagues[36] report a prevalence of 13.6% in summer and 16.7% in late winter. Similar trends have been reported by others.[2, 28, 30]

DISTRIBUTION OF DIGITAL LESIONS

Reports on the distribution of digital lesions within a population of cattle shed some light on disease trends and importance. The conditions listed in the first five rows of Table 1–1 are allegedly associated with the occurrence of subclinical laminitis. A decrease in the reported incidence of interdigital phlegmon since 1980 may not represent an absolute reduction. This statistic could denote greater adoption of (unreported) treatment by farmers but more likely is a reflection of the increased incidence of other lesions during the period. The high incidence of pododermatitis circumscripta reported by Choquette-Levy and colleagues[6] is also an interesting statistic because these workers examined all of the digits in a population, not only those of lame animals.

The compilation of Table 1–1 is confused by problems of terminology. Underrunning of the sole[17] in current terminology would be termed a *double sole*. Reference to overworn soles in a clinical context possibly indicates bruising of the sole. It is extremely important that terminology be expanded to describe an increased range of lesions and permit greater precision (see Fig. 1–2(3), Classification of Lesion).

PRODUCTION LOSSES AND THE COST OF LAMENESS

Lameness results in decreased performance measured in various parameters:

TABLE 1–1. DISTRIBUTION OF DIGITAL LESIONS

Description of Lesions	Clarkson et al[8]	McLennan[21a]	Choquette-Levy et al[6]	Russell et al[30]	Eddy and Scott[12]
Pododermatitis circumscripta (sole ulcer)	28	2.3	48.5	12	11.4
White line disease	22	8.4	11.8	16.6	34.9
Heel erosion	4	3.3	11.8		
Double or underrun sole	3			6.8	1.9
Laminitis	1.5	1.4	1.2	3.2	
Interdigital hyperplasia	5	2.3	1.6	4.2	1.7
Footrot	5	15	7.3	15.8	14.4
Bruising	8				
Retroarticular abscess	3	5.1	1.6	3.9	
Septic arthritis of distal interphalangeal joint					
Vertical fissure (sand crack)	0.5	4.7	2		3.4
Claw deformity	2				
Digital dermatitis	8				
Foreign body	5	2	8.5	14.3	27.4
Interdigital dermatitis	1				
Other	4		5.7		

Clarkson et al[8]: UK; Lancashire, Cheshire, Wales, Somerset
McLennan[21a]: Australia
Choquette-Levy et al[6]: Quebec
Russell et al[30]: UK; 40 practices
Eddy and Scott[12]: UK; Somerset

TABLE 1–2 COST OF A CASE OF SOLE ULCER

	$	£
Cost of treatments including veterinarian's time	65.00	40.54
(1 @ $40.00 [£25.00], 1 @ $19.00 [£12.00], 2 @ $2.80 [£1.77] turnout)		
Herdsman's time (5 hours @ $6.40 [£4.00]/hour)	32.00	20.00
Costs of culling, 18% of $1380 (£862)*	248.00	155.16
Cost of longer to conception (40 days @ $5.36 [£3.35])	214.00	134.00
Cost of extra service, 0.72 @ $32.00 (£20.00)	23.00	14.40
Yield reduction (180 liters @ $0.26 [0.1623]/liter)	47.00	29.21
Milk withdrawal (180 liters @ $0.35 [£0.1967]/liter)	22.00	13.78
Cost of extra 0.4 case	47.00	29.73
Costs of 1.4 cases per cow	699.00	436.82

*See footnote, Table 1–3.

- Decreased feed intake from impaired ambulation and increased recumbency
- Decreased body weight as a direct effect of the reduced feed intake
- Decreased milk production
- Decreased sexual activity (e.g., reduced signs of estrus), and, resulting from this, decreased fertility

Economic losses are directly related to:

- Decreased production (milk, meat), poorer reproductive performance (prolonged calving interval)
- Increased culling rate with possible partial or total carcass condemnation at slaughter
- Higher veterinary costs
- Increased labor demand for management and treatment of lame cattle

Several workers have estimated the annual cost of lameness in various countries. Whitaker and colleagues[38] thought that in the United Kingdom each farmer is faced with a loss of $280 (£175) for every 100 cows. Other workers place the annual cost of lameness to the dairy industry in the United Kingdom at $24,000,000 (£15,000,000) annually.[3, 27] Digital disease in dairy cattle in Quebec[6] is estimated to cost $10,000,000 per annum. In Australian herds, the estimated cost was $45 per cow per annum.[18] The annual cost of digital dermatitis in California[29] is estimated at $12 million.

Tables 1–2 to 1–5 demonstrate the economic effect of lameness on herd efficiency. These data suggest that the national estimates for losses due to lameness may be grossly underestimated if all costs are added in. Note that the major items are reduced fertility and cull costs, which include cost of a replacement. These two items account for 55% to 67% of the total costs of clinical lameness. The veterinary costs are a minor item in comparison. Such information is useful in encouraging farmers to undertake preventive measures. These figures do not take ac-

TABLE 1–3 COST OF A CASE OF DIGITAL LAMENESS

	$	£		
Costs of treatments including veterinarian's time (1 @ $32 [£20], 2 @ $12 [£7.50], plus $2.80 [£1.77] turnout)	58.00	36.77		
Herdsman's time (3 hours @ $6.40 [£4]/hour)	19.00	12.00		
Cost of culling, 11% of $1368 [£862]*	151.00	94.82		
Cost of longer calving to conception (9 days @ $5.36 [£3.35])	48.00	30.15		
Cost of extra services, 0.39 @ $32 [£20]	12.00	7.80		
Yield reduction (120 liters @ $0.26 [£0.1623])	31.00	19.48		
Milk withdrawal (30 liters @ $0.315 [£0.1967])	28.00	17.70		
Cost of extra 0.4 case	42.00	26.59		
Cost of 1.4 cases per cow	389.00	245.31		
*Cost of an extra cull	$		£	
Sale of cull at 520 Kg at $1.12 (£0.70)/kg	582		364	
Heifer cost to buy	1600		1000	
Difference		1018		636
Reduced production from heifers: 1000 liters × $0.26 (16.23 p)	259		162	
Lower value of calf from heifer	102		64	
		361		226
Total net cost		1379		862

TABLE 1–4. COST OF A CASE OF INTERDIGITAL LAMENESS

	$	£
Costs of treatments (1 @ $12 [£7.50], 1 @ $11 [£7], turnout)	34.00	21.13
Herdsman's time (1 hour)	5.60	3.50
Cost of longer calving to conception (17 days @ $5.36 [£3.35]/day)	79.00	49.64
Cost of extra service 0.2 @ $32 (£20)	6.00	4.00
Yield reduction (60 liters @ $0.135 [£0.196]/liter)	18.00	11.76
Single case total	138.00	90.03
Cost of extra 0.4 of a case	16.00	9.85
Cost of 1.4 cases per cow	154.60	99.88

count of the unquantifiable subclinical cases of lameness.

Schepers and Dijkhuisen[31] stated that when calculating disease losses, it is necessary to ask three questions:

- To what extent does the disease in its various forms occur?

- What are the quantitative and qualitative effects of production, culling, and so on?

- How can these physical effects be expressed in financial terms?

CAUSES OF LOSS

Treatment. In the United Kingdom in 1994, an animal needing veterinary attention incurs a daytime call-out fee of $26 (£16) (or proportion of it) and time at $96 (£60) per hour, as well as the costs of treatment. On average, a cow that becomes lame once has a 1.6 times greater chance of having another problem during the same lactation, thus further increasing treatment costs.

Discarded Milk. Discarded milk due to drug treatment is charged at $0.31 (19.67 pence) per lost liter.

Yield Reduction. The reduction in milk production depends on the severity and duration of the lameness and the period during the lactation when the incident occurs. The marginal net loss (value of milk less purchased feed) would be $0.26 (16.23 pence) per liter. Although it is assumed that the farmer would feed to the level of production, thus reducing concentrate consumption, in many cases the lame cows are in fact fed concentrates at an unchanged rate, thus further inflating costs.

Feed Intake. Reluctance to walk reduces an animal's ability to forage or compete for feed. Lame cows at summer grass lie down longer and graze less than normal cows.[19] A painful lameness causes a reduction in appetite. The cow produces less milk and loses weight, using up fat and even muscle reserves to survive. In a small study,[35] body condition score dropped by an average of 0.8 unit in 30 of 35 cows with a digital lameness (range 0.5 to 2.0). The cow may be 100 to 200 kg lower in weight than normal, and this severely affects market value.

Reproductive Problems. The effect of negative energy balance increases the likelihood of failure to conceive. Decreased sexual activity at a postpartum estrus due to reluctance to move and to mount and an increased lying time all are likely to prolong the calving-conception interval. If anestrus is present, a cow not only fails to be inseminated but may also be treated by a veterinarian. Cows in poor condition are not likely to respond to treatment. Lowered fertility requires more inseminations, which, irrespective of the outcome, involve the additional cost of $32 (£20) per insemination. The cost of an extra day on the calving index may be $5.35 (£3.35) per day beyond 365 days.

The incidence of lameness has been correlated with reduced fertility.[9] Mean days open were increased by 28 days in a Pennsylvania study.[20] This would today be equivalent to $93 (£58) loss on each cow.

TABLE 1–5. AVERAGE COST OF A CASE OF LAMENESS

	Prevalence	$	£
Cost of a case of interdigital lameness @ $160 (£99.88)	0.33	53.00	32.96
Cost of a case of digital lameness @ $392 (£245.31)	0.33	129.00	80.95
Cost of a case of sole ulcer @ $700 (£436.82)	0.33	230.00	144.1
Average cost of a case of lameness		412.00	258.0

Opportunistic Cost. When herdsmen spend time with lame cows, some say that no cost should be added because that is their job. However, these workers have other even more valuable tasks that are being neglected. Perhaps they could be better employed watching for cows coming in heat or attending to feeding. They could miss some essential time off. Whatever the "opportunistic cost," a lame cow demands extra time, costing about $6.40 (£4) per hour, from the stockperson in respect to both treatment and general management.

Culling. Even if a cow does conceive, it may be culled if the dry period is calculated to be uneconomical. Involuntary culling due to lameness can lead to a reduced rate of genetic gain, which reduces the long-term efficiency of the herd. Culling for lameness usually ranks after infertility, udder problems, and low production, which may in some cases mask a primary lameness problem resulting in a poor yield. "Feet and legs" accounted for only 1.2% of culls in New York State herds,[22] 7.7% in a Swiss study,[16] and 14% in German Holstein-Friesians.[11]

Cows should live productively for six or seven lactations (not the four we almost achieve). The cost of losing a cow early includes the difference between the cull price and the cost of replacement. The replacement cost should be determined as the cost of rearing including feed, labor, buildings, and interest. Today (1996) this amounts to $1680 (£1050). If the replacements are on land that could be better used for producing milk (or something else), then another opportunity cost should be added. This amounts to another $320 (£200) per replacement. To this cost should be added the cost of profit forgone on the animal that has been culled, which, had she stayed healthy for two or three more lactations, would have made higher net profits for the herd than the lactation yields of the replacement.

It is assumed that the cost of an extra cull due to severe lameness is high because the cow may reach a sale weight of only 520 kg, achieving a price of $590 (£370).

Susceptibility to Other Diseases. Lame cows have been shown to be more susceptible to other diseases (usually indirectly) such as mastitis.[25]

The cost of lameness in a 100-cow herd (cost per herd and cost per cow in herd) can reach very large sums, adding up to $21,150 (£13,219) in a herd in which 56% of the animals were lame. This herd is in the worst quartile in the country, with about 40% of the lame cows incurring costs of $15,488 (£9680). The top quartile of herds loses approximately $3450 (£2150), and thus the benefit of improving the herd from the worst quartile to the best is $12,050 (£7530) per herd per year. Once the improvement is brought about by good housing and husbandry, this benefit should accrue each year that good management continues.

RECORDS

CODING AND CLASSIFICATION

A lesion coding system is summarized in the data capture form (Fig. 1–2). A lameness record should include fields such as the following:

- Herd ID (identity)
- ID of the animal, either ear tag, tattoo, or freezebrand
- Severity of lameness (score 1 to 5)
- Date of incident (lameness)
- Region affected (limb, claw)
- Region of the sole (1 to 7)
- Diagnosis of lesion (selection from list)
- Degree of severity of lesion (score 1 to 5)
- Body condition score and weight
- Treatment

The term *lameness score* was introduced by Manson and Leaver[21] in observational studies of the effect of different concentrate-to-roughage ratios on the degree of lameness. In their lameness assessment scale, each cow was judged when walking away from an observer who stood at a distance of 5 to 10 meters. The severity of lameness is scored from 1 to 5 (see Fig. 1–2 legend, #1, for explanation). It was claimed that this new approach to locomotion scoring was a precise and sensitive measure of foot problems. The repeatability of these locomotion scoring estimates was good, within-observer repeatability being 0.89 and between-observer repeatability 0.84.

In the United Kingdom, it is probable that only a minority of farmers keep lameness records. This is partly because of their practical nature, partly because of their lack of experience or training in record keeping, and partly because they think that they can manage perfectly well without them. In the future, they will be unable to manage serious lameness problems effectively unless they keep adequate records.

Computerized systems for dairy farmers have not generally been very good at covering disease records, but there are exceptions. These systems have the advantage that they are integrated databases each linked to the other by common fields such as herd ID and animal ID. In order to avoid repeated data entry, one database stores invariable data about an animal, its birth date, breed, sex, genealogy, date of death, or culling. Other databases contain lifetime details on all fertility events (calving, heats, services, pregnancy diagnosis) and other diseases. Different databases within the system usually contain information on production, milk quality, or growth.

Future databases might contain information about changes in nutrition. Claw scoring (shape and size) might be another useful parameter to explore.[8] There is no reason why veterinarians using an integrated computerized recording system should not record a

LAMENESS DATA CAPTURE FORM

Animal ID Ear Tag_____ Tatoo_____ FARM ID_____
Examination Date DD___MM___YY____ Body Score_____ Weight_____Kg

Date of Birth DD___MM___YY__   Sex: Male ¦ Female ¦ Steer¦   Date of Disposal DD___MM___YY__
      Reason for Disposal Lame ¦ Production ¦ Infertility ¦ Mastitis ¦ Death ¦ Other_____

① LAMENESS SCORE

1 NORMAL

2 SLIGHT ABNORMALITY
    Uneven gait, stiff, tender.
3 SLIGHT LAMENESS
    Moderate and consistent lameness
4 OBVIOUS LAMENESS
    Obvious lameness affecting behavior
5 SEVERE LAMENESS
    Very marked lameness.

② LIMB/CLAW AFFECTED

Lesions of sole
01. Hemorrhage of sole
02. Sole ulcer
03. White line disease
04. Heel erosion
05. Worn/bruised sole
06. Double sole
07. Sole trauma
08. Sole abscess
Interdigital lesions
10. Foot rot/foul
11. Interdig dermatitis
12. Interdig hyperplasia
13. Foreign body
Digital Lesions
20. Digital dermatitis
21. Septic Arthritis
22. Retroartic abscess
Fissures of the Claw Wall
30. Vert fissure Type I
31. Vertical fissure Type II
32. Vertical fissure Type III
33. Vertical fissure Type IV
34. Horizontal Groove
        (Severity = cm)
38. Hor fissure/thimble
39. Hor fiss broken toe
Abnormalities of Wall
40. Normal overgrowth
41. Slipper foot (Chr Lam)
42. Corkscrew claw
43. Scissor claw
44. Hook claw
45. Reaction Ridge
        (Severity = cm)
46. Change Coronary Band
Lesion of Proximal Limb
50. Fracture/rupture
51. Hematoma

01. Scapula or Pelvis
02. Humerus or Femur
03. Radius or Tibia
04. Carpus of Tarsus
05. Metacarpus or Metatarsus
06. Proximal Phalanx
07. Intermediate Phalanx
08. Distal Phalanx
09. Distal Sessamoid
10. Interdigital

01. Hoof Sole   07. Skin
02. Hoof Wall   08. Nerve
03. Hoof Heel   09. Tendon
04. Bone   10. Ligament
05. Muscle
06. Joint

⑧ TISSUE →

⑦

BODY REGION →

PHOTOGRAPH	
YES	NO
MARK	cm

LESION NUMBER

	LEFT FORE	RIGHT FORE	LEFT HIND	RIGHT HIND		1	2	3	4
	12	34	56	78					

LAT	MED	MED	LAT	LAT	MED	MED	LAT
1	2	3	4	5	6	7	8 →

④ SEVERITY OF LESION →

1. Mild, Trace.
2. Distinct diagnostic sign
3. Marked clinical lesion
4. Complicated or serious
   or infected

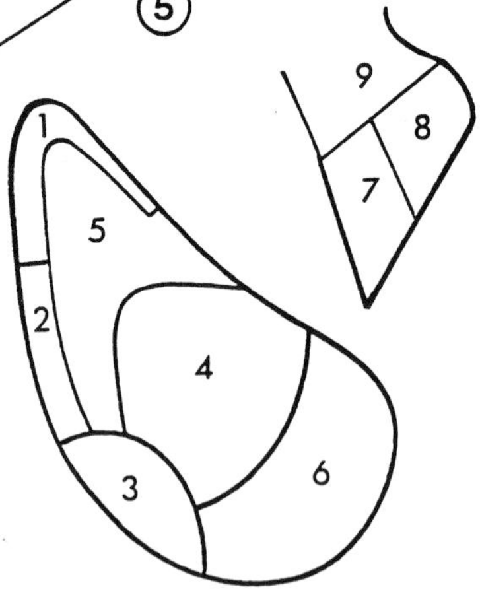

③ CLASSIFICATION OF LESION

⑤ ZONE OF CLAW

⑥ TREATMENT

01. Topical
10. Penicillin G Procaine
11. Penicillin G Benzathine
12. Lincomycin
13. Tetracycline
14. Oxytetracycline
15. Erythromycin
16. Tylosin
30. Sulfadimethoxine
31. Sulfachlorpyridazine
32. Sulfadiazine
40. Analgesic
45. Phenylbutazone
46. Dexamethasone
47. Prednisolone
50. Bandage/Boot
60. Amputation
61. Resection
62. Arthrodesis
70. Hoof Trim
71. Block/lift
90. Veterinarian
91. Stockman
92. Technician/student

Treatment: Date of Recovery DD___MM___YY__
DrugUsed_____ Dosage_____ Frequency per day_____ #Days_____

Drug Use_____ Dosage_____ Frequency per day_____ #Days_____
Other Treatments_____

Figure 1–2 *See legend on opposite page*

score for cubicle design, accessibility, and comfort, as well as for the texture of indoor and outdoor walking surfaces.[8] Poor bedding and comfort scores have been associated with more lameness or higher locomotion scores.

The computer can be programmed to compare the same field in successive records or list a field such as a lesion across animals in one or more herds, adding qualifiers such as animal age or season of the year. Provided the records are noted in the basic written record and are keyed into the computer, trends can be spotted and early action taken to control the problem. For example, what quantity of lameness would warrant a full-scale ecopathological or epidemiological study of the herd? This awareness might be triggered at a herd lameness incidence of 10% or a 5% prevalence of sole ulcers. These criteria wait to be finally determined, but the study by Clarkson and colleagues[8] provides a wealth of information on which such data can be logically based.

Computer programs will be adapted to meet future veterinary needs and are able to display good graphical information, so that data entry can be extremely user friendly. Many veterinarians need more training to enable them to tackle herd problems and to be confident and competent with management and information systems. Records need to be used so that solutions can be formulated, costed with their benefits valued so that farmers can be persuaded to invest in the future rather than rue the expenses of the past.

Lameness data usually cannot be effectively recorded on a computer located in the barn or milking parlor. A written record is therefore required. These records (data capture records) are most valuable if standard terminology (see p. 219), internationally accepted descriptions of lesion severity (see p. 10), lameness scores, and so on are used. The excellent Compton data capture sheet[17, 30] has been modified and is illustrated in Figure 1–2. At first sight, this data capture record may seem too complicated. However, it is implicit in the system that the individual

---

Figure 1–2. Instructions for using the Lameness Data Capture Form. Enter animal ID, date of examination, and a herd ID (the herd ID should consist of a three-letter identifier for the person conducting the investigation, plus a number). Then complete the form from field to field, following the numerical order.

1. LAMENESS SCORE (after Manson and Leaver[21])

    1.0 Minimal abduction/adduction, no unevenness of gait, no tenderness
    1.5 Slight abduction/adduction, no unevenness or tenderness
    2.0 Abduction/adduction present, uneven gait, perhaps tender
    2.5 Abduction/adduction present, uneven gait, tenderness of feet
    3.0 Slight lameness, not affecting behavior
    3.5 Obvious lameness, difficulty in turning, not affecting behavior
    4.0 Obvious lameness, difficulty in turning, behavior affected
    4.5 Some difficulty in rising, difficulty in walking, behavior affected
    5.0 Extreme difficulty in rising, difficulty walking, behavior affected

The examiner may use the full score or a simplified modification. In the lameness data capture form, the following abbreviation is used:

    1 Normal—Not lame
    2 Slight abnormality—Uneven gait, stiff, tender
    3 Slight lameness—Moderate and consistent lameness
    4 Obvious lameness—Obvious lameness affecting behavior
    5 Severe lameness—Very marked lameness

2. LIMB/CLAW AFFECTED

Claws are numbered clockwise, commencing at the left fore lateral. The numbers appropriate to the two claws are used to designate the limb affected—i.e., fore left = 12, fore right = 34, hind right = 78, and hind left = 56.

3. CLASSIFICATION OF LESION

If the lameness score is entered, the causal lesion number must appear in the first column (first lesion number). Lesions (horizontal fissures, overgrowth, abnormal coronary band, and reaction ridge) that are present in several claws need only be scored as affecting one claw. Space is provided for up to four lesions, which should be entered in order of importance. A new lesion is recorded if it occurs in a different claw or in the same claw after more than 28 days.

4. SEVERITY OF LESION

Most degrees of severity are scored from 1 to 4 or 5. In the case of a horizontal fissure and a reaction ridge, the figure entered should be the distance in centimeters from the skin-horn junction. The field in the database can be formulated to calculate automatically the date of insult—i.e., exam date − (measurement in cm + 2.5).

5. ZONE OF CLAW

Zones used are those agreed at the 6th International Symposium on Diseases of the Ruminant Digit, Liverpool, UK, 1990.

6. TREATMENT

This field allows for flexibility in entering treatments, some of which are designated in the appropriate region of the text. Recovery date is useful when dealing with phlegmon, because if improvement is not noted in 3 days, the diagnosis may be questionable.

7. BODY REGION (Usually Optional)

This field in combination with the limb field designates the anatomical region. Used mainly for conditions affecting the proximal limb. Note that "interdigital" is included here.

8. BODY TISSUE (Usually Optional)

This field is used mostly in combination with body region. A joint or ligament is identified as that most proximal to a bone, a muscle or tendon to its insertion.

Note: If photographs are taken, make the appropriate note in the box at the top right-hand corner of the form. In the same box, measurements for claw growth can be made by creating a mark 3 cm from the skin-horn junction on the dorsal surface of the claw, and from subsequent records a formula can automatically calculate the rate of growth. This is a useful strategy to check the rate of claw horn growth.

completing the record be forced to make consistent and correct observations. This should result in an improvement in knowledge about lameness. *Ad hoc* record keeping has proved to be useless for herd evaluation owing to incomplete data and inconsistency between individual recorders. Dairy farmers surveyed on their recognition of lameness revealed that not one overestimated the number of lame cows in their herd, when compared with the number detected by a veterinary observer on the same day.[34] Also, those farmers most aware of lame cows had the lowest prevalence of lameness in their herd (P < 0.001). A repeat survey on a further 14 farms confirmed this result.[23]

CONCLUSIONS

The incidence of lameness is probably increasing. Certainly there is a heightened awareness. It is widely believed that this increase is associated with high production and the associated intensive management and nutrition. Hence, lameness is regarded as a production disease. Ecopathology and epidemiology are the disciplines that by appropriate and efficient recording systems can relate a disease (e.g., lesions causing lameness) to associated risk factors. These multiple risk factors are related to the ability of the farmer, the building design, nutrition, genetics, and animal behavior. Computerized herd data management will enable the industry to respond rationally by making informed decisions that achieve optimal production in an environment of cow comfort and conditions of optimal animal welfare.

REFERENCES

1. Animal Welfare Foundation Annual Review 1993–4. London, British Veterinary Association, 1994, p 10.
2. Arkins S: Lameness in dairy cows. Parts I & II. Ir Vet J 35:135–140, 163–170, 1981.
3. Baggott DG, Russell AM: Lameness in cattle. Br Vet J 137:113–132, 1981.
4. Bargai U, Levin D: Lameness in the Israeli dairy herd; a national survey of incidence, distribution and estimated costs (first report). Isr J Vet Med 48:88–92, 1992.
5. Beemster CMT, Quiros T, Burger R, et al: Epidemiological study of foot lesions in dairy cattle in the Poas Region, Costa Rica. Ciencias Veterinarias (Heredia) 14(1):13–22, 1992. (Abstr Vet Bull 64:1202, 1994).
6. Choquette-Lévy L, Baril J, Lévy M, et al: A study of foot diseases of dairy cattle in Quebec. Can Vet J 26:278–281, 1985.
7. Clarkson MJ: Method of data evaluations in studies on lameness. Proceedings of the 6th International Symposium on Diseases of the Ruminant Digit. Liverpool, England, 1990, pp 177–183.
8. Clarkson MJ, Downham, DT, Faull WB, et al: An epidemiological study to determine the risk factors of lameness in dairy cows. (University of Liverpool Veterinary Faculty [UK] CSA 1370) Final report, 1993.
9. Collick DW, Ward WR, Dobson H: Associations between types of lameness and fertility. Vet Rec 25: 103–106, 1989.
10. Donaldson AI, Gloster JD, Harvey LDJ, et al: Use of prediction models to forecast and analyse airborne spread during the foot-and-mouth disease outbreaks in Brittany, Jersey and the Isle of Wight in 1981. Vet Rec 110:53–57, 1989.
11. Düring F: Zur Eignung von Daten zu Abgangshäufigkeiten für die Beurteilung des Gesundheitsstatus in Milchviehherden. Berl Muench Tieraerztl Wochenschr 101:203–208, 1988.
12. Eddy RG, Scott CP: Some observations on the incidence of lameness in dairy cattle in Somerset. Vet Rec 113:140–144, 1980.
13. Enevoldsen C, Mortensen K: Epidemiologic analyses of digital disorders in cattle: Relevance for research and herd health management. Proceedings of the 2nd International Congress for Orthopedics in Hoof and Clawed Animals. Vienna, Austria, October 6–9, 1993, p 32.
14. Espinasse J, Savey M, Thorley CM, et al: Colour Atlas on Disorders of Cattle and Sheep Digit. Maisons-Alfort, France, Editions du Point Vétérinaire, 1984.
15. Esslemont RJ, Spincer I: The incidence and costs of diseases in dairy herds. DAISY Report 2. Dept. of Agriculture, University of Reading, UK, 1993.
16. Frey R, Berchtold M: Analyse vorzeitiger Ausmerzungen. Zuchthygiene 18(5):203–209, 1983.
17. Greenough PR, MacCallum FJ, Weaver AD: Lameness in Cattle, 2nd ed. Bristol, England, Wright Scientechnica, 1981.
18. Harris CD, Hilburt GA, Anderson GA, et al: The incidence, cost and factors associated with foot lameness in dairy cattle in South-Western Victoria. Aust Vet J 65:171–176, 1988.
19. Hassall SA, Ward WR, Murray RD: Effects of lameness on the behaviour of cows during the summer. Vet Rec 132:578–580, 1993.
20. Lee LA, Ferguson JD, Galligan DT: Effect of disease on days open assessed by survival analysis. J Dairy Sci 72:1020–1026, 1989.
21. Manson FJ, Leaver JD: The influence of concentrate amount on locomotion and clinical lameness in dairy cattle. Anim Prod 47:185–190, 1988.
21a. McLennan MW: Incidence of lameness requiring veterinary treatment in dairy cattle in Queensland. Aust Vet J 65:144–147, 1988.
22. Milian-Suazo F, Erb HN, Smith RD: Descriptive epidemiology of culling in dairy cows from 34 herds in New York State. Prev Vet Med 6:243–251, 1988.
23. Mill JM, Ward WR: Lameness in dairy cows and farmers' knowledge, training and awareness. Vet Rec 134:162–164, 1994.
24. Murphy PA: Diseases of beef cattle housed intensively on slatted floors. Vet Update 1(8):25–29, 1985.
25. Peeler EJ, Otte MJ, Esslemont RJ: Inter-relationships of peri-parturient diseases in dairy cows. Vet Rec 134:129–132, 1994.
26. Philipot JM, Pluvinage P, Cimarosti I, et al: On indicators of laminitis and heel erosion in dairy cattle: Research on observation of digital lesions in the course of an ecopathological survey. Proceedings of the 6th International Symposium on Disorders of the Ruminant Digit. Liverpool, UK, 1990, pp 184–198.
27. Pinsent PJN: The management and husbandry aspects of foot lameness in dairy cattle. Bovine Pract 16:61–64, 1981.
28. Prentice DE, Neal PA: Some observations on the incidence of lameness in dairy cattle in west Cheshire. Vet Rec 91:1–7, 1972.
29. Read DH, Walker RL: Papillomatous digital dermatitis of dairy cattle in California: Clinical characteristics. Proceedings of the 8th International Symposium on Disorders of the Ruminant Digit. Banff, Canada, 1994, pp 159–163.
30. Russell AM, Rowlands GJ, Shaw SR, Weaver AD: Survey of lameness in British dairy cattle. Vet Rec 111:155–160, 1982.
31. Schepers JA, Dijkhuisen AA: The economics of mastitis and mastitis control in dairy cattle: A critical analysis of estimates published since 1970. Prev Vet Med 10(3):213–224, 1991.
32. Smits MCJ, Frankena K, Metz JHM, et al: Prevalence of digital disorders in zero-grazed dairy cows. Livest Prod Sci 32:231–244, 1992.
33. Tranter WP, Morris R: A case study of lameness in three dairy herds. N Z Vet J 39:88–96, 1991.
34. Ward WR: The role of stockmanship in foot lameness in UK

dairy cattle. Proceedings of the 8th International Symposium on Disorders of the Ruminant Digit. Banff, Canada, 1994, pp 301–302.

35. Weaver AD: Long-term observations on dairy herd lameness. Proceedings of the 6th International Symposium on Disorders of the Ruminant Digit, Liverpool, UK, 1990, pp 59–61.

36. Wells SJ, Trent AM, Marsh WE, Robinson RA: Prevalence and severity of lameness in lactating dairy cows in a sample of Minnesota and Wisconsin herds. J Am Vet Med Assoc 202:78–82, 1993.

37. Wells SJ, Trent AM, Robinson RA: Prevalence of clinical lameness in dairy cows in the Midwestern United States. Proceedings of the 6th International Symposium on Disorders of the Ruminant Digit, Liverpool, UK, 1990, p 55.

38. Whitaker DA, Kelly JM, Smith EJ: Incidence of lameness in dairy cows. Vet Rec 113:60–62, 1983.

39. Yoshitani K, Suzuki T, Kaseki K: Investigation on the incidence of digital disease in dairy cows in Awa, Japan. Proceedings of the 6th International Symposium on Disorders of the Ruminant Digit, Liverpool, UK, 1990, 58.

2

Examination of the Locomotor System

RESTRAINT

GENERAL PRINCIPLES

Dairy cows are accustomed to daily physical contact with an attendant and to limited restraint in milking parlors. For this reason, lifting a limb for the purpose of examining the sole of a digit is easier than with bulls, dairy heifers, or beef cattle. With the latter animals, supplementary control through chemical restraint is often required (see p. 47). Devices such as a mobile crush (restraining cage) or tipping-table can be used (see pp. 127–129).

Lifting a pelvic limb by hand is inappropriate for anything but a cursory inspection because effective restraint is impossible. Some individuals raise a pelvic limb by hand to save time, but this ultimately leads to mistakes—for example, incorrect diagnoses such as an unrecognized penetrating solar foreign body. It is usually practicable to elevate a thoracic limb manually.

It is essential when lifting a limb of a standing animal to restrict the movement of its body in all directions—forward, backward, and sideways. Clearly, restraint in a chute/crush fulfils this requirement. In its absence, applying a halter and lifting the nose upward disorients some animals sufficiently to permit manipulation of the limb.

In production units with a high lameness incidence, special facilities should be created or suitable restraining equipment purchased. The site should be carefully selected. It should be under cover, well lit, easily cleaned, and with access and exit attractive to cows. Ideally, the crush should be adjustable for different sizes of cattle. It should be designed to avoid potential injury to stock and handlers (no sharp corners). It should be relatively quiet in operation and firmly secured and should have a non-slip base. Provision should be available to fix ropes to the framework high above the back of the cow. Crushes for bulls usually incorporate leather slings that are placed around the ventral portion of the abdomen to stop an animal's falling. A clean water source and hose of adequate length to reach the feet are also desirable. In some countries (e.g., Netherlands), veterinarians routinely use a mobile crush for lameness

work with dairy herds (see Chapter 9). Nevertheless, situations arise in which veterinarians are required to lift a limb with the assistance of mechanical equipment. Lifting a limb in a dairy parlor is not advocated because control is minimal and the risks to the operator are considerable. Also, some animals become apprehensive about entering the parlor afterward, and milk letdown could be affected.

Unsuitable forms of restraint include elevation of the tail (uncertain and then effective for only a short period), the use of hock clamps (unwieldy, dangerous, and by their nature maintain the pelvic limb in an extended position), casting by Reuffs method (additional roping of each limb is then necessary), and use of the halter and nose lead method (doubtful efficacy, and the assistant is remote from the hindquarters).

With quiet dairy herds, an experienced claw trimmer alone can handle six to eight cows per hour using a lightweight portable tilt table (see Figs. 9–13 and 9–14) equipped with two body slings and four hobbles. This procedure permits excellent visualization and operation on all four limbs.

LIFTING A THORACIC LIMB

The thoracic limbs are less frequently examined, and restraint is awkward. An assistant standing slightly in front of the animal's shoulder and facing the rear should elevate the limb. The assistant should clasp his or her hands around the limb just below the carpus, aiming to flex both carpal and elbow joints. The limb should be pulled gently forward while the assistant leans into the animal's shoulder to give additional support and to transfer the maximum weight to the contralateral limb, thus aiding elevation. The main weight is taken by the assistant, freeing the veterinarian to manipulate the digits (Fig. 2–1). It is wise not to bend too low because some cattle can strike forward with the pelvic limb even if the thoracic limb is raised.

Some animals tend to sink to the ground when a thoracic limb is raised. A bale of straw placed below the sternum is usually sufficient to correct this problem.

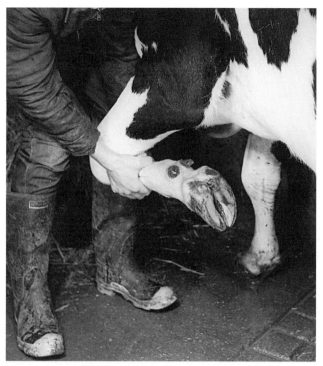

Figure 2–1. The thoracic limb is best elevated manually. The limb is supported by an assistant standing in front of the shoulder and gripping the metacarpus with both hands.

LIFTING A PELVIC LIMB

Rope or Pulley

The widespread use of free stall (cubicle) housing systems has made it difficult to provide facilities for using a mechanical device to elevate a pelvic limb. Nevertheless, hospital or examination stalls should be provided with adequate facilities for restraining an animal. Such facilities would include either a head gate or rings set in the walls at different heights together with one or more rails to restrict lateral movement. An open beam or a U-bolt attached to a roof rafter at a suitable point above an animal's body is one other device that is appropriate. A do-it-yourself automotive pulley is inexpensive and can be left permanently attached to the overhead fixture. A heavy-gauge nylon noose may be looped around the hock and hooked into the lifting attachment of the pulley. Alternatively, a rope may be applied to the hock and passed around the overhead device. Two important principles follow:

1 The rope or pulley must be inclined in a forward direction such that the line of the suspension system passes over the hip. Optimal elevation then ensures that the stifle is firmly flexed beneath the hock and gives the animal a sense of security against falling. If the rope is not so directed, the animal can extend the limb and perhaps struggle violently.

2 A noose must be placed around the hock (Fig. 2–2). This exerts pressure on the tendon of the gastrocnemius muscle, thus reducing the ability to extend the limb.

A rope should not be placed around the pastern to pull the limb directly backward. Such a manipulation inevitably provokes a violent reaction, potentially leading to limb injury.

Elevating a pelvic limb of an intractable beef cow can be very difficult. Chemical sedation is commonly used. Casting the animal with side lines may then be done if the examination or procedure is likely to be prolonged. If a sedated beef cow is in a crush/chute, the increased risk of recumbency can lead to potential asphyxia if the head cannot be rapidly released from the head catch.

The Hoofnak

A Hoofnak is a portable device that can be applied to pipe railings (Fig. 2–3). The lifting is made possible with a lever and ratchet system. This method is very appropriate for veterinarians engaged in dairy practice.

EXAMINATION

The examination must be systematic. Superficial and hasty examination of a lame cow does little to impress a farmer (who may have treated the cow empirically) because an incorrect diagnosis can be embarrassing when the error is revealed at a second visit a few days later ("the cow's still lame"). Descriptive records should be kept for each case (see p. 9). This enables the operator to match treatment to the disease progression. It also provides valuable historical information about the herd incidence. In more than 80% of dairy cow lameness, the seat of lameness is found in the digital region. The overall four-phase protocol for conducting a lameness examination is outlined in Table 2–1.

PHASE ONE—COLLECTION OF DATA

BASIC RECORDS

Specific Identification

Even for individual cases of lameness, it is becoming increasingly necessary to keep detailed case records. A record must contain fields that are exclusive to a particular animal at a particular time. These fields do not change (e.g., date of birth, farm identification, breed, sex, and identification number (ear tags, collars, tattoos, skin brands, transponders).

Variable Records

Once the specific identification of an animal is established, each subsequent record varies according to

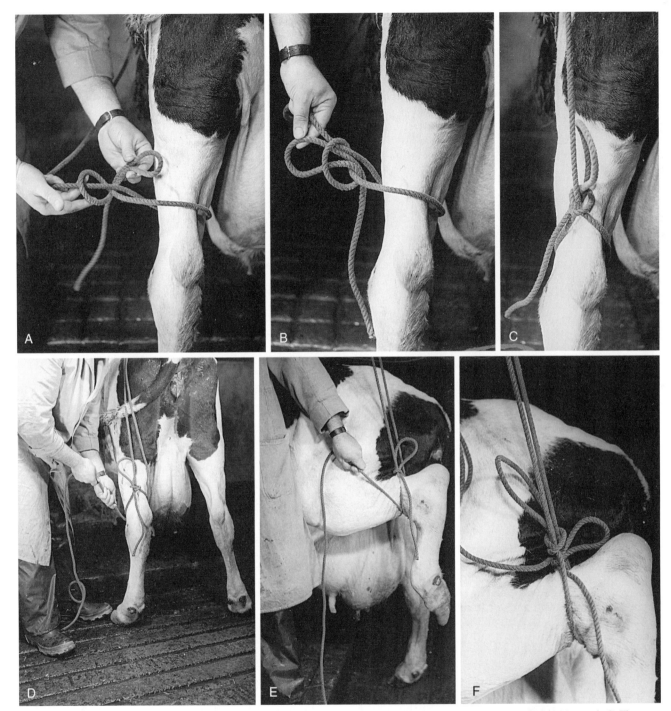

Figure 2–2. *A,* A rope is attached around the gastrocnemius tendon just above the hock. *B,* A quick-release slipknot is used. *C,* The noose is drawn tight, and the free end passed over a beam or other supporting structure above the cow. *D,* The free end is then passed beneath the hock and used as a means of lifting the limb. *E,* It is important to note that the rope is passed forward over the hip. If the rope inclines behind the animal, the animal usually resists restraint by kicking. *F,* The limb may be restrained in the elevated position by applying a quick-release knot.

the date of the examination. Height, body condition score, and weight may be measured or estimated.

Case History

At the time the case is presented, circumstances may suggest a prioritization of risk factors. Animals of

certain ages and types have a greater than average risk of specific disease problems. For example, old bulls used for artificial insemination and old cows are more likely to have an arthrosis of the tarsal or the digital joints or spondyloarthrotic changes. First-calving heifers are prone to pododermatitis circumscripta (sole ulcer) under intensive feeding conditions. Acute, subacute, or subclinical laminitis is frequently encountered in intensively fed feedlot cattle. The pattern of lameness can then be studied from well-recorded herds.

The information about the lame animal in the period preceding the onset of clinical signs noted by a competent animal attendant is invaluable and may suggest a possible line of investigation. The urge to jump to conclusions must be avoided. Considerable care is required in evaluating the quality of the information given by the stockperson. Guilt and ignorance can distort the truth about the time of onset of the lameness as well as any care (or treatment) that may or may not have been given. The following questions are suggested:

- How long has the animal been lame?

  Sudden onset may indicate an acute infection such as phlegmon, sole abscess, or sudden trauma (e.g., a foreign body penetrating the sole or a fractured distal phalanx). Acute laminitis has a sudden onset, but if the condition affects only single claws, the clinical signs may be bizarre.

  Slow onset usually suggests a progressive disease process such as occurs in a sole ulcer, an arthritic condition, or infections of the heel region.

- Has there been any variation in the clinical signs observed?

  A rapid increase in the severity of the pain probably indicates a reaction to an infection. An insidious onset followed by a rapid increase in pain suggests a sudden change in the pathology such as septic infection of a vertical fissure or a white line lesion. In other conditions such as laminitis and

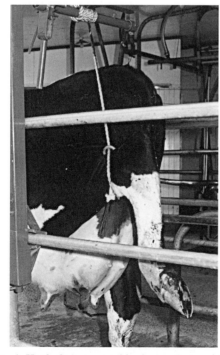

Figure 2–3. A Hoofnak is a portable device that can be fixed to horizontal piping. The hock is elevated by a rope around the hock, and the free end of it can be reeled in by means of a ratchet system fixed to the cantilever over the animal's hip.

TABLE 2–1. FOUR-PHASE PROTOCOL FOR LAMENESS EXAMINATION

Examination	Activity
Phase One	***Collection of Data***
Signalment	Breed, age, sex, identification number, weight, special characteristics
Case history	Duration of lameness, limb/region affected, body condition score (BCS), special observations of owner
Herd history	Condition of facilities, status of hygiene, level of nutrition, management and administrative skills, breeding policy
Phase Two	***General Examination of Patient***
Observe the animal standing	Abnormal posture or behavior, recumbency, obvious pathology including decubital lesions and claw lesions, muscle atrophy
Observe the animal walking	Severity of the lameness, limb(s) affected, altered gait (adduction, abduction, protraction, retraction) and incoordination; identification of the seat of lameness
Phase Three	***Physical Examination of Limbs***
Examine each digit starting with the affected claw (provocative testing)	Identification of the painful area, applying pressure by hand or hoof pincers
Examine the soles of the claws and make invasive tests	Identification of lesions and the region affected; physical exploration of lesions
Phase Four	***Conduct Specific Tests***
Regional or intra-articular anesthesia	Localize pain
Radiography	Obtain details of changes
Ultrasonography	Identify abnormalities
Laboratory tests on body fluids or tissues	Confirmation or exclusion of clinical findings

arthritis, pain may resolve naturally in a few days only to recur later.

- Has the animal had any treatment?

  Treatment administered by a stockperson or another veterinarian may mask clinical signs. In some countries, the purchase and administration of antibiotics by a stockperson are permitted. It is important to ensure that the product has been correctly stored, is uncontaminated, and has been correctly administered (dose, route, and frequency). Recording a recovery date is useful for record keeping. Animals that have been correctly treated for interdigital phlegmon should show signs of recovery within 3 days. If this is not the case, the animal should be re-examined.

- What is the reproductive status of the animal?

  The peak incidence of many types of lameness is about 8 weeks postpartum. The majority occur in the first 3 months postpartum. If outside this period, it may be useful to inquire if other animals have a similar lameness history. If so, these cases may have a common and unusual etiology. Lameness associated with recent estrus (or transport) may be related to proximal limb trauma.

Herd History

- Is the lameness related to changed or exceptional nutrition?

  Sudden changes in the composition of rations occur as a result of economic pressures. Turnout onto spring pastures causes a radical feeding change. The introduction of a new stockperson or management system also can be associated with problems (adaption problems in heifers).

- When was claw trimming last performed?

  Iatrogenic lameness may occur after claw trimming.

- Is the housing causing unusual stress?

  Certain characteristics of housing have been identified as being stressful to cattle. The following are some of the features for evaluation: the construction of the floor, the amount of slurry present, the loafing space for each animal, dimensions of cubicles, the type and quality of bedding, footbath use, and building changes.

- Do the animals have access to pasture?

  If animals walk to and from pasture, the characteristics of the roadways are important. The maintenance of the pastures is also important. Areas of high traffic density tend to become infected with organisms that may be involved in digital diseases. Pastures may be heavily manured or treated with nitrogenous fertilizers, both of which can increase the risk of nitrite toxicity.

- Is nutrition likely to be a problem?

  The frequency of feeding concentrates, levels of energy and protein, and the percentage of fiber in the ration may have an impact on the incidence of lameness (see p. 297).

- Is production stress likely to be an issue?

  High milk yields, short calving intervals, use of bovine somatotropin (BST), winter calving, and poor body condition in dry cows may be indicators of a herd under stress.

- What is the general disease history of the herd?

  Increasing evidence links lameness to an increased incidence of other conditions such as reproductive disorders and mastitis (see p. 308). Specific problems such as septic arthritis or osteomyelitis in calves are of special interest. Laboratory reports may be available.

- What are the main reasons for culling, and how many animals are culled each year?

  Information about culling provides an indication of the severity of disease problems, particularly those associated with trauma. It also identifies the source of replacement stock, which may be involved in the introduction of genetic or disease problems. Most animals are usually culled because of infertility ("barren"), mastitis, or poor milk yield. Lameness is usually the fourth major reason for culling.

PHASE TWO—GENERAL EXAMINATION

OBSERVE THE ANIMAL STANDING

- Body size, condition, and conformation?

  Large-framed, heavy animals with straight pelvic limbs and small claws are especially susceptible to trauma of the sole or joints. This evaluation should be made from the sides as well as the front and rear of the animal (see p. 73).

- Posture?

  The significance of posture is described in Chapter 6 and cannot be underestimated in the evaluation. The way in which a recumbent cow attempts to rise may be significant but may also be related to cubicle design.

  The veterinarian should evaluate claw conformation and toe angles of thoracic and pelvic limbs as well as the width of the interdigital space. Inspection should start by viewing from the front, then from the side, and finally from behind. The occurrence of swelling, atrophy, wounds, and so on should be noted. A description of normal claw conformation is found in Chapters 6 and 14.

OBSERVE THE ANIMAL AT A WALK

Lameness is defined as a disturbance of the physiological locomotor pattern of one or more limbs. Lameness is usually caused by pain. Mechanical factors can cause lameness, such as locking of a joint or paralysis of a muscle. A combination of these two factors is possible. A painful process in one limb leads to compensatory movements of other limbs and of the head. Such movements are normally slight and should be differentiated from movements directly resulting from lameness.

An altered/abnormal gait is defined as disturbance of the physiological locomotor pattern of one pair of limbs. Such a gait can be caused by pain or mechanical alterations. An inexperienced investigator may find this type of bilateral locomotor disturbance difficult to confirm. Do not overlook a minor problem in a less-affected digit.

Lameness should not be confused with abnormal gait caused by non-painful factors. Some animals are nervous about walking on slippery or slatted floors. Others may need a claw trim. The patient should be observed during conditions that permit locomotion to be as unstressed as possible. It is essential that the animal be observed walking on hard, non-slip surfaces.

Animals conventionally kept tied or confined to a box move less freely than cattle kept on pasture. On slatted floors, animals move cautiously and with short steps. A young calf moves differently from a mature bull.

The affected animal should be observed at a walk, from the front, rear, and side. The following factors should be evaluated:

1 *Arc of digital flight.* From behind or in front, view the arc of flight outward or inward. In sound cattle, the arc is symmetrical. Unequal arcs usually indicate lameness or compensatory movements.

2 *Weight-bearing.* Equal weight distribution should be found on both claws of each limb. With a painful claw, the animal tries to put less weight on the claw in which a lesion is present. In fracture of the medial distal phalanx of the pelvic limb, some animals cross their legs in overadduction.

3 *Line of progression.* The spine is normally parallel to the line of progression. In cases of severe pelvic limb lameness, the digits of the non-affected side are placed toward the midline to maintain balance. This avoids placing too much pressure on the affected side. The spine is oblique relative to the direction of travel.

4 *Alteration in the phases of gait.* Each stride commences from the stance position, when the full weight is taken by the bearing surface of the abaxial wall. Movement from and back to the stance phase is the swing phase, subdivided into retraction and protraction phases. As the animal moves forward, the digits provide traction until the heel leaves the ground and the retraction phase ends. The digits are then thrown forward in the protraction phase and touch the ground heel first, more obviously with the hind digits, after which the soles resume the weight-bearing position. Pain or mechanical interference causes changes in this pattern.

The metacarpus is closer to the vertical than is the metatarsus, and flexion of the carpus allows a wider range of movement in the thoracic than the pelvic limbs. The thoracic limb acts as a prop for the body while the pelvic limb, which bears a smaller percentage of the body weight (about 48%), propels the body forward. The stride of the thoracic limb is comparable to that of the pelvic limb.

EVALUATE THE SEAT OF LAMENESS

Supporting Limb Lameness. An obviously shortened weight-bearing phase and a quick swing phase are seen. This change is typical of many very painful types of lameness in which the causal lesion is located in the claw.

A prolonged protraction phase may indicate that a painful lesion is present in the toe. Conversely, a prolonged retraction phase suggests a heel lesion (e.g., ulceration of the sole or severe heel erosion). The changes in stride with very overgrown claws may mimic those seen in a true lameness.

An animal may abduct a limb to avoid weight-bearing on the lateral claw.

Swinging Limb Lameness. As the term implies, the affected limb swings and remains stiff. Pain results from joint flexion, indicating that the lameness originates in the proximal limb.

EVALUATE THE SEVERITY OF THE LAMENESS

The severity of lameness should be evaluated using the scoring system provided in Figure 1–2.

PHASE THREE—PHYSICAL EXAMINATION OF THE LIMBS

- Physical examination commences with the most affected limb.

- The limb, especially the claws, should be cleaned.

- The claws should always be examined first even when obvious changes are seen elsewhere in the limbs.

- The contralateral limb must *always* be examined.

- The examination should not stop if only one lesion is found.

Flexion tests in cattle are limited to selected cases in such suspect conditions as ruptured cranial cruciate ligament and gonitis, degenerative joint disease, and distortion or intra-articular fractures. Some degree of cooperation from the animal is necessary, and aggression and resistance are limiting factors.

EXAMINATION OF THE DIGITS

Visually Inspect the Claws with the Animal Standing

Claw wall characteristics can be noted with the animal standing. They may be missed if the operator concentrates on the sole:

- The coronary band, its color and texture (laminitis, see p. 285)

- Wall, rugae, grooves, thimbles, or ridges (see p. 111)

- Dorsal surface, concavity and length (chronic laminitis; see p. 279)

- Fissures (see pp. 109–113)
- Exungulation (see p. 110)
- Soft tissue swelling (phlegmon, see p. 90; retroarticular abscess, see pp. 92–93; septic arthritis, see p. 103; deep flexor tendon necrosis, see p. 103)

The interdigital space should be narrow. If it is wider than normal, possible explanations include

- Septic arthritis of the distal interphalangeal (DIP) joint (see p. 104)
- Phlegmon (see p. 90)
- Interdigital hyperplasia (see p. 119)

Examine the Elevated Claw

The *sole* should be lightly pared (Fig. 2–4), even if no horn overgrowth is present, in order to expose unstained horn. The presence and severity of lesions may be mapped and scored in accordance with the international system for bovine sole lesion evaluation (see Fig. 1–2).

A normal sole is concave, with weight-bearing taking place on the distal surface of the abaxial wall. In concrete yards and cubicle housing, the sole is often flat. All blemishes on the surface should be explored with a hoof knife. The average thickness of sole horn is between 6 and 10 mm at any location. Firm thumb pressure should be applied to the center of the sole (region 4). Never more than a very slight depression of the horn should be possible.

- Flatness, excessive wear (see p. 286) or laminitis (see p. 277)
- Yellow waxlike appearance (laminitis, see p. 277)
- Hemorrhages, generalized or localized, in the horn (laminitis, see p. 286)

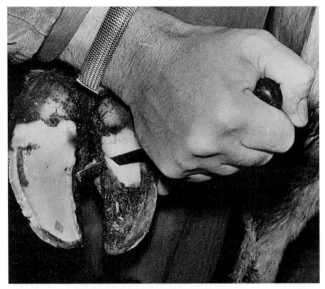

Figure 2–4. A search knife is drawn across the sole to expose clean horn in which grooves may be exposed for further exploration.

- Hemorrhage, extensive *under* the horn (bruising, see p. 114)
- Pododermatitis circumscripta, region 4 (sole ulcer, see p. 101)
- Foreign body or tract (see p. 114)
- Double sole (see p. 287)

The *zona alba (white line)* is best explored with the tip of a hoof knife, although care must be taken to avoid damaging the horn of the wall unnecessarily.

- Separation (avulsion) of the zona alba (subsolar abscess, see pp. 104–107; or sinus, see p. 104)

The *bulb (heel)* should be normal in animals younger than 2 years. Thereafter, changes are inevitable, particularly in animals that are housed.

- Erosion, ridging or discoloration, erosio ungulae (heel erosion, see p. 116)
- Hypertrophy of the heel, overburdening (see p. 124)
- Atrophy of the heel, chronic laminitis (see p. 288)

The *coronary band* should be examined carefully both visually and by palpation for swelling or any other signs of infection. Apply firm pressure with the thumb, starting on the dorsal surface and proceeding abaxially to the heel; then repeat the process on the axial surface. This is essential in a complete digital examination.

- Vertical fissure (see p. 109) and septic arthritis of the DIP joint (see p. 105)
- Abscess in the heel (ascending infection from the zona alba, see p. 92; or foreign body of the heel, see pp. 104–106)
- Abscess, axial, abaxial, or dorsal coronary band (septic arthritis of the DIP joint, see pp. 104 and 250)
- Fistulas (septic arthritis or retroarticular abscess, see pp. 92–93)
- Partial exungulation (see p. 116)
- Separation of the coronary band (septic pododermatitis, see p. 104)
- Vesicles (foot and mouth disease, bovine virus diarrhea/mucosal disease [BVD/MD]) (see p. 90)

Examine the Interdigital Space

Separate the claws as far apart as possible and inspect the region visually and by palpation.

- Interdigital hyperplasia (see p. 119)
- Interdigital phlegmon (see p. 89)
- Wounds or foreign bodies (see p. 114)
- Vesicles (foot and mouth disease, BVD/MD) (see p. 90)
- Interdigital or digital dermatitis (see pp. 94 and 96)

Manipulate the Distal Interphalangeal Joint

With the limb still elevated, grasp one claw and stress the DIP joint and the interdigital ligaments by extending, flexing, and rotating the digit. Repeat the procedure with the contralateral phalanx. Finally move both claws apart, stressing the distal interdigital ligament. Pain on extension and flexion without other signs can be found in fracture of the distal phalanx or distortion of the DIP joint.

To localize a painful aseptic process in one digit, it may help to elevate the unaffected claw by temporarily fixing a wooden block to the trimmed normal claw with strong adhesive tape. In the case of fracture of the distal phalanx or severe distortion of the DIP joint, a considerable decrease in lameness is observed. A septic process should be precluded through careful examination in every case.

Test the Sensitivity of the Corium

Both claws should be subjected to the pressure applied with a hoof tester. An equine tester may be used, but a model with one straight and one curved jaw is preferred. First apply pressure to various parts of the sole, with one branch of the tester applied to the abaxial wall and the other applied to the sole. Next compress the axial and the abaxial wall. Pain is generated in such conditions as subsolar abscessation, involvement of the DIP joint, or fracture of the distal phalanx. When using hoof testers, avoid placing pressure on the coronary band. Percussion with a small hammer is a very sensitive method for locating painful areas.

EXAMINATION OF THE PROXIMAL LIMB

Examination of the Pastern

Examination of the pastern should take place with the limb elevated. Inspect the plantar/palmar skin for signs of digital dermatitis or eczema. Starting at the heel, gently palpate the plantar/palmar region of the pastern, including the portion of the flexor tendon sheath extending to the bulbs.

Next proceed dorsally to palpate the location of the dorsal pouch of the DIP joint located on either side of the extensor process. Palpating up to the fetlock joint, differentiate the extensor tendons, the tendon sheaths of which start about 7 to 10 cm above the coronary band.

Examination of the Fetlock

The metatarso/metacarpophalangeal joint should also be examined with the limb elevated. Palpate the fetlock joint, starting dorsally. The joint space and the adjacent joint surfaces normally can be easily palpated. The fetlock joint of the third digit communicates with that of the fourth digit via a slot in the intertrochanteric area. Excess joint fluid can be detected by simultaneous palpation of the dorsal and the palmar/plantar recesses. On the plantar/palmar aspect, the recesses can be palpated in the triangle formed by the distal part of metatarsus/metacarpus, the interosseous muscle, and the proximal sesamoid bones. Proximal to the interosseous muscle, the proximal compartment of the digital flexor tendon sheath can be palpated. It should be noted that if a purulent infection is present in the sheaths, it is impossible or difficult to determine if the joint is also involved. Manipulate the fetlock by extending, flexing, and rotating the digit.

Check the dewclaws for exungulation, bandage pressure, and digital dermatitis.

Examination of the Metatarsus/Metacarpus (Cannon Bone)

Examine the metatarsus/metacarpus and the surrounding structures both visually and by palpation.

- Diaphyseal fractures (see p. 265)
- Tendon lacerations (see p. 188)
- Epiphysitis, nutritional or infective (see p. 230)
- Chronic osteomyelitis (see p. 243)
- Salter-Harris fracture of the distal carpal/tarsal growth plates (see p. 231)

Examination of the Tarsal Joint (Hock)

No connection normally exists between the synovial cavities of the talocrural joint and the distal tarsal joints.

- Firm, diffuse swelling on the medial aspect of the joint (bone spavin, see pp. 171 and 191)
- Acute or chronic septic arthritis/osteomyelitis (see p. 166)
- Restricted movement, periarticular exostoses (see p. 191)
- Decubital lesions (see p. 191)
- Tarsal periarthritis (see p. 190)

To evaluate any distention of the joint capsule, place one hand in the angle formed by the distal border of the tibia and the anterior aspect of the calcaneus on the lateral and medial surfaces of the joint. Place the other hand on the dorsal surface of the joint where the joint capsule can be palpated on either side of the extensor tendons.

- Serous tarsitis or bog spavin (see p. 191)

To palpate the calcaneus, start distally and proceed proximally. Pain or distention of the bursa calcanea subcutanea or the bursa calcanea subtendinea may be detected.

Examination of the Tibia

The whole area should be palpated after careful observation.

- Distal growth plate, metastatic infection
- Tibial fracture (see p. 266)
- Achilles (gastrocnemius) tendon or muscle tendon, trauma (see p. 197)
- Rupture of the peroneus muscle

Examination of the Stifle

The stifle should be observed for swelling, wounds, and other abnormalities. Enlargement of the stifle joint is often best appreciated from a lateral view. Palpation should commence at the medial tibial condyle, proceeding to the tuberositas tibiae and then to the lateral tibial condyle. Evaluate the patellar ligaments inserting at the tuberositas tibiae. By deep palpation in the gap formed by the straight patellar ligaments, distention of the capsules of the medial or lateral femorotibial joint can be appreciated. Proceeding to the patella, the joint capsule of the femoropatellar joint can be identified. All femorotibial joint cavities in the ox are interconnected in most animals. Palpate the femorotibial collateral ligaments. Abduction and adduction of the whole extremity provokes joint instability, caused by rupture of a femorotibial ligament (usually the medial). In some cases of rupture of the cruciate ligaments, instability can be provoked by pulling the tibia caudally while the examiner stabilizes the hock with his or her knee ("drawer forward sign"). Move the calcaneus medially and laterally while palpating the stifle for signs of crepitus. The pelvic limb flexion test is carried out like a spavin test in horses. This test is restricted to very cooperative animals.

Examination of the Femur and the Hip

The femoral region is observed for muscle atrophy and asymmetry. Stand behind the animal, locate the trochanter major, and relate its position to the tuber ischiadicum and the tuber coxae. Compare these bony points on each side as an indication of femoral luxation. Upward luxation is the most common form of hip dislocation. The adductor group of muscles should be palpated and compared for evidence of swelling.

The hip joint itself is not accessible by palpation; therefore, the status of this joint cannot be evaluated except by skilled arthrocentesis. A stethoscope placed over the great trochanter may reveal crepitation as an assistant rotates the femur.

Rectal examination is obligatory in the investigation of hip and pelvic problems, especially in the case of a "downer cow." This internal examination should check for pelvic asymmetry, swelling, and the abnormal movement of bones when the animal is rocked from side to side by an assistant. Crepitation is sometimes palpable only when the animal is moving or when one extremity is lifted. The obturator foramen may have an abnormal contour owing to the pressure of the caudally luxated femoral head. The iliopsoas and pelvic muscles as well as the sacroiliac joints are palpated for abnormal swelling, edema, and painful points. During a rectal examination, particularly in older bulls, the ventral aspect of the lumbosacral vertebral column should be palpated.

- Neonatal fracture, femur (see p. 271)
- Luxation of the hip (see p. 175)
- Rupture or hematoma of adductors (see p. 196)
- Fracture of the femoral head or neck (see p. 272)
- Spondylosis
- Pelvic fracture or iliosacral strain

Examination of the Carpal Joint

The carpus is examined visually and by palpation for soft tissue swelling, joint capsule distention, and pain. The carpus should be flexed and extended to define more precisely the location of the lesion. The tendon sheaths of the common and lateral digital extensor muscles and the extensor carpi radialis muscle should be evaluated for swelling. Deep palpation of the carpal bones may promote pain. The routine palpation should commence with the distal row (os carpale secundum et tertium, os carpale quartum) and continue to the proximal row (ossa carpi radiale, ossa carpi intermedium, ossa carpi ulnare). Palpate the radial epiphysis.

- Precarpal bursitis (see p. 192)
- Septic carpitis (see p. 262)
- Osteomyelitis of calves (see p. 166)

Examination of the Forearm and Cubital Region

Deep palpation of the forearm should proceed proximally to the level of the elbow joint. One hand follows the contour of the radius on the medial aspect of the limb while the other palpates the soft tissue and the muscles up to the joint space and the collateral ligaments. Only a massive fluid distention of the elbow joint is detectable by palpation. Continue upward to the olecranon with the outer hand. The inner hand palpates the pectoralis region.

Examination of the Humerus, the Shoulder, and the Scapula

The humerus and associated muscles should be checked for swelling, pain, and crepitation. The contours of the biceps muscle should be palpated up to the point of the shoulder. In a case of traumatic bursitis of the bicipital bursa, pain and edema are present at the cranial aspect of the shoulder joint. The joint capsule cannot be evaluated under normal conditions.

- Rupture of the ventral serrate muscle (see p. 195)

- Fracture of the scapula (see p. 265)

- Luxation of the shoulder (see p. 265)

- Penetrating wounds (see p. 183)

For a flexion test of a thoracic limb, the examiner should stand just in front of the shoulder, facing backward grasping the metacarpal region with both hands. The limb should be elevated to flex the digital joints and carpus until the claws approach the elbow. In this position, the metacarpus is almost parallel to the radius when the carpal joint has been flexed to the maximum. After 2 minutes, the animal is walked ahead. Increased lameness indicates a painful process in one or more of the flexed joints. Any restricted range of motion or a painful response should be noted during flexion of the joints.

EXAMINATION OF THE BACK

The back should be inspected with the animal standing. Palpation of the spinous and transverse processes should check for irregularities; obvious swellings; the occurrence of kyphosis, lordosis, and scoliosis; painful zones; abnormal rigidity; and edema. Skin sensation and pain reactions should be tested, starting at the withers region and proceeding to the pelvic region and tail.

PHASE FOUR—CONDUCT SPECIAL TESTS

DIAGNOSTIC ANESTHESIA

Diagnostic anesthesia is rarely performed but is useful to differentiate a painful lesion from one associated with mechanical failure. It is also used to confirm or disprove that the seat of lameness is located in the digital region in cases in which no obvious lesion can be identified. To a limited extent, regional anesthesia can be used to locate a painful condition in an area supplied by one specific nerve or branch of a nerve.

Nerve blocks need an exact technique, as described in Chapter 4. Complete anesthesia is sometimes difficult to obtain if significant inflammatory edema is present.

Intra-articular anesthesia is useful if a painful arthritic condition is suspected. The indications for this form of diagnostic aid are described in Chapter 11. The sites of joint puncture are described in Chapter 14, dealing with applied anatomy (see p. 227).

RADIOGRAPHY

Radiography is discussed in Chapter 3.

ULTRASONOGRAPHY

Ultrasonography, currently underused in clinics, will become increasingly valuable for examining large animals (see p. 38).

LABORATORY TESTS

The value of microbiological samples is discussed in Chapter 15, and blood and synovial fluids are addressed in Chapter 11.

John W. Pharr *Canada*

Uri Bargai *Israel*

3

Radiology

EQUIPMENT FOR FIELD RADIOGRAPHY

Although the basic x-ray machine has changed little from the days of Konrad Roentgen, certain improvements have made veterinary radiography more feasible and safer. The typical modern portable machine (Fig. 3–1A) now has a high-quality electronic (rather than mechanical) exposure timer and is usually equipped with a collimator (rather than a cone or diaphragm) to limit the radiation field. These are important factors.

An *electronic timer* ensures rapid, accurate exposure times as low as 1/120 second, compared with 1/10 second for a mechanical timer.

The *collimator* can be adjusted in size to shape a radiation field that exposes only the required part of a patient and incorporates a light source that illuminates the exposure field to make alignment of the radiation beam with the patient's part and the x-ray cassette more reliable. Some machines also have aiming devices similar to those used in range-finder cameras to aid alignment of the radiation beam.

Portable x-ray machines of 20 or 30 mA output are available, as well as those of 10 or 15 mA output. These higher-output machines offer greater flexibility, although at a cost of greater weight. The recent development of high-frequency generators has made possible the production of lightweight portable x-ray machines (Fig. 3–1B) of considerable power. Although these new machines are good, it is by no means necessary to purchase a new x-ray machine to perform high-quality field radiography, because older machines may also have or may be retrofitted with a collimator and an electronic timer. It may even be possible to purchase a used machine with a limited warranty, although a warranty increases the cost. The x-ray tube itself is the part of a used machine that is most likely to fail, and the amount of life left in a tube cannot be accurately measured. Thus, it is wise to budget for the possibility of tube replacement if a warranty is not available.

Intensifying screens and x-ray film are two parts of what may be called the *imaging system*, the third part being the film-processing technology. Significant improvement has taken place in the area of intensifying screen and x-ray film technology. It has always been desirable in veterinary medicine to use the fastest possible screen-film combinations in order to minimize exposure times using x-ray machines with much lower outputs than the machines commonly used for human radiography. The disadvantage of doing this is that image quality using older high-speed systems is less than optimal, sometimes greatly so.

Rare earth intensifying screens represent a major leap forward for veterinary radiography. Rare earth screens are so much more efficient than standard calcium tungstate screens at converting x-rays into visible light to expose the x-ray film that excellent detail can be preserved with very fast exposure times. This advantage is so great that it can be convincingly argued that one's money would be better spent by investing in cassettes with rare earth screens even if it means buying a used x-ray machine. Also, using exposure times that are still practical, a portable x-ray machine can be used with rare earth screens to radiograph larger patient parts (e.g., the bovine stifle) than could be readily managed with conventional screens. Rare earth screens have now been available for many years, but this technology is constantly being developed and improved.

X-ray films as well have been markedly improved in the past 10 years, offering higher speed and better image quality than ever before. Continued improvement can be expected in these areas of radiographic technology, driven by the desire for reduced patient exposures in human medicine. One caution must be observed: *The components of the imaging system must be matched or compatible for optimum performance.*

Unlike large-volume users (hospitals, veterinary colleges), most veterinarians purchase x-ray supplies from an independent distributor rather than from a manufacturer (e.g., DuPont, Kodak, Fuji, Agfa) and may sometimes be tempted to purchase supplies without considering component compatibility. Intensifying screen phosphors may emit either blue, green, or ultraviolet light to expose the x-ray film sandwiched between the screens in the cassette. *The x-ray film used must be sensitive to the light emitted by*

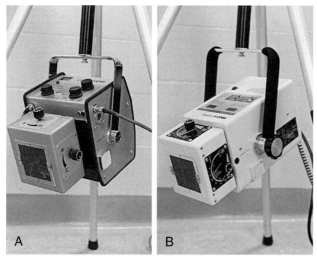

Figure 3–1. *A,* Modern portable x-ray machine (MinXray 803G; MinXray, Inc, Northbrook, IL) mounted on a tripod. Weighing 17.6 kg, this machine is equipped with a collimator and an electronic timer capable of exposures as short as 0.02 second (1/50 second) and can produce up to 30 mA (at 50 kVp) or 20 mA (at 80 kVp). *B,* High-frequency portable x-ray machine (MinXray HF80; MinXray, Inc, Northbrook, IL). This machine, equipped with a collimator and an electronic timer capable of exposures as short as 0.02 second, produces 10 mA at 50 to 80 kVp and weighs only 10 kg. (Equipment courtesy of MedTec Marketing, Ltd, Edmonton, AB, Canada.)

the screens, or poor results will be obtained. Also, a change in x-ray film when modifying one's imaging system may require a change in darkroom safe light bulbs and film-processing technology.

One small but important item that every veterinarian should have in addition to standard x-ray viewboxes or illuminators is a high-intensity lamp or bright-light. To examine dark (overexposed or overdeveloped) films or darker film areas this simple device is essential; using it can often make taking repeat films unnecessary.

It is generally accepted that x-ray films or radiographs are a valid part of an animal's veterinary medical record, as long as they are identified in an acceptable manner. Proper medicolegal identification of a radiograph specifies (1) the veterinarian who made the film, (2) the date the film was made, and (3) the animal. A logbook code number may suffice to identify the film date and the animal. A radiographic orientation marker is also essential for most films, including all orthopedic films in which the limb must be identified (right versus left; fore versus hind). All of this information should be indelibly marked in the emulsion of the x-ray film; added adhesive labels are not acceptable.

RADIATION SAFETY IN BOVINE RADIOGRAPHY

Recent reassessments of the risks inherent in chronic exposure to low-dose ionizing radiation, such as x-radiation, have resulted in revised radiation health and safety laws in many countries. However, al-though the allowable occupational total-body exposure dose of x-radiation has typically been lowered from 50 millisieverts per year to 20 millisieverts per year, it is still possible to practice veterinary radiography and keep exposure doses well within these new limits. Using a modern x-ray machine and an imaging system as described earlier does enhance one's ability to perform radiography in veterinary practice with optimum safety.

The fundamental precautions of veterinary radiation safety remain unchanged:

• Use the minimum possible exposure time.

• Keep the maximal distance away from sources of radiation.

• Use appropriate radiation shielding.

Minimum Exposure Time. The most important rationale for using minimum exposure time is that the number of retakes is minimized. If the animal moves during an exposure, the x-ray image is blurred, usually so much so that the radiograph is non-diagnostic and has to be repeated. Not only is this usually inconvenient, but it means that the personnel involved were exposed while accomplishing nothing and have to be exposed again to obtain a diagnostic radiograph. With a modern imaging system and x-ray machine, the shortest possible exposure times can be achieved.

Distance. Distance reduces radiation exposure because of the inverse square law (the intensity of radiation decreases proportional to the square of the distance from the radiation source). The principal source of x-radiation exposure in veterinary medicine is normally scatter radiation from the body of the patient. Anyone whose presence is not required to assist in the radiographic procedure should vacate the area or move at least 10 meters away. Those who do participate in the procedure should make an effort to position themselves as far as possible from the part of the animal being radiographed; even a small added distance, such as achieved by leaning away from the patient, is beneficial. Most of the scatter radiation arises on the tube side of the patient; thus, even if distances are equal, a person standing on the cassette side of the part being exposed receives less radiation exposure. This does not mean standing directly behind the cassette, however, because this would place the person in the path of the primary x-ray beam, a considerable proportion of which passes through a standard (i.e., not lead backed) cassette. Exposure to the primary x-ray beam should be avoided at all costs. Also, when working in the field, one must take extra care that persons not in the immediate vicinity of the radiographic procedure are not standing in the path of the primary beam.

Shielding. Shielding for radiation protection means at least wearing lead aprons, and lead gloves or mittens should be worn by anyone who is near the primary beam holding a cassette, cassette holder, or part of the patient. Protective thyroid collars and eyewear are also recommended. It must be borne in mind that such protective gear is designed to protect the wearer from scatter radiation, *not* from the primary x-ray beam. In particular, gloved hands must be kept out of the field of the primary beam; an ungloved hand near but outside the primary beam receives less radiation exposure than a gloved hand inside the primary beam. For this reason, the use of cassette holders (either brackets, hand-held or on mobile stands, or slotted wooden blocks) is strongly recommended; these function very well with smaller cassettes (8 × 10 inches; 10 × 12 inches). When the study requires the use of a larger field (e.g., for elbow or stifle films) and the use of a cassette holder is not possible, one may use a cassette larger than the required field and collimate the primary beam so that only a portion of the cassette is exposed; gloved hands can then be used to grasp the unexposed portion of the cassette.

INTRODUCTION TO RADIOLOGY

The effective and accurate use of radiological knowledge is a stepwise, logical process. This process is based on an understanding of both the anatomy of the species being examined and the physical principles of radiography, such as film contrast and image geometry. The basic steps of the process are as follows:

- Technical analysis—exposure, positioning, artifacts, identification

- Analysis for roentgenographic signs of abnormality

- Interpretation of the roentgenographic signs

Technical Analysis. The clinician's first step must be a technical analysis of the films. This includes assessing the quality of film exposure and film processing, the accuracy of anatomical positioning, and the presence or absence of any complicating factors (e.g., patient motion blur, dirt on the foot, questionable identification markers). A film or film series does not have to be perfect to be diagnostic, but it is important to identify technical defects in order to recognize the effects that such defects may have on the image. One can then proceed to further analysis with the appropriate level of confidence.

Identification of Signs of Abnormality. The second step is the analysis of the films for roentgenographic or radiographic signs of abnormality. There are five basic roentgenographic signs:

- Change in opacity

- Change in size

- Change in shape

- Change in location

- Change in number

Individually and in combination, these signs can be used to recognize and describe every possible radiographic lesion. However, neither individual signs nor combinations of signs are necessarily specific for a single disease; for example, periosteal new bone production and soft tissue swelling occur both with trauma and with osteomyelitis. Radiological analysis includes assessing the pattern and magnitude of the radiographic lesions and sometimes assessing change over time with serial films. One should note every roentgenographic sign visible; some findings may only be incidental lesions, but others may alter the treatment or prognosis for a case.

Interpretation of Signs. When both steps of analysis are complete and a list of the visible roentgenographic signs has been assembled, one may then proceed to the final step, which is interpretation of these signs. One should interpret the roentgenographic signs by using all information available, including signalment, history, physical examination, and any other diagnostic tests, to make the radiological diagnosis most logically based on this information. At times no single diagnosis conclusively explains all clinical findings. In such cases, radiology should at least narrow the differential diagnosis, and radiology often suggests what additional diagnostic tests (e.g., arthrocentesis) to perform when seeking a definitive diagnosis.

It is important for inexperienced veterinarians to approach radiology in this stepwise fashion to avoid making incorrect or inaccurate diagnoses. Although this process can proceed very quickly when the reader of the radiograph is experienced, appearing to an observer to be almost instantaneous, stepwise film analysis and interpretation are fundamental to the sound practice of radiology.

RADIOLOGY OF THE DIGITAL REGION

Radiographic Technique. A major proportion of bovine radiology involves the digital region (distal metacarpus/metatarsus through the distal phalanx) because numerous diseases affect this region. Clinical findings may indicate disease in a specific part of the foot, such as the distal interphalangeal joint and distal phalanx, and if so the radiographic study should be centered on this part. In cattle, however, such localization is not possible as frequently as in horses, so the entire foot is often radiographed in a single study.

The claws and interdigital space should be cleaned thoroughly before radiography. Shadows created by mud, manure, matted hair, or medications applied to the region make image analysis difficult. Previous treatment, in particular paring away portions of the hoof, also alters the soft tissue images superimposed over the bones and joints, and this must be borne in mind when analyzing the films.

The Dorsopalmar/Plantar Projection. This projection provides the single most useful view of the digital region. This image shows all of the major bones and joints without overlap, and many diseases of the bovine foot can be correctly diagnosed using this view alone. Additional views, however, provide yet more specificity in diagnosis, thus improving accuracy in prognosis and decisions on treatment.

Oblique Projection. Because the ox has two digits, oblique views are often of critical importance. A pair of matched 45° oblique views (dorsolateral to palmaro/plantaromedial and dorsomedial to palmaro/plantarolateral) are extremely helpful in detecting bone and joint lesions. There is some superimposition of structures, especially proximally, but comparison of the two oblique views enables the reader of the radiograph to define the extent of lesions with greater confidence and frequently reveals lesions that could not be detected on the dorsopalmar/plantar view.

Lateromedial or Mediolateral Projection. Because of the superimposition of digits, the lateromedial or mediolateral view of the bovine foot is far more confusing than that of an equine foot and is of much less value. This view is important for the assessment of fractures and fracture repairs, but it adds little information in many other conditions.

Axial Projection. An important exception is the lateromedial or mediolateral view of a single claw made by placing a non-screen film (paper cassette) between the digits; this view produces a good image of the affected distal phalanx and, if interdigital soft tissue swelling is not too great, the distal interphalangeal joint.

NORMAL RADIOGRAPHIC ANATOMY—ADULT

On a well-positioned dorsopalmar/dorsoplantar view (Fig. 3–2), the digits appear symmetrical. The proximal and distal sesamoid bones are superimposed on, respectively, the distal metacarpus/metatarsus and the distal portion of the middle phalanx. If the study is made with the animal weight-bearing, the distal phalanges appear slightly foreshortened.

On oblique views (Fig. 3–3), the sesamoid bones are seen with less superimposition, and their articulations can be appreciated. Because each digit is projected differently on an oblique view, it is advisable to compare two obliques made at comparable but opposite angles.

On the lateromedial or mediolateral view (Fig. 3–4), the digits are superimposed but foot alignment can be appreciated. This view is most useful in cases of severe trauma, such as fractures or luxations.

On all of the views just mentioned, the small bones of the rudimentary digits (dewclaws) can be noted.

On the interdigital view (Fig. 3–5), most of a single distal phalanx and a portion of the distal interphalangeal joint can be examined without superimposition.

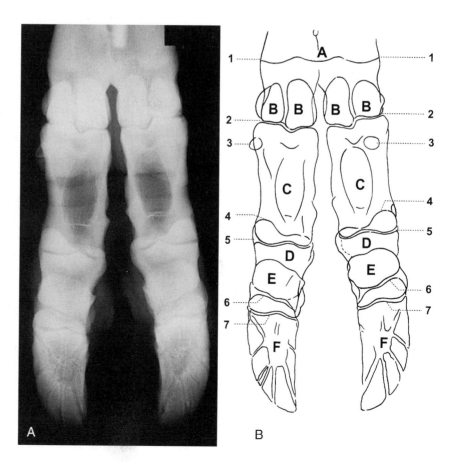

Figure 3–2. *A,* Dorsopalmar/dorsoplantar view of normal bovine digits in a Holstein-Friesian cow, 3 years old, not weight-bearing on radiography. *B, A,* Distal metacarpus/metatarsus; B, proximal sesamoid bones; C, proximal phalanges (P1); D, middle phalanges (P2); E, distal sesamoid bones (navicular bones); F, distal phalanges (P3); 1, sites of distal metacarpal (metatarsal) physes; 2, metacarpo-(metatarso)-phalangeal joints, 3, bones of rudimentary digits (dewclaws); 4, proximal palmar/plantar borders of middle phalanges; 5, proximal interphalangeal joints; 6, proximal palmar/plantar borders of distal phalanges; 7, distal interphalangeal joints, dorsal borders.

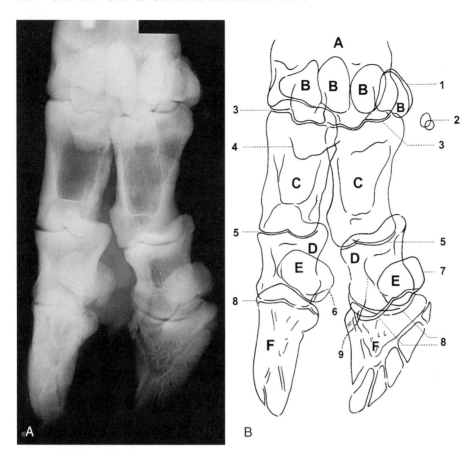

Figure 3–3. *A*, Dorsolateral-palmaro-(plantaro)-medial oblique view of normal bovine digits in a Holstein-Friesian cow, 3 years old, not weight-bearing on radiography. *B*, A, Distal metacarpus/metatarsus; B, proximal sesamoid bones; C, proximal phalanges (P1); D, middle phalanges (P2); E, distal sesamoid bones (navicular bones); F, distal phalanges (P3); 1, abaxial border of abaxial sesamoid bone, lateral digit; 2, bones of lateral rudimentary digit (dew claw); 3, metacarpo(metatarso)-phalangeal joints; 4, soft tissue shadow created by medial dew claw; 5, proximal interphalangeal joints; 6, axial border of navicular bone, medial digit; 7, abaxial border of navicular bone, lateral digit; 8, distal interphalangeal joints; 9, soft tissue shadow created by heel of medial digit.

Figure 3–4. *A*, Lateromedial view of a normal bovine foot in a Holstein-Friesian cow, 3 years old, not weight-bearing on radiography. *B*, A, Distal metacarpus/metatarsus; B, proximal sesamoid bones, superimposed; C, proximal phalanges (P1), superimposed; D, middle phalanges (P2), superimposed; E, distal sesamoid bones (navicular bones), superimposed; F, distal phalanges (P3), superimposed; 1, distal interphalangeal joints; 2, rudimentary bones of dewclaws, superimposed; 3, proximal interphalangeal joints; 4, proximal palmar/plantar eminences of middle phalanges; 5, distal interphalangeal joints.

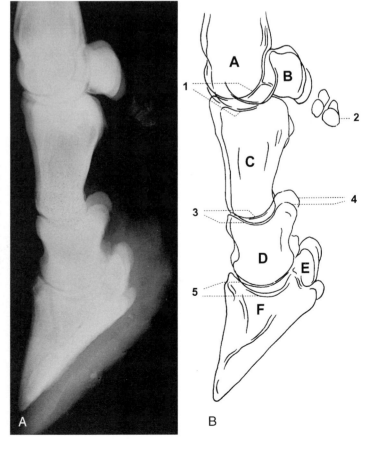

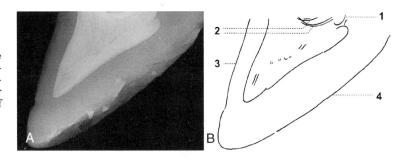

Figure 3–5. *A*, Lateromedial view of a normal bovine digit, made with interdigital non-screen film. Holstein-Friesian cow, 3 years old. Not weight-bearing on radiography. *B*, 1, distal palmar/plantar border of navicular bone; 2, distal interphalangeal joint; 3, dorsal aspect of claw; 4, sole of claw.

NORMAL RADIOGRAPHIC ANATOMY—JUVENILE

The digital region of a calf is similar to that of an adult, but growth plates (physes) are present in the distal metacarpus/metatarsus and at the proximal ends of the proximal and middle phalanges (Fig. 3–6). In a very young calf, the distal phalanges may be incompletely ossified, and thus the bones appear small and their distal ends rounded and indistinct. Also in young calves, particularly those of large and late-maturing breeds, the subchondral bone may not have completed enchondral ossification and may thus appear indistinct and finely irregular; this should not be mistaken for the subchondral bone lysis that occurs in septic arthropathy.

RADIOLOGY OF THE CARPUS

Only two views (dorsopalmar and lateromedial) usually are made of the bovine carpus, and these suffice for diagnosis in most cases. Occasionally, if a soft tissue swelling is present only over one particular aspect of the carpus, an oblique view silhouetting this swelling may be very useful in revealing any underlying bone or joint lesions.

NORMAL RADIOGRAPHIC ANATOMY

The carpus is a complex assemblage of bones, and considerable structural superimposition is unavoidable. It is important to analyze carefully each aspect of each bone, even though superimposition is present, in order to detect subtle but clinically significant lesions such as small areas of subchondral bone lysis.

On the dorsopalmar view (Fig. 3–7), the accessory carpal bone and the distal ulna are superimposed over other structures, whereas on the lateromedial view (Fig. 3–8) these bones are more clearly visible.

In a young animal, the growth plates (physes) of

Figure 3–6. *A*, Dorsopalmar/dorsoplantar view of a normal immature bovine foot in a Simmental calf, 2 months old, not weight-bearing on radiography. *B*, A, Distal metacarpus/metatarsus; B, proximal sesamoid bones; C, proximal phalanges (P1); D, middle phalanges (P2); E, distal sesamoid bones (navicular bones); F, distal phalanges (P3); 1, distal metacarpal (metatarsal) physes; 2, metacarpo(metatarso)-phalangeal joints; 3, physes of proximal phalanges; 4, proximal interphalangeal joints; 5, physes of middle phalanges; 6, distal interphalangeal joints.

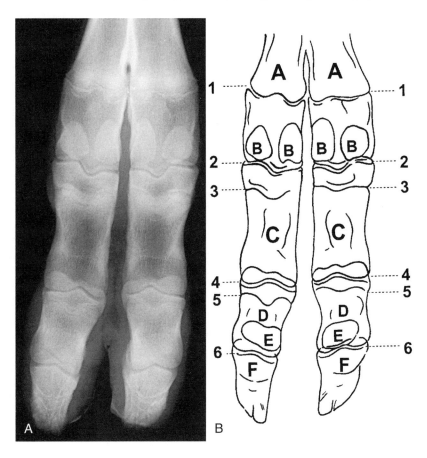

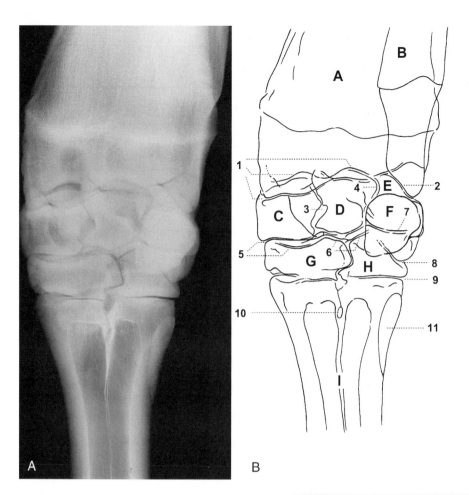

Figure 3–7. *A,* Dorsopalmar view of a normal bovine carpus in a Holstein-Friesian cow, 3 years old. *B,* A, Distal radius; B, distal ulna; C, radial carpal bone; D, intermediate carpal bone; E, ulnar carpal bone; F, accessory carpal bone (superimposed); G, third carpal bone; H, fourth carpal bone; I, fused third and fourth metacarpal bones; 1, antebrachiocarpal joint, with radius; 2, antebrachiocarpal joint, with ulna; 3, intercarpal joint between radial and intermediate carpal bones; 4, intercarpal joint between intermediate and ulnar carpal bones; 5, middle carpal joint, between radial and third carpal bones; 6, middle carpal joint, between intermediate and third and fourth carpal bones; 7, middle carpal joint, between ulnar and fourth carpal bones—dorsal part; 8, middle carpal joint, between ulnar and fourth carpal bones—palmar part; 9, carpometacarpal joint; 10, nutrient foramen; 11, rudimentary fifth metacarpal bone (superimposed).

Figure 3–8. *A,* Lateromedial view of a normal bovine carpus in a Holstein-Friesian cow, 3 years old. *B,* A, Distal radius; B, distal ulna; C, proximal row of carpal bones, superimposed; D, accessory carpal bone; E, distal row of carpal bones, superimposed; F, fused third and fourth metacarpal bones; 1, radioulnar joint; 2, antebrachiocarpal joint; 3, intercarpal joint between ulnar and accessory carpal bones; 4, middle carpal joint; 5, palmarodistal border of ulnar carpal bone; 6, carpometacarpal joint; 7, palmar border of fourth carpal bone; 8, rudimentary fifth carpal bone.

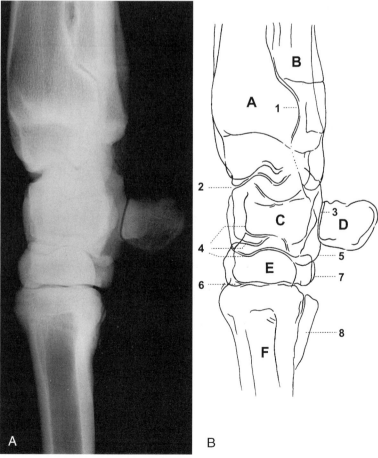

the distal radius and ulna are visible as transverse lucent lines separating the metaphyses and epiphyses. In a young calf, the physes are wide, especially at the periphery, and the adjacent actively ossifying bone, especially in the metaphysis, appears indistinctly marginated. As an animal matures, the physes narrow and become more distinctly marginated and the radial physis undulates.

RADIOLOGY OF THE TARSUS

Only two views (dorsoplantar and lateromedial) usually are made of the bovine tarsus, and these suffice for diagnosis in most cases. Additional views may occasionally be made, usually to further define lesions identified on the standard views. The following are among the additional views that may be useful in a particular case:

- Oblique views at 45° or to silhouette a local soft tissue swelling

- Angled craniocaudal views to highlight certain aspects of articular surfaces, particularly those of the talus

- A skyline (dorsoplantar) view of the calcaneus made with the tarsus flexed

NORMAL RADIOGRAPHIC ANATOMY

On the dorsoplantar view (Fig. 3–9), much of the calcaneus, including all of the tuber calcis, is superimposed over the distal tibia and the talus. The lateral malleolus of the talocrural (tibiotarsal) joint is a separate bone, representing the remnant of the distal fibula. On the lateromedial view (Fig. 3–10), the curved proximal and distal articular surfaces of the talus are more readily appreciated.

In a young animal, growth plates (physes) are visible in the distal tibia and in the proximal tip of the calcaneus. As with all physes, these are wider and less well marginated in younger animals. Because of the tension applied to the epiphysis of the calcaneus through the gastrocnemius tendon, the plantar portion of the calcaneal physis (the part opposite the tendon insertion) is the last to undergo enchondral ossification and may remain quite wide even when most of this physis has become narrow. This normal feature should not be mistaken for an avulsion fracture.

RADIOLOGY OF THE PROXIMAL LIMBS

Radiology may be an important aid to diagnosis in diseases affecting the bovine forelimb proximal to the

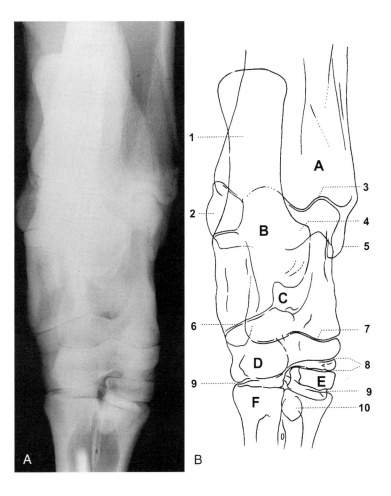

Figure 3–9. *A,* Dorsoplantar view of a normal bovine tarsus in a Holstein-Friesian cow, 3 years old. *B,* A, Distal tibia; B, calcaneus; C, talus; D, fused central and fourth tarsal bones; E, fused second and third tarsal bones; F, fused third and fourth metatarsal bones; 1, calcaneal process; 2, lateral malleolus (rudimentary distal fibula); 3, talocrural joint; 4, sustentaculum tali; 5, medial malleolus; 6, calcaneoquartal joint; 7, talocalcaneocentral (proximal intertarsal) joint; 8, centrodistal (distal intertarsal) joint; 9, tarsometatarsal joint; 10, rudimentary second metatarsal bone.

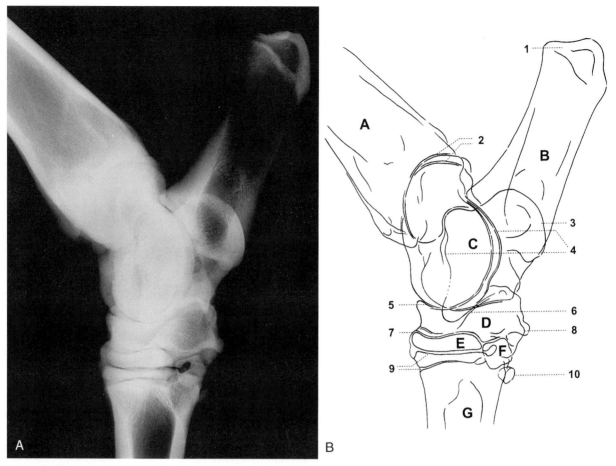

Figure 3–10. *A,* Lateromedial view of a normal bovine tarsus in a Holstein-Friesian cow, 3 years old. *B, A,* Distal tibia; B, calcaneus; C, talus; D, fused central and fourth tarsal bones; E, fused second and third tarsal bones; F, first tarsal bone; G, fused third and fourth metatarsal bones; 1, tuber calcanei; 2, talocrural joint; 3, sustentaculum tali; 4, intertarsal joint between talus and calcaneus; 5, talocalcaneocentral (proximal intertarsal) joint; 6, calcaneoquartal joint; 7, centrodistal (distal intertarsal) joint; 8, plantar tuberosity of fourth tarsal bone; 9, tarsometatarsal joint; 10, rudimentary second metatarsal bone.

carpus and the hind limb proximal to the tarsus, especially in calves injured during forced extraction at parturition. In such young animals, upper limb radiography may be quite feasible in the field.

Upper hind limb injuries may occur in adult cattle as well, particularly stifle joint injuries, but the practical limitations of adult upper hind limb radiography in the field are considerable. With higher-powered portable equipment and a high-speed imaging system, it may be possible to make lateromedial radiographs of some adult bovine stifles, but this area of bovine radiology is most often handled at referral centers with high-powered mobile or fixed x-ray equipment. Under such conditions, especially if general anesthesia is possible, satisfactory radiographs of the stifle region and pelvis of adult cattle may be obtained.

Even referral centers have difficulty dealing with upper forelimb problems in adult cattle, particularly in the shoulder. Anatomy, both soft tissue thickness and the relative immobility of the upper limb, simply precludes making useful radiographs of the adult bovine shoulder in most cases, particularly in bulls. The elbow region can be radiographed more easily,

but in a standing animal the soft tissue anatomy of the axilla prevents placing the cassette high enough to see much of the distal humerus; satisfactory radiographs of the elbow may only be obtainable if the animal is radiographed in a recumbent position with the limb extended.

The clinical dilemma of examining, for instance, a bull with a suspected humeral fracture can thus be very trying. Anesthetizing the animal for radiography may permit a diagnosis, but afterward the animal may never be able to regain its feet for treatment or transport to slaughter. It is sometimes necessary in such cases to rely on less than optimal radiographs such as, to use the same example, an oblique view that shows only the craniolateral aspect of the humerus. It still may be possible, even under such conditions, to make a diagnosis sufficient for determining what to do with the patient. If one is certain of the anatomy, detecting an abnormal contour or shape of one surface of a bone on a single suboptimal view may be enough to make the diagnosis of a fracture. Diagnosis of lesions more subtle than displaced fractures, however, in most cases is impossible.

RADIOLOGICAL ANALYSIS AND INTERPRETATION

Because specific disease problems, including radiological features, are dealt with elsewhere in this book, radiological analysis and interpretation are discussed here in broad general terms, emphasizing certain pitfalls that must be avoided.

The highly reactive *periosteum* of a bovine is a characteristic that influences the radiographic signs seen in many diseases, particularly trauma and infection. Diseases stimulating the production of periosteal new bone in cattle can cause marked changes in bone contour and increased bone opacity.

Osteophytes at *articular margins* (Fig. 3–11) and enthesiophytes at musculotendinous attachments are commonly seen on radiographs of older cattle and may only be incidental findings unrelated to the lameness under examination. One goal of radiological analysis is to assess the duration or age of a lesion, in order to correlate this information with the history.

Reactive new bone (osteophyte, enthesiophyte, or exostosis) that is chronic in duration is distinctly marginated and relatively homogeneous in opacity; however, it may not be smooth in surface contour but can be quite irregular or rough (Fig. 3–12). This surface irregularity should not be mistaken for a sign of recent or current bone activity.

Active new bone production is characterized by indistinct margins, non-homogeneous opacity, and an irregular outline (Fig. 3–13).

Diffuse loss of bone opacity occurs in metabolic or nutritional bone disease and with limb immobilization.

Focal or localized loss of bone opacity occurs in bone infection (osteomyelitis) or inflammation (osteitis), in early fracture healing, and with defects in enchondral ossification (osteochondrosis).

Soft tissue swelling is demonstrated on radiographs only in the early stages of a septic disease.

The absence of visible bone lesions cannot be taken as firm evidence that joints or bones are not involved. A considerable proportion of mineral must be lost from bone before a decrease in opacity is detectable radiographically. This is one reason why overexposed or overdeveloped radiographs, with the resultant low film contrast, are particularly unreliable for detecting subtle bone lesions. Also, overexposed films prevent reliable analysis of soft tissue shadows.

Increase in joint width, caused by effusion, may be the earliest detectable roentgenographic sign of septic joint disease (see Fig. 3–13). The affected joint should be compared with the same joint in the adjacent digit. One caution is that the two digits should be in similar positions and bearing similar weight; placing a block under only one claw makes

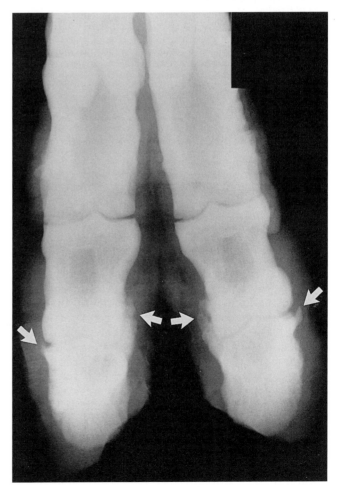

Figure 3–11. Chronic osteophytosis. This polled Hereford bull, 6 years old, became acutely lame on its left hind limb 2 days previously; no previous lameness was observed. Dorsoplantar view. Mature, chronic osteophytes (arrows) are seen at the axial and abaxial margins of both distal interphalangeal joints. No soft tissue swelling or acute bone lesions are visible.

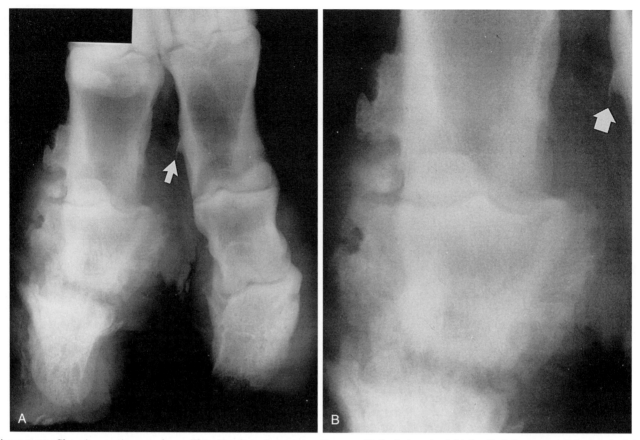

Figure 3–12. Chronic reactive new bone. This Aberdeen-Angus cow, 6 years old, had chronic right forelimb lameness. It had a draining tract in the digit 2 months earlier. *A*, Dorsopalmar view. *B*, Closeup of lateral digit in *A*. Extensive new bone proliferation is seen, especially on the middle phalanx and the abaxial aspect of the proximal phalanx. Although very irregular or rough in contour, this new bone is homogeneous and opaque and has distinct margins. Also seen is extensive destruction of subchondral bone with indistinct margination on both sides of the distal interphalangeal joint, indicating active osteomyelitis. An incidental finding is mature enthesiophytes projecting from the axial aspects of the proximal phalanges (arrows).

analysis difficult. This sign is more often detected in calves, which are usually radiographed in non–weight-bearing positions. In adult cattle radiographed in the standing position, this sign may not be evident.

Indistinctness and loss of opacity of the subchondral bone may be subtle in early septic arthropathy, requiring optimal radiographs to detect. Because a focal loss of opacity in early septic arthritis may affect only a small part of the subchondral bone of a joint, careful analysis of multiple views, comparing all projected aspects of each joint, is the most reliable means of detecting early disease. The more views that are made of a suspect joint, the more likely one is to be able to detect early signs of septic arthropathy (see Fig. 3–13; Fig. 3–14). In calves, one must remember that the subchondral region is the last portion of many bones to undergo endochondral ossification and thus may be indistinct in a young animal. In such cases, radiographing the contralateral limb for comparison is a valid technique. If the disease progresses unchecked, bone loss and alteration of the subchondral bone contour become marked and easily detected (see Figs. 3–12 and 3–14), and periosteal new bone proliferation develops.

Radiographic assessment of *fracture healing* is im-

portant to determine the success of fixation. Immediate postfixation radiographs should always be made of fracture repairs, for medicolegal reasons as well as to provide a true baseline on which to judge subsequent progress. Immediate postfixation alignment and apposition of all bone fragments, location of internal implants, and the condition of the soft tissues are factors that may subsequently prove very important in assessing healing, and they should be documented. Fractures that heal without complications (Fig. 3–15) pose no diagnostic problem, but questions are often raised when fracture healing does not proceed optimally. The distinctions between delayed union and non-union and between infected and normal bone healing are sometimes difficult to make on one particular set of follow-up films, and comparison with a subsequent follow-up may be necessary in some cases (Figs. 3–16 and 3–17).

Metabolic and nutritional diseases that cause a generalized rather than a focal loss of bone opacity are more difficult to diagnose radiographically, because disease cannot be detected by comparing one part of the limb with another as can be done with localized diseases. Loss of opacity of the subchondral bone, changing from a thick band of opacity fading gradually into the cancellous bone of the epiphysis to

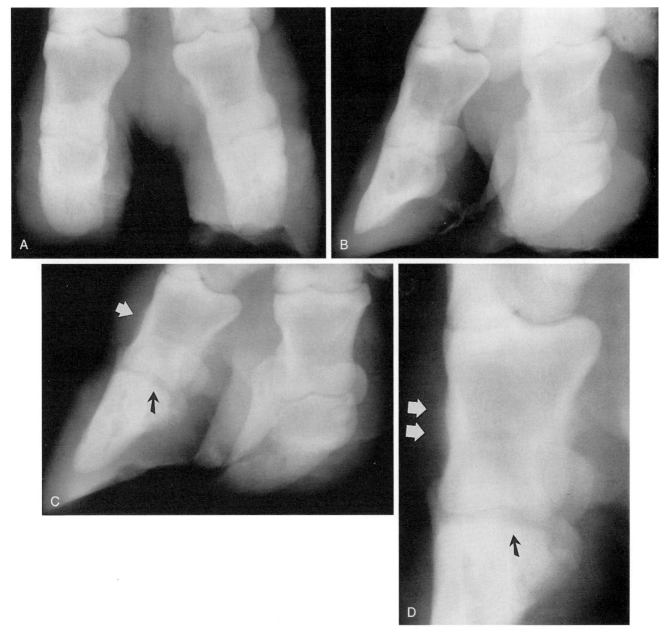

Figure 3–13. Subacute reactive new bone. This Holstein-Friesian cow, 7 years old, had left hind limb lameness for 3 weeks. Temporary improvement occurred after the sole ulcer was trimmed, but lameness is now severe. *A*, Dorsoplantar view. *B*, Dorsolateral-plantaromedial oblique view. *C*. Dorsomedial-plantarolateral view (reversed for comparison with *B*). *D*, Closeup of lateral digit in *C*. The lateral digit is swollen above the coronary band. The reactive new bone on the middle phalanx is not highly opaque, and its margins are indistinct, especially dorsolaterally (white arrows). The distal interphalangeal joint of the lateral digit is slightly widened on all views, and on the dorsomedial-plantarolateral oblique view a subtle loss of subchondral bone opacity is visible (black arrows).

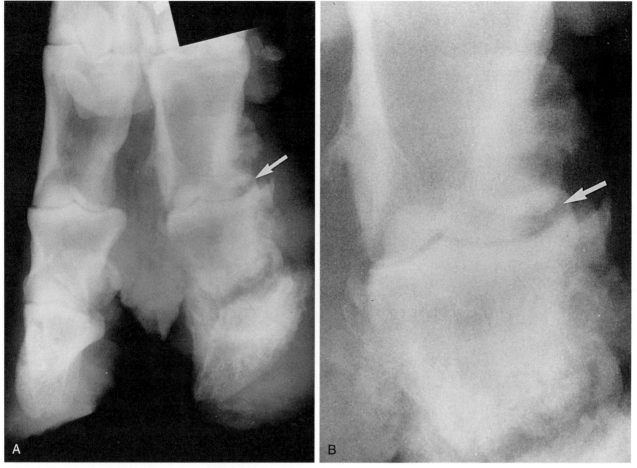

Figure 3–14. Focal subchondral bone loss. Same animal as in Fig. 3–12 had chronic right forelimb lameness. *A*, Dorsolateral-palmaromedial view. *B*, Closeup of lateral digit in *A*. A subchondral bone lucency is seen in the distal palmarolateral aspect of the middle phalanx (arrows), indicating septic arthropathy involving the proximal interphalangeal joint in addition to the extensively damaged distal interphalangeal joint. This very focal lucency is not clearly visible on the dorsopalmar view (see Fig. 3–12).

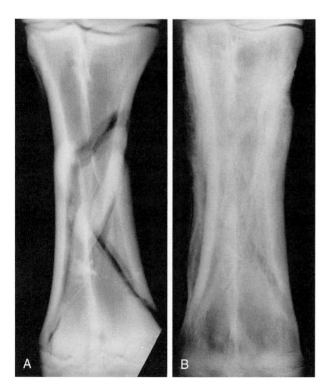

Figure 3–15. Uncomplicated fracture healing. This Angus calf, 6 months old, had a fractured left metacarpus, stabilized by a cast. *A*, One day after injury. *B*, Two months after injury. Dorsopalmar views. Although there were multiple fragments, none were greatly displaced. Fracture lines are still faintly visible on follow-up but are bridged by well-developed internal and external callus.

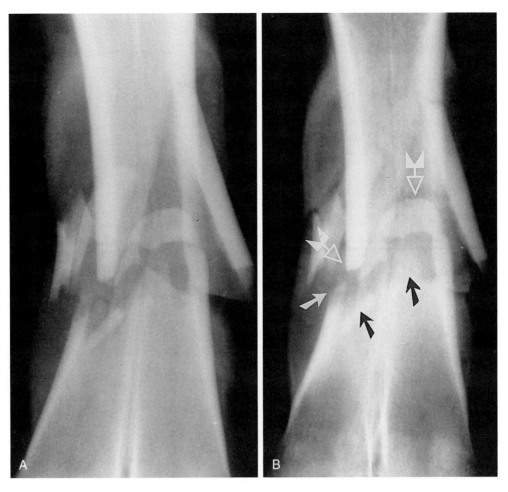

Figure 3–16. Delayed fracture healing. This Simmental-Charolais calf, 9 months old, had a fractured left metatarsus, stabilized by a cast. *A,* 2.5 weeks after injury. *B,* 6.5 weeks after injury. Dorsoplantar views. At 2.5 weeks (*A*), satisfactory periosteal callus has been produced, but the fracture margins of all fragments remain as distinct as at presentation, indicating delayed healing consistent with vascular injury (sequestration). At 6.5 weeks (*B*), healing is still suboptimal but there has been a modest increase in callus, both internal and external, and some fracture margins (solid arrows) have become less distinct, indicating early healing as the fragments revascularize. Some fracture margins (open arrows) remain unreactive, but there has been enough progress to indicate a guardedly fair prognosis.

a thin discrete line, is one of the more reliable signs. In a young animal, a similar change occurs in the metaphyses, normally a broad band of opacity with a somewhat indistinct margin toward the diaphysis. In metabolic/nutritional bone disease, the metaphyseal opacity may become a very narrow and distinct band immediately adjacent to the physis (growth plate). In an adult animal, cancellous regions in the bone ends may become coarser or granular in appearance as smaller bone trabeculae are resorbed. In the diaphysis of a normal bone in both immature and adult animals, the cortex is thickest at midshaft and becomes thinner toward both ends. If the cortex at midshaft approaches the thinness of the proximal and distal diaphyses, generalized osteopenia must be suspected. Radiographically, the osteopenia that occurs with limb immobilization is indistinguishable from that occurring in metabolic or nutritional bone diseases (Fig. 3–18).

Soft tissue lesions that are visible radiographically are often overlooked, attention being focused on the bones and joints. Soft tissue shadows can be very useful in directing attention toward the affected bone or joint (Fig. 3–19). This is particularly true in animals that have multiple bone lesions. By examining the nature of the soft tissues overlying a bone lesion, one may be able to determine the significance of the skeletal abnormality.

As noted earlier, chronic bone lesions are homogeneous and well marginated; however, such a chronic lesion may not be clinically silent just because an injury occurred previously at that site. One potential way of determining whether reinjury has occurred in a region with a chronic proliferative bone lesion is to examine the soft tissue shadows. If the overlying soft tissues are merely deformed by the bone lesion and conform to the contour of the underlying bone, the bone lesion is less likely to be the cause of recent lameness, and one should at least look for another, less chronic lesion. However, if the soft tissues overlying a chronic bone lesion are frankly swollen or thickened, reinjury may well have occurred at the same site.

The soft tissues should also be examined on every radiograph, even where there are no visible bone lesions. The contour and character of soft tissue swellings may indicate both where a disease process lies and the structures involved. A relatively discrete circumferential swelling centered over a joint suggests joint disease. A lengthy soft tissue swelling in one aspect of a limb, such as the palmar metacarpal region, signals muscle or tendon disease. Diffuse regional soft tissue swelling denotes diffuse soft tissue disease such as cellulitis or edema. In areas where infection with gas-forming organisms is present or where a sinus tract or laceration provides communi-

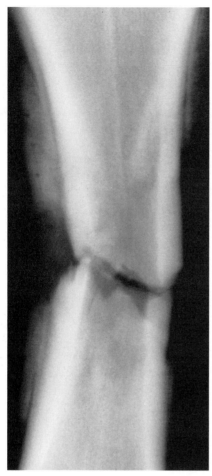

Figure 3–17. Delayed union, severe. This Simmental calf, 3 months old, had an open, overriding fracture of the left metatarsus with extensive soft tissue injury, stabilized by a cast. Four weeks after injury. Dorsoplantar view. There is suboptimal periosteal new bone production, with little in the immediate area of the fracture. The fracture margins and most of the adjacent cortical surfaces are unreactive. There was ongoing soft tissue infection as well as chronic vascular injury, creating a delayed union, which could become a non-union through sequestration of the fracture ends.

cation with the atmosphere, dark gas shadows may be detectable on radiographs (Fig. 3–20). Gas may be present as linear shadows in tendon sheaths or fascial planes, as multiple pockets of variable size and shape in a sinus tract, or even as a semi-spherical gas-capped fluid pocket in a discrete abscess.

In summary, radiology can play an important part in the diagnosis of bovine lameness. It simply must be practiced with care and common sense, bearing in mind its limitations and the undeniable fact that the quality of radiological diagnosis is directly proportional to the quality of the radiographs.

ULTRASONOGRAPHY IN BOVINE LAMENESS

Ultrasonography (diagnostic ultrasound imaging) is a feasible, if not inherently practical, ancillary imaging modality that may be applied to the investigation of bovine lameness.

The use of ultrasonography in lameness examination is well established in horses, especially in the evaluation of injuries to the tendons and ligaments of the palmar metacarpal and plantar metatarsal regions. Ultrasonography has also been successfully used in the identification and presurgical location of radiolucent foreign bodies such as wood fragments and in the mapping of draining sinus tracts and deep abscesses, particularly within large muscle masses such as the thigh (see p. 183).

Ultrasonography also has potential, especially in combination with radiography, in the evaluation of joints. Unless highly abnormal (highly cellular), synovial fluid is hypoechoic enough to outline intra-articular structures that cannot be seen radiographically, including articular cartilage, ligaments, and synovial surfaces. In horses, joint ultrasonography has been used to diagnose villonodular synovitis, pa-

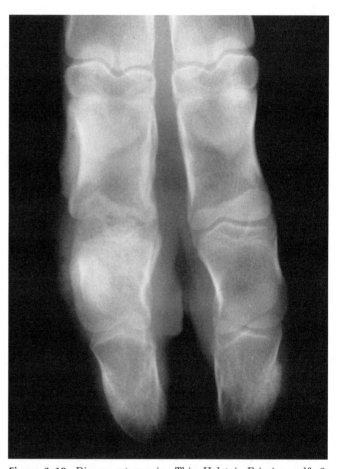

Figure 3–18. Disuse osteopenia. This Holstein-Friesian calf, 3 months old, had septic arthritis of the proximal interphalangeal joint of the left front medial digit, treated surgically. It has been in a cast for 3.5 weeks. Dorsopalmar view. In addition to a subtle overall decrease in bone opacity, the subchondral bone opacities at the unaffected joints have become thin distinct lines, and the mid-diaphyseal cortices of the proximal and middle phalanges have become thinner (compare with Fig. 3–5A). There is early chronic periosteal new bone production on the proximal and middle phalanges of the medial digit, fairly homogeneous and distinctly marginated but not highly opaque. The osteomyelitis was deemed to be healing, in that the subchondral bone destruction had not increased and appeared somewhat more marginated. Also, soft tissue swelling had decreased.

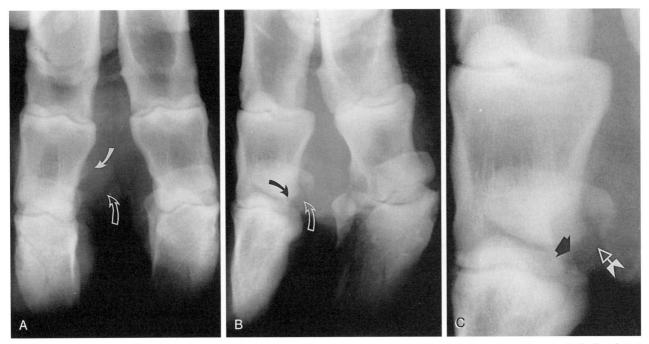

Figure 3–19. Focal osteomyelitis. This Charolais cow, 7 years old, was lame on its right hind limb for 2 to 3 weeks. It had a draining tract on the axial aspect of the lateral claw. *A*, Dorsoplantar view. *B*, Dorsomedial-plantarolateral oblique view. *C*, Closeup of lateral digit in *B*. On the dorsoplantar view (*A*), soft tissue swelling (open arrow) on the axial aspect of the lateral claw and periosteal new bone (solid arrow) on the diaphysis of the middle phalanx indicate cellulitis and periostitis, but there is no visible sign of osteomyelitis. On the oblique views (*B* and *C*), focal destruction of the distal axial portion of the lateral navicular bone (open arrows) and the adjacent portion of the articular condyle of the middle phalanx (solid arrows) confirms osteomyelitis and distal interphalangeal joint involvement (compare with Fig. 3–13 *C* and *D*).

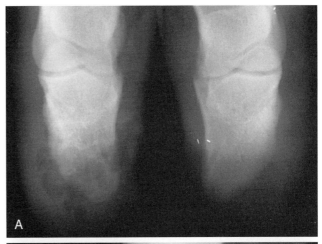

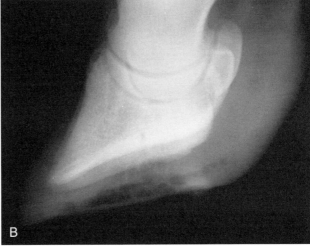

Figure 3–20. Subsolar abscess. This Charolais cow, 1 year old, had recent left forelimb lameness. *A*, On this dorsopalmar view, an aggregate of gas pockets is superimposed over the distal phalanx of the medial digit. Based on this view alone, the gas pockets could be either dorsal or palmar to the phalanx, or both. *B*, On this later-omedial view, although superimposition prevents determining which claw is involved, the gas pockets can be localized to the subsolar soft tissues. Superimposed gas shadows complicate analysis of underlying structures, but analysis of all views made, including obliques, revealed no conclusive bone involvement.

tella and patellar ligament displacement, and injuries to stifle joint ligaments and menisci.

Although it is principally a soft tissue imaging tool, ultrasonography may also be used in the proximal limb regions, such as the shoulder or hip, to confirm bone lesions that cannot be easily identified on radiographs because of the thickness of these regions. Avulsion fractures of the humeral tubercle in horses have been diagnosed sonographically by noting alteration in the contours of the bone surface echoes created by the fracture. Other fractures (e.g., scapular, pelvic, greater trochanteric) may potentially also be diagnosed in this manner. If the normal contours of the bone surface echoes are known for a specific anatomical location or can be determined by scanning the contralateral limb, significant alteration in those bone contours in the lame leg may be inferred

to confirm a fracture. Because only the surface of the bone nearest the transducer (scanner head) is imaged, one must remember that lesions other than recent fractures may alter the contour of a bone surface. To infer that a fracture is present and causing the lameness, all other information (historical and clinical) should point to that diagnosis.

BIBLIOGRAPHY

Bargai U: Radiology of the Bovine Foot: An Approach for the Practitioner. Veterinary Annual 33:62–74, 1993.

Bargai U, Pharr J, Morgan JP: Bovine Radiology. Ames, IA, Iowa State University Press, 1989.

Morgan JP: Techniques in Veterinary Radiology. Ames, IA, Iowa State University Press, 1993, pp 384–442.

Singh AP, Singh J: Veterinary Radiology. Delhi, India, CBS Publishers and Distributers, 1994, pp 217–241.

John C. Thurmon   *United States*
Jeff C. H. Ko

4

Anesthesia and Chemical Restraint

Mechanical restraint (see p. 14) is adequate for physical examination of most dairy cattle. Forceful restraint may occasionally compound the injury causing the lameness. It may sometimes be safer for the patient and the veterinarian to use chemical immobilization for examination purposes.

Immobilization and analgesia are essential for surgical treatment of many conditions. Technology has improved with the availability of new local analgesic techniques and better mechanical restraint devices (e.g., head catches, tilt tables, squeeze chutes, and so on). Many effective drugs and drug combinations (but relatively few approved by the United States Food and Drug Administration) are available for this purpose. It should be clearly understood that veterinarians using unapproved products are responsible for ensuring that cattle receiving them are not slaughtered until the drug has cleared the animal. Similarly, milk should not be permitted to be placed on the market until all drug residues have been cleared.

PAIN

Surgical intervention, trauma, inflammation, and neoplasia cause pain, as do other entities perceived in the central nervous system (CNS) as damaging to body tissues and an animal's well-being. The response to pain is important for short-term survival, but if prolonged, it becomes harmful. The stress response to pain increases myocardial work and total-body oxygen consumption. Ischemia and tissue hypoxia are associated with oxidative radical release (superoxides), which further increases tissue damage and depresses myocardial function. Intense vasoconstriction diminishes blood flow to vital tissues and can lead to vital organ failure (e.g., renal or hepatic). Prolonged stress increases nutrient requirements, which are met by catabolism of body tissues, resulting in a negative nitrogen balance. In many patients with severe posttraumatic or postsurgical pain, neuroendocrine responses may initiate the onset of circulatory shock, terminating in a patient's death if not properly treated.

The use of corticosteroids and non-steroidal anti-inflammatory drugs (NSAIDs) is controversial, but they may help ameliorate the cascade of inflammatory substances resulting from tissue degradation that contribute to the shock syndrome (see p. 164). Attenuation of the stress response through adequate pain relief and supportive therapy promotes healing and speeds patients' recovery. Pain can be controlled initially by systemic administration of analgesics. Opioids and alpha$_2$-adrenergic agonists seem to be the most effective. Long-term control of pain may include epidural or spinal injection of one or more of these drugs or long-acting local anesthetics (e.g., bupivacaine). They can also be used effectively for short-term relief of pain. A brief respite from pain may be all that is required to stimulate a desire to eat and to diminish production of catabolic substances.

Peculiar to the alpha$_2$-adrenergic agonists may be their endocrine effects in addition to their sedative and analgesic actions. Specifically, these drugs decrease sympathetic tone and inhibit cortisol and release of antidiuretic hormone while enhancing release of growth hormone. Thus, they may be of value in maintaining renal function, countering tissue catabolism, and decreasing the stress/distress responses so very injurious to circulatory function.

The NSAIDs are useful for relief of pain resulting, in part, from continued release of substances such as prostaglandins from injured and inflamed tissues. Non-pharmacological treatments including supportive bandaging and splinting should be considered. These techniques can prevent further tissue damage and injury to other body structures, promoting rapid return to normal/painless body function.

Pain is often described as *acute* or *chronic*. These clinical descriptions only serve to designate rapidity of onset and duration as perceived by patients afflicted with developing, existing, or potential tissue destruction.

Pain is perceived in the CNS as a signal that tissue destruction is occurring or has occurred. It causes an animal to avoid activities that would lead to further tissue/structural damage.

Acute pain can result from tissue damage due to any cause such as accidental or surgical trauma.

41

Acute pain is of rapid onset and short duration and can be controlled by local analgesics, general anesthetics, opioids, or alpha$_2$-agonists. The action of opioids and alpha$_2$-agonists acting on specific receptors can be terminated with specific antagonists (e.g., nalorphine [opioids], tolazoline or yohimbine [alpha$_2$-agonists]).

Chronic pain, as the term implies, is generally of several weeks' duration but may be somewhat protective in the early stages of the healing process. It can be a result of many physical disorders. According to severity, it is characterized by all the body changes that accompany stress/distress. Analgesics generally fail to relieve chronic pain permanently, yet these drugs often restore body function and a sense of well-being, promoting eating.

Pain tolerance defines the greatest amount of pain that a subject can tolerate. Tolerance varies considerably among species, individual animals, and anatomical location. It is influenced greatly by an individual's prior experience, environment, and stress/distress level, as well as by drugs.

When pain is intense and acute, opioids are among the most efficacious analgesics available, but these drugs are not always tolerated well by ruminants. Unless pain is severe or opioid administration is preceded by a tranquilizer or a sedative (e.g., acepromazine or xylazine), an excitatory response may occur. The agonist opioids have a relatively short half-life and require supplemental dosing. Most provide analgesia within 30 minutes after administration. Duration of action varies but ranges from 2 to 4 hours. The agonist-antagonists butorphanol and buprenorphine provide longer periods of analgesia (i.e., 4 to 5 hours for butorphanol). Analgesia up to 12 hours has been observed after buprenorphine injection, in some species. These drugs are expensive; therefore, their use in cattle cannot be justified on economic grounds alone. Nevertheless, veterinarians may wish to offer clients an option of reducing pain and suffering of animals despite the costs. Amelioration of postoperative pain may require the use of opioids for 24 to 48 hours.

The NSAIDs are often ineffective for complete relief of severe postoperative pain. They do have a place in treating pain associated with inflammation, particularly in articulations of the extremities (e.g., degenerative joint disease). In ruminants, NSAIDs should not be given for an extended period, as may be required to control chronic pain, because major side effects may accompany their use. These side effects are characterized by uncontrolled hydrochloric acid secretion, decreased mucus secretion, decreased bicarbonate levels, decreased blood flow, and delayed epithelization. Ruminant species are exceptionally prone to abomasal mucosal irritation or ulceration with prolonged NSAID therapy. Ulcerations may give rise to abomasal mucosal hemorrhage, hypovolemia, and death. Abomasal wall perforation with contents leaking into the abdominal cavity and peritonitis is a real possibility.

In cattle, the NSAID phenylbutazone has a 36 to 72-hour half-life, whereas in horses the half-life is only 3 to 6 hours. Clearly, phenylbutazone should not be administered more often than once each 36 to 48 hours and not repeated more than two to three times. In order to avoid severe side effects, treatment with NSAIDs must be followed by a reasonable respite from therapy to avoid cataclysmic side effects.

When using unapproved drugs for control of pain—or for any other purpose, for that matter—it is the veterinarian's responsibility to ensure that neither meat, milk, nor other products from these treated animals enter the human food chain until all drug or drug residues have cleared.

Veterinarians have a moral obligation to attempt to control pain and suffering in their animal patients. Practice based purely on economic considerations is unable to justify the cost of pain control but only at the expense of patients' well-being.

The following discussion lists doses of selected analgesic drugs proved to be effective in controlling various types of pain in ruminants.

OPIOIDS

Agonists

Morphine, 0.2 to 0.4 mg/kg IM
Meperidine, 1.0 to 2.0 mg/kg IM
Oxymorphone, 0.05 to 0.1 mg/kg IM

Agonists-Antagonists

Pentazocine, 1 to 2 mg/kg IM
Butorphanol, 0.1 to 0.2 mg/kg IM or IV
Buprenorphine, 0.005 to 0.008 mg/kg IM or IV

Analgesic drugs should be administered to effect rather than relying only on dosage recommendations, because various factors can affect their efficacy.

LOCAL ANALGESICS

Analgesics commonly used in cattle include procaine, tetracaine (esters), and lidocaine, bupivacaine, and mepivacaine (amides).

Lidocaine, not to exceed 12 mg/kg. If it is administered as a regional intravenous block, the dose should not exceed 9 mg/kg.
Bupivacaine, not to exceed 6 mg/kg. This drug is four times more potent than lidocaine; therefore, care must be taken not to exceed the recommended dose.

Either drug should be administered to effect and as frequently as required, bearing in mind that side effects may occur. The rapidity of tissue diffusion can be increased with hyaluronidase and slowed with epinephrine. Lidocaine toxicity (see Intravenous Regional Analgesia, p. 46) can be treated with a sedative dose of a barbiturate (2 to 4 mg/kg IV) or benzodiazepine (e.g., diazepam, 0.2 mg/kg IV) and respiratory support with oxygen.

NON-STEROIDAL ANTI-INFLAMMATORY DRUGS

Aspirin, 100 mg/kg PO every 12 hours
Flunixin meglumine, 1.1 to 2.2 mg/kg IV or IM
Phenylbutazone, 10 mg/kg IV or PO every 48 hours
Dipyrone, 20 mg/kg IV, IM, SC every 8 to 12 hours.

OTHER ANTI-INFLAMMATORY PRODUCTS

Dimethyl sulfoxide (DMSO). Apply over affected area.

SPINAL ANALGESIA

Spinal analgesia is classified as epidural analgesia or subarachnoid analgesia. This section refers to injection of the analgesic drug into the epidural space.

Lidocaine injected into the epidural space affects the motor nerves of the rear limbs and, depending on the dose, reduces the patient's ability to remain standing. The nerves of the autonomic nervous system will be affected. In hypotensive patients, high epidural analgesia is therefore unacceptable unless hypotension is corrected before drug injection; otherwise, irreversible shock may follow. Severe hypotension is treated with a balanced electrolyte solution by rapid intravenous fluid loading (20 to 40 mL/kg). Ephedrine (0.15 to 0.2 mg/kg) helps to restore blood pressure. Half of the dose should be slowly administered initially, with the remainder given in divided doses as required over minutes. Epinephrine is contraindicated.

It is essential that strict asepsis be maintained in epidural injection. The hair should be clipped and the skin scrubbed and prepared as for aseptic surgery. A local analgesic intended for epidural injection should not be taken from a partly used multidose vial because of likely bacterial contamination. Failure to follow strict rules of asepsis can result in necrosis, loss or paralysis of the tail, osteomyelitis, or ultimately meningitis.

The dose of 2% lidocaine required for complete immobilization of the posterior extremities of a 450-kg heifer in caudal epidural analgesia (Fig. 4–1) is approximately 60 mL. With procaine, 1.5 to 2 times the lidocaine dose is required. A dose greater than 10 mL will cause ataxia, from which injury may result.

Recent clinical observations have confirmed that xylazine is not only a potent sedative-analgesic but also a local anesthetic. Xylazine may be injected alone into the epidural space or combined with lidocaine. Clinical experience has shown that 20–25 mL of 2% lidocaine combined with 0.05–0.1 mg/kg of xylazine, when injected into the lumbosacral epidural

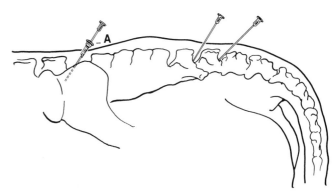

Figure 4–1. Sites for epidural injection. To decrease needle–skin drag, a short needle (1 or 2 cm) serves as a cannula through which the injection needle is passed into the lumbosacral epidural space (A). The two more caudal sites (sacrococcygeal and first intercoccygeal) are commonly used.

space, induces recumbency, mild sedation, and profound analgesia. In cows, xylazine alone injected into the epidural space at a dose of 0.06 mg/kg induces profound analgesia as well as overt sedation. Xylazine analgesia persists for approximately 1.5 hours.

The sedative but not the analgesic responses to epidural xylazine can be antagonized with yohimbine, 0.12 mg/kg plus 0.5 mg/kg of doxapram IV or 1 to 2 mg/kg of tolazoline. Atipamezole is also an effective sedative antagonist.

When using epidural analgesia for hind limb surgery, it is preferable to allow spontaneous recumbency after the administration of xylazine. If epidural analgesia is performed in a standing animal, an awkward and potentially hazardous period of ataxia may ensue before the animal falls. To avoid this possibility, the animal may be cast on soft bedding and epidural analgesia administered in recumbency. The sidelines or hobbles should remain in place until the analgesia has taken effect.

LOCAL ANALGESIA OF THE EXTREMITIES

PELVIC LIMB ANALGESIA

Pelvic limb analgesia extending from immediately below the hock and including the digital region can be induced by desensitizing the common peroneal and tibial extensions of the sciatic nerve.

The peroneal nerve is approached immediately caudal to the posterior edge of the lateral condyle of the femur as it courses anteriorly. This large nerve can be readily palpated in cattle with thin skin, making the injection site easy to identify (Fig. 4–2).

The site for desensitizing the *tibial nerve* is about 10 cm proximal to the tuber calcanei craniad to the deep flexor and gastrocnemius tendons. The tibial nerve is highly myelinated, and although it lies closer to the medial aspect of the limb, it requires injection from both medial and lateral sides.

Common peroneal block is characterized by the inability to extend the digits, or knuckling. In a ma-

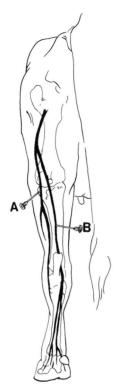

Figure 4–2. Location for blocking the common peroneal (A) and tibial (B) nerves.

ture cow, 20 mL of 2% lidocaine around the common peroneal nerve and 30 to 40 mL equally divided on the medial and lateral side of the tibial nerve effectively induces analgesia. An 18- to 20-gauge (1 mm diameter), 2.5-cm needle should be used. Onset of analgesia usually occurs in 15 to 20 minutes and lasts for 45 to 90 minutes.

THORACIC LIMB ANALGESIA

Thoracic limb analgesia can be induced by blocking the median, musculocutaneous, and ulnar nerves, but the technique is difficult and results are inconsistent (Fig. 4–3). The former and latter nerves are large in diameter and require a minimum of 10 to 20 mL of 2% lidocaine injected under the skin and fascia. When blocking these nerves, one expects to achieve analgesia from the carpus distally. Practitioners often resort to a *ring block* just distal to the carpus. Neither ring block nor individual nerve blocks immobilize the limb, which must be fixed by ropes.

The *median nerve* lies deep and requires an 18- to 20-gauge (1 mm diameter), 4- to 6-cm needle. It is located on the posterior aspect of the radius, 5 to 8 cm distal to the elbow and anterior to the flexor carpi radialis muscle. Desensitization requires 10 to 20 mL of 2% lidocaine. Complete blockade requires several minutes to take effect owing to the large size of this nerve.

The *ulnar nerve* site is 10 to 12 cm proximal to the accessory carpal bone in a groove between the ulnaris lateralis and flexor carpi ulnaris tendons. The nerve is located just under the skin and fascia. Failure occurs when the drug is deposited too deeply. Only a 20-gauge (0.9 mm diameter), 2.5-cm needle should be used. Eight to 10 mL of 2% lidocaine is sufficient, and complete blockade results in 10 to 15 minutes.

The *musculocutaneous nerve* is blocked immediately anterior to the cephalic vein. In thin-skinned cattle, the nerve can be palpated as it courses over the anterior aspect of the radius, where it lies just below the skin and fascia. Five to 10 mL of 2% lidocaine is injected through a small-gauge needle. With minimal restraint, a cow does not object to the procedure.

Brachial Plexus Block

A brachial plexus block (Fig. 4–4) is very useful for analgesia and immobilization of a thoracic limb, especially under field conditions. This block immobilizes the limb and induces complete analgesia from above the carpus distally, permitting manipulation and traction on the affected limb. This procedure is not recommended for general use by practitioners. Before this block is administered, the animal should be immobilized with a light level of general anesthesia or even deep sedation with xylazine.

A brachial plexus block is best performed with a cow positioned on her back. An 18 to 20-gauge (1.2

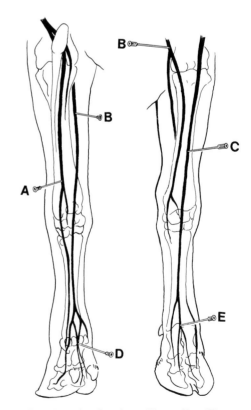

Figure 4–3. Locations for the ulnar (A), median (B), musculocutaneous (C), and interdigital (D, E) injections. Anterior and posterior views of the front limb.

mm diameter), 15 to 20-cm needle is used to inject 25 to 40 mL of 2% lidocaine into the area around the plexus. The plexus is approached by locating the tips of the transverse processes of the three distal cervical vertebrae. At this site, the needle is inserted horizontally through the skin and directed caudally until the tip contacts the anterior lateral edge of the first rib. The plunger of the syringe is slightly withdrawn to ensure that the tip of the needle is not located in an air space or blood vessel. Ten milliliters of lidocaine is injected at this site. As the needle is withdrawn, the remainder of the dose is injected slowly. If the needle is correctly placed, blockade develops in 15 to 20 minutes and persists for 90 to 120 minutes. A brachial plexus block is verified by complete flaccidity and analgesia of the limb. Although the procedure is technically more difficult in large adult cattle than calves, it is easily learned. Incorrect technique can lead to pneumothorax or pyothorax.

DISTAL DIGITAL ANALGESIA

The nerves supplying sensory innervation to the digit may be blocked with four separate injections, but this is technically more difficult than the common peroneal and tibial nerve blocks. Under field conditions, it is often considered easier and simpler to perform a ring block in the metatarsal (or corresponding metacarpal) region. The technique is illustrated in Figures 4–5 and 4–6.

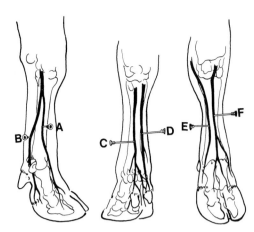

Figure 4–5. Locations for blocking sensory innervation of the digits of the forelimb and mid-metacarpus. Lateral branch of the ulnar (A), posterior branch of the ulnar (B), lateral palmar branch of the ulnar (C), medial palmar branch of the ulnar (D), dorsal branch of the ulnar (E), and dorsal metacarpal nerve (F).

When anesthetizing the digit of either the thoracic or pelvic limbs for surgical procedures, precise blocks can be administered at any of the four sites discussed next.

The *dorsal site* is located on the dorsal axis proximal to interdigital space close to the metacarpal/tarsal-phalangeal joint. Care should be taken in placing the needle in the dorsal site, because the proper digital artery can be encountered at this location. Ten milliliters of 2% lidocaine is injected with an 18- to 20-gauge (1 mm diameter), 10-cm needle. If the needle is inserted deep into the interdigital space, the nerves of the flexor surface can be reached. This obviates the need for a flexor site block for simple procedures. If the needle travels too far, it may encounter resistance from the cartilaginous plate of the annular ligament of the fetlock.

The distribution of the nerve supply to the axial

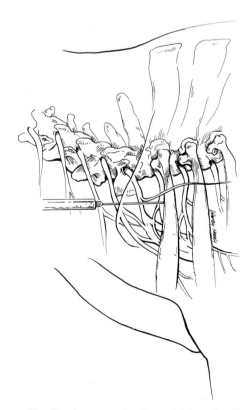

Figure 4–4. Needle placement for desensitizing the distal three cervical nerves and the first thoracic nerve, a brachial plexus nerve block. Lateral view.

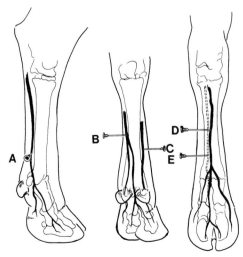

Figure 4–6. Locations for blocking sensory innervation to the hind digits. Lateral plantar (A), lateral (B) and medial (C) plantar nerves, superficial peroneal nerves (D), and deep peroneal nerve (E).

aspect of the digits of the thoracic limb is not constant. Thus, this technique is unreliable for digital analgesia of the thoracic limb.

The *flexor site* (if used) that is preferred is a little lower than the dorsal counterpart because it is difficult to pass a needle through the partially cartilaginous palmar/plantar ligament. Five to 8 mL of 2% lidocaine is injected with an 18 to 20-gauge (1.2 mm diameter), 5-cm needle.

Medial and lateral sites are located at the level of the dewclaws. A subcutaneous tract of 5 to 8 mL of 2% lidocaine is injected with an 18- to 20-gauge (1 mm diameter), 7 to 10-cm needle dorsally (horizontal in the standing animal) from a point 2.5 cm slightly proximal to the dewclaws.

- For surgery of the digit, such as amputation, the dorsal, palmar/plantar, and medial *or* lateral sites are used, depending on the claw requiring the intervention.

- For interdigital surgery (e.g., removal of corns), both the dorsal and palmar/plantar sites are used.

INTRAVENOUS REGIONAL ANALGESIA

Intravenous regional analgesia has become the preferred analgesic technique for the bovine digit. As with other local techniques, the limb is not immobilized and should be restrained to prevent movement during surgery.

The procedure, which is safe and simple, has been described in the literature.[1, 12, 19]

1 The patient is restrained in lateral recumbency, manually or chemically, although the procedure can be performed in the standing position in tractable patients.

2 A strong rubber tourniquet or inflatable cuff is placed around the limb proximal to the intended site of intravenous injection. A properly applied tourniquet appears to be more effective than an inflatable cuff. Placement of the tourniquet and injection of the local analgesic can be at any level at which the venous system can be compressed. Analgesia distal to the tourniquet and lidocaine injection site develops in about 10 minutes. One or more gauze rolls (depending on the site and number of veins) placed beneath the tourniquet and directly over the vein(s) being injected improve the effectiveness of hemostasis, promoting retrograde movement of the lidocaine and contact with nerve endings.

3 It is immaterial which vein is chosen for injection. Injection into the saphenous vein or any of its branches is effective as long as the tourniquet is secure and the dose is adequate. The same applies for palmar, metacarpal, radial, or other thoracic limb veins. The objective is to occlude venous blood outflow and induce retrograde movement of the local analgesic (Fig. 4–7). Measurement of the local (limb) and systemic intravenous (jugular) concentrations of lidocaine demonstrates some diffusion through tissues at the level of the tourniquet, because a measurable systemic concentration remains. It is probable that this results from diffusion along intraosseous routes.

In a mature bull or cow, a 20 to 22-gauge (1.2 mm diameter) needle should be used for intravenous injection of the local analgesic. Scalp vein needles or butterfly trocars are useful. Large needles may result in a hematoma when the needle is removed while the tourniquet remains in place. The dose of lidocaine without epinephrine ranges from 10 to 30 mL, depending on the animal's size, the position of the tourniquet, and the site of injection. In calves, 5 to 10 mL suffices. Despite the overall effectiveness of this technique, incomplete analgesia has been noted in the interdigital tissues in some patients. This is easily corrected by injecting 5 to 10 mL of 2% lidocaine into the tissues just proximal to the interdigital space from both the dorsal and flexor aspects.

Adverse reactions to lidocaine are rare in mature

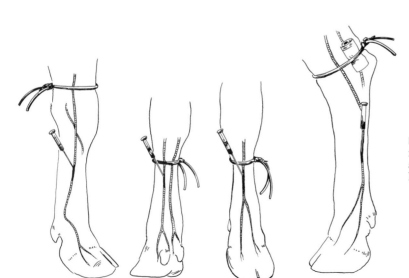

Figure 4–7. Tourniquet placement and injection technique for intravenous regional analgesia in the front and rear limbs. Note the gauze roll used on the rear limb to improve the tourniquet effect.

cattle. At completion of surgery, the tourniquet is released slowly and then retightened, then a few minutes later again released. This maneuver avoids possible local analgesic toxicity. Because ischemic necrosis has been reported when venous blood flow was occluded for 2 or more hours,[12] the tourniquet should not be left in place for more than 90 minutes.

CHEMICAL RESTRAINT AND SEDATION

Cattle that are unaccustomed to being handled for limb and foot examination may require chemical restraint with tranquilizers or sedatives. Furthermore, cattle may be sedated before general anesthesia or in conjunction with a local or regional analgesic when a painful surgical procedure is required. Consideration should be given to several environmental and systemic factors such as the need for clean, soft bedding in potentially recumbent cattle, adequate lighting, protection from risk of heat stroke in prolonged recumbency, and supportive fluid therapy.

Phenothiazine derivatives include promazine, acepromazine, chlorpromazine, triflupromazine, and propiopromazine. Acepromazine is the most commonly used phenothiazine derivative. The dose is 0.03 to 0.05 mg/kg IV or 0.1 to 0.2 mg/kg IM. Tranquilizers are not widely used in cattle for the following reasons:

- Slow onset of action
- Induce mild sedation only
- Lack of measurable analgesia
- Hypotensive properties
- Risk of prolapse of the penis in bulls and subsequent traumatization

Alpha$_2$-adrenoceptor agonists are much more effective than the phenothiazines and are commonly used in cattle as preanesthetic medication, for chemical restraint, analgesia, and sedation. They include xylazine, detomidine, and medetomidine. Xylazine is widely used, although it is not approved for use in cattle in the United States. Detomidine and medetomidine are more recent additions to the list of alpha$_2$-adrenoceptor agonists. Their use has been explored in cattle.[5, 11] The advantages of alpha$_2$-adrenoceptor agonists for chemical restraint and sedation in cattle are

- Rapid onset of action
- Reliable calming, sedation, analgesia, and muscle relaxation

Sedation can be antagonized rapidly with an alpha$_2$-adrenoceptor antagonist (e.g., atipamezole, tolazoline). Of importance to practitioners is the sedative effect of alpha$_2$-adrenoceptor agonists, which may exceed their duration of analgesic activity.[11]

Xylazine in low doses has a calming effect on cattle. When the dose is increased, various stages of sedation and eventually recumbency occur.[10] Cattle are among the domestic species most sensitive to xylazine. The Brahmin breed is very sensitive and responds favorably to as little as 1/10 the xylazine dose used in domestic breeds.[2] Dose rates are given in Table 4–1.

The use of xylazine in pregnant cows is debatable. Xylazine induces bovine uterine contractility in vitro[6] and in vivo.[9] The increase in uterine contractility is dose dependent in vitro.[6] The mechanism of action seems to be mediated through alpha$_2$-adrenoceptors located in the myometrium.[6, 9] It has been reported that xylazine given to cows in the last trimester of pregnancy can cause premature parturition and retention of fetal membranes.[16] However, we are not aware of any controlled studies demonstrating that xylazine does or does not cause pregnant cows to abort. Informal practitioner surveys indicate very few reports of abortions in the third trimester in cows given xylazine. Clinically, we have used xylazine alone and in combination with ketamine in mid- and late-term pregnant cows without complications. However, xylazine increases urine production in cows by as much as six-fold 2 hours after a single IM injection (0.22 mg/kg). Therefore, care should be taken in using xylazine in dehydrated animals. Furthermore, xylazine should not be used to sedate steers with retained urinary calculi, otherwise the increase in urine output can easily cause bladder rupture.

Detomidine administered intravenously at a rate of 10 μg/kg induces sedation characterized by drooping of the head and marked ataxia. The onset of sedation occurs 1 to 10 minutes after intravenous administration and 5 to 15 minutes after intramuscular injection. The intramuscular dose of detomidine in a clinical setting is 30 to 80 μg/kg.[6, 11] Within this dose range, approximately 12% of cattle become recumbent. Bulls and young heifers are more likely to lie down than mature cows. The duration of sedation and recovery is dose dependent. When compared with either xylazine or medetomidine, detomidine-treated cattle are more likely to continue to stand.[11] Detomidine (20 μg/kg IV) has not been associated with complications in cows in their last trimester of pregnancy.[5] However, some investigators have cautioned against the use of any alpha$_2$-adrenoceptor agonist in pregnant cows.[2]

Medetomidine, when compared with either xyla-

TABLE 4–1. TRANQUILIZERS, SEDATIVES, AND ALPHA$_2$-ADRENOCEPTOR ANTAGONISTS DOSE RATES IN CATTLE

Drugs	IV Dose	IM Dose
Xylazine	0.05–0.15 mg/kg	0.1–0.33 mg/kg
Detomidine	10–20 μg/kg	40–60 μg/kg
Medetomidine	10–20 μg/kg	30–40 μg/kg
Yohimbine	0.12 mg/kg	0.1–0.2 mg/kg
Idazoxan	30–50 μg/kg	50–100 μg/kg
Tolazoline	1.0–2.0 mg/kg	2–3 mg/kg
Atipamezole	30–60 μg/kg	60–120 μg/kg

zine or detomidine, has greater specificity for alpha$_2$-adrenoceptors and is more of a hypnotic in cattle.[11] Intravenous administration of 5 μg/kg induces profound sedation, whereas 10 μg/kg causes recumbency. Medetomidine has not yet been thoroughly investigated in calves.

Alpha$_2$-adrenoceptor antagonists include yohimbine, idazoxan, tolazoline, and atipamezole.[4] The effects of yohimbine, idazoxan, and tolazoline on xylazine-induced respiratory changes and CNS depression have been studied in ruminants. Idazoxan is a useful antagonist of xylazine-induced bradycardia and CNS depressions in calves.[15] Tolazoline (1.1 mg/kg IV) also has been shown to be an effective antagonist of xylazine-induced (0.1 mg/kg IV) sedation in cattle.[14] Tolazoline doses as high as 2 to 4 mg/kg have been used to antagonize xylazine sedation without measurable side effects. Clearly, tolazoline is more effective in reversing xylazine-induced sedation than yohimbine. In ruminants, the sedative-antagonizing effect of yohimbine can be improved when doxapram (0.5 to 1.0 mg/kg IV) is given shortly after yohimbine. The two drugs may also be combined in the same syringe. Atipamezole, the most specific alpha$_2$-adrenoceptor antagonist, effectively antagonizes the sedative action of detomidine and medetomidine in cattle and is also an effective antagonist of sedation accompanying medetomidine-ketamine anesthesia in calves.[8]

GENERAL ANESTHESIA

General anesthesia is required for surgery on lame cattle when local or regional analgesia is inappropriate, as in extensive surgery of the forelimb (e.g., fracture reduction and fixation) or hindquarters (e.g., coxofemoral luxation, femoral and tibial fractures) or whenever the temperament of the patient contraindicates local or regional analgesia.

In mature cattle, general anesthesia can be induced and maintained with injectable drugs or an inhalant. Hazards associated with general anesthesia in ruminants are well recognized and are discussed in standard textbooks.[3, 7, 13] These hazards include active and passive regurgitation, ruminal tympany or bloat, and excessive salivation. Preventive measures should be instituted to avoid these potential problems.

CARE DURING GENERAL ANESTHESIA

Cattle do not appear to be as susceptible as are horses to generalized myositis. Nevertheless, 5 to 7.5 cm of foam rubber padding, an air mattress, or a substantial thickness of bedding should be provided if lateral recumbency may be prolonged.

Radial nerve paralysis has been observed in heavy cattle kept deeply anesthetized for prolonged periods. An inflated automobile tire inner tube strategically placed beneath an adult cow's shoulder may prevent radial nerve paralysis. The inner tube is prepared by wrapping duct tape around at least one half of its circumference (Fig. 4–8). For proper placement of an inflated inner tube, the patient is rolled onto its back and the dependent leg is passed through the tube opening. The patient is turned back onto its side. The tape prevents that portion of the tube positioned between the patient's front limbs from inflating and the portion surrounding the shoulder (i.e., scapula) from deflating when the patient is returned to a lateral position. The scapula is permitted to fall away from the rib cage, taking body weight off the plexus that lies between the scapula and rib cage. The lower forelimb should be pulled forward, and the upper hindlimb elevated. Even under field conditions, cattle should always be anesthetized on a soft, clean surface.

FLUID THERAPY

In healthy patients subjected to short-term light surgical anesthesia and undergoing a procedure that is only mildly traumatic, intravenous fluid administration is not absolutely necessary unless the animal has been starved of food and water for 24 hours or more.

Prolonged deep surgical anesthesia, on the other hand, is best managed with fluid support. Cannulating the jugular vein with a large-bore catheter (i.e., 10 to 13 gauge) allows rapid delivery of large amounts of fluid. At the same time, a route is established for administering emergency drugs (e.g., cardiotonic or antidysrhythmics). Balanced electrolyte solutions (e.g., lactated Ringer's) are best suited for this purpose. If serum electrolyte analysis is unavailable, balanced electrolyte solutions should be used because they tend to return either low or high serum electrolyte concentrations toward normal.

For maintenance purpose, fluids are generally given at a rate of 4 to 8 mL/kg/hour. In an emergency situation (e.g., shock, acute blood loss, hypotension),

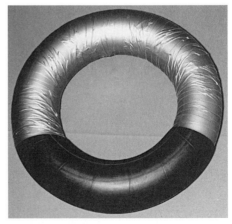

Figure 4–8. An automobile tire inner tube can be used to prevent radial nerve paralysis in heavy cows or bulls. Note how the tube has been prepared by wrapping the portion that will rest between the patient's front limbs with heavy duct tape.

rapid administration is required. A volume of 4 to 8 liters is usually adequate to arrest falling blood pressure in an adult cow. Larger volumes are required in mature patients in shock. Continuous monitoring of cardiopulmonary function is vital when large amounts of fluid are infused.

Hematocrit and serum protein values, if they can be determined, should be used to evaluate response to fluid volume expansion. When the hematocrit values decrease below 20%, blood transfusion is necessary. Serum protein concentrations less than 4.5 grams/dL indicate excessive blood dilution. Under such circumstances, continued administration of a crystalloid solution can easily result in pulmonary edema.

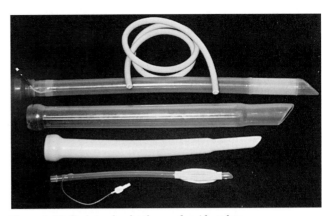

Figure 4–10. Endotracheal tubes and guide tubes.

ENDOTRACHEAL INTUBATION

Endotracheal intubation is essential whenever ruminants are anesthetized. It ensures a patent airway (preventing aspiration of saliva and regurgitant), provides a rapid and safe means for controlling or assisting ventilation in apneic patients, and establishes a route for delivery of oxygen or inhaled anesthetic.

Death during general anesthesia occurs most often as a result of respiratory arrest. When the trachea is intubated and the patient connected to an anesthetic machine, ventilation can be controlled by squeezing the reservoir bag. A hand-operated resuscitator (Fig. 4–9) is an effective device for supporting ventilation with room air.

Cuffed tubes, when inflated, provide an airtight seal between the tube and tracheal wall (Fig. 4–10). The cuff should be inflated to a pressure that just prevents escape of gas between the cuff and tracheal wall when 20 to 25 cm H_2O of positive pressure (2.0 to 2.5 kPa) is applied. Most foreign material (i.e., saliva, regurgitant) accumulating in the trachea anterior to the cuff is extracted to the oropharynx when the tube is removed with the cuff inflated. It is for this reason that cuffed tubes are generally used.

Tube Size. The largest-diameter tube that can be placed in the trachea without injury to the delicate airway tissues should be used. It is the tube's internal diameter that determines the amount of resistance to breathing. Thin-walled tubes are desirable, but if the wall is too thin, the tube can easily become

kinked if the patient's neck is flexed. Overinflation of the cuff can cause tubes with thin walls to collapse, creating airway obstruction. Endotracheal tube sizes for cattle are listed in Table 4–2.

The length of tube may be excessive in some animals. A tube that is too long may occlude the lateral bronchus, and too much tube outside of the animal constitutes mechanical dead space. Disposable tubes for human or canine use are satisfactory for calves. It is wise to have three tubes on hand: one the size judged to be appropriate by tracheal palpation, one a size larger, and another one size smaller.

Technique. In calves, intubation is easily accomplished with the aid of a laryngoscope. A large standard human blade (at least 205 mm in length) is adequate in young calves (Fig. 4–11). Older calves may require a longer blade, which can be fashioned by attaching an extension to the standard-size blade.

In adult cattle, a dental wedge prevents injury to the anesthetist's hand and damage to the endotracheal tube by the animal's teeth. It should be left in place during anesthesia and until extubation. Adhesive tape or gauze placed around the animal's muzzle in front of the mouth wedge prevents its dislodgment.

The animal's head is extended to minimize the orotracheal angle, thereby creating a straight pathway from mouth to trachea. The tongue is drawn out of the mouth, and the anesthetist's hand is passed between the dental arcades until the fingers contact the epiglottis and arytenoid cartilages. The tube is

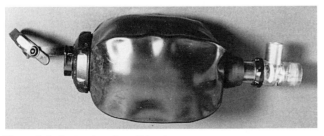

Figure 4–9. A simple rebreathing bag.

TABLE 4–2. CATTLE CUFFED ENDOTRACHEAL TUBE SIZES

	Internal Diameter (mm)	Approximate External Diameter (mm)	Length (cm)
Large bulls and cows	30	38	95–100
Average cows	25	31	75–80
Yearling cattle	20	26	65–75
Calves 6 months	18	22	55–60
Calves 3 months	14	18	45–50

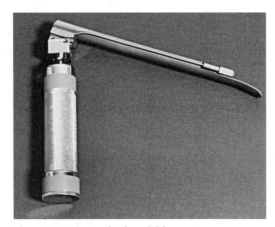

Figure 4–11. A standard-model laryngoscope.

then passed alongside or beneath the anesthetist's arm and gently guided with fingertips through the laryngeal opening and into the trachea (Fig. 4–12).

Alternatively, a small, stiff tube (e.g., an equine stomach tube three times the length of the endotracheal tube, Fig. 4–13) is passed through the larynx and into the trachea. The anesthetist's hand is withdrawn from the patient's mouth, and the endotracheal tube is passed over the guide tube and into the trachea. The guide tube is removed.

PATIENT MONITORING

All anesthetized patients should be closely monitored to ensure proper depth of anesthesia and adequate

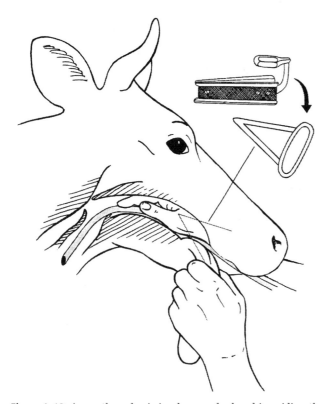

Figure 4–12. A mouth wedge is in place, and a hand is guiding the tube into the trachea.

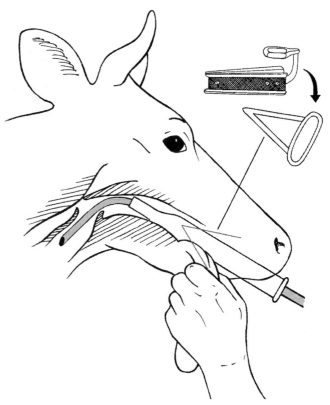

Figure 4–13. A Coles tube being passed through the guide tube and into the trachea.

cardiorespiratory function. Most commonly, heart rate, respiration rate, body temperature, arterial blood pressure, and the electrocardiogram reading are monitored. In acutely ill patients, acid-base status should be determined and corrected if required. Values for these variables provide accurate information for assessing anesthetic depth and physiological response to anesthesia.

- Palpate the peripheral pulse
- Auscultate the heart
- Evaluate mucous membrane color and capillary refill time (2 to 4 seconds)
- A respiratory rate of 25 to 30 breaths per minute is not uncommon in anesthetized adult cattle. In halothane-anesthetized cattle, respiration rate, pulse rate, and arterial blood pressure tend to increase over time.

INJECTABLE ANESTHESIA

Injectable anesthesia is useful in field and hospital for short-duration surgery (e.g., claw amputation in fractious patients).

Xylazine-Ketamine

Xylazine (0.1 to 0.2 mg/kg) and ketamine (2 to 3 mg/kg), given sequentially or combined in the same syringe and injected intravenously as a bolus, is a useful and safe anesthetic regimen. This drug combination is well adapted to use under field conditions to anesthetize adult cattle for foot trimming and other procedures. A smaller dose of xylazine (0.06 to 0.08 mg/kg) is suggested in cattle heavier than 700 kg.

This rapid induction technique has several advantages:

- Rapid immobilization with a smooth transition to anesthesia
- Little or no excitement that may accompany a slow rate of injection
- Reasonable cardiorespiratory stability, small drug volume, and a smooth recovery

Disadvantages may include

- A short duration of surgical anesthesia (15 to 20 minutes), although supplementary doses can prolong anesthesia
- Increased muscle rigidity in the extremities and jaw
- Increased salivation

The duration of surgical anesthesia can be prolonged by 10 to 20 minutes by redosing the patient with one third to one half of the initial dose of each drug

(Table 4–3). Alternatively, after xylazine-ketamine induction, cattle can be maintained with guaifenesin-ketamine-xylazine continuous infusion (see Table 4–3).

Other drugs can be added to the basic regimen to improve anesthesia. Injection of diazepam (0.22 mg/kg) or acepromazine (0.03 to 0.05 mg/kg) intramuscularly 20 to 30 minutes before xylazine and ketamine administration or intravenous diazepam (0.02 mg/kg) followed by ketamine 3 to 5 minutes after injecting xylazine improves muscle relaxation and the quality of induction. These combinations are useful in large bulls or debilitated cattle. The major drawback is expense and the probable legal requirement (depending on country) for accurate record keeping of use of controlled substances.

Butorphanol as an Adjunct

Butorphanol is a synthetic opioid with agonist and antagonist properties. The analgesic action of butorphanol is approximately three to five times greater than that of morphine.[7] We have used butorphanol (0.05 to 0.1 mg/kg IV) with xylazine (0.1 mg/kg IV) for joint flush procedures in calves. Sedation and analgesia are provided in adult cattle given butorphanol (0.02 to 0.04 mg/kg) in the same syringe with

TABLE 4–3. INDUCTION AND MAINTENANCE OF ANESTHESIA USING INJECTABLE DRUGS IN CATTLE

Premedication	Induction	Duration of Surgical Anesthesia (Minutes)	Methods of Extending the Duration of Anesthesia
Xylazine (0.1–0.2 mg/kg IV)*†‡	Ketamine (2–3 mg/kg IV)	15–20	Readminister xylazine and ketamine at half the initial doses or infuse triple drip§ as described to effect.
Xylazine (0.05–0.1 mg/kg IV) and butorphanol (0.05 mg/kg IV)*†	Ketamine (2 mg/kg IV)	20–30	Readminister xylazine and ketamine at one third the initial doses or infuse triple drip§ as described earlier.
Xylazine (0.05–0.1 mg/kg IV) and butorphanol (0.05 mg/kg IV)*†	Telazol (1 mg/kg IV)	15–20	Administer ketamine and xylazine. More telazol can cause prolonged recovery.
Xylazine (0.05–0.1 mg/kg IV)*†	Telazol (1 mg/kg IV)	15–20	Administer more xylazine and telazol at half the initial dose.
Xylazine (0.02 mg/kg IV),* then wait 3 minutes	Guaifenesin (5%)–ketamine (2 mg/mL)–xylazine (0.1 mg/mL)–triple drip to effect§	5–10†	Slowly administer remainder of triple drip§ to effect.
Xylazine (0.02 mg/kg IV),* then wait 3 minutes	1 L of 5% guaifenesin mixed with 3 grams of thiamylal, administer to effect	5–10†	Slowly administer remainder of guaifenesin and thiamylal.
Xylazine (0.02 mg/kg IV),* then wait 3 minutes	1 L of 5% guaifenesin mixed with 2–3 grams of ketamine	5–10†	Slowly administer remainder of guaifenesin and ketamine.

*Premedication can be given IM at twice the IV dose.
†Length of anesthesia if only induction dose is given. Anesthesia may be safely prolonged by appropriate IV infusion.
‡Premedication can be given simultaneously with induction drugs in the same syringe.
§Calculation for *triple drip* using a standard IV administration set (15 drops = 1 mL); maintenance: 30 × kg (body wt) ÷ 60 = drop/min ÷ 60 = drops/sec; large animals may require the use of two IV administration sets.

xylazine (0.01 to 0.02 mg/kg) injected intravenously. Not only is butorphanol a rather effective analgesic when combined with xylazine or detomidine, but it also improves the quality and prolongs the duration of xylazine-ketamine anesthesia for procedures performed on the extremities of cattle. Dose rates of butorphanol with xylazine-ketamine and xylazine-Telazol for induction and maintenance of anesthesia in cattle are listed in Table 4–3.

Telazol-Xylazine

Telazol, a 1:1 proprietary combination of tiletamine and zolazepam, is a useful anesthetic in cattle when combined with xylazine. Intramuscular injection of Telazol, 4 mg/kg, and xylazine, 0.1 to 0.2 mg/kg, in 75-kg calves induces anesthesia in approximately 2.5 minutes and persists for approximately 2.5 hours. Analgesia and muscle relaxation are excellent.[17] Telazol (1 mg/kg) and xylazine (0.05 to 0.1 mg/kg) injected intravenously from the same syringe smoothly induce anesthesia in cattle. Duration of anesthesia is greater than that of a xylazine-ketamine combination.

For capture of free-ranging cattle (using small syringe darts) for lameness examination and treatment, Telazol (500 mg powder in a 5-mL vial) can be reconstituted with 1 mL of 10% xylazine. The resulting solution contains 500 mg of Telazol and 100 mg of xylazine. The intramuscular dose of this special reconstituted Telazol-xylazine is 1 mL/500 kg. The immobilizing power can be increased when 2 mL of 10% xylazine is used to solubilize Telazol. Adding butorphanol to Telazol and xylazine increases analgesia (see Table 4–3).[16]

Human safety in the use of these products under field conditions is of considerable importance. The availability of antidotes to counteract accidental self-injection is mandatory.

Other Alpha$_2$-Agonists

Although these drug combinations have not yet been studied extensively, we believe the use of detomidine or medetomidine with drugs such as ketamine, Telazol, and butorphanol will provide a drug regimen for anesthetizing lame cattle under field and hospital conditions.

Guaifenesin-Ketamine-Xylazine ("Triple Drip")

Anesthesia can be induced and maintained in cattle of all ages with 5% guaifenesin prepared in 5% dextrose containing 1 to 2 mg/mL of ketamine and 0.1 mg/mL of xylazine (triple drip). Extensive clinical experience has shown that this drug combination, given by intravenous infusion, induces safe and reliable general anesthesia in adult cattle and in calves. The major advantage of this regimen, compared with other bolus injectable techniques (e.g., xylazine-ketamine), is that induction and maintenance of anesthesia can be precisely controlled. An intravenous catheter is required for continuous infusion. The dose is 0.5 to 1.0 mL of solution per kilogram. If infused slowly, the higher dose is required. For maintenance of anesthesia, triple drip is given at a rate of 2.2 mL/kg/hour (for calculation see footnote [§], Table 4–3). As with any general anesthetic regimen, the trachea should be intubated and oxygen should be available.

Guaifenesin-Thiobarbiturates and Guaifenesin-Ketamine

Other injectable anesthetic regimens for induction and maintenance of general anesthesia include infusion of 5% to 10% guaifenesin in 5% dextrose in combination with thiobarbiturates (see Table 4–3). Before induction, patients are often given a tranquilizer (acepromazine) or a sedative (xylazine). Placement of an intravenous catheter is highly recommended because thiobarbiturates in high concentration cause tissue necrosis if injected perivascularly. Anesthesia can be maintained by continued slow infusion as described earlier. Recovery from guaifenesin-thiobarbiturate anesthesia is relatively slow but smooth.

Chloral Hydrate

Chloral hydrate anesthesia is only recommended for use in countries in which the low value of cattle does not warrant the use of barbiturates or inhalation anesthesia. However, in countries in which cost or availability prohibits the use of more sophisticated drugs, chloral hydrate still has a place for general anesthesia. On humane grounds, for painful surgical procedures it is preferable to use chloral hydrate than no general anesthesia at all.

The drug is highly soluble in either oil or water. One gram is easily dissolved in 0.25 mL of water. As a result, it is often prepared as a 10% to 30% solution. Chloral hydrate is extremely caustic and causes hemolysis when prepared in a high concentration and given intravenously. If injected perivascularly, severe tissue irritation occurs, resulting in tissue slough. For this reason, chloral hydrate solution should not be injected into an abdominal milk vein of milking cows or goats. Oral administration causes abomasal irritation, and peritoneal injection results in peritonitis. As an anesthetic, chloral hydrate has only a limited place in veterinary anesthesia today because many more efficacious and safer drugs are available.

In safe doses, chloral hydrate is a good sedative-hypnotic but provides little or no analgesia. Doses that induce general anesthesia closely approach the lethal dose. Many drugs have been combined with chloral hydrate to enhance its anesthetic action, the two most popular being magnesium sulfate, a muscle relaxant, and pentobarbital, a sedative in low doses. In large doses, pentobarbital is an anesthetic, but when used alone, the anesthetic/analgesic dose is, as with chloral hydrate, close to the lethal dose. These drugs should not be used to induce and maintain general anesthesia in neonates. It is appropriate to say that because of its narrow safety margin, chloral hydrate–magnesium sulfate–pentobarbital is a dangerous anesthetic drug combination in the hands of the inexperienced. This does not suggest that these drugs cannot be used effectively in cattle. Veterinarians should be aware of their narrow safety margin and use extreme caution and vigilance when giving these drugs either alone or in combination to immobilize cattle.

Generally, a sedative dose of chloral hydrate or a chloral hydrate–magnesium sulfate–pentobarbital combination is supplemented with local or regional analgesia for surgery or other painful procedures.

In improperly fasted cattle, an anesthetic dose of chloral hydrate is often associated with ruminal bloat, regurgitation, tracheal aspiration, and either immediate suffocation or a subsequent foreign body pneumonia. Tracheal intubation is thus essential, as is oxygen supplementation, during the course of general anesthesia. Chloral hydrate crosses the blood-brain barrier slowly, requiring approximately 5 minutes to induce its full effect. Thus, rapid administration until surgical anesthesia is achieved results in an actual overdose. When given to induce sedation-hypnosis or anesthesia in healthy adult cattle, the dose ranges from 5 to 7 grams/100 kg or 10 to 18 grams/100 kg of body weight, respectively. When combined with magnesium sulfate and pentobarbital, the dose of chloral hydrate is decreased by one third to one half. A mixture of chloral hydrate (30 grams), magnesium sulfate (15 grams), and thiopental (2.5 grams) solubilized in 1 liter of distilled water given intravenously at a dose of 2 mL/kg of body weight has been used successfully to anesthetize adult cattle for 20 to 30 minutes. Maintaining surgical anesthesia for a prolonged period with this mixture results in a protracted and often rough recovery.

INHALATION ANESTHESIA

If properly performed, inhalation anesthesia is the safest and most satisfactory method of maintaining prolonged surgical anesthesia in cattle. Disadvantages of inhalation anesthesia in field practice include

- Equipment cost
- Cost of the drugs
- Time required and inconvenience of transporting equipment to the field

Halothane and Isoflurane

Potent volatile anesthetics such as halothane and isoflurane have a rather broad safety margin. The depth of anesthesia can be precisely and quickly regulated because halothane and isoflurane have a low solubility and are highly volatile. Recovery is relatively rapid compared with injectable anesthesia. Excitement and rough recovery are extremely rare.

Halothane and isoflurane readily cross the placental barrier, resulting in fetal depression. However, once breathing is initiated in a neonate, anesthetic blood concentrations decrease and CNS depression diminishes rapidly, especially with isoflurane. Because of their potency and high volatility, halothane or isoflurane is unsafe and too costly to use as an open drip. Safety can be ensured only when these anesthetics are administered with a precision vaporizer, using a circle or to-and-fro rebreathing system.

Equipment

Human or small-animal-size machines are satisfactory for calves weighing up to 200 kg. Machines should be equipped with a precision (calibrated) halothane vaporizer located out of the breathing circuit. With this arrangement, a precise amount of anesthetic vapor can be delivered to the breathing circuit each minute.

An *out-of-circuit vaporizer* uses a circle breathing system that routes exhaled gases through an absorbent for extraction of carbon dioxide. The breathing circuit may be used as a semi-closed or closed delivery system. The *semi-closed system* delivers more fresh gas to the breathing system each minute than the patient's metabolic requirement for oxygen. The excessive gas is exhausted through a pop-off valve and scavenge system to prevent overfilling of the breathing circuit, excessive airway pressure, and ambient pollution. This system is preferred for large patients. The *closed system* provides a fresh flow of gas to just meet a patient's metabolic requirement for oxygen. This method is more economical but requires closer monitoring to ensure safe and stable anesthesia. However, hypercapnia is no more likely with a closed system than with a semi-closed system, provided the carbon dioxide absorbent is active. Hypoxia does not occur provided the rebreathing bag contains an amount of oxygen that exceeds the patient's tidal volume.

Oxygen Flow Rate and Anesthetic Vapor Concentration

The concentration of nitrogen in the lungs is approximately 80% in resting cattle breathing ambient air. High oxygen flow rates are necessary in the induction period for rapid nitrogen washout. An alternate method is to flush the breathing system and the patient's lungs several times with oxygen as soon as the endotracheal tube is connected to the anesthetic machine. The purpose of nitrogen washout is to avoid hypoxia during induction and to facilitate induction of anesthesia by replacing the nitrogen with oxygen and anesthetic vapor.

After induction with an injectable anesthetic (see Table 4–3), the oxygen flow should be set at 5 to 8 L/minute in adult cattle and 2 to 4 L/minute in calves. The out-of-circuit vaporizer is adjusted to deliver 3% to 5% halothane or isoflurane, depending on the desired rate of induction. When a 5% setting is used, particularly in calves, patients should be closely observed to prevent anesthetic overdose. The oxygen flows and vaporizer settings are gradually decreased as a patient approaches surgical anesthesia, which usually requires 15 to 20 minutes. When surgical anesthesia is present, the oxygen flow should be decreased to 3 to 5 L/minute in adult cattle and 1 to 2 L/minute in calves. Vaporizer settings of 1.5% to 3% are required to maintain surgical anesthesia in most cattle. In adult cattle, the higher vaporizer setting is required with low oxygen flow rates. Because of individual patient variation, it is more appropriate to rely on a patient's response than on specific oxygen flow and vaporizer settings when determining induction rate and anesthetic depth.

Rotation of the eyeball of cattle under inhalation anesthesia was first described in detail by Thurmon and colleagues[18] and has proved to be reliable for monitoring anesthetic depth as well as progression of recovery from inhalation anesthesia. The eyeball is normally centered between the eyelids in an unanesthetized cow in lateral recumbency (Fig. 4–14A). As anesthesia is induced, the eyeball begins a ventral rotation (Fig. 4–14B). When the cornea has become partially obscured by the lower eyelid, light surgical anesthesia is present (Fig. 4–14C). When the cornea is completely hidden by the lower eyelid, a medium depth of surgical anesthesia exists (Fig. 4–14D). A further increase in anesthetic depth is characterized by dorsal rotation of the eyeball. Dorsal movement is complete when the cornea is centered between the eyelids (Fig. 4–14E). This sign indicates deep surgical anesthesia with profound muscle relaxation. With this depth of anesthesia, vital signs must be monitored closely and the anesthetic dose must be decreased to a maintenance level.

During recovery, eyeball rotation occurs in reverse order of that observed during induction.[16] When the eyeball is centered between the eyelids, deep anesthesia is characterized by drying of the cornea and loss of the corneal and palpebral reflexes. Centering of the cornea between the eyelids during the recovery process is accompanied by a return of the corneal and palpebral reflexes, and the cornea appears moist.

Approximately 5 minutes before completion of the surgery, the anesthetic vapor concentration should be decreased to about one half that required for maintenance. Immediately before completion of surgery, anesthetic administration should be discontinued. The rebreathing system should be flushed with oxygen. The patient should remain connected to the anesthetic machine and should breathe oxygen until signs of recovery are observed.

The endotracheal tube should not be removed until strong airway protective reflexes have returned. If a cuffed endotracheal tube was used, it should be re-

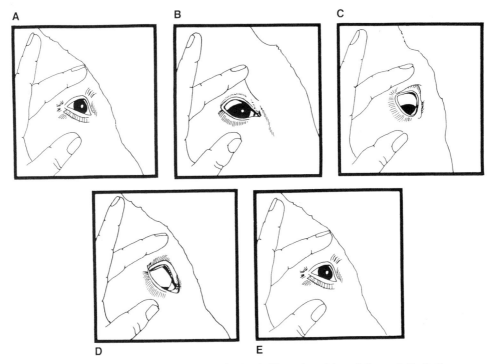

Figure 4–14. Eyeball rotation during induction of gaseous anesthesia. *A,* Normal position of the eyeball. *B,* Commencement of downward rotation during induction. *C,* Light surgical anesthesia. *D,* Complete ventral rotation indicates medium surgical anesthesia. *E,* Dorsal rotation is an indication of deep anesthesia.

moved with the cuff inflated in order to withdraw foreign material that may have accumulated in the trachea proximal to the cuff.

REFERENCES

1. Benson GJ, Thurmon JC: Regional analgesia. *In* Howard JL (ed): Current Veterinary Medicine 3: Food Animal Practice. Philadelphia, WB Saunders, 1993, pp 77–88.
2. Greene SA, Thurmon JC: Xylazine—a review of its pharmacology and use in veterinary medicine. J Vet Pharmacol Ther 11:295–313, 1988.
3. Hall LW, Clark KW (eds.): Anaesthesia of the ox. *In* Veterinary Anaesthesia, 9th ed. London, Bailliere Tindall, 1991, pp 236–259.
4. Hsu WH, Hanson CE, Hembrough B, Schaffer DD: Effects of idazoxan, tolazoline, and yohimbine on xylazine induced respiratory changes and central nervous system depression in ewes. Am J Vet Res 50:1570–1573, 1989.
5. Jedruch J, Gajewski Z: The effect of detomidine hydrochloride (Domosedan) on electrical activity of the uterus in cows. Acta Vet Scand 82:189–192, 1986.
6. Ko JCH, Hsu WH, Evans LE: The effects of xylazine and alpha-adrenoceptor antagonists on bovine uterine contractility in vitro. Theriogenology 33:601–611, 1990.
7. Lumb WV, Jones EW (eds.): Preanesthetic agents. *In* Veterinary Anesthesia, 2nd ed. Philadelphia, Lea & Febiger, 1984, pp 165–197.
8. Raekallio M, Kivalo M, Jalanka H, Vainio O: Medetomidine/ketamine sedation in calves and its reversal with atipamezole. J Vet Anaesth 18:45–47, 1991.
9. Rodrigues-Martinez H, McKenna D, Weston PG, et al: Uterine motility in the cow during the estrous cycle. III. Effect of oxytocin, xylazine, and adrenoceptor blocks. Theriogenology 27:350–367, 1987.
10. Rosenberger G, Hempel E, Baumeister M: Contributions to the effect and applicability of Rompun in cattle. Vet Med Rev 2:137–142, 1969.
11. Short CE (ed.): Alpha$_2$-adrenergic agonists/antagonists in ruminants. *In* Alpha$_2$-Agents in Animals. Santa Barbara, CA, Brilling Hill, 1992, pp 71–77.
12. Skarda RT: Techniques of local analgesia in ruminants and swine. Vet Clin North Am Food Anim Pract 2:621–663, 1986.
13. Steffey EP: Some characteristics of ruminants and swine that complicate management of general anesthesia. Vet Clin North Am Food Anim Pract 2:507–516, 1986.
14. Takase K, Hikasa Y, Ogasa-Wara S: Tolazoline as an antagonist of xylazine in cattle. Jpn J Vet Sci 48:859–862, 1986.
15. Thompson JR, Hsu WH, Kersting KW: Antagonistic effect of idazoxan on xylazine-induced central nervous system depression and bradycardia in calves. Am J Vet Res 50:734–736, 1989.
16. Thurmon JC, Benson GJ: Anesthesia in ruminants and swine. *In* Howard JL (ed): Current Veterinary Therapy 3: Food Animal Practice. Philadelphia, WB Saunders, 1993, pp 58–76.
17. Thurmon JC, Lin HC, Benson GJ, et al: Combining Telazol and xylazine for anesthesia in calves. Vet Med 84:824–830, 1989.
18. Thurmon JC, Romack FE, Garner HE: Excursions of the bovine eyeball during gaseous anesthesia. Vet Med 63:967–970, 1968.
19. Weaver AD: Intravenous local anesthesia of the lower limb in cattle. J Am Vet Med Assoc 160:55–57, 1972.

Ava M. Trent   *United States*
Kimberly A. Redic-Kill

5

Clinical Pharmacology

PRINCIPLES OF TREATMENT

Lameness usually results from pain caused by inflammation initiated by infectious or non-infectious stimuli. Pharmacological agents are generally used in treatment of lameness to achieve one or more of three goals: to eliminate infectious stimuli, to prevent secondary involvement of infectious agents in compromised tissue, and to control the host inflammatory response.

The choice of drug therapy should be guided by pharmacokinetic and pharmacodynamic factors, as well as by issues relating to the health and status of the patient, government regulation, client concerns, patient management issues, and economics. Treatment failure or client dissatisfaction commonly results when these factors are not fully considered. Treatment failure may occur from selection of a drug that is ineffective against a specific agent, is not administered at a therapeutic level, does not reach the site or pathogen in adequate levels, results in adverse reactions that prevent effective use, or cannot be administered at therapeutic levels by the owner. Avoidable therapeutic failure and excessive or unexpected cost of drug therapy are common sources of client dissatisfaction.

Pharmacokinetics is described as the mathematical relationship between dose and plasma concentration-time profiles.

Pharmacodynamics is the study of the relationship between the plasma concentration and the pharmacological effect of a drug.

FACTORS AFFECTING DRUG TRANSFER ACROSS MEMBRANES

Physicochemical characteristics of drugs that affect the transfer across cell membranes include molecular size and shape, solubility at the site of administration, degree of ionization, and relative lipid solubility of the ionized and non-ionized forms. Drugs that are ionized and highly water soluble (e.g., many antibiotics) are easily transported via the vasculature and interstitial fluid.

Degree of ionization is determined by a molecule's pKa (dissociation rate constant) value relative to the pH of the environment. Basic drugs tend to accumulate in fluids that are acidic relative to the plasma (e.g., milk), whereas acidic drugs tend to concentrate in fluids that are basic relative to the plasma (e.g., ruminant urine). The pKa values and acidic or alkaline nature of common drugs are presented in Table 5–1.

Relative lipid solubility determines the ease with which drugs can cross lipophilic membranes to enter cells. These membrane barriers may be a single cell thick (intestinal epithelium or capillary endothelium) or several layers of cells thick (skin). The lipid solubility of a drug can be clinically important in treating lameness, because drugs must be absorbed from a site of administration and delivered to target tissues by crossing several membranes. Drugs with high lipid solubility may have superior access to target tissues such as the central nervous system (CNS), in which the blood-brain barrier is highly lipophilic. Conversely, lipid solubility is less of a factor in drug delivery into muscle, bone, or joint.

PHARMACOKINETIC PARAMETERS

Bioavailability is the rate and extent of active drug transfer to its site of action. Bioavailability is dependent on methods of absorption, distribution, and clearance, as well as inherent properties of each drug.

Absorption describes drug transfer from the site of administration and is affected by the physicochemical factors that affect transport across membranes. Regardless of the site of administration, drug solubility is a key factor. Drugs given in aqueous solution (e.g., aqueous penicillin G) are more rapidly absorbed than those given in oily vehicles, solid form (e.g., penicillin oral tablets), or suspensions (e.g., procaine penicillin G), because they mix more readily with the aqueous phase at the absorption site. For solid dosage forms, dissolution is often the rate-limiting step in drug absorption.

Route of administration is a consideration because

TABLE 5–1. CHARACTERISTICS OF PHARMACOLOGICAL AGENTS USED IN THE TREATMENT OF LAMENESS

Drug Class (Acidic or Basic) (pKa)	Mechanism of Action	Absorption	Distribution	Elimination	Side Effects and Cautions, Additional Information
Penicillins Acidic 2.7–2.8	Bactericidal: Inhibit mucopeptide synthesis in the cell wall	Var PO Var IM Var SC	ECF Var CNS Good synov fl Good bone	Glomerular filtration Tubular secretion	Hypersensitivity reactions; oral dosing—N/V/D; SC dosing—local reactions; site of injection may influence serum levels; long-acting forms generally produce lower serum levels than short-acting forms
Cephalosporins Acidic 1–4.1	Bactericidal: Inhibit mucopeptide synthesis in the cell wall	Fair PO Good IM Good SC	ECF Var CNS Good synov fl Good bone	Glomerular filtraton Tubular secretion	Hypersensitivity reactions, drug fever, immune reactions
Aminoglycosides Basic 7.5–7.8	Bactericidal: Bind to 30S ribosomal subunit	None PO Good IM Good SC	ECF Not CNS Good synov fl Good bone	Glomerular filtration	Nephrotoxicity (gentamicin > amikacin); vestibular toxicity (gentamicin > amikacin); cochlear toxicity (amikacin > gentamicin); neuromuscular blockade; decreased activity in acidic environment or pus; *monitor serum levels if possible and avoid other nephrotoxins*
Lincosamides Basic 7.45–7.6	Bacteriostatic/ bactericidal: Bind to 50S ribosomal subunit	Var PO	TBW Var CNS Good synov fl Good bone	Hepatic tubular secretion	IM dosing—pain at injection site; rapid IV dosing—hypotension; elevations of liver enzymes
Tetracyclines Basic na	Bacteriostatic: Bind to 30S and 50S ribosomal subunits	Var PO Good IM Good SC	TBW Poor CNS Good synov fl Good bone	Glomerular filtration	Oral dosing—depression of ruminal microflora and ruminoreticular stasis; rapid IV dosing—hemolysis; cardiodepressant effects in calves; IM dosing—local reactions and tissue necrosis; nephrotoxicity
Sulfonamides Acidic 4.79–8.56	Bactericidal (if potentiated): Inhibit folic acid pathways	Good PO Good IM Good SC	ECF, TBW Fair CNS Good synov fl Good bone	Hepatic Glomerular filtration Tubular secretion	Nephrotoxicity, rash, hypersensitivity reactions; IM dosing—local reactions; hemolytic anemia; inactivated by pus or necrotic tissue; rapid resistance develops in unpotentiated forms
Macrolides Basic 7.1–8.9	Bacteriostatic/ bactericidal: Bind to 50S ribosomal subunit	Var PO Fair IM	TBW Poor CNS Good intracellular	Biliary Hepatic	Myocardial depression; neuromuscular blockade; IM dosing—local reactions; PO dosing—N/V/D, avoid in ruminants as severe diarrhea may result
Fluoroquinolones Basic 6.0–8.8	Bactericidal: Inhibit DNA gyrase	Good PO Good IM	TBW Poor CNS Good synov fl Good bone	Hepatic Glomerular filtration Tubular secretion	PO dosing—N/V/D; cartilage damage in juvenile animals
Metronidazole Basic 2.6	Bactericidal: Unknown	Var PO	TBW Good CNS Good bone	Hepatic	Neurological disorders, neutropenias, hepatotoxicity, N/V/D
Chloramphenicol Basic 5.5	Bacteriostatic/ bactericidal: Bind to 50S ribosomal subunit	Var PO	Widely distributed Good CNS Good bone Good joint	Hepatic	Bone marrow depression, idiosyncratic aplastic anemia, N/V/D, hepatotoxicity; *should not be considered first-line agent because of human health risk of aplastic anemia*
Antifungals Varies Varies	Fungistatic/ fungicidal: Interference with sterol synthesis	Var PO	Var CNS Good synov fl Good bone	Hepatic	Hepatotoxicity; topical dosing—local reactions rare
Non-steroidal Anti-inflammatory Acidic 3.5–4.4	Inhibition of cyclooxygenase	Good PO	TBW	Hepatic glomerular filtration Tubular secretion	Blood dyscrasias (phenylbutazone); GI irritation and bleeding; hypersensitivities; IM dosing—local reactions; highly protein bound
Corticosteroids Acidic na	Varied and complex effects on virtually all cell types and systems in mammals	Good IM	TBW	Hepatic	Minimal when used short term; IM, intra-articular dosing—local reactions

CNS, central nervous system; ECF, extracellular fluid; GI, gastrointestinal; N/V/D, nausea, vomiting, diarrhea; Synov fl, synovial fluid; TBW, total body water; Var, variable; na, no information available.

local conditions at the site of drug administration, such as tissue pH and fluid volume, alter solubility. The surface area to which a drug is exposed depends in large part on the route of administration. Some characteristics of the major routes of administration used when treating lameness are summarized in Table 5–2.

Distribution is described as the movement of a drug from the site of administration into tissues.

Volume of distribution refers to the apparent space in the systemic circulation, interstitial fluids, and cellular fluids that contain the drug. The specific pattern of distribution within the available space is a function of physiological factors and physicochemical

TABLE 5–2. CHARACTERISTICS OF COMMON ROUTES OF DRUG ADMINISTRATION

Route	Absorption Pattern	Advantages and Clinical Utility	Disadvantages and Precautions
Intramuscular	Prompt from aqueous solution Slow and sustained from repository forms (oil vehicle or suspension) Dependent on perfusion of injection site Dependent on drug solubility at local tissue pH	Suitable for moderate volumes Suitable for oily vehicles Suitable for some irritating substances	Possible pain or inflammation from irritating drugs Suspension formulation may affect bioavailability Injection location may affect bioavailability Precluded during anticoagulation therapy Drug peaks and durations variable May cause local tissue necrosis
Intra-articular	Variable Systemic levels generally low	Higher drug levels in synovial fluid Minimal systemic side effects Suitable as adjunct to systemic therapy	Chemical synovitis Fibrin deposition may compartmentalize intra-articular space
Intravenous	Absorption circumvented Potentially immediate effects	Valuable for emergency use Permits titration of dose Suitable for large volumes Suitable for irritating substances (when diluted) Most consistent level of drug delivery	Increased risk of adverse effects Must generally inject solutions slowly Not suitable for oil vehicles or insoluble drugs Requires venous access Requires close monitoring
Oral	Dependent on drug release from dosage form Dependent on drug stability in the rumen May be affected by gastrointestinal motility Dependent on drug solubility in rumen pH	Most convenient Usually most economical Well suited for young animals (functional monogastics)	Gastric irritation Destruction of drugs by ruminal pH or enzymes May alter ruminal microflora Drugs may undergo significant metabolism in intestinal mucosa or liver before reaching system
Regional infiltration	High local levels, especially in interstitial fluid Systemic levels generally low	Suitable for antibiotic delivery at incision closure Higher drug levels in local tissues Minimal systemic side effects	Possible pain or inflammation from irritating drugs Diffusion to adjacent tissues limited Short duration of high local levels
Regional intravenous	Absorption circumvented distal to tourniquet High local levels Systemic levels generally low	Higher drug levels in local tissues Minimal systemic side effects Suitable as adjunct to systemic therapy	Requires venous access Requires animal restraint for several minutes Requires high degree of technical skill
Subcutaneous	Prompt from aqueous solution Slow and sustained from repository forms (oil vehicle or suspension) Dependent on perfusion of injection site Dependent on drug solubility at local tissue pH	Suitable for some insoluble suspensions Suitable for implantation of solid pellets	Not suitable for large volumes Possible pain or inflammation from irritating drugs Drug peaks and durations variable Emaciated patients may exhibit erratic absorption Obese patients may exhibit erratic absorption
Topical	Dependent on drug release from vehicle Penetration through stratum corneum variable Enhanced by oily vehicle, surfactants, DMSO Systemic absorption greater through abraded skin	Suitable for conditions limited to superficial layers of dermis or epidermis Suitable as adjunct to systemic therapy Minimal systemic side effects	Most drugs penetrate poorly to deep layers of dermis or epidermis

properties of the drug. Delivery to muscle, bone, fat, viscera, and structures primarily composed of connective tissues such as skin, tendon, and ligament is slower than delivery to well-perfused organs such as the heart, lungs, liver, and brain. It may take minutes to hours for tissue and plasma levels to equilibrate. Equilibration is most rapid and predictable after intravenous administration.

Bone is a complex tissue of organic matrices, minerals, and osteogenic cells and contains substantial extracellular and intracellular fluid spaces. Drugs in the circulation must cross the osseous capillaries to distribute to bone. Electron microscopy studies have discounted the idea of a blood-bone barrier for either normal or infected bone.[11] Cortical bone has relatively slow blood flow, which may explain why peak drug levels in cortical bone lag behind those of other more vascular body tissues. Most antibiotics are considered to distribute well to bone under normal conditions. Local conditions, such as ischemia, alkaline or acidic pH, the presence of abscesses or necrotic debris, and elevated temperature, all may diminish clinical efficacy of some drugs.

Joints are usually accessed by drugs via a synovial membrane, where they are distributed in the synovial fluid. Studies of neonatal calves have demonstrated that typical systemic doses of most antibiotics (except aminoglycosides and erythromycins) provide adequate synovial fluid levels to treat infections caused by susceptible organisms.[6, 14, 22] Infection or irritation initiates a marked inflammatory response resulting in the accumulation of fibrin, neutrophils, and inflammatory exudate within the closed space of the joint cavity. Fibrin deposition may compartmentalize the intra-articular space. The effect of these responses on the absorptive capacity of the synovial membrane is debated, but it is generally held that absorption increases during acute inflammation and decreases during chronic inflammation.[18]

CNS penetration by systemically administered drugs requires that the agents cross a membrane with a predominance of tight junctions. Drugs that are lipophilic cross this membrane readily, whereas drugs that are polar at physiological pH cross into the CNS poorly. Although inflammation increases distribution of non-lipophilic drugs into the CNS during the acute inflammatory phase of a disease, restoration of membrane integrity occurs as inflammation diminishes, and selection of a lipophilic drug is preferable for long-term therapy.

Elimination is the process by which active drugs are physically or functionally removed from the body.

Clearance measures the ability of the body to eliminate a drug and is expressed in units of flow (e.g., mL/minute). *Half-life* is the time required for 50% of a drug to be cleared from a tissue or fluid. Renal elimination is the most important process for removal of drugs and their metabolites. Excretion of drugs into the milk is important, not because of the quantity of drug removed but because of the concern over drugs in the commercial milk supply and the effects of drugs on nursing young. Lipid-soluble drugs must typically be metabolized to more water-soluble forms before elimination. This process is relatively rapid in ruminants, preventing direct extrapolation of clearance rates from studies performed in other species.

PHARMACODYNAMIC FACTORS

AGE

The age of an animal determines probable mechanisms of disease and typical pathogens. It also affects pharmacokinetic and pharmacodynamic profiles and places economic limitations on the selected drugs.

Neonates typically experience an increase in intensity and duration of drug activity compared with adults, attributed to differences in drug disposition. Neonates typically exhibit better absorption from the gastrointestinal tract, increased volumes of distribution for drugs that distribute in extracellular fluid or total-body water, increased permeability of the blood-brain barrier, and slower elimination.[4] Consequently, small or less frequent doses are necessary during the neonatal period (generally the first 6 weeks of life in calves). Neonates and preruminant calves are relatively susceptible to septicemic spread of disease, and the potential for multifocal infection of bone and joint should be considered when lameness is observed (p. 61).

PHYSICAL CONDITION

Alterations in an individual animal's physical condition (e.g., emaciation, obesity, shock, dehydration, septicemia) can affect its pharmacokinetic profile and the potential for adverse effects of drug therapy. The potential for economic recovery of costs through sale of milk or meat also influences treatment choice, placing pressure on the selection of agents with shorter milk or meat withdrawal time or those that can be administered by routes that do not cause carcass damage (oral, intravenous, or subcutaneous as opposed to intramuscular).

LESION-SPECIFIC FACTORS

Characteristics of the lesion affect the distribution of drugs to the target site, pharmacodynamics of the drug at the site of action, the route of drug administration, the ability to remove the deleterious material from the lesion, and the ability of tissue to recover function after treatment.

The maturation of a lesion often proceeds in a predictable manner, regardless of site, characterized by an initial increase in vascular supply and tissue permeability during acute inflammation, followed by a relative decrease as fibrous tissue or sclerosis develops.[4] Early increased permeability may allow lesion access for some systemic agents that are not normally considered permeable for a given tissue, but the reverse may occur in later stages. Lesion factors that can alter drug efficacy include changes in pathogen growth patterns or structure, altered lesion pH, and the presence of inflammatory or therapeutic substances at the lesion site that alter drug activity.

An organized abscess presents several therapeutic challenges: decreased penetration through the abscess walls; an acidic pH, which decreases the activity of drugs such as the aminoglycosides; changes in microbial membranes, which may decrease activity of cell wall–active drugs such as the beta-lactam agents; and a slowed microbial growth rate, which may decrease the efficacy of agents, such as the beta-lactams, which are most active against dividing cells. External drainage of abscesses can often offset the potential decrease in efficacy of systemically administered drugs by physically removing organisms and inflammatory debris, altering the pH, and improving access to systemic drugs. Therefore, the ease of drainage is a lesion-specific factor that should be assessed for each case.

ANTIMICROBIAL PHARMACODYNAMICS

Several pharmacodynamic characteristics apply specifically to antimicrobial therapy. These factors affect how the agents interact with the host and pathogens, as well as with each other.

SUSCEPTIBILITY AND ANTIMICROBIAL SENSITIVITY

Causative organisms can include a wide variety of bacteria and, less commonly, fungi and spirochetes. Collection of a specimen for culture and sensitivity testing is a crucial step in developing the most effective treatment. When possible, a Gram stain should guide initial empirical antibiotic therapy. Culture and sensitivity data should be used to narrow and target antibiotic therapy. *In vitro* antimicrobial susceptibility testing is a predictor of sensitivity but does not ensure *in vivo* efficacy against the infectious organism. Unfavorable local conditions can affect growth characteristics of the organism or the activity of the drug and so alter the anticipated effect.

Minimum inhibitory concentration (MIC) data indicate the lowest concentration of drug that prevents visible growth after 18 to 24 hours. For susceptible organisms with high MICs, higher or more frequent dosing may be necessary to eradicate the infection. It may seem reasonable to attempt to maintain drug concentrations at the site of infection that exceed the MIC throughout the entire dosing interval. In reality, a controversy exists about whether it is clinically more effective to achieve relatively constant antibacterial levels or to achieve high peak concentrations followed by periods of subinhibitory levels to allow persistent organisms to re-enter an antimicrobial-susceptible phase.

POSTANTIBIOTIC EFFECT

Many antibiotics exhibit a postantibiotic effect (PAE) against some microorganisms. This effect is a quiescence in cell growth and division, even though drug levels are below the organism's MIC. In general, maximal PAE occurs *in vitro* after 2 hours of exposure to drug levels of 5 to 10 times the MIC. Under these circumstances, agents that inhibit protein and nucleic acid synthesis (chloramphenicol, tetracyclines, lincosamides, aminoglycosides, rifampin, and quinolones) induce a PAE of 2 to 6 hours across most organisms in their spectrums of activity.[12] In contrast, cell wall agents (penicillins, cephalosporins) and trimethoprim induce a PAE of about 2 hours against gram-positive organisms but have short or no PAE against gram-negative organisms.[12]

COMBINATION REGIMENS

The goal of antimicrobial therapy should always be to use the most selectively active agent that produces the fewest adverse effects. Nevertheless, *in vivo* and *in vitro* evidence shows that simultaneous use of multiple antimicrobials has potential clinical benefit. Selection of an appropriate combination requires an understanding of the potential interaction between the agents. Because of differing mechanisms of action, drug combinations may be either synergistic or antagonistic. Likewise, combinations may either lower or raise the potential for toxicities.

Clinical indications for the concurrent use of multiple antimicrobial agents include the treatment of mixed bacterial infections, the initial empirical treatment of severe infections until causative organisms can be identified, the need to combat antibacterial synergy in polymicrobial infections, and deterrence of bacterial resistance to some antibiotics (rifampin, sulfas). However, inappropriate use of combinations can lead to prolonged administration of toxic or expensive drugs. This is due to failure to obtain adequate cultures before therapy or failure to reduce the number of agents based on susceptibility data. Indiscriminate use of multiple drugs can also increase exposure of microbes to antibiotics, promoting emergence of resistant bacteria within the environment. *In vitro* data also suggest that antagonism of antibacterial effects results when bacteriostatic and bactericidal agents are given concurrently.

DURATION OF ADMINISTRATION

The duration of antibiotic administration is determined by whether the agent is being used prophylactically or therapeutically.

Therapeutic antibiotic administration should generally be continued for at least 3 days after the last sign of infection is detected to ensure that low levels of persistent organisms are not left to multiply at the infection site. Infections at sites that are known to harbor subclinical infection or for which signs are not easily detected may require treatment for several weeks after cessation of clinical signs (e.g., bone and joint). Patients with impaired host defenses may also require a longer duration of therapy, because any persistent organisms may be better able to survive.

Bone and joint infections are, with few exceptions, treated successfully only if an appropriate antimicrobial is administered for an effective length of time. Parenteral antimicrobial therapy is recommended in osteomyelitis or septic arthritis for 2 to 6 weeks or for 1 to 2 weeks after clinical improvement.[18, 28] Although parenteral therapy, preferably by an intravenous route, provides the optimum chance of maximum recovery, economic or client compliance considerations in food animals often restrict parenteral therapy (e.g., 10 to 14 days). This may be followed by an additional short course of oral agents for 2 to 3 weeks. Consideration of this regimen should be limited to those cases in which oral antibiotics are bioavailable (calves younger than 4 weeks), the specific etiological agent has been identified, and a favorable clinical response to parenteral therapy has been demonstrated.

Prophylactic antibiotics should only be administered long enough to ensure high circulating or local tissue levels during the period of risk for contamination. When a specific onset of contamination can be predicted, as for scheduled surgeries, a single systemic preoperative dose of antibiotics far enough in advance (10 to 30 minutes preoperatively for most intravenous antibiotics; 30 to 90 minutes preoperatively for most intramuscular antibiotics) to achieve high circulating and tissue levels at the time of incision, followed by any additional doses needed to maintain high levels until the incision has a fibrin seal (4 to 8 hours postoperatively), is an optimal dosing regimen for prophylaxis in most cases. Prolonged preoperative or postoperative administration does not further decrease the incidence of infection resulting from the surgical procedure and may increase the risks of infection with resistant flora and of drug-related complications. In cases of unanticipated contamination, such as in traumatic injuries, some prophylactic effect can still be achieved by obtaining high circulating drug levels at any time within the "golden period" of 4 to 6 hours after contamination before organisms have invaded tissue and established an infection. Infection can result despite appropriate use of prophylactic antibiotics if the amount of contamination and tissue damage exceeds the combined host and antimicrobial defenses. If such a situation occurs or is anticipated, a therapeutic antibiotic regimen should be initiated as described earlier.

ANTIMICROBIAL FAILURES

Confirmation or reasonable suspicion of an infectious agent and application of the antimicrobial principles provide a foundation for appropriate drug use. In reality, these agents are frequently misused, and clinical failures may result. The lack of complete bovine pharmacokinetic data, the variations in reported dosing regimens for cattle, and the economic constraints of drug dosing in this population all may adversely affect the selection of an appropriate antimicrobial dose and lead to therapeutic failure. These poor outcomes may often be explained by the following:

1 Lack of or incorrect identification of the causative organisms

2 Presence or emergence of resistant organisms

3 Reliance on drugs with the omission of appropriate surgical drainage

4 Inappropriate dosing or duration of therapy

5 Treatment of inaccessible infections

6 Delay of treatment beyond the stage of permanent tissue damage

OTHER CONSIDERATIONS

ADVERSE EFFECTS

Adverse effects are a concern with any drug therapy, and each drug has its own set of potential side effects. The risk increases when prolonged therapy is needed, and concern may be sufficient to change the drug selection. For example, the potential for nephrotoxicity with aminoglycosides with prolonged therapy may make other drugs with similar spectrums (such as cephalosporins or fluoroquinolones) a more appropriate antibiotic choice in cases requiring extended treatment. Similarly, the risk of adverse side effects may increase in animals with specific physiological changes (e.g., hypovolemic patients are at increased risk of renal toxicity with non-steroidal anti-inflammatory drugs [NSAIDs] as well as aminoglycosides).

PUBLIC HEALTH AND REGULATORY CONCERNS

Drugs not approved by national regulation agencies for use in cattle present further considerations. Some, such as chloramphenicol, are absolutely contraindicated for use in food animals owing to the potential human health hazard. Others, such as flunixine meglumine and aspirin, are used frequently as unapproved drugs or as approved drugs in other countries and have established a precedent for use. Finally, many agents are approved for use in limited circumstances in cattle or at specific doses but are frequently used in circumstances or at doses beyond that for which they have been approved.

WITHDRAWAL TIMES

Withdrawal times of sufficient duration should be recommended in all cases. Table 5–3 lists drug with-

TABLE 5–3. DOSING GUIDELINES FOR PHARMACOLOGICAL AGENTS USED IN THE TREATMENT OF LAMENESS

Drug	Dose (mg/kg or units/kg)	Route	Bacterial Spectrum				Withdraw Times		Reference (for Dose Only)
			G+ Aer	G– Aer	Anaerobe	Other	Meat	Milk	
Penicillins									
Amoxicillin	11 mg/kg q 12–24 h	IM, SC	+ +	+ +	+		25 d	96 h	Beech[5]
Amoxicillin	7 mg/kg q 8 h	PO†	+ +	+ +	+		20 d	na	Baggot[3]
Amoxicillin + clavulanic acid	10 mg/kg q 8 h	PO†	+ + +	+ +	+ +		na	na	Prescott and Baggot[21]
Amoxicillin + clavulanic acid	8.75 mg/kg q 24 h	IM	+ + +	+ +	+ +		na	na	Prescott and Baggot[21]
Ampicillin + sulbactam	10 mg/kg q 24 h	IM	+ +	+ + +	+ +		na	na	Prescott and Baggot[21]
Ampicillin Na	22 mg/kg q 12 h	IM, IV, SC, PO†	+ +	+ +	+		6 d	48 h	Beech[5]
Ampicillin trihydrate	15–22 mg/kg q 8 h	IM, SC	+ +	+ +	+		6 d	48 h	Beech[5]
Penicillin G Benzathine	44,000–66,000 U/kg q 48 h	IM, SC	+ + +	+	+ +		30 d	non-lact	Upson[25]
Penicillin G Na or K	10,000–50,000 U/kg q 6–8 h	IM, IV	+ + +	+	+ +	S	14 d	5 d	Upson[25]
Penicillin G Procaine	44,000–66,000 U/kg q 24 h	IM, SC	+ + +	+	+ +	S	10–30 d	72 h–5 d	Upson[25]
Ticarcillin	50–75 mg/kg q 6–8 h	IM, IV	+	+ + +	+	S	na	na	Prescott and Baggot[21]
Cephalosporins									
Cefadroxil	35 mg/kg q 12 h	PO†	+ + +	+	+		na	na	Prescott and Baggot[21]
Cefazolin	22 mg/kg q 8 h	IM	+ + +	+	+		30 d	na	Allen et al[1]
Cefoperazone	30 mg/kg q 6–8 h	IM	+ + +	+ +	+ +		na	na	Prescott and Baggot[21]
Cefoxitin	20–30 mg/kg q 4–6 h	IM, IV	+	+ + +	+ +		na	na	Prescott and Baggot[21]
Ceftazidime	20–40 mg/kg q 12–24 h	IM, IV	+	+ + +	+		na	na	Prescott and Baggot[21]
Ceftiofur	1.1 mg/kg q 24 h	IM	+	+ +	+		0 d	0 d	
Cephadrine	7 mg/kg q 12 h	PO†	+ + +	+	+		na	na	Prescott and Baggot[21]
Cephalothin	55 mg/kg q 6 h	SC	+ + +	+	+		30 d	na	Beech[5]
Aminoglycosides									
Amikacin	10 mg/kg q 8 h–25 mg/kg q 12 h	IM	+	+ + +	–		na	na	Beech[5]
Gentamicin	2.2 mg/kg q 8–12 h	IM, IV	+	+ + +	–		180–360 d*	5 d	Upson[25]
Neomycin	4.4–22 mg/kg q 8–12 h	IM	+	+ + +	–		120 d*	96 h	Beech[5]
Spectinomycin	7–13 mg/kg q 8 h	IM	+	+ +	–		30–60 d	96 h	Upson[25]

Drug	Dose	Route					Meat	Milk	Reference
Lincosamides									
Lincomycin	15–25 mg/kg q 8–12 h	PO†	+ +	–	+ +	M	na	na	Prescott and Baggot[21]
Lincomycin	10–20 mg/kg q 12–24 h	IM, IV	+ +	–	+ +	M	na	na	Prescott and Baggot[21]
Tetracyclines									
Tetracycline	6–11 mg/kg q 12–24 h	IV	+ +	+ +	+	C, R, M, S	4–14 d	non-lact	Howard[15]
Tetracycline	11–15 mg/kg q 6 h	PO†	+ +	+ +	+	C, R, M, S	4–14 d	non-lact	Prescott and Baggot,[21] Howard[15]
Oxytetracycline	6–11 mg/kg q 12–24 h	IM, SC, IV	+ +	+ +	+	C, R, M, S	15–28 d	non-lact	Howard[15]
Oxytetracycline-long acting	20–40 mg/kg q 48 h	IM	+ +	+ +	+	C, R, M, S	15–28 d	non-lact	Upson,[25] Prescott and Baggot[21]
Sulfonamides									
Sulfadimethoxine	55 mg/kg q 12–24 h	IM, IV, SC, PO†	+	+	–	Co, T	5–7 d	60 h	Prescott and Baggot[21]
Sulfachlorpyridazine	88–110 mg/kg q 12–24 h	IV	+	+ +	–	Co, T	5–7 d	56 h	Upson[25]
Sulfadiazine + trimethoprim	25–44 mg/kg q 12–24 h	IM, IV, PO†	+ +	+ +	–	Co, T	5–7 d	56 h	Upson[25]
Sulfamethoxazole + trimethoprim	25–44 mg q 12–24 h	IM, IV, PO†	+ +	+ +	–	Co, T	5–7 d	56 h	Upson[25]
Macrolides									
Erythromycin	4–8 mg/kg q 12–24 h	IM, IV, SC, PO†	+ +	–	–	M, R	14 d	72 h	Jenkins[16]
Tilmicosin	10 mg/kg q 72 h	SC	+ +	–	–		28 d	non-lact	Prescott and Baggot[21]
Tylosin	20–30 mg/kg q 8–12 h	IM	+ +	–			21 d	non-lact	Prescott and Baggot[21]
Fluoroquinolones									
Enrofloxacin	2.5–5 mg/kg q 12–24 h	IM, PO†	+ +	+ + +	–	C, M, R	na	na	Prescott and Baggot[21]
Miscellaneous									
Isoniazid	11–22 mg/kg q 24 h	PO†	+ +	–	–	M	na	na	Prescott and Baggot[21]
Chloramphenicol	25 mg/kg q 8–12 h	IM, IV	+ +	+ +	+ +	C, M, R	do not use	non-lact	Prescott and Baggot[21]
Metronidazole	28 mg/kg × 1; 26 mg/kg q 8 h	IV	–	–	+ + +		na	na	Bhavsar and Malik[7]
Rifampin	20 mg/kg q 24 h	PO†	+ +	–	–	M	na	na	Prescott and Baggot[21]
Rifampin	10 mg/kg q 24 h	IM, IV	+ +	–	–	M	na	na	Prescott and Baggot[21]

Table continued on following page

TABLE 5–3. DOSING GUIDELINES FOR PHARMACOLOGICAL AGENTS USED IN THE TREATMENT OF LAMENESS *Continued*

Drug	Dose (mg/kg or units/kg)	Route	Bacterial Spectrum				Withdraw Times		Reference (for Dose Only)
			G+ Aer	G− Aer	Anaerobe	Other	Meat	Milk	
Antifungals									
Griseofulvin	10–20 mg/kg q 24 h	PO†	−	−	−	F	na	na	Pier[19]
Ketoconazole	10 mg/kg q 12–24 h	PO†	−	−	−	F	na	na	Prescott and Baggot[21]
Amphotericin B	0.5% solution locally	Topical	−	−	−	F	na	na	
Miconazole	1% solution locally QID	Topical	−	−	−	F	na	na	
Topical Agents									
Copper sulfate	10%–20% solution 20 min BID	Topical	+	+	+				
Dimethyl sulfoxide (DMSO)	90% gel or solution locally	Topical	−	−	−				
Formaldehyde	3%–10% solution 20 min BID	Topical	+ +	+ +	+ +	F			
Mupirocin	2% ointment locally TID	Topical	+ + +	+ +	−				Prescott and Baggot[21]
Nitrofurazone	0.2% solution locally	Topical	+ +	+ +	+ +				
Povidone-iodine	5%–10% solution locally	Topical	+ +	+ +	+ +	F			
Tetracycline	1% solution locally or lavage	Topical	+ +	+ +	+	C, M, R, S			
Tris (1.34 mM) EDTA (0.01M)	Locally or lavage	Topical	+ +	+ +	−				Ashworth and Nelson[2]
Zinc sulfate	10%–20% solution 20 min BID	Topical	+	+	+				
Non-Steroidal Anti-Inflammatory Agents									
Aspirin	15–100 mg/kg BID–TID	PO					24 h*	24 h*	Jenkins[17]
Dipyrone	50 mg/kg	IM, IV, SC					na	na	Howard[15]
Flunixin	2.2 mg/kg × 1; 1.1 mg/kg q 8 h	IV					do not use	non-lact	Jenkins[17]
Phenylbutazone	10–20 mg/kg × 1; 2–5 mg/kg q 24 h	IV, PO					do not use	non-lact	Jenkins[17]
	9 mg/kg × 1; 4.5 mg/kg q 48 h	IV, PO							Eberhardson[12a]
Corticosteroids									
Dexamethasone	5–20 mg q 24 h	IM					0 d	0 d	Berg[7]
Prednisolone	10–200 mg q 24 h	IM, IV					0 d	0 d	Berg[7]
Isoflupredone	10–20 mg q 12–24 h	IM, IA					0 d	0 d	Allen et al[1]
Triamcinolone	6–18 mg × 1	IA					0 d	0 d	Howard[15]
Triamcinolone	0.02–0.04 mg/kg	IM					0 d	0 d	Howard[15]

*Dosage cited is taken from the corresponding reference.
†PO in preruminants only.
C, *Chlamydia*; Co, coccidia; F, various fungal species; M, *Mycoplasma*; R, *Rickettsia*; S, *Spirochaeta*; T, *Toxoplasma*.
All withdrawal times taken from Sundlof et al[23]; d, days; h, hours; na, no information available; non-lact, use in non-lactating animals only; do not use, should not be used in animals intended for slaughter.

64

drawal times when available. These times are based on specific drug doses and regimens in healthy animals. The margin for error in any given animal may be high; therefore, these times should be considered the minimum appropriate times, especially when drugs are not used according to their label. Estimation of withdrawal times in milk and meat for non-approved use is often based on a standard length of time (e.g., 30 days) or a minimum number of plasma half-lives (e.g., 10); however, neither system can consistently predict drug clearance from milk or tissues, and the veterinarian and owner assume the responsibility for any residues present.

CLIENT-SPECIFIC FACTORS

Client expectations for the animal and the herd, price limitations, previous experience with similar problems, and ability to comply with treatment recommendations all may affect choice of therapy. In food animal practice, the choice of agent, the duration of administration, and the dose are often ultimately determined by the drug's cost and availability. Although this approach is not ideal, it is the reality for most food animal patients. For example, penicillin G, oxytetracycline, and the aminoglycosides are considerably less expensive therapy than the cephalosporins and quinolones and are frequently chosen for therapy in the presence of potential inferiority with respect to spectrum of activity, withdrawal times, or risk of toxicity.

The need for a specific diagnosis as a guide for individual animal treatment or as a basis for herd management must be weighed against the value of rapid initiation of antibiotic or anti-inflammatory therapy. The owner must be clearly informed of anticipated duration of therapy, cost, and prognosis before treatment begins. For food animals, the owner's economic interest in recouping costs through slaughter must be related to withdrawal times of potential therapies. The value of systemic drug treatment for mild or chronic lameness must be weighed against the value of maintaining cows in the milk line. In all cases, clients must make the final choice, and veterinarians are obligated to provide owners with the information necessary for them to make an informed choice.

MANAGEMENT FACTORS

Patient management issues are frequently important in selecting for treatment of lameness in cattle. Lack of facilities or equipment may preclude topical treatment with footbaths for conditions such as superficial digital dermatitis, and improved topical hygiene may be difficult to accomplish for similar reasons. Conversely, topical therapy may be more easily achieved than systemic treatment of multiple animals when herd problems exist. Conditions requiring long-term therapy, such as osteomyelitis, present particular

problems for operations that lack a convenient area for confinement and treatment of individual animals. Lack of personnel may also present a challenge for continued drug treatment of animals. The need to preserve public safety places unique restrictions on veterinarians, who may have to select drugs that may persist as meat or milk residues, particularly when adequate medical therapy requires the use of drugs at higher doses or for longer periods than approved by label.

ANTIMICROBIAL CLASSES

Mechanisms of action, quality of absorption, method of elimination, side effects, and precautions for the major classes of antimicrobial agents are described in Table 5–2. Doses, routes of administration, spectrum of activity, and withdrawal times for specific antibiotics currently or potentially used in cattle are provided in Table 5–3.

BETA-LACTAM ANTIBIOTICS

The beta-lactam antibiotics include the penicillins and cephalosporins. These are weak acids used either as the free bases or as the sodium or potassium salts. Penicillins and cephalosporins are usually bactericidal against susceptible organisms and act by inhibiting mucopeptide synthesis in the cell wall. Beta-lactam antibiotics have no effect on existing cell walls; therefore, susceptible organisms must be actively multiplying to be affected. The beta-lactam antibiotics achieve levels in bone and joints above the MICs for susceptible organisms. The presence of inflammation generally enhances diffusion into various tissues, including the cerebrospinal fluid, abscesses, and synovial fluids.

The penicillins encompass several distinct classes of compounds with various spectrums of activity: the natural penicillins, the penicillinase-resistant penicillins, the aminopenicillins, the extended-spectrum penicillins, and the potentiated penicillins. Aqueous procaine penicillin G and ampicillin trihydrate are the beta-lactam agents most commonly used in food animals; however, their respective sodium or potassium salts generally attain higher levels in blood, bone, and joints and should be considered for use, particularly early in therapy. Disadvantages of sodium or potassium salts include frequent administration (every 6 to 8 hours) and greater expense.

The cephalosporin antibiotics comprise several different classes of compounds with dissimilar spectrums of activity and pharmacokinetic profiles. The cephalosporin class is usually divided into three classifications or generations. The first-generation cephalosporins generally possess excellent coverage against most gram-positive pathogens and variable to poor coverage against most gram-negative pathogens. The second-generation cephalosporins have expanded gram-negative coverage at the expense of some of the gram-positive coverage provided by the first-generation agents. The third-generation cephalosporins have extended activity against gram-negative organisms but less activity against the gram-positive organisms, particularly *Staphylococcus* spp. Enough variability exists with individual bacterial sensitivities that susceptibility testing is necessary.

AMINOGLYCOSIDES

The aminoglycoside antibiotics act on susceptible bacteria by irreversibly binding to the 30S ribosomal subunit of microorganisms, thereby inhibiting protein synthesis. They are considered to be bactericidal. Considering toxicity, cost, and efficacy factors, gentamicin and amikacin are therapeutically useful agents available for food animal medicine. The spectrum of activity for gentamicin and amikacin includes coverage against many aerobic gram-negative and some aerobic gram-positive bacteria.

Aminoglycosides are generally distributed into bones and joints in sufficient levels to achieve therapeutic efficacy against susceptible bacteria. However, the activity of the aminoglycosides is decreased in acidic environments and sites with extensive tissue damage, conditions that typically exist in bone and joint infections. Aminoglycosides also penetrate fibrin poorly and have decreased activity in the presence of necrotic debris.

The aminoglycosides are infamous for their nephrotoxic and ototoxic effects. Ototoxicity is rare in cattle; however, nephrotoxicity is a clinical concern. The volume of distribution and rate of clearance can vary substantially in individual animals, and monitoring of plasma levels should be considered to adjust doses and minimize the risk of toxicity in valuable animals.

LINCOSAMIDES

The lincosamides include the agents lincomycin and clindamycin. These agents have excellent gram-positive activity and also have activity against many mycoplasmas and some anaerobes. Clindamycin is considered to be more active against susceptible organisms but is considerably more expensive than lincomycin.

Lincomycin's use in ruminants is controversial, because the drug has reportedly caused acute gastroenteritis in ruminants and death in sheep after oral ingestion.[10] Lincomycin has been used to treat joint infections in both cattle and sheep. No gastrointestinal adverse effects were reported.[20]

TETRACYCLINES

Tetracyclines generally act as bacteriostatic antibiotics. They inhibit protein synthesis by reversibly binding to 30S ribosomal subunits of susceptible organisms, thereby preventing binding to those ribosomes of aminoacyl transfer RNA. Tetracyclines also are believed to bind reversibly to 50S ribosomes and alter cytoplasmic membrane permeability in susceptible organisms.

As a class, the tetracyclines have activity against some gram-positive and gram-negative bacteria, most *Mycoplasma*, spirochetes (including the Lyme disease organism), *Chlamydia*, and *Rickettsia*. Oxytetracycline and tetracycline share nearly identical spectrums of activity and patterns of cross-resistance, and a tetracycline susceptibility disk is usually used for *in vitro* testing for oxytetracycline susceptibility. Tetracyclines are widely distributed in the body, including the synovial fluid and bone, particularly in active sites of ossification. Oxytetracycline and tetracycline given to young animals can cause bones and teeth to become yellow, brown, or gray, and high doses or long-term administration may delay bone growth and healing. Efficacy in bone infections with systemic administration may be limited by inactivation via chelation with calcium or other divalent or trivalent cations. However, experimentally induced osteomyelitis in dogs has resolved after surgical intervention and tetracycline lavage.[26]

Rapid intravenous injection of undiluted propylene glycol–based products can cause intravascular hemolysis with resultant hemoglobinuria. Propylene glycol–based products have also caused cardiodepressant effects when administered to calves. When administered intramuscularly, local reactions, yellow staining, and necrosis may be seen at the injection site.

SULFONAMIDES, POTENTIATED SULFONAMIDES

Sulfonamides are usually bacteriostatic agents when used alone. They are thought to prevent bacterial replication by competing with para-aminobenzoic acid in the biosynthesis of tetrahydrofolic acid in the pathway to form folic acid. Only microorganisms that synthesize their own folic acid are affected by sulfas.

Sulfonamides are reportedly distributed throughout most body tissues and fluids, including synovial fluid. Sulfonamides have been a mainstay of therapy of *Nocardia* osteomyelitis in humans and in cattle. The sulfas are less efficacious in pus, necrotic tissue, or areas with extensive cellular debris.

Microorganisms that are usually susceptible to sulfonamides include some gram-positive and gram-negative species. As development of strains of bacteria resistant to sulfonamides has increased, the addition of trimethoprim to the sulfonamide has expanded the spectrum of activity of the combination over sulfonamides alone. Many strains of staphylococci, most streptococci, and several species or strains of Enterobacteriaceae are susceptible, but not *Pseudomonas aeruginosa*.

MACROLIDES

The macrolide antibiotics include erythromycin and tylosin. Usually considered to be bacteriostatic agents, they may be bactericidal in high concentrations or against highly susceptible organisms. The macrolides are believed to act by binding to the 50S ribosomal subunit of susceptible bacteria, thereby inhibiting peptide bond formation.

Macrolides have *in vitro* activity against gram-positive cocci and bacilli and some strains of gram-negative bacilli.

Absorption is very slow after intramuscular or subcutaneous injection of the polyethylene-based veterinary product in cattle. Bioavailability is only about 40% after subcutaneous injection and 65% after intramuscular injection. It is also unknown how well the drug penetrates into bone, and it has been reported that it does not enter synovial fluid easily.

Adverse effects are relatively infrequent. Intravenous injections should be given very slowly, because the intravenous forms can readily cause thrombophlebitis.

FLUOROQUINOLONES

The mechanism of action of enrofloxacin and other fluoroquinolones is not thoroughly understood, but they are believed to act by inhibiting bacterial DNA, thereby preventing DNA supercoiling and DNA synthesis. Considered bactericidal, these agents have good activity against many gram-negative bacilli and cocci, variable activity against most streptococci, and weak activity against most anaerobes.

Fluoroquinolones are distributed throughout the body. Highest concentrations are found in the bile, kidneys, liver, lungs, and reproductive system (including prostatic fluid and tissue). Therapeutic levels are also attained in bone, synovial fluid, skin, muscle, aqueous humor, and pleural fluid. With the exception of potential cartilage abnormalities in young animals, the adverse effect profile of these drugs appears to be minimal.

MISCELLANEOUS ANTIBIOTICS

Metronidazole has good bone penetration and has activity against many anaerobic bacteria, including penicillin-resistant varieties of *Bacteroides*. It is a potentially useful antibiotic for treating anaerobic bone or joint infections in food animals, and its pharmacokinetics have been described in calves.[8]

Rifampin is active against various *Mycobacterium* spp and gram-positive organisms. Bacterial resistance occurs rapidly when the drug is used alone. After oral administration, rifampin is relatively well absorbed from the gastrointestinal tract in species studied. Oral administration results in variable absorption. Rifampin is very lipophilic and penetrates most body tissues, cells, and fluids (including cerebrospinal fluid) well. It also penetrates abscesses and caseous material.

Chloramphenicol is a bacteriostatic agent with wide tissue distribution, including the CNS. It has a low incidence of side effects and a broad spectrum of activity. Clinical utility is limited by the potential for idiosyncratic fatal aplastic anemia in humans exposed to chloramphenicol, either through milk or meat or during administration of the drug to patients. The drug is absolutely contraindicated in animals potentially used for human consumption.

ANTIFUNGAL AGENTS

Fungal infections affecting bone or joint tissue occur rarely in the normal immunocompetent food animal population. Therapeutic choices for systemic antifungal treatment of bone or joint infections are very limited, and the lack of either research data or clinical experience with potential therapeutic agents in target species severely limits clinicians' available treatment options. Superficial fungal infections of skin may respond to topical hygiene without use of specific antifungal drugs.

TOPICAL AGENTS

Astringents precipitate proteins and, when applied to mucous membranes or to damaged skin, form a superficial protective layer and are not generally absorbed. They may be used to harden the skin and to decrease exudative secretions and minor bleeding. Zinc sulfate and copper sulfate are effective astringents and may be used as footbaths. These agents are also mildly antiseptic. Frequent changes of solution or antecedent use of a cleansing footbath may increase efficacy by improving direct contact of the agent with damaged tissue and by minimizing drug inactivation by inorganic materials.

Antiseptics are generally used to destroy or inhibit the growth of pathogenic microorganisms in the non-sporulating or vegetative state. They are typically used to limit or prevent infection and are useful primarily as an adjunct to systemic therapy in serious conditions. Povidone-iodine is a loose complex of iodine and a carrier polymer, which slowly releases iodine to exert an effect on most bacteria, fungi, protozoa, cysts, and spores. It is less potent than preparations containing free iodine but also is less toxic. Formaldehyde is effective against vegetative bacteria, fungi, and many viruses but is much less effective against bacterial spores. It does not penetrate the skin well, and when applied to unbroken skin, it hardens the epidermis and produces a local anesthetic effect.

Topical antibiotics such as tetracyclines and nitrofurans are suitable for wound lavage and footbaths and are effective against a broad spectrum of bacteria.

Dimethyl sulfoxide (DMSO) has a wide spectrum

of pharmacological effects, including membrane penetration, anti-inflammatory effects, local analgesia, weak bacteriostasis, diuresis, vasodilation, and dissolution of collagen. It is also useful for enhancing drug penetration of the skin. DMSO should not be used in lactating animals or in those intended for slaughter.

Tris-EDTA solution added to antimicrobial irrigation solutions may potentiate their efficacy. Tris-EDTA acts by decreasing the stability and increasing the permeability of some bacterial cell walls to the antimicrobial agents. Positive outcomes have been reported in non-responsive fracture osteomyelitis and coffin joint abscesses in cattle.[2]

ANTI-INFLAMMATORY AGENTS

Control of inflammation is an essential part of treatment for lameness due to most causes. Early and aggressive anti-inflammatory therapy is particularly important in treatment of diseases involving joints and the CNS, where the inflammatory response itself can be the principal source of permanent tissue damage. Steroids and NSAIDs are the principal anti-inflammatory agents used systemically. Characteristics of these drugs are listed in Tables 5–2 and 5–3, as well as in Chapter 4 (see pp. 41). Topical therapy of inflammation with topical vasodilating agents (e.g., alcohol, glycerin) or compression bandages are also potentially useful in dealing with edema or, more controversially, cellulitis. Adjunct therapy should include immobilization of unstable tissues, decompression of swollen compartments such as joints or abscesses, and removal of inflammatory stimuli.

RECOMMENDATIONS BY SYSTEM

JOINT-RELATED LAMENESS

Joint diseases that commonly result in bovine lameness include infectious arthritis, traumatic arthritis (acute), and degenerative joint disease (chronic) (see pp. 166–172). When mobile diarthrodial joints such as the fetlock, proximal hock, and stifle are affected, therapy must result in preservation of pain-free motion in order to be effective. Therefore, elimination of infectious agents and rapid control of inflammation are critical to prevent irreparable damage to articular cartilage. In treatment of disease of relatively low-motion joints, such as those of the distal hock and coffin joint, treatment may be directed either toward preservation of normal function or toward elimination of painful motion through arthrodesis. The approach to pharmacological therapy depends to a large extent on the nature of the disease process.

Infectious arthritis is a disease process that can rapidly result in permanent loss of function owing to damage to the articular cartilage. In human infants and neonates, irreversible damage can occur within 48 to 72 hours of symptom onset if left untreated.[27] A similar time frame is probable for calves. Much of the damage to articular structures results from the rapid influx of inflammatory mediators and white blood cells, which are part of the normal host response to joint infection. Therapeutic priorities include elimination of infectious agents, control of the host inflammatory process, and prevention of further damage. Systemic antibiotics and anti-inflammatory agents are commonly crucial parts of initial therapy in addition to joint decompression or lavage to remove inflammatory products. Intra-articular antibiotics may also have value in treating infected joints, although their use is controversial. Antibiotics should be continued at high levels after the last sign of infection, which often necessitates a prolonged parenteral course of 4 to 6 weeks. Immobilization may help to relieve pain and its associated release of inflammatory mediators during the acute stage of infection. Controlled joint use is important after infection and acute inflammation are under control in order to combat intra-articular and periarticular adhesions, which can permanently decrease the range of motion.

Achievement of therapeutic goals can be strongly affected by lesion, patient, and management factors. Lesion-specific factors have perhaps the greatest impact on the treatment approach and efficacy. Infectious arthritis in cattle is most commonly caused by bacteria, with rare involvement by *Chlamydia*, spirochetes, viruses, and fungi. Evaluation of each case should include collection of a sample of joint fluid for Gram stain and culture and sensitivity testing. However, certain bacteria are recognized to be more common pathogens in bovine joints.[24] *Actinomyces* (formerly *Corynebacterium*) *pyogenes* is the most commonly recognized pathogen of joints in cattle of all ages. Other commonly reported bacterial pathogens include *Streptococcus* spp. (G+), *Salmonella* spp. (G−), *Escherichia coli* (G−), *Proteus* spp. (G−), and *Fusobacterium necrophorum* (G− anaerobe). Less commonly reported bacterial joint pathogens in cattle include *Staphylococcus* spp. (G+), *Erysipelothrix* spp. (G+), *Pseudomonas* spp. (G−), *Pasteurella* spp. (G−), *Haemophilus* spp. (G−), *Bacteroides* spp. (G− anaerobe), *Brucella* spp. (anaerobe), and *Mycoplasma* spp. Mixed infections with gram-negative aerobes plus either anaerobes or gram-positive aerobes are also common.

Infection of the joint typically results in a decreased local pH, an accumulation of proteolytic enzymes from bacteria and host inflammatory cells, and an accumulation of fibrin, all of which decrease the penetration and activity of a number of antibiotics including aminoglycosides and sulfonamides. Early and aggressive joint lavage can decrease the amount of debris and fibrin, presumably increasing the efficacy of systemically administered antibiotics. The presence of fibrin may allow the persistence of viable organisms within the fibrin matrix for weeks, contributing to the recommendation for extended antimicrobial therapy for 4 to 6 weeks.

Of the patient-specific factors, age has a particularly important role in selection of pharmacological therapy in that it allows prediction of probable mechanisms of disease and typical pathogens, and places potential pharmacokinetic and economical limitations on the chosen drugs. Infectious arthritis in neonates is typically associated with septicemic spread, and consequently, it is not only often found in multiple joints but may concurrently affect other systems. Septicemic spread of infection steadily decreases in frequency as age increases over 4 to 6 months and is uncommon in mature animals. Certain organisms are also more common in some age groups. As an example, polyarthritis due to *Salmonella* spp. is typically encountered in neonatal calves younger than 12 weeks, whereas polyarthridites due to *A. pyogenes* are more common in slightly older calves.[9, 13]

The frequency with which preruminant calves are affected expands the options for antimicrobial agents to drugs only given orally, although intravenous or intramuscular therapy is preferred for at least the first 10 to 14 days of therapy in order to achieve optimal blood and tissue levels. The potential effects of poor physical condition and the presence of concurrent disease on drug pharmacokinetics and potential toxicities should also be considered in therapeutic planning.

BONE-RELATED LAMENESS

Bone is a complex, dense connective tissue that is characterized by a restricted blood supply with variable penetration of different drugs depending on their pharmacokinetic characteristics and with limited routes for removal of necrotic material. The slow lymphatic and venous drainage systems and the normally buried location of bones limit natural drainage routes and make surgical debridement an important adjunct to pharmacological treatment for established infections of bone. Although bone has enormous regenerative capacity, healing requires time, and continued damage must be prevented until healing has occurred. Use of anti-inflammatory agents may be an important part of treatment to prevent continued damage, but their potential value must be weighed against the risk of promoting increased activity leading to further mechanical trauma.

SKIN-RELATED LAMENESS

Lesions restricted to the superficial layers of skin, such as interdigital dermatitis, cause lameness due to inflammation and pain. Such lesions are characterized by a limited systemic blood supply, restricted permeability to topical agents, excellent drainage, constant exposure to contamination, and a high tolerance of tissue loss due to a rapid regenerative capacity. The role of antibiotics is probably secondary to topical hygiene. Providing a dry, clean environment and the use of topical astringent disinfectants in footbaths are typically as important in successful

treatment as is a decision about systemic antibiotics. When an environmental change is not possible, antibiotics may help limit spread of the infection until such changes can be made.

As lesions extend to involve the deeper layers of the skin, antibiotics become a more crucial part of management, both as a part of therapy and as prophylaxis. Unless the superficial layers of skin have been lost, topical antimicrobial therapy may be less valuable than systemic therapy. If abscessation has occurred, antibiotic selection must address the need for drug penetration of fibrin and retention of activity in the presence of necrotic debris. However, as a general rule, drainage should be the primary goal for treatment of established abscesses, with antibiotic therapy serving as a method to help minimize damage to tissue along a drainage route or as an alternative to drainage when a safe portal for drainage is not available.

LIGAMENT/TENDON-RELATED LAMENESS

Treatment of lesions involving injury of ligaments and tendons must contend with a limited blood supply, limited ability to regenerate functional tissue, limited capacity for self-debridement, and, specifically for tendons, a need for preservation of maximal function. In addition to use of systemic antibiotic therapy and, for many traumatic injuries, surgical debridement, early control of inflammation with anti-inflammatory agents and controlled mobilization are important parts of treatment to minimize adhesion formation.

MUSCLE-RELATED LAMENESS

Muscle is a highly vascularized tissue that regenerates poorly but can tolerate a greater amount of functional tissue loss without affecting daily activities than can other tissues. Replacement of large amounts of muscle with fibrous scar tissue can permanently impair function in some sites. Therefore, anti-inflammatory treatment is an important part of therapy. Most antimicrobial and anti-inflammatory agents reach adequate levels in muscle when administered systemically. Because of the highly vascularized nature of muscle, drainage is not as commonly a part of treatment for infections in muscle as it might be in other tissues. The exception to this rule is clostridial infection, in which rapid exposure of the anaerobic organisms to air can slow local tissue destruction and the systemic spread of what can be a rapidly fatal infection.

NEUROLOGICAL-RELATED LAMENESS

Lameness or altered gait resulting from lesions of the neurological system presents special challenges for pharmacological therapy. Nervous tissue has very limited regenerative capacity and is susceptible to inflammation and compression. Initial therapy must include aggressive anti-inflammatory medication and, if appropriate for peripheral neuropathies, physical decompression.

REFERENCES

1. Allen DG, Pringle JK, Smith D: Handbook of Veterinary Drugs. Philadelphia, JB Lippincott, 1993.
2. Ashworth CD, Nelson DR: Antimicrobial protention of irrigation solutions containing tris-(hydroxymethyl) aminomethane-EDTA. J Am Vet Med Assoc 197:1513–1514, 1990.
3. Baggot JD: Systemic antimicrobial therapy in large animals. In Bogan JA, Lees P, Yoxall AT (eds): Pharmacological Basis of Large Animal Medicine. Oxford, Blackwell Scientific Publications, 1983, pp 45–69.
4. Baggot JD: Clinical pharmacokinetics in veterinary medicine. Clin Pharmacokinet 22:254–273, 1992.
5. Beech J: Respiratory tract—horse, cow. In Johnston DE (ed): The Bristol Handbook of Antimicrobial Therapy. Evansville, IN, Veterinary Learning Systems, 1987, pp 88–109.
6. Bengtsson B, Franklin A, Luthman J, et al: Concentrations of sulphadimidine, oxytetracycline, and penicillin G in serum, synovial fluid and tissue cage fluid after parenteral administration to calves. J Vet Pharmacol Ther 12:37–45, 1989.
7. Berg JN: Aseptic laminitis in cattle. In Howard JL (ed): Current Veterinary Therapy: Food Animal Practice 2. Philadelphia, WB Saunders, 1986, pp 896–898.
8. Bhavsar SK, Malik JK: Pharmacokinetics of metronidazole in calves. Br Vet J 150:389–393, 1994.
9. Blood DC, Radostits OM (eds): Veterinary Medicine, 7th ed. London, Baillière Tindall, 1989, pp 463–472.
10. Bulgin MS: Losses related to the ingestion of lincomycin-medicated feed in a range sheep flock. J Am Vet Med Assoc 192:1083–1085, 1988.
11. Cooper RR, Milgram JW, Robinson RA: Morphology of the osteon: An electron microscopic study. J Bone Joint Surg 48A:1239–1271, 1966.
12. Craig WA, Vogelman B: The post-antibiotic effect. Ann Intern Med 106:900–902, 1987.
12a. Eberhardson B, Olsson G, Appelgrew LE, et al: Pharmacokinetic studies of phenylbutazone in cattle. J Vet Pharmacol Ther 2:31–37, 1979.
13. Firth EC, Kersjhes AW, Dik KJ, et al: Haematogenous osteomyelitis in cattle. Vet Rec 120:148–152, 1987.
14. Guard CL, Byman KW, Schwark WS: Effect of experimental synovitis on disposition of penicillin and oxytetracycline in neonatal calves. Cornell Vet 79:161–171, 1989.
15. Howard JL (ed): Current Veterinary Therapy: Food Animal Practice 2. Philadelphia, WB Saunders, 1986.
16. Jenkins WL: Chloramphenicol, macrolides, lincosamides, vancomycin, polymyxins, rifamycins. In Johnston DE (ed): The Bristol Handbook of Antimicrobial Therapy. Evansville, IN, Veterinary Learning Systems, 1987, pp 261–265.
17. Jenkins WL: Pharmacologic aspects of analgesic drugs in animals: An overview. J Am Vet Med Assoc 191:1231–1240, 1987.
18. Orsini JA: Strategies for treatment of bone and joint infections in large animals. J Am Vet Med Assoc 185:1190–1193, 1984.
19. Pier AC: Dermatophytosis. In Howard JL (ed) Current Veterinary Therapy: Food Animal Practice 2. Philadelphia, WB Saunders, 1986, pp 924–927.
20. Plenderleith RWJ: Treatment of cattle, sheep and horses with lincomycin: Case studies. Vet Rec 122:112–113, 1988.
21. Prescott JF, Baggot JD: Antimicrobial Therapy in Veterinary Medicine, 2nd ed. Ames, IA, Iowa State University Press, 1993.
22. Shoaf SE, Schwark WS, Guard CL, et al: Pharmacokinetics of trimethoprim/sulfadiazine in neonatal calves: Influence, of synovitis. J Vet Pharmacol Ther 9:446–454, 1986.
23. Sundlof SF, Riviere JE, Craigmill AL: Food Animal Residue Avoidance Databank Tradename File: A Comprehensive Compendium of Dairy Cattle Drugs. Gainesville, FL, Institute of Food and Agricultural Sciences, University of Florida, 1992.
24. Trent AM, Plumb D: Treatment of infectious arthritis and osteomyelitis. Vet Clin North Am Food Anim Pract 7:747–778, 1991.
25. Upson DW: Handbook of Clinical Veterinary Pharmacology, 3rd ed. Manhattan, KS, Dan Upson Enterprises, 1988.
26. Varshney A, Harpal-Singh, Gupta RS, Singh SP: Microbiological aspects of experimental osteomyelitis in dogs. Indian J Anim Sci 60:946–948, 1990.
27. Welkon CJ, Long SS, Fisher MC, et al: Pyogenic arthritis in infants and children: A review of 95 cases. Pediatr Infect Dis 5:669–676, 1986.
28. Wingfield WE: Surgical treatment of chronic osteomyelitis in dogs. J Am Anim Hosp Assoc 11:568–569, 1975.

Paul R. Greenough *Canada*

Ben T. McDaniel *United States*
Horst W. Leipoldt†

6

Conformation, Growth, and Heritable Factors

Conformation

Paul R. Greenough

DEFINITIONS OF CONFORMATION AND POSTURE

The dimensions and shape of an animal are referred to collectively as its *conformation*.

Posture is the manner in which an animal stands, as distinct from its shape.

Objective physical measurements of bone length and fixed points (see p. 72), as well as angles between the long bones and the pelvis, permit scientific recording of conformation.

Abnormal posture is acquired in an attempt to relieve pain or to adjust to a mechanical influence. The posture may become habitual after the cause is no longer present. Posture is important, first, as an indication of the seat of pain, and, second, because individuals who are evaluating body characteristics confuse abnormal posture with abnormal conformation.

ANATOMICAL MEASUREMENTS

Anatomical Landmarks of the Body

The following 10 anatomical points are appropriate for objective linear measurements of conformation or body shape and size (Fig. 6–1). The terminology is taken from the Nomina Anatomica Veterinaria (1994).[39]

1 The cranial spine of the crest of the sacrum

2 The ventrolateral process of the tuber ischiadicum (pin)

3 The center of the lateral surface of the trochanter major (thurl)

4 The ventrolateral process of the tuber coxae (hook)

5 The femorotibial articulation caudal to the patellar ligament (stifle)

6 The tuber calcanei (point of the hock)

7 The tubercle on the lateral aspect of the metatarsus immediately distal to the tarsometatarsal joint

8 The dorsal surface of the center of the metatarsus

9 The extremity of the spine of the third thoracic vertebra (withers)

10 The cranial extremity of the major tubercle of the humerus (point of the shoulder)

Common body measurements are as follows (Fig. 6–2):

Loin height (hip height) (A)	(1) to ground
Withers height (B)	(9) to ground
Shoulder height (C)	(10) to ground
Body length (D)	(2) to (10)
Pelvic length (E)	(2) to (4)
Pelvic inclination (rump) = angle made by pelvic length to ground	
Pelvic angle	(2) to (3) to (4)
Hock angle	(5) to (7) to (8)

The tuber calcanei, in a normal stance, is located vertically below the tuber ischiadicum, whether viewed from the rear or the side.

†deceased

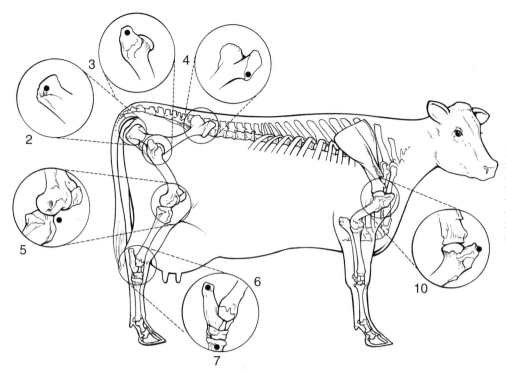

Figure 6–1. Anatomical landmarks of the body. Tuber ischiadicum (2), trochanter major (3), tuber coxae (4), ligamentum patellae laterale (5), tuber calcanei (6), lateral tubercle of the proximal end of the metatarsus (7), and tuberculum majus (10).

Anatomical Landmarks of the Claw

1 The skin-horn junction at the bulb

2 The skin-horn junction (limbus), dorsal surface of the claw

3 The apex (point of the toe) of the claw

Common claw measurements are as follows (Fig. 6–3):

Claw angle, the angle between the dorsal wall and the ground

Claw height	(2) to ground
Claw diagonal	(3) to (2)
Heel height	(2) to ground

Bearing Surface of the Claw

An approximation of the bearing surface of a claw can be calculated for claws free of acquired defects by using the following formula (units are square inches or square centimeters):

$$\text{Claw diagonal} \times \text{width of both digits taken at widest point} \times 0.5$$

The true bearing surface of the claw is the wall plus approximately 2 cm of the adjacent solar surface. The true bearing surface is variable depending on wear; therefore, the approximation formula is appropriate for purposes of comparison.

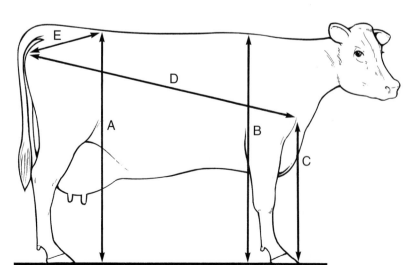

Figure 6–2. Common body measurements. Loin height (A), withers height (B), shoulder height (C), body length (D), and pelvic length and slope of rump (E).

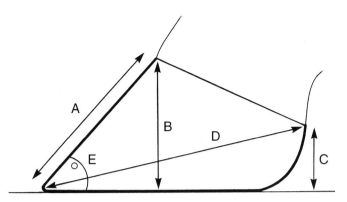

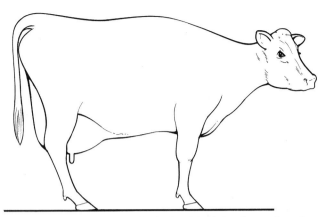

Figure 6–4. Camping forward. The hind limb is advanced so that the tuber calcanei is located in a vertical plane anterior to the tuber ischiadicum. A similar imbalance of the forelimb is referred to as *protraction* of the limb.

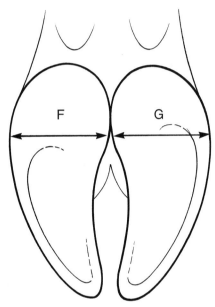

Figure 6–3. Common claw measurements. Claw length (A), claw height (B), heel height (C), claw diagonal (D), toe angle (E), claw width (F and G). F + G = digit width.

POSTURE AND GAIT

Protraction of the Limb (Camping Forward)

Camping forward is defined as the posture or gait of an animal that carries its hind feet farther under its body than normal (Fig. 6–4). This posture suggests that the seat of lameness (pain) is in the toe region. The back may be arched.

If pain is present in the toe of one claw, the first and second phases of the limb strides are unequal. The affected extremity is carried farther forward than the contralateral sound limb. When both claws are affected equally, both limbs are carried well forward in the first phase. Protraction of the limb, typical of laminitis, is frequently confused with the conformation characteristic of *sickle hock*.

Retraction of the Limb (Camping Back)

An animal that stands camped back holds its hind feet well behind the vertical (Fig. 6–5). This may

indicate pain in the heel region and is a typical stance or posture in animals with ulceration of the sole or severe erosion of the heel. It can also be associated with a spinal lesion.

An animal with a sore heel is reluctant to bear weight during the first phase of the stride. It does not carry the limb as far forward as normal, and the second phase tends to be prolonged. It must be emphasized that camping back is not a conformation defect but an acquired characteristic.

Adduction (Standing Narrow)

When viewed from behind, cattle walk with the limbs and extremities close together. To an untrained observer, it may appear that the animal is bowlegged (poor conformation). However, pain in the inside claws (e.g., laminitis) is usually the cause of adduction.

Severe pain in the inner hind claw(s) sometimes results in a cross-legged stance (see p. 249).

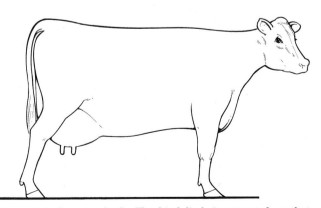

Figure 6–5. Camping back. The hind limb is retracted so that the tuber calcanei is located in a vertical plane posterior to the ischiadicum. A similar imbalance of the forelimb is referred to as *retraction* of the limb.

Flexion of the Metatarsophalangeal Joint (Knuckling Over)

Flexion of the metatarsophalangeal joint is a posture (or gait) that usually indicates heel pain. Normally, the hind limb heel touches the ground first, and during initial weight-bearing, the fetlock and pastern joints are held fixed until the second or lift-off stage of the stride (Fig. 6–6). An animal with a sore heel sometimes brings the toe to the ground first. This is possible only if the fetlock is slightly bent during the first phase of the stride. The act of knuckling over is performed extremely rapidly. Animals affected with tibial or peroneal paralysis also display knuckling.

Supination of the Tarsus (Cow Hock)

An animal with supination of the tarsus stands with the tuber calcanei directed medially and the points of the claws directed laterally (outward rotation) (Fig. 6–7). This posture usually results from the increased horn depth (overburdening) beneath the bulb of the lateral digits. It may result from pain in the lateral digit and the reduction of weight-bearing on the claw. The condition is reversible after therapeutic hoof trimming (see Chapter 9).

FUNCTIONAL EFFICIENCY

Functional efficiency is an animal's ability to perform the functions for which it was intended for a prolonged period.[6] Functional efficiency is therefore related to productivity as well as to the following factors:

- Fertility
- Calving ease (size and shape of the pelvis)
- Longevity (usually refers to the length of useful life)

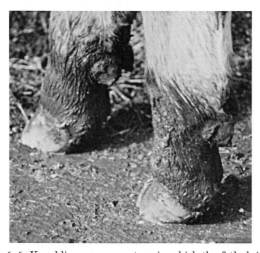

Figure 6–6. Knuckling over, a posture in which the fetlock is held slightly flexed to relieve pain in the heel. A comparable adaptation occurs during locomotion.

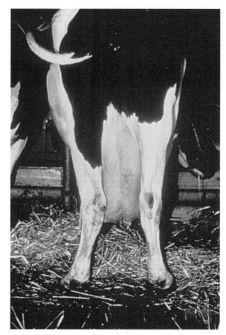

Figure 6–7. Cow hock, an acquired posture in which the point of the hock is rotated medially (supination), usually caused by a buildup of horn beneath the bulb of the lateral claw (overburdening). The posture is reversible with appropriate therapeutic trimming (see Chapter 9).

- Carcass merit (beef cattle)
- Frame score
- Freedom from diseases of the musculoskeletal system

Research reports that have demonstrated a positive correlation between objective measurements and a desired characteristic have implications for improving the cost effectiveness of the livestock industry. However, conformation has traditionally been judged on aesthetic qualities or on the anecdotal association of a given trait with performance. Aesthetic qualities are influenced by the muscularity and the distribution of subcutaneous fat. The show ring may perpetuate an unscientific and purely subjective system. Judgment based only on fashion, tradition, or the personal bias of a judge is contrary to the interests of the commercial producer. Changes in production systems render a formerly desirable conformation less reliable or even worthless under present conditions.

STATURE

Size differences between and within breeds in cows of the same age and in the same environment demonstrate the effect of genetics on conformation. Traits closely correlated to fitness are relatively little influenced by genetics owing to the effects of natural selection, but those traits unrelated to natural fitness have more genetic variation, especially of the additive type. The large differences in body size and shape demonstrate that their variety is unrelated to natural fitness.

The most highly heritable traits within breeds are stature (tallness) and body length. Even data based on visual appraisal give high heritabilities. Traits prone to measurement errors, such as rump and leg angles, are considerably less heritable. These lower heritabilities may result more from measurement errors than from a true lack of genetic variation.

Many genes influence several body size traits simultaneously. The genetic correlations among size traits are highly positive. This means that selection for a single trait such as growth rate usually increases stature and body length to some extent.

In dairy cattle, stature (withers height) is reported to be a highly heritable characteristic. The Holstein industry suggests that guidelines for the stature of an ideal Holstein cow are 137 cm (54 inches) at 24 months or 142 cm (56 inches) after 60 months. However, the size of a Holstein cow is generally measured as its weight, 527 kg (1170 pounds) being desired at 24 months and 675 kg (1500 pounds) after 60 months of age. These criteria can be important when considering the rearing of replacement animals (see p. 84 and Chapter 20).

In the past, when beef cattle with large frame sizes were desired, breeders selected animals with straight hocks as a means of increasing the animal's stature in the erroneous belief that stature was a reflection of frame size. Selection for higher hock angles usually increases stature but does not affect body weight much. In beef cattle, the bone-to-meat ratio remains constant irrespective of the angulation of the hind limb.[5]

The stature of beef cattle is measured at the hip. The term *hip height* does not refer to the height of the coxofemoral joint (thurl) but to the height of the tuber coxae (hook). Unfortunately, the position of the tuber coxae relative to the dorsal surface of the animal is variable. The tuber coxae is about 7 cm long. The part of the tuber from which measurements are taken is usually not specified, adding to the inaccuracy of hip height measurement. A consistent landmark, the lower external tubercle, is used, not as a measure of height but to determine pelvic length and external angles of the pelvis. The *true* height should be referred to as *loin height*, which is the distance from the bearing surface to the cranial spine of the crest of the sacrum.

CONFORMATION AND FERTILITY

The increase in length of long bones occurs at physeal plates. Each bone has a pattern or time for growth, which means that animals of different ages have characteristic conformations. A sudden growth spurt occurs at puberty. Thereafter, the physeal plates start to close, and increases in the bone length finally cease. This process is controlled endocrinologically by the thyroid's acting synergistically with somatotropic hormone. Full bone maturation requires additional influences of reproductive hormones. However, the closure of physeal plates is delayed in castrated males. Unqualified selection for improving stature can produce animals with low fertility.[6]

The majority of workers define body length as the distance from the tuber ischiadicum (pin) to the point of the shoulder. The point that is recommended for identification is the most lateral and lowest part of the tuber ischiadicum.

South African workers have reported that for beef cattle, "highly significant positive correlations were established between shoulder height and body length with average daily gain per day of age and final mass. Partial correlations showed that body length exercised greater influence on performance traits than shoulder height."[45]

Sadly, the relationship between body conformation, body weight, and skeletal disease resulting in clinical lameness has never been systematically investigated. This failure is partially attributable to the multiplicity of confounding factors, which make statistical evaluation difficult or impossible unless a large cohort is selected for study.

Nebulous and anecdotal reports, which are impossible to verify or to reproduce in repeated studies, lack scientific validity.

Genetics of Conformation

Ben T. McDaniel

REVIEW OF THE LITERATURE

The validity of visual appraisal is not guaranteed because "the skill to evaluate conformation with consistent accuracy is shared by a limited number of individuals."[19] Nevertheless, many individuals who are trained in the use of scientific principles can become highly competent in the skill.

Research reports indicate that a better understanding of conformation and its heritability is of great economic importance.

The dairy industry uses a so-called nine-point linear scale for evaluating conformation. Some traits relate to production; others such as hock or claw angle are termed *non-production traits* (NPTs). Other traits are descriptive and are evaluated subjectively. Some descriptive traits can be evaluated relatively accurately even by untrained evaluators. The attractiveness of using linear traits is the sheer number of records; for example, the Holstein Friesian Society of Great Britain and Ireland has a database of 220,000 records.

The term *linear measurement* in beef cattle refers to a specific measurement between two anatomical points. Workers in the beef industry report that positive correlations exist between linear measurements and desirable characteristics of production and longevity in beef cattle.[27, 31, 45] However, many reports lack specific anatomical criteria for linear measurements, whereas in others they are vague. The measurements used in research must be precisely defined and comparable between workers.

LINEAR TRAITS OF DAIRY CATTLE

Traits are scored on a nine-point scale that indicates the desirability or undesirability of a particular characteristic. Claws may vary in color from black to white. A descriptive trait such as *feet and legs* contains many variables. An accurate general assessment is not possible by even a trained observer unless individual parts are scored in combination with a standard set of weighting factors. Nevertheless, this trait has been used extensively by research workers who report that *feet and legs* have low heritability. Ideally, the combined trait should be evaluated as two separate components, (1) claws and (2) limbs. The heritability of individual characteristics might be found to be quite different, as in the case of Habel,[25] who demonstrated high heritability in the slope of the metatarsus. Some evaluation programs actually score each trait separately but combine them with a properly derived formula.

Linear traits involved with locomotion that are widely scored in dairy cattle are claw angle, legs side view, and legs rear view.

Trait	Scoring	Desirable
Claw angle	Low to high	High to 60°
Rear leg, side view	Posty to sickled	Intermediate
Rear leg, rear view	Close to straight	Straight

A biomechanical relationship exists between body weight, the angulation of the limb joints, the size and quality of the claw, the degree to which the claw is affected by disease, and the environment in which the animal is maintained.

If the total weight-bearing area of the soles is disproportionately small relative to the weight of the animal, giving a high value of kilograms per square centimeter of sole area, the claw functions poorly in absorbing the mechanical stresses of weight-bearing. The resulting trauma is a factor to be considered in laminitis, bruising, white line disease, and ulceration of the sole.

If claw size is to be used as a criterion for genetic selection, measurements should be taken before or soon after the first calving. The shape of the claw can change in accordance with an animal's age and as a result of the effects of diseases such as laminitis

and heel erosion. Claw shape is also affected by the amount of wear, which is influenced by the floor surfaces and moisture. Productive cows that have maintained a normal claw shape throughout several years' production under conditions in which many of their contemporaries' claws have become misshapen have obviously desirable genetics.

Two claw measurements, length and diagonal, have been extensively investigated.

Claw Length and Claw Diagonal

Although the length of the bearing surface of claws is a valuable measurement,[4, 14, 41, 42, 44] breeding organizations have been reluctant to use such data owing to the potential bias caused by trimming (see Fig. 6–3A).

A different score used in the Netherlands is the claw diagonal (see Fig. 6–3D). This distance is easy to measure accurately. The measurement is highly repeatable, and the distance is heritable.[4, 42] As scored, it includes both claw angle and length of claws. Analyses of Dutch data show that the eye scores are adequately heritable for accurate sire evaluations. The heritability of claw diagonal based on actual measurements was the highest obtained for any measured claw trait.

Heel Height

One weakness in measuring heel height is that it is extremely difficult to measure accurately[26] (see Fig. 6–3C). Another is that the ratio between claw length and heel height is affected by measurement errors in both heel height and toe length rather than just one. Ral[41] found the ratio of toe length to heel height to be the least repeatable of all claw measurements taken. However, the ratio was the most highly correlated with a combined score for deformities plus diseases in his small sample of data.[41]

In a mature cow, the vertical distance between the skin-horn junction over the bulb and the bearing surface (heel height) ideally averages approximately 3.75 cm. The desired heel height is considered to be 3.8 cm. Workers in the United States[14] have reported a positive phenotypical correlation between heel height and high milk production in *first lactation*. Care should be taken in interpreting this observation. Mature cows may be low at the heel because of wear; others may have high heels because of overburdening. In either case, they may or may not be high producers. The state of the heel of mature cows (older than 5 years) is likely to be an *acquired* characteristic unrelated to the level of production. The genetic correlation of heel height to milk production was near zero according to Choi and McDaniel,[14] supporting this observation.

TABLE 6–1. A COMPOSITE OF RECENT HERITABILITY ESTIMATES BASED ON EYE SCORES

| | Heritabilities of Scored Claw and Leg Traits in Holsteins on a Single-Cow Basis | |
	North America	Britain
Claw angle	0.08 to 0.10	0.18
Rear leg, side view	0.12 to 0.16	0.15
Rear leg, rear view	0.08 to 0.10	0.12
Front leg toe out		0.10
Weak pasterns		0.31
Open toes		0.21
Corkscrew claw		0.07

From Brotherstone S, Hill WG: Dairy herd life in relation to linear type traits and production. 2. Genetic analyses for pedigree and non-pedigree cows. Anim Prod 53:289–297, 1991.

Heritabilities of Claw and Limb Traits

Measured values on an individual cow are not a reliable indicator of her genetic merit for the trait, but 0.10 is adequate to obtain a reliable estimate of the breeding value of a bull or cow with many offspring.

Heritabilities for hind limbs viewed from the rear are slightly lower than those for hind limbs viewed from the side (Table 6–1). The major contributor to low heritabilities for limb traits appears to be variation in the posture of a cow when she is scored. Scores or even actual measures of individual cows often show large changes after a cow moves a few steps.[47] Accuracy of categorizing an individual cow can be improved by scoring her multiple times and averaging the scores. These results emphasize the worth of using breeding values from a progeny test of bulls with little emphasis on scores of individual cows when selecting to improve locomotion traits.

The low heritabilities of claw and limb scores of individual cows listed in Table 6–1 illustrate the low accuracy of selection of individual cows based on only a single score. To be successful in making genetic improvement, selection should be based as far as possible on progeny tests of 50 or more daughters.

Relative selection accuracies of individual and progeny tests for different heritabilities are listed in Table 6–2. Values show that accurate breeding values

of bulls for low-heritability traits are possible when adequate numbers of progeny are available. The general rule is that six progeny are needed to equal the accuracy of individual selection for the same trait and heritability.

Practically all scoring for conformation of claw and leg traits is based only on the pelvic limb. Characteristics of front legs and claws are generally ignored because variation in them is not considered to be a cause of many locomotor disorders; however, genetic variation in front claws seems as large as that in back claws.[4, 26] Traits of front legs were also more heritable than those of rear legs in one study.[4] This study also showed that four of the six front leg or claw traits were more heritable than their rear counterpart. Their scores, when added to those for rear claws, might make it easier to recognize genetic differences among individual cows.

If and when it is important to have more accurate breeding values for claw traits of an individual cow, the values may be obtained by combining her values with those for her sire. Actually, data from other related animals also contribute to more accurate breeding values. Use of an animal model that includes the genetic relationships among all animals evaluated provides more reliable genetic values for individual females as well as bulls. Even with the extra information provided by relatives, the reliability of the claw and limb information is of limited value in predicting what a cow will transmit to her offspring.

Relationship of Linear Traits to Foot Problems and Survival

Progeny tests of bulls for conformation of feet and legs of their daughters have been associated with longevity of daughters in both North America and Europe. This was especially true when claws and legs were scored independently. Correlations of genetic values of sires for claw angles have been more closely related to survival than those of leg traits. Results are summarized in Table 6–3.

Breeding values, which are unbiased measures of a bull's true genetic value, should be the selection criteria rather than the actual progeny averages so often used. It is imperative that genetic values for

TABLE 6–2. ACCURACIES OF BREEDING VALUES FOR INDIVIDUALS AND PROGENY TESTS AT DIFFERENT HERITABILITIES

| Heritability | Record on Cow | Number of Progeny | | | | |
		10	20	50	100	200
0.05	0.22	0.33	0.45	0.62	0.75	0.85
0.10	0.31	0.45	0.58	0.75	0.85	0.91
0.20	0.44	0.59	0.71	0.85	0.91	0.95
0.30	0.54	0.67	0.78	0.90	0.94	0.97

TABLE 6–3. SUMMARY OF ASSOCIATIONS OF SCORES OF LOCOMOTION TRAITS AND SURVIVAL

Trait	Relation to Survival
Foot or claw angle	Higher angles, longer survival
Rear leg, side view	Mildly straight leg, longer survival
Rear leg, rear view	Straighter from rear, longer survival

claw and limb traits be computed as accurately as possible on bulls for effective genetic improvement.

Most studies of the relationship of foot and limb linear scores to survival were in the desirable direction.[9, 10, 15, 20, 43] All studies showed that higher claw angles (>45°) were positively correlated with increased survival (see Table 6–3). This was especially true when milk was included as a covariate to remove the effects of early culling of low-yielding first-lactation cows.

Much of the value of claw angle seems to be differences in survival of cows with extremely high or low claw angles. There is little difference in the longevity of cows with claws scored for 11 through 33 on a 50-point scale, but those with scores of 34 to 50 lived 162 days longer. Conversely, cows with low scores of 1 to 10 lived 54 days less than those with intermediate scores.

Legs were less correlated with longevity than claw angle in most studies. In these same studies, sire evaluations of bulls transmitting straighter limbs from the rear view (less hocking in) were positively associated with higher survival rates. Values indicated that limbs straighter from the side (higher hock angles), considered optimum by the various agencies doing the scoring, were associated with longer lives. In most studies, the degrees of straightness that predicted the longest lives still were limbs with considerable set (straightness) to the hock. Generally, scores of rear limbs (rear view) have been more highly correlated with survival than those of rear legs (side).

The regression of herd life on claw angle is higher in tie stalls than in free stalls or loose housing. Also, the association of claw angle and herd life is lower in herds with claws that are never trimmed than those routinely trimmed. Perhaps in herds in which claws are never trimmed, the environment does not stress claws as much as do tie stalls. Effects on limbs do not differ except in loose housing, where they had only half as much impact as in free or tie stalls. Time on concrete, bedding type, heifer housing, amount of exercise, or use of footbaths does not affect the relationships.

Breeding values for claw traits scored in first lactation have generally been negatively correlated with those for milk production.[10] Actual measurements have shown similar trends.[14, 42] These results mean that positive selection pressure must be placed on claw traits, or they will deteriorate when selection is based on milk or protein yields.[17]

Studies of relationships of measured claw traits and survival have given similar results even though they were based on much smaller samples of data. The genetic correlation of average claw angle and last age was 0.87 in one study,[14] with smaller differences detected in another.[42] In both investigations, first-lactation cows with shorter claws lived longer.

Genetic Basis of Claw Disorders

Inappropriate genetic selection—namely, selection that relies on criteria that have no rational basis—can lead to an increased incidence of characteristics with negative health implications (properly referred to as *sublethal traits*).

Several claw disorders seem to have a partially genetic basis. The heritability of laminitis was reported to vary from 0.14[28] to 0.22.[42] The estimates for the heritability of erosion of heel horn have been consistent, 0.13[28] and 0.15.[4] Values for interdigital dermatitis have been variable: 0.04,[28] 0.09,[42] 0.13[4] and 0.27.[40] Only single estimates of 0.21 for sole contusion and 0.31 for hyperplasia interdigitalis are available.[4] The heritability of sole ulcer has varied from 0.03 to 0.39, depending on the method of scoring and the stage of lactation. The heritability for white line separation has varied from 0.08[28] to 0.17.[4]

Genetic correlations between claw measurements and claw disorders have been moderate. As angle of the dorsal wall (foot angle) increased, laminitis, dermatitis digitalis, and sole contusion decreased. These values suggest that selection for higher claw angles should decrease the frequency of these disorders. Correlations of claw angle with heel horn erosion and hyperplasia interdigitalis were low but positive (see Distl and colleagues[17] for individual references).

Several workers[1, 3, 21] have reported that animals with straight hocks are susceptible to arthritis. Serous tarsitis (bog spavin) is observed in cattle with straight hind limb conformation and is considered to be heritable. Straight hocks may also predispose an animal to spastic paresis.

Claw Color

White skin above the coronary band (white socks), which is a trait preferred by breeders of Holstein cattle and required for registration in the herd book, is usually associated with light-colored claw horn. Almost all registered Holsteins now have white claws. White horn may be softer than dark-colored horn and more prone to damage.[13, 16] Dark-pigmented (melanin) horn is about 30% harder than white horn. This provides a good example of fashion conflicting with considerations of health.

Growth

Paul R. Greenough

WEIGHT GAIN AND FEEDING INTENSITY

Dairy advisors commonly recommend that producers should aim to calve dairy heifers for the first time at 24 months of age or younger. It has been demonstrated that first calving at more than 25 months of age decreases productive life.[46]

The average daily weight gain usually recommended for dairy heifers between the ages of 3 and 20 months is 650 grams. It has been demonstrated[23] that heifers gaining weight at more than 800 grams/day are likely to have sole hemorrhages, a sign that is characteristic of early laminitis. Although accelerated growth rates can be achieved through feeding, it is not without risk. It is unwise to establish policies for calving dairy heifers before 25 months if the standards include some specific criteria for weight or height at the withers.

Research with beef steers[24] has demonstrated conclusively that serious damage to the claws occurs in calves that are fed intensively when they are younger than 13 months. Similar changes were not observed in older animals subjected to the same treatment. Danish workers[37] found that feeding dairy heifers high levels of dietary carbohydrates leads to a higher incidence of laminitis and that most overfed heifers did not achieve their full milking potential.

EFFECT OF CLAW OVERGROWTH ON GAIT AND POSTURE

Beef cattle with high daily weight gains produce sole horn at rates up to 2.5 times greater than normal. The presence of overgrown claws in young bulls may be used to justify culling. Sole horn is also produced more rapidly in very cold weather because the blood flow through the claw is increased to keep the tissues warm. In other words, it may not be wise to cull *young cattle* only because they have overgrown claws. With older cattle, the situation may be quite different. Workers in Colorado[8] have shown that certain lines of older beef bulls do transmit a predisposition to claw overgrowth.

Congenital Defects of the Musculoskeletal System

Horst W. Leipold

Congenital defects, defined as abnormalities of structure or function, are encountered with great frequency in cattle and cause locomotion problems. Many are due to single or multiple genes. The skeletal system may be affected in its entirety or with single isolated defects.[34–36]

GENERALIZED SKELETAL DEFECTS

Four conditions are of concern here: dwarfism, osteopetrosis, chondrodysplasia, and arachnomelia.

Dwarfism

Dwarfism, a generalized skeletal disorder affecting many beef breeds, is due to homozygosity of a single recessive gene. A discussion of the various types of dwarfism and their genetic relationship is beyond the scope of a book on lameness in cattle. Dwarfism was once a big problem in the American beef-breeding industry, but few dwarfs are encountered today. Dwarfism needs to be carefully distinguished from cases of intrauterine growth retardation and other environmentally caused conditions.[34] Dwarfism affects mainly Dexter, German, Shorthorn, Friesian, Angus, and Hereford cattle and at one time contributed 12.6% of all skeletal defects reported in the United States and 1.4% of all congenital defects reported in the United Kingdom during a 2-year period. Dwarfism is characterized by small stature, a prominent frontal bone, brachycephaly, small and short limbs, and a large abdomen (Fig. 6–8).

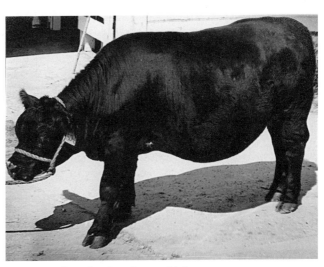

Figure 6–8. Dwarfism in a 2-year-old Angus.

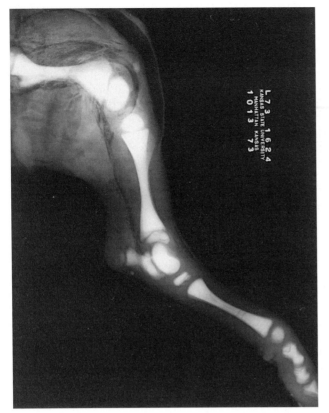

Figure 6–9. Radiograph of the left hind leg of an Angus calf with osteopetrosis.

Osteopetrosis

Osteopetrosis is a generalized skeletal problem in Angus cattle. It is due to homozygosity of a simple autosomal recessive gene. It is characterized grossly by lack of bone remodeling and therefore persistence of chondro-osseous tissue throughout bones where bone marrow cavities should have developed.[7] In addition, brachygnathia and impaction of molar teeth occur. Figure 6–9 depicts a radiograph of a typical case of osteopetrosis, showing solid bone within bone. Calves are born dead prematurely around 260 days of gestation. They are easily recognizable by their external features such as a short lower jaw. Long bones are fractured easily on pressure.

Chondrodysplasia

Chondrodysplasia is a generalized skeletal problem that is characterized by disturbance of the conversion of the cartilage model to bone. It is encountered in various breeds of dairy and beef cattle. In many cases, afflicted calves are aborted late in gestation. Chondrodysplasia is a genetic defect.[34]

Arachnomelia

Arachnomelia is due to homozygosity of a simple autosomal recessive gene and has occurred in Sim-

mental and Brown Swiss calves. The calves have long, thin, slender legs and bones that fracture easily. The muscles are smaller than normal. Associated defects are a short lower jaw and kyphoscoliosis.[32, 33] Preterminal cesarean section is used to test bulls for heterozygosity of arachnomelia.[32]

REGIONAL SKELETAL DEFECTS

Various facial defects that occur are of no concern here. A few defects of the axial skeleton may cause locomotion problems, such as kyphoscoliotic deformities of the thoracolumbar area in calves. Some of these kyphoscoliotic deformities may be severe and cause lateral recumbency of a calf. Little is known about the etiology of these axial skeletal defects.[34]

Another axial defect of more frequent occurrence is atlanto-occipital fusion in Holstein, Charolais, and polled Hereford calves. It is suspected to be of genetic origin. Calves affected with atlanto-occipital fusion may be recumbent at birth or may develop gait changes or become recumbent after minor trauma late in life.[18]

APPENDICULAR SKELETAL DEFECTS

Adactyly

Adactyly is defined as absence of all or part of a digital structure including the hoof. Affected calves lack development of one or more toes (Figs. 6–10 and 6–11). The condition is not very common but is of genetic cause.

Tibial Hemimelia

Hemimelia is characterized by bilateral agenesis or hypoplasia of the tibias (Fig. 6–12). It is due to homozygosity of a simple autosomal recessive gene and occurs most frequently in Galloway calves. Associated defects in Galloway calves are non-union of the

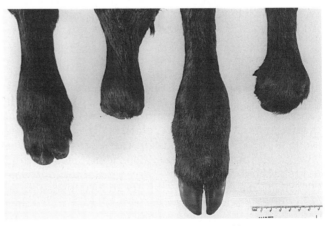

Figure 6–10. Adactyly in a neonatal Brangus calf.

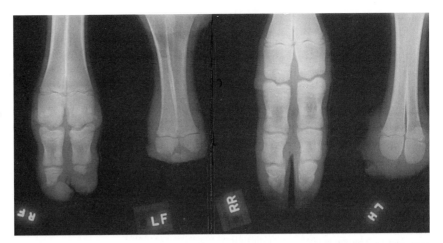

Figure 6–11. Radiograph of the feet of the calf shown in Figure 6–10. Note the variable degree of expressivity of adactyly.

pelvic symphysis, meningocele, and cryptorchidism or non-union of the müllerian ducts. Afflicted calves are unable to rise. Tibial hemimelia of presumably genetic origin also occurs in other breeds.[34]

Polymelia

Duplication of a whole limb, or polymelia, may involve one or more legs. The cause is unknown. In heterotopic polymelia, one or two additional legs are attached to various body regions.

Abrachia and Apodia

Reduction of the number of extremities is uncommon and is of unknown cause in cattle. It severely interferes with locomotion of afflicted calves, which usually have to be destroyed. *Abrachia* is agenesis of both front legs, and *apodia* designates the same process involving hind legs. *Monobrachia* and *monopodia* are used to characterize a calf with lack of development of one front or hind leg (Fig. 6–13).

Polydactyly

Polydactyly is an increased number of digits. It is seen in various breeds of cattle and is of genetic origin. Most commonly, both front feet are afflicted with polydactyly. The second digit is developed and frequently fused to the third digit. With advancing weight and age (usually by 6 months of age), cattle with polydactyly develop marked lameness. Figures 6–14 and 6–15 depict external appearance and radiographic features. It is a genetic condition in Simmental cattle and other breeds and requires a dominant gene at one locus and recessive genes at another locus.[30]

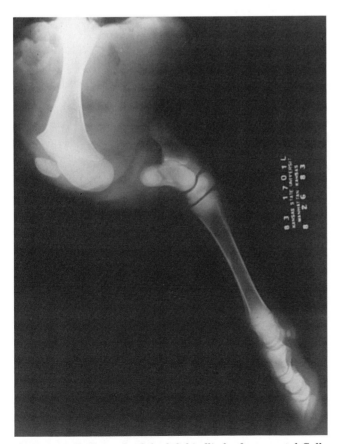

Figure 6–12. Radiograph of the left hindlimb of a neonatal Galloway calf with tibial hemimelia.

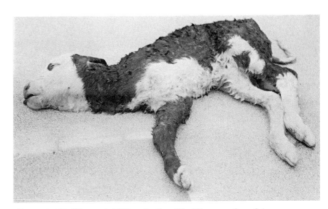

Figure 6–13. Neonatal Hereford calf with monobrachia.

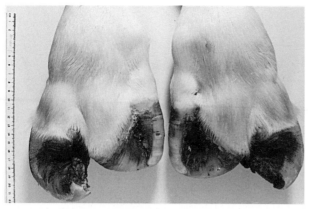

Figure 6–14. Polydactyly of both forelimbs in a Simmental heifer. Note the development of the second digits.

Syndactyly

Syndactyly is fusion or non-division of functional digits. It is due to homozygosity of a simple autosomal recessive gene with complete penetrance, various degrees of expressivity, and pleiotropic effect. It is the single most important defect in Holstein cattle. The various degrees of expressivity mean that the right front foot is most commonly afflicted, followed by the left front foot, then the right hind, but rarely are all

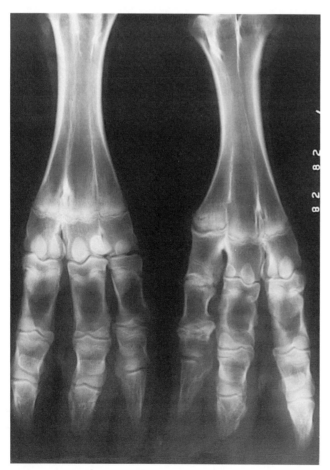

Figure 6–15. Radiograph of forelimbs affected with polydactyly.

four feet involved (Fig. 6–16). If two front feet are affected, the right one has more advanced degrees of synostosis than the left, but the front feet show the same condition as the hind feet. An occasional calf that has a syndactylous genotype escapes affliction and has externally normal feet (incomplete penetrance). *Pleiotropic effect* refers to the extreme susceptibility of syndactylous Holstein cattle to succumb to environmental temperature stress.

Syndactylous Holstein cattle are severely handicapped and have locomotion problems. With more feet afflicted and more advanced degrees of fusion, calves are unable to move about effectively. With advancing weight and age, syndactylous cattle also develop degenerative arthritis in the phalangeal joints. The single most important aspect of the diagnosis of syndactyly is verification of the defect supported by radiographs and parentage verification by blood typing if changes in breeding programs are involved.

Syndactyly has also occurred in Chianina, Charolais, Hereford, Angus, Simmental, and other breeds.

In our experience, the defect has been much more severe in beef breeds and usually involves all four feet. Syndactylous beef calves are severely lame. In cases associated with contractures of the feet, calves may be unable to get up. Syndactyly can be diagnosed easily in 60-day-old fetuses. Superovulation of syndactylous cows, embryo transfer, and early gestation cesarean sections have been used to test bulls or cows for the presence or absence of this gene.

Monodactyly

Monodactyly looks confusingly similar externally to syndactyly. At least one foot has a single claw. However, radiographs reliably establish a diagnosis by the agenesis of a digital structure (Figs. 6–17 and 6–18). Furthermore, monodactyly does not have an expressivity pattern and may afflict any foot at random. It is of unknown cause.[34]

Congenital Defects of the Joints

Congenital defects of the joints may afflict a single or several joints or may be generalized.

OSTEOARTHRITIS OF THE STIFLE
Osteoarthritis of the stifle has been reported as a simple autosomal recessive trait in Jersey and Holstein cattle.

HIP DYSPLASIA
Hip dysplasia (see p. 173) appears to be a genetic problem in various beef breeds, particularly Hereford and Charolais cattle. Degenerative hip joint disease has been reported in Hereford and Charolais but may occur in other breeds.[12] Marked lameness is present, cattle taking short steps and being reluctant to walk. They have difficulties in rising and eventually may

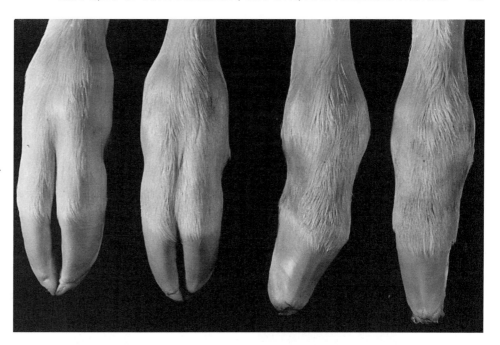

Figure 6–16. Syndactyly in a neonatal Holstein calf. Note syndactyly of both forelimbs and partial syndactyly of the right rear foot.

be recumbent. Crepitus of the hip joints occurs. Muscles of the hind legs may undergo atrophy. A genetic cause has been postulated.

GENERALIZED JOINT DEFECTS

A generalized condition afflicting all major joints of the body has been reported in the offspring of one Angus bull. Affected calves were born in various states and at different seasons. The only common link was the sire.

Soon after birth, the Angus calves developed lameness and had swollen joints. The joint degeneration progressed within a few weeks to recumbency. Necropsy examination revealed degeneration of all major joints. In addition, the head was characterized by facial dysplasia.[29] We have encountered similar cases in the offspring of one Limousin bull.

MUSCULAR SYSTEM DEFECTS

Congenital muscular defects are common in cattle, and some traits are of considerable economic significance.[34]

Congenital Flexure of the Pastern

Congenital flexure of the pastern has been reported in Jersey cattle as a simple autosomal recessive trait. It also occurs in other breeds. Calves usually are affected bilaterally and knuckle over in the front pasterns. The hind legs may occasionally be affected. The trait is reversible, and calves usually become normal within 2 to 8 weeks of birth. Splinting of affected legs is sometimes performed, and surgery is occasionally performed to alleviate this problem.

Arthrogryposis

Arthrogryposis occurs worldwide. It is characterized by permanent joint contracture of multiple joints and is present at birth. It has known causes but frequently is of unknown cause.[34] It is one of a heterogenous group of defects that have in common limita-

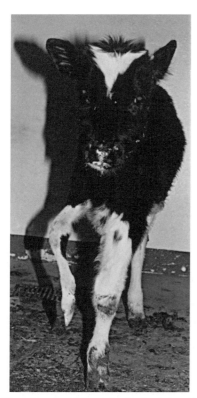

Figure 6–17. Monodactyly of the right forelimb in a Holstein calf.

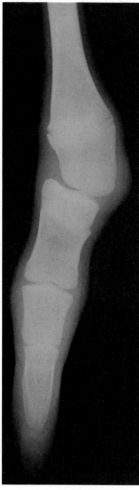

Figure 6–18. Radiograph of a monodactylous claw.

tions of joint movement. Associated skeletal defects such as cleft palate, axial deformities such as kyphosis and scoliosis, and their combinations may also occur. In those of viral etiology, such as Akabane or bluetongue infection *in utero*, arthrogryposis is combined with severe central nervous system defects such as hydranencephaly. Arthrogryposis caused by ingestion of lupine between days 40 and 70 of gestation is characterized by non-symmetrical multiple joint contractures. Cleft palate may be present and of variable severity. Axial skeletal defects are also present.

Arthrogryposis in Charolais cattle is inherited and due to homozygosity of a simple autosomal recessive gene. It has several characteristic features.[38] Calves are usually recumbent, and if they are aided to stand, locomotion is severely restricted by bilateral symmetrical joint contractures involving major joints of all four legs. Rarely is involvement confined to front or hind legs only. In addition, most Charolais calves afflicted with this genetic syndrome have a bilateral complete cleft palate. Furthermore, both patellas are hypoplastic and consist entirely of cartilage. This feature can be readily demonstrated by a lateral radiograph or by necropsy examination. Some calves

have hypermobile fetlock joints, a feature typical of this syndrome.

Many more genetic types of arthrogryposis exist in cattle and await careful description of their pathology and etiology.

Muscular Hypertrophy

Many different names have been applied to genetic muscular hypertrophy, such as double muscling, muscular hyperplasia, and Doppellender. Most major beef breeds seem to have this trait as a simple autosomal recessive.[2]

Stance and external appearance of these cattle are abnormal. Difficulty in locomotion may occur, particularly if secondary problems of joint and bone pathology are induced.

Muscular hypertrophy varies widely, and few calves have all features typical of it. The hindquarters usually have a round outline (hamlike), and the muscles are separated by deep grooves. The tail is attached higher or more cranially. The muscles of the neck are separated by deep septa. The neck appears wider and shorter, and the head smaller and lighter. The limb bones appear slender and shorter than normal. In addition, macroglossia may be present. Furthermore, infantile impaired reproductive delay of sexual maturity and high birth weight and dystocia may occur.

Limber Leg

Limber leg in Jersey calves is characterized by lateral recumbency, and calves are unable to rise after birth. They lack control of their legs, which may be moved passively with ease. It is a simple autosomal recessive trait.

RECOMMENDATIONS FOR GENETIC SELECTION[22]

1 Make a thorough routine evaluation of the pelvic limb of any animal intended for breeding at 22 to 26 months of age. Record the following parameters:

   • Angle of the hock

   • Legs rear

   • Toe angle

   • Claw diagonal

   • Claw shape/balance

2 Consider the following to be heritable unsoundness:

   • Serous tarsitis (bog spavin)

   • Corkscrew claw

- Interdigital skin hyperplasia (fibroma) in beef cattle
- Obvious imbalance of the convexity of the axial surface of the medial claw of the thoracic limb versus that of the lateral claw
- Obvious imbalance of the convexity of the axial surface of the lateral claw of the pelvic limb versus that of the medial claw
- Imbalance (worse than 3:2) of the relative width of any two claws

3 Select in favor of

- Hock angles between 155° and 160°
- Dark or black claw horn
- Toe height to heel height ratio 2:1 at 24 months
- Toe angle (pelvic limb) greater than 45°

4 Do not cull animals for the following reasons:

- Normally overgrown claws in young (<20 months) animals
- Interdigital skin hyperplasia (fibroma) in Holsteins/Friesians

5 Make recommendations to avoid reoccurrence of genetic conditions causing locomotion problems

- Document defect and parentage verification by blood typing or DNA studies
- Note that most conditions are due to homozygosity of a simple autosomal recessive gene

6 Select for claw angles greater than 45°

REFERENCES

1. Amstutz HE: Prevention and control of lameness in dairy cattle. Vet Clin North Am Food Anim Pract 1:25–37, 1985.
2. Arthur PF, Makarechian M, Price MA: Incidence of dystocia and perinatal calf mortality resulting from reciprocal crossing of double-muscled and normal cattle. Can Vet J 29:163–167, 1988.
3. Bailey JV: Bovine arthritides; classification, diagnosis, prognosis and treatment. Vet Clin North Am Food Anim Pract 1:39–51, 1985.
4. Baumgartner C, Distl O: Correlation between sires and daughters and selection for improved structural claw soundness. Proceedings of the 6th International Symposium on the Diseases of the Ruminant Digit. Liverpool, UK, 1990, pp 199–218.
5. Berg JN, Butterfield RM: New concepts of cattle growth. New York, John Wiley & Sons, 1976.
6. Bonsma JC: Factors Affecting Calf Crop (Cunha, TJ, Warwick AC, Koger AC, eds.) Gainesville, FL, University of Florida Press, 1973, pp 197–231.
7. Brem G, Wanke R, Hondele J: Zum Auftreten des Arachnomelie-Syndroms in der Brown-Swiss x Braunvieh Population Bayerns. Berl Muench Tieraerztl Wochenschr 97:393–397, 1984.
8. Brinks J: Hoof health is inherited. Cattleman September:86–88, 1984.
9. Brotherstone S, Hill WG: Dairy herd life in relation to linear type traits and production. 1. Phenotypic and genetic analyses for pedigree type classified herds. Anim Prod 53:279–287, 1991.
10. Brotherstone S, Hill WG: Dairy herd life in relation to linear type traits and production. 2. Genetic analyses for pedigree and non-pedigree cows. Anim Prod 53:289–297, 1991.
11. Brotherstone S, McManus CM, Hill WG: Estimation of genetic parameters for linear and miscellaneous type traits in Holstein-Friesian dairy cattle. Livest Prod Sci 26:177–192, 1990.
12. Carroll AG: Degenerative joint disease of the hip joint in Hereford bullocks. Aust Vet J 60:316, 1983.
13. Chesterton RN, Pfeiffer DU, Morris RS, Tanner CM: Environment and behavioural factors affecting the prevalence of foot lameness. N Z Vet J 37:135–142, 1989.
14. Choi YS, McDaniel BT: Heritabilities of measures of hooves and their relation to other traits of Holsteins. J Dairy Sci 76:1989–1993, 1993.
15. Dekkers JCM, Jairath LK, Lawrence BH: Relationships between sire genetic evaluations for comformation and functional herd life of daughters. J Dairy Sci 77:844–854, 1994.
16. Dietz O, Prietz G: Klauenhornqualität—Klauenhornstatus. Berl Muench Tieraerztl Wochenschr 36:419–422, 1981.
17. Distl O, Koorn DS, McDaniel BT, et al: Claw traits in cattle breeding programs: Report of the EAAP working group "claw quality in cattle." Livest Prod Sci 25:1–13, 1990.
18. Engleken TJ, Leipold HW, Spire MF, Cash WC: Atlanto-occipital fusion in two polled Hereford calves. J Vet Med Ser A 39:236–238, 1992.
19. Fisher AV, Harries JM, Robinson JM: Sensory assessment of fatness and conformation of beef steers. Meat Sci 5:283–295, 1980–81.
20. Foster WW, Freeman AE, Berger PJ, Kuck A: Association of type trait scored linearly with production and herdlife in holsteins. J Dairy Sci 72:2651–2664, 1989.
21. Greenough PR: A review: The conformation of cattle. Bovine Pract 1:20–34, 1980.
22. Greenough PR: A review of factors predisposing to lameness in cattle. *In* Owen JB, Axford RFE (eds): Breeding for Disease Resistance in Farm Animals. Wallingford, UK, C.A.B. International, 1991, pp 371–393.
23. Greenough PR, Vermunt JJ: Evaluation of subclinical laminitis in a dairy herd and observations on associated nutritional and management factors. Vet Rec 128:11–17, 1991.
24. Greenough PR, Vermunt JJ, McKinnon JJ, et al: Laminitis-like changes in the claws of feedlot cattle. Can Vet J 31:202–208, 1990.
25. Habel RE: On the inheritance of metatarsal inclination in Ayrshire cattle. Am J Vet Res 3:131–139, 1984.
26. Hahn MV, McDaniel BT, Wilk JC: Description and evaluation of objective hoof measurements of dairy cattle. J Dairy Sci 67:229–236, 1984.
27. Hand RK, Gould SR, Basarab JA, Engstrom DF: Condition score, body weight and hip height as predictors of gain in various breed crosses of yearling steers on pasture. Can J Anim Sci 63:447–452, 1986.
28. Huang Y, Shanks R: Within herd estimates of heritabilities of hoof characteristics (abstract). J Dairy Sci 76(Suppl 1):148, 1993.
29. Jayo MJ, Leipold HW, Dennis SM: Brachygnathia superior and degenerative joint disease: A new lethal syndrome in Angus calves. Vet Pathol 24:148–155, 1987.
30. Johnson JL, Leipold HW, Schalles RR: Hereditary polydactyly in Simmental cattle. J Hered 72:205–208, 1981.
31. Kempster AJ, Cuthbertson A, Harrington G: The relationship between conformation and the yield and distribution of lean meat in the carcasses of British pigs, cattle, and sheep: A review. Meat Sci 6:37–53, 1982.
32. König H, Gaillard C, Chavaz J: Prufung von Schweizer Braunvieh-Bullen auf das vererbte Syndrom der Arachnomelie und Arthrogrypose (SAA) durch Untersuchung der Nachkommen im Fetalstadium. Tieraerztl Umsch 42:692–697, 1987.
33. Leipold HW, Dennis SM, Schalles R: Osteopetrosis in cattle. Bovine Pract 21:96–101, 1986.
34. Leipold HW, Hiraga T, Dennis SM: Congenital defects of the bovine musculoskeletal system and joints. Vet Clin North Am Food Anim Pract 9:93–104, 1993.
35. Leipold HW, Huston K, Dennis SM: Bovine congenital defects. Adv Vet Sci Comp Med 27:197–271, 1983.

36. Leipold HW, Woollen N, Saperstein G: Congenital defects in ruminants. *In* Smith B (ed): Large Animal Internal Medicine. St Louis, CV Mosby, 1990, pp 1544–1566.
37. Mortensen K, Hesselholt M, Basse A: Pathogenesis of bovine laminitis (diffuse aseptic pododermatitis): Experimental models. Proceedings of the 14th World Congress on Diseases of Cattle. Dublin, Ireland, 1986, pp 1025–1030.
38. Nawrot PS, Howell WE, Leipold HW: Arthrogryposis: An inherited defect in newborn calves. Aust Vet J 56:359–364, 1980.
39. Nomina Anatomica Veterinaria, 4th ed. International Committee on Veterinary Gross Anatomical Nomenclature. NAV, World Association of Veterinary Anatomists, Ithaca, NY, 1994.
40. Petersen PH, Van Vuuren AS, Buchwald E, Thysen I: Genetic studies on hoof characters in dairy cows. Z Tierz Zuechtungsbiol 99:286–291, 1982.
41. Ral G: Hoof and leg traits in dairy cattle. Proceedings of the 6th International Symposium on Diseases of the Ruminant Digit. Liverpool, UK, 1990, pp 219–231.
42. Reurink A, Arendonk J: Relationships of claw disorders and claw measurements with efficiency of production in dairy cattle. Proceedings of the 38th Annual Meeting of the European Association for Animal Production, Lisbon, Portugal, 1987.
43. Rogers GW, McDaniel BT, Dentine MR, Funk DA: Genetic correlations between survival and linear type traits measured in first lactation. J Dairy Sci 72:523–527, 1989.
44. Smit H, Verbeek B, Peterse DJ, et al: The effect of herd characteristics on claw disorders and claw measurements in Friesians. Livest Prod Sci 15:1–9, 1986.
45. Swanepoel FJC, Heyns H: The relationship between body measurements and growth test results of Simmentaler bulls. South Afr J Anim Sci 16:31–35, 1986.
46. Tabbaa MJ, McDaniel BT: Factors affecting length of production life of Holsteins in the southeastern United States. American Dairy Science and Northeast ADSA and ASAS meeting. Abstract pp 46 and 162, 1993.
47. Te Plate HAM, McDaniel BT: Description and evaluation of measuring rear legs side and rear view using photogrammetry in Holstein Friesians (manuscript). Raleigh, NC, Department of Animal Science, North Carolina State University, 1990.

Conditions Affecting the Distal Region

7

Infectious Diseases of the Digits

INTRODUCTION

Several major systemic diseases can be associated with digital lesions potentially leading, as a result of localized pain, to stiffness and lameness. They include foot-and-mouth disease (FMD), mucosal disease/bovine virus diarrhea (MD/BVD) complex, bovine malignant catarrh, salmonellosis, vesicular stomatitis, and bluetongue. The initial signs at presentation may include lameness, which may be overshadowed by other features. It is therefore wise on every farm visit to cases of bovine lameness, and especially in group problems, first to eliminate the possibility of a systemic infectious disease. The scope of the symptomatology and appropriate control measures in these conditions, which may develop into major outbreaks of massive economic importance, is quite outside the scope of this text. Table 7–1 very briefly summarizes some clinical features of six such systemic conditions.

This chapter is otherwise devoted to major specific infections of the digits: interdigital phlegmon (foot rot), interdigital dermatitis (ID), and digital dermatitis (DD).

INTERDIGITAL PHLEGMON (FOOT ROT)

DEFINITION

Interdigital phlegmon (phlegmona interdigitalis, foot rot, foul in the foot) is a subacute or acute necrotic infection originating from a lesion in the interdigital skin. Pain, pyrexia, and partial anorexia leading to mild or severe lameness are major signs of the disease. Meat and milk production is affected. The anaerobic bacterium *Fusobacterium necrophorum* can often be isolated from the lesion, which produces a characteristic foul odor. The infection spreads rapidly into the soft tissues. Complications can result in septic digital arthritis and tendovaginitis.[4, 20]

INCIDENCE

Interdigital phlegmon has a worldwide distribution, is usually sporadic, but may be endemic in high-intensity beef or dairy cattle production units. Epizootics sometimes occur when animals are moved, mixed together, or exposed to new environments.[12, 15] The incidence varies depending on climate, weather, season of the year, grazing periods, housing system, breed, and age. In British,[36] French,[21] and Australian[28] surveys, interdigital phlegmon was the most common separate lesion in lame cows treated by practicing veterinary surgeons. It accounted for about 15% of claw diseases, although there was a great variation among veterinary practices.

In temperate areas, interdigital phlegmon is encountered in animals grazed all year as well as in animals pastured seasonally or kept indoors. Phlegmon is most common in wet weather or under conditions with high soil moisture, which often occur during the autumn months,[3, 29, 46] but an increased incidence has also been observed on extremely dry pastures. In pasture-fed dairy cows, interdigital phlegmon was the third most common lesion.[24]

In stanchion stalls, the interdigital skin generally stays drier than in loose housing systems. In loose housing, the risk of an outbreak is also higher because of more frequent contacts between animals. Interdigital phlegmon in beef cattle is found to be more frequent in straw yards than in systems with slatted floors.[31, 41] The Jersey breed seems to be less susceptible than other breeds.[28] Calves seem to be more resistant during the first months of life owing to maternal immunity.[18] The incidence in older cows is decreased.[24]

Regular foot trimming decreases the frequency, although the majority of animals treated for interdigital phlegmon have a normal claw shape.

LITERATURE

Years after agreement on recommended nomenclature of digital diseases, different designations of the same disease still exist in papers and textbooks, causing confusion. Interdigital phlegmon is probably the disease with the most synonyms in literature: infectious pododermatitis, interdigital necrobacillosis, foot abscess, foot rot, foul in the foot, panaritium,

TABLE 7–1. MAJOR SYSTEMIC INFECTIOUS DISEASES OF CATTLE IN WHICH LAMENESS MAY BE A PRESENTING SIGN

Disease	Incidence	Age	Etiology	Incubation Period	Signs Related to Lameness	Major signs	Diagnosis	Differential	Treatment Control
Foot-and-mouth (FMD)	Endemic in parts of Africa, Asia, Europe, South America. Not known in New Zealand, eradicated in 1929 in United States, 1953 in Canada	All ages	Aphthovirus of Picornaviridae	2–14 days	Vesicles on coronary band and interdigital space, rupturing after 2–3 days to leave shallow red granular eroded areas. Secondary bacterial infection delays healing. Sequelae, including chronic interdigital infection and hoof deformities ("thimbling")	Pyrexia, vesicles on tongue, hard palate, lips, muzzle, teats; loss of condition, lowered yield	Virus isolation. Antibody titers in non-vaccinated stock	Digital trauma, necrobacillosis, malignant catarrh, BVD/mucosal disease, vesicular stomatitis	National vaccination or slaughter control programs. Individual treatment rarely given as virus is extremely infectious and widespread dissemination easy
Mucosal disease BVD (BVD/MD)	Endemic subclinical infection in many countries of Europe and North America	Young cattle (1–18 months) develop mucosal disease; older animals, BVD	Pestivirus of Togaviridae	Very variable	Erythema of coronary band, shallow interdigital ulcers usually on several limbs, laminitic signs; chronic interdigital and coronary skin hyperplasia	Oral and nasal mucosal erosions, salivation, diarrhea, weight and condition loss	Virus isolation from blood, other tissue	FMD, Rinderpest	Eradication of viremic animals, possibly vaccination
Bovine malignant catarrh	Endemic in Africa, sporadic elsewhere	All ages	Herpes virus	3–8 weeks	Necrosis of skin-born junction at back of pastern, rarely sloughing of claw horn	Pyrexia, lymphadenopathy, widespread mucosal necrosis, various manifestations (e.g., "head and eye" and peracute forms)	Clinical signs and gross pathology	Rinderpest, BVD/MD	Isolation; slaughter, vaccination
Salmonellosis	Widespread	All ages	Various strains of Salmonella, e.g., Dublin	1–2 days	Occasionally dry gangrene of extremities from fetlock distally in calves (also tail, ears); more commonly in young calves polyarthritis (hock, carpus, stifle)	Septicemia, enteritis	Clinical signs, bacterial isolation	Colibacillosis in calfhood, fescue or ergot toxicity	Chemotherapy
Vesicular stomatitis	Sporadic North, Central, and South America	All ages	Vesiculovirus of Rhabdoviridae	2–4 days	Vesicles on coronary band, rupturing to leave ulcers, secondary infection	Vesicles on tongue, lips, gums, teats	Clinical signs, virus isolation	FMD	Vaccines in development and trial; general nursing
Bluetongue	Widespread, sporadic North America, South Africa, Israel, Portugal	Any age	Orbivirus of Reoviridae	Variable	Usually subclinical stiffness, coronary band erythema; skin sloughing as secondary sign in severe cases	Pyrexia, hyperemia of oral, nasal, and teat mucosae with eventual sloughing	Enzyme-linked immunosorbent assay, virus isolation	FMD, Rinderpest, BVD/MD, vesicular stomatitis	Specific serotype vaccination, elimination of Culicoides vector

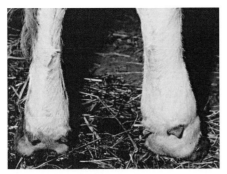

Figure 7–1. Interdigital phlegmon of the right hind foot, with swelling extending to the pastern and fetlock.

and others. Foot rot is often used when the diagnosis is unclear. Interdigital phlegmon has therefore probably been overdiagnosed. In detailed studies, interdigital phlegmon has been found to be a minor problem compared with other diseases of the hoof horn.[3, 43]

ETIOLOGY AND PATHOGENESIS

Local injury of the claw skin is a prerequisite for an infection. Traumatic lesions, caused by a stone, straw, stubble, piece of wood, and so on, are the most common causes. Uneven ground, extremely dry pastures, a rough floor, or slats can also cause lesions in the skin. Maceration of the skin by water, feces, and urine may predispose the claw to injuries. A systemic infection by microorganisms may cause skin lesions, as may local infections by *Dichelobacter (Bacteroides) nodosus*.

F. necrophorum, the predominant isolate in interdigital phlegmon, is an obligate anaerobic gram-negative bacterium. It is an opportunistic pathogen, hosted by cattle and sheep.[19] Three different strains of the bacterium have been identified. Isolates from interdigital phlegmon most often reveal biotypes A and AB. Biotype B, which is regarded as non-pathogenic, is the predominating biotype in the rumen and the gastrointestinal tract. Biotypes A and AB produce a potent endotoxin, as well as an exotoxin

with leukocidal and hemolytic properties, inducing necrotic cellulitis.[19] An infective dose of biotype A can be dramatically reduced when mixed with other bacteria, such as *Staphylococcus aureus, Escherichia coli, Actinomyces pyogenes*, and others.[37] In mixed infections, *F. necrophorum* seems to be able to act synergistically. Whether synergism occurs between *F. necrophorum* and *Bacteroides melaninogenicus* in the pathogenesis of interdigital phlegmon is questionable. In non-specific bovine foot infections, *F. necrophorum* and *A. pyogenes* have been shown to act synergistically, *A. pyogenes* being largely responsible for the suppurative reaction.[26] Moreover, in interdigital phlegmon, several saprophytic bacteria, which are thought capable of enhancing the inflammatory process, can often be isolated (i.e., species of *Spirochetes, Bacteroides, Staphylococcus, Streptococcus*, and *Bacillus*).

CLINICAL SIGNS

The infection can affect either the foredigits or, more commonly, the hind digits, but it is rare that more than one claw is affected at the same time in dairy cows.[3, 24, 28] However, the disease can occasionally occur in several claws in calves.

The first sign is swelling and erythema of the soft tissues of the interdigital space and the adjacent coronary band. The inflammation may extend to the pastern and fetlock (Fig. 7–1). The claws typically are markedly separated, and the inflammatory edema is uniformly distributed between the two digits (Figs. 7–2 and 7–3).

The onset of the disease is rapid, and the extreme pain leads to increasing lameness. The animal tries to avoid contact with the ground if the digital region

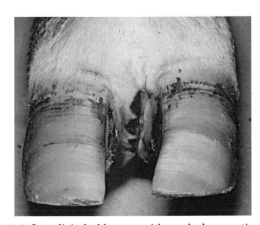

Figure 7–2. Interdigital phlegmon with marked separation of the digits.

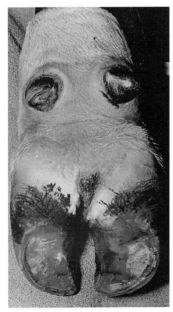

Figure 7–3. Uniformly distributed inflammatory edema (interdigital phlegmon).

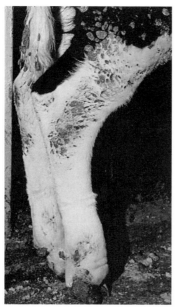

Figure 7–4. This animal avoids ground contact with the severely affected digits (interdigital phlegmon).

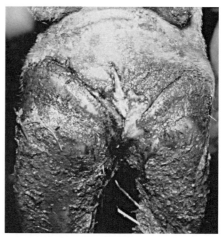

Figure 7–6. Fissures and necrosis of the skin around the bulb (interdigital phlegmon).

is severely affected (Fig. 7–4). The body temperature is raised, and the appetite is reduced. The process can originate from any part of the interdigital skin.

On close examination of the swollen interdigital space, the skin appears discolored, and fissures are observed later. Exudate is present, the tissues become necrotic, and sloughing of the skin is likely to follow (Figs. 7–5 and 7–6). Interdigital phlegmon is characterized by a foul odor.

If the disease proceeds unchecked, the affected animal suffers severe weight loss and has a significant reduction in milk yield. Milk production may not recover during that lactation. The open lesion can be infected with secondary invaders. Depending on circumstances, infection of the distal interphalangeal (DIP) joint can result (Fig. 7–7). Involvement of the navicular bursa, the flexor tendon sheath, the distal

ligaments, and the phalangeal bones may produce a retroarticular abscess. Osteomyelitis or infectious arthritis may result (see Chapter 11). Severe digital cellulitis occasionally leads to septicemia and toxemia.

In recent years, a peracute form, *super foul*, has become more common in the United Kingdom[7, 14, 48] (Fig. 7–8). In this more severe form of the disease, the symptoms are more extensive and the severe interdigital necrosis and ulceration may progress uncontrollably despite adequate therapy. *Blind foul* is interdigital phlegmon in which no skin lesion of the interdigital space is present initially, although typical lameness is evident.

DIAGNOSIS

When antibiotics are freely available, producers may routinely assume that any digital lameness is caused

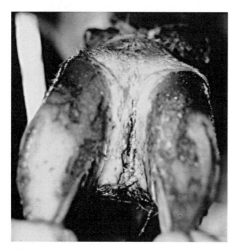

Figure 7–5. Necrosis of the interdigital tissue with sloughing of the skin (interdigital phlegmon).

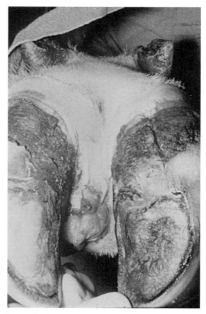

Figure 7–7. Granulation tissue associated with a joint fistula following a severe case of interdigital dermatitis.

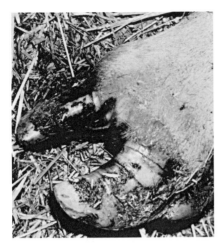

Figure 7–8. Super foul.

by interdigital phlegmon. Therefore, a careful examination is often not made, with the result that in a minority of cases the misdiagnosis results in serious consequences. For veterinarians, it is mandatory that they make a reliable clinical diagnosis and distinguish this condition from other diseases causing lameness. The claws and the interdigital skin have to be carefully examined after the region has been restrained and washed.

The characteristic clinical signs are as follows:

• Sudden lameness (most often in only one limb)

• Elevated body temperature

• Swelling of the digital region with claw separation

• Typical lesion of the interdigital skin

A bacteriological identification of *F. necrophorum* is rarely used to confirm the clinical diagnosis.

The lesion most consistently confused with interdigital phlegmon is a retroarticular abscess or septic arthritis in the DIP joint. The cause of these conditions is unrelated to interdigital phlegmon (Fig. 7–9). In this case, however, the clinical signs are confined to one claw, with inflammatory edema being the diagnostic feature. This phenomenon is most frequently a complication of a sole ulcer, sole abscess, white line disease, or a vertical fissure. The presence of an interdigital foreign body produces a clinical picture very similar to that of interdigital phlegmon.

Advanced cases of digital dermatitis or interdigital dermatitis (ID) can produce a comparable clinical picture. However, close careful examination of the interdigital space permits an accurate diagnosis.

TREATMENT

Most treated animals recover in a few days.[43] Spontaneous recovery or recovery after only local treatment with disinfectants or antibiotics may occur in mild cases but is rare. *F. necrophorum* and most other bacteria usually isolated from the process are sensitive to most antibiotics and sulfonamides (see Chapter 5).

Good results are obtained with systemic treatment with penicillin G intramuscularly for 3 days. It is particularly important that the treatment be administered as soon as signs are observed. It should be noted, however, that the label dose may be inadequate to bring about a rapid resolution on some farms. Veterinarians are therefore advised to use discretion in substantially increasing the dose. Clients must be advised about the increased withdrawal times. The treatment of super foul has to be particularly aggressive. Early cases responded well to single doses of long-acting oxytetracycline. More advanced cases recovered after tylosin administered parenterally for 4 days and chlortetracycline and clindamycin ointment applied topically to the debrided interdigital lesion.

Sodium sulfadimidine solution intravenously[4] or trimethoprim-sulfadoxine given intravenously or intramuscularly twice a day for 3 days may also be a primary choice. A single oral administration of a long-acting bolus containing baquiloprim-sulfadimidine may be suitable for treating beef cattle.

Other possible antibiotics, such as amoxicillin, ampicillin, cephaloridine, cephalosporin, clindamycin, erythromycin, gentamicin, lincomycin, oxytetracycline, streptomycin, or tylosin, are alternatives when a satisfactory result has not been achieved with other therapy.[9]

High concentration of an active substance in the claw can be achieved by a regional intravenous injection (see Chapter 4). Positive results have been obtained with penicillin or oxytetracycline.

Local treatment is beneficial but requires restraint to deal with the painful area. The lesion must be

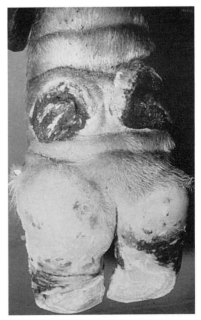

Figure 7–9. Swelling of the bulb region associated with a retroarticular abscess is frequently confused with interdigital phlegmon.

cleansed with warm soapy water and necrotic tissue removed. A non-irritant bacteriostatic agent such as Furacin or a sulfa preparation should be used. If a bandage is applied to protect the wound, it is important to ensure that the wound can drain. The bandage should be replaced frequently.

In the event of serious complications, surgical procedures may be used to save valuable animals. Early recognition of the complication is essential to avoid excessive tissue loss (see Chapter 16).

PREVENTION AND CONTROL

Animals that are actively shedding infection should be isolated until signs of lameness have disappeared. If this is not possible, a waterproof dressing or protective boot should be applied to affected animals. Protective boots must, however, be carefully supervised to avoid additional damage and should be disinfected between farm visits.

Busy traffic areas are invariably heavily contaminated. Therefore, steps should be taken to ensure that areas around drinking troughs, gateways, and tracks are adequately drained. Animals at pasture might be moved to a clean, dry area, or it may be possible to house them during periods of heavy rainfall. During enzootic outbreaks, it may be necessary to shift pasture or to confine the animals indoors. Contaminated concrete areas must be frequently cleaned and scraped free of manure.

Prophylactic use of a footbath with an antiseptic and astringent solution is recommended. Copper sulfate or zinc sulfate (7% to 10% in water) is normally advised. Formaldehyde solution (3% to 5% in water) can also be used but can be hazardous to handle (see Chapter 9).

Ethylenediamine dihydroiodide has been used for prevention with positive results,[5] but in a Swedish study, severe side effects were reported.[1]

Efforts made to produce a reliable vaccine against *F. necrophorum* have failed because of the weak immune response to the bacterium.[38] The best result (a protective effect of about 60%) has been achieved in Australia with a vaccine containing a concentrated culture supernatant of a toxigenic strain of *F. necrophorum*.

INTERDIGITAL DERMATITIS

DEFINITION

Dermatitis interdigitalis (ID) is an inflammation of the interdigital epidermis caused by a bacterial infection. *D. nodosus (B. nodosus)* is the most frequently isolated infectious agent. In most acute cases, the inflammation is superficial and no clinical symptoms occur. In chronic cases, infection tends to involve the claw horn and develop into heel horn erosion (*erosio ungulae*, see Chapter 8), which thus can be viewed as a more severe and late form of ID. This form can give rise to severe lameness.

INCIDENCE

ID has a worldwide distribution, being most prevalent under poor hygienic conditions in intensive dairy production. A very high prevalence has been reported from a Dutch investigation in which more than 50% of female calves and indoor-fed dairy cows showed signs of ID.[22] Fewer than 1% of the animals in this study were lame. A much lower disease incidence has been reported in other countries.

The morbidity is high; as many as 100% of the animals within affected herds may show signs of infection, with the prevalence being highest at the end of the indoor season. In other studies, the prevalence seems to be highest shortly after housing for calving.[6, 44] Spontaneous resolution of the superficial inflammation of the interdigital epidermis has been observed. The prevalence of heel horn erosion may increase in herds affected with ID,[42] thus suggesting a close relationship between the two diseases.

In tied systems, the hind limbs are more often affected by ID than the front limbs. In loose house systems, the distribution between front and hind limbs is about equal. Animals on slatted floors are less affected than animals on a solid floor.[40]

LITERATURE

ID has often not been clearly defined. It might earlier have been described by such terms as *foot rot, slurry heel, stinky foot,* or *scald.* More relevant descriptions later applied were *bovine contagious* ID[25] and *heel horn erosion* stages I and II.[42] Confusion in interpreting information in the literature may occur for one or more reasons:

• The disease is not associated with obvious clinical symptoms in its early stages.

• It is easily ignored when found together with the more obvious heel horn erosions.

• Other laboratories have been consistently unable to isolate *D. nodosus* from typical active cases of ID in the United Kingdom.[7]

• It is intimately associated with some outbreaks of digital dermatitis.

ETIOLOGY AND PATHOGENESIS

ID is caused by a mixed bacterial infection. The obligate anaerobe gram-negative *D. nodosus* is alleged to be the predominant agent.[27, 33, 39] Experimentally, *D. nodosus* can be transmitted from one bovine animal to another and from cattle to sheep.[45] Different bacterial pilation and the production of proteolytic enzymes explain differences in pathogenicity and

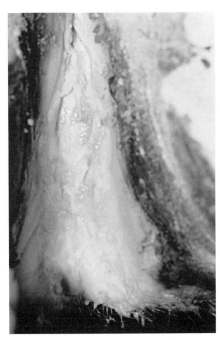

Figure 7–10. Initial stage of interdigital dermatitis in the interdigital space.

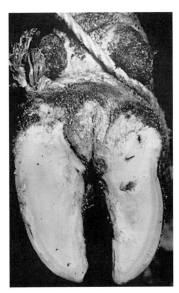

Figure 7–12. Chronic progressive interdigital dermatitis in which the skin is hyperplastic with a subcutaneous soft tissue reaction.

variations between species.[17] Synergism with other agents, *F. necrophorum* in particular, has also been discussed.[13, 25]

The disease is strongly associated with high relative humidity, temperate climates, and poor hygienic conditions, especially in housed dairy cattle. The source of the infection is the cow itself, and the infection spreads from affected to non-affected animals through the environment. *D. nodosus* cannot survive for more than 4 days on the ground. Manure mixed with finely chopped bedding material (e.g., straw) adheres to the claws and can therefore produce an environment that favors growth of the bacterium.

The bacteria colonize and cause loss of integrity of the epidermal cells but do not pass the basement membrane.[16] As the infection proceeds, the border

between the skin and soft heel horn is destroyed by proteolytic activity.

CLINICAL SIGNS AND COURSE OF DISEASE

In mild cases or in the initial stages, the interdigital skin, including the dorsal or palmar/plantar areas, becomes hyperemic. Superficial erosion and ulceration appear with a serous or grayish exudate (Fig. 7–10). The course of the disease is usually not dramatic (Figs. 7–11, 7–12 and 7–13). More aggressive forms interfere with horn formation in the bulbs, where fissures, hemorrhages, and necrosis can arise (Fig. 7–13). The subcutaneous tissue can then be

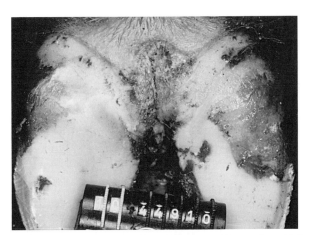

Figure 7–11. Early stage of the chronic palmar/plantar interdigital lesion. Similar in appearance to digital dermatitis, there is no white border or raised areas. The lesion healed spontaneously.

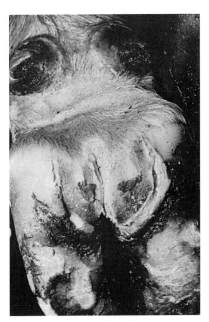

Figure 7–13. Erosion of skin horn junction is a common result of prolonged interdigital dermatitis.

secondarily inflamed. Swelling and, in a more chronic stage, hyperkeratosis may develop. Such interdigital irritation may cause slight to severe interdigital hyperplasia *(hyperplasia interdigitalis)* (Fig. 7–14). A papillomatous process causing verrucose dermatitis *(dermatitis verrucosa)* was thought to be a chronic manifestation of ID. Today it is believed that verrucose dermatitis and the proliferative type of digital dermatitis are indistinguishable. ID has also been discussed as an initial phase of interdigital phlegmon *(phlegmona interdigitalis)*.[12, 16, 25, 42] The most common complication is, however, heel horn erosion.

DIAGNOSIS

ID is diagnosed, after cleansing, by the characteristic superficial lesions of the interdigital epidermis. Confirmation by isolation of *D. nodosus* is possible by identifying the causal agent by microscopic examination and the fluorescent antibody technique.

The principal problem in differential diagnosis is the coexistence of DD *(dermatitis digitalis)*. The most obvious differences between the two diseases are the clinical symptoms and the greater contagious nature of DD. However, in mild cases or in early stages of DD, this differentiation may be dubious (Fig. 7–15). Some systemic virus infections (foot-and-mouth disease, mucosal disease, and malignant catarrhal fever) also can give rise to local lesions resembling ID.

TREATMENT

ID should be treated topically. The lesions should be cleaned, necrotic tissue removed by a clean dry swab, and a topical bacteriostatic agent applied, such as a

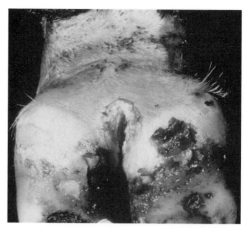

Figure 7–15. The initial stages of digital dermatitis. Some thickening and sclerosis of the skin borders the interdigital space between the bulbs. (Photo courtesy of Carlo Maria Mortellaro, Milan, Italy.)

50% mixture of sulfamezathine powder and anhydrous copper sulfate. Foot bathing is usually recommended to keep the infection under control (see Chapter 9). Systemic treatment with antibiotics has little effect. Skin lesions usually regress spontaneously if the environment is improved. Electric cow trainers, about which ethical and welfare issues have been raised, can help to provide a cleaner environment in tie stalls.

CONTROL

Good management and housing systems to keep claws dry and clean are most important. Regular foot trimming helps to avoid complications. Foot bathing, commencing in the late fall and before clinical cases can be identified during high-risk periods, is essential in herds known to be infected with ID (see Chapter 9). Bathing the feet weekly may be sufficient in the late fall, but the frequency may have to be increased in late winter. Vaccination with *D. nodosus* has been of little benefit in cattle.[13] Oral administration of zinc sulfate has not been shown to have any prophylactic effect.

DIGITAL DERMATITIS

Digital dermatitis (DD) is a contagious superficial inflammation of the epidermis proximal to the coronal margin or the interdigital space. Two types of lesions have been reported: One is a circumscribed erosive/reactive condition, and the other is a proliferative wartlike lesion. Both forms cause various degrees of discomfort and may give rise to severe lameness. The cause is unclear, but the tendency for the disease to spread within a herd indicates that infectious agents are involved.

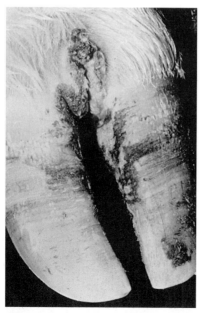

Figure 7–14. Chronic irritation is associated with interdigital hyperplasia development in dairy cattle.

INCIDENCE

When a herd becomes affected, the disease can rapidly spread within the herd and the morbidity may reach 90%.[10, 34, 35] Animals of all ages and breeds are susceptible, but it is most commonly encountered in heifers when they first enter the milking herd. This suggests that an immunological factor may be involved. DD is also spread from animals newly introduced into a herd or by any other means that brings infected manure from one location into contact with unaffected animals. All limbs can be affected but most commonly the pelvic limbs.

Outbreaks are most frequent in loose-housed herds. In tie stalls, single cases can be observed. However, if the stalls are not kept clean, a high incidence of the condition is likely. In housed animals, the prevalence is highest in the fall and winter and decreases when the animals are pastured. DD is usually associated with an unhygienic environment. However, epidemic outbreaks have sometimes been reported in well-managed herds. Under field conditions, the disease may be transmitted to healthy herds through apparently clinically healthy animals from affected herds.

LITERATURE

Since first described in Italy in 1974,[11] DD has been diagnosed and reported in the majority of European countries, the United States, and the Middle East. The literature is reviewed comprehensively in various reports.[8, 34, 35, 47]

ETIOLOGY AND PATHOGENESIS

The lesions of DD can be of at least two distinct types, erosive/reactive (strawberry-like) and proliferative (wartlike) forms. One or the other of these morphological variations may be seen more frequently in a particular geographical region than another. On the other hand, both types can be seen on different animals on the same farm. It may be that these two forms merely reflect differences in the stages of the disease process.[10, 23] It has also been suggested that there are associations and similarities between ID and a mild form of DD.

The most reasonable explanation is that this is a multifactorial disease[30, 47] in which spirochetes, together with either bacteria or viruses, may develop an opportunistic pattern of pathogenesis. The different types of the disease may also be influenced by the environment or the age of the animal and its level of immunity.

Deep in the epidermis of erosive/reactive lesions, two spirochetes can be demonstrated using Warthin and Starry stains. One is a long, spiral, filamentous organism 12 μm long and 0.3 μm wide, and the other is a shorter spirochete 5 to 6 μm long and 0.1 μm wide.[8] Although most workers have identified the presence of spirochetes (*Treponema* spp.) from different types of lesions, it has not been possible to reproduce the condition artificially. The primary changes closely resemble those associated with bovine papillomas caused by different types of papovavirus, but the role of a virus has not yet been confirmed.[47] The possible involvement of *D. (Bacteroides) nodosus* has been suggested.[32]

The histopathological criteria of the proliferative type are parakeratotic hyperkeratosis with profuse colonization by spirochetes; absence of the stratum granulosum; confluent acanthosis with invasion of the outer stratum spinosum by spirochetes; absence of deep ulceration; invasion of neutrophils into the outer dermal papillae and stratum spinosum; perivascular infiltration of the reticular dermis by mononuclear leukocytes; and absence of dermal fibromatous change.[35]

CLINICAL FEATURES AND COMPLICATIONS

A circular lesion 1 to 4 cm in diameter is generally seen in the plantar (or palmar) skin adjacent to the heel or, less commonly, in the proximal part of the interdigital space.

In the mild form of DD, the skin is hyperemic, producing a serous exudate. In early stages, the hairs of the diseased areas are usually erect, and they later disappear (see Fig. 7–15). In the erosive form, the skin is covered with a purulent, pungent-smelling exudate. Cleansing exposes reddish granulation tissue (strawberry) with a concave profile. The area is circumscribed by a whitened epithelial border (Figs. 7–16 and 7–17). The lesion is very sensitive and easily bleeds, but the soft tissue is not swollen. The animal is often lame.

The proliferative type may give rise to the papillomatous (verrucous) type, which is characterized by a mass of hard, fine tendrils that can be several centimeters in length and cover a considerable area

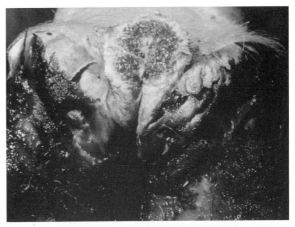

Figure 7–16. A granulating round lesion, often referred to as a *strawberry*. Note the white border around the lesion. (Photo courtesy of Carlo Maria Mortellaro, Milan, Italy.)

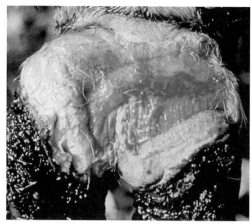

Figure 7–17. Erosive/ulcerative lesion. The first lesion was photographed in 1976. (Photo courtesy of Carlo Maria Mortellaro, Milan, Italy.)

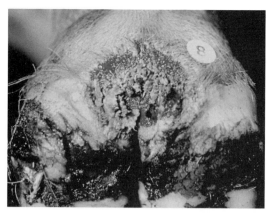

Figure 7–19. A mixed lesion showing both granulation and proliferative changes. (Photo courtesy of Carlo Maria Mortellaro, Milan, Italy.)

(Figs. 7–18, 7–19, and 7–20). These proliferations easily bleed if traumatized.

Complications are uncommon. However, when the skin lesion is adjacent to the growing heel horn, horn production can be disturbed and heel horn erosion *(erosio ungulae)* may result (see Chapter 8). Rarely the disease progresses radially into the heel horn, severely damaging the underlying corium, which may lead to the development of a sole ulcer *(pododermatitis circumscripta)* (see Chapter 8). A lesion at the coronary margin can disturb perioplic horn production and cause a vertical fissure of the horn wall *(fissura ungulae verticalis)* (see Chapter 8).

DIAGNOSIS

The diagnosis of DD is often based on a history of an epidemic onset of discomfort and lameness in a herd.

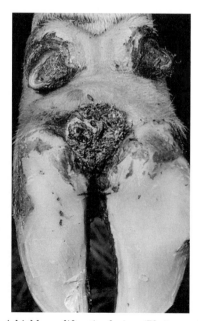

Figure 7–18. A highly proliferative lesion. (Photo courtesy of Carlo Maria Mortellaro, Milan, Italy.)

Diseased animals should be examined with the limb lifted and restrained. The affected area should be washed carefully. The characteristic circular lesion, often with a strawberry surface, is very painful. A pungent odor is often noted.

In contrast to interdigital phlegmon, DD causes no interdigital fissures, swelling of the digital region, or fever. Mild forms of DD located close to the interdigital space may be confused with ID. However, typical lesions of ID are not associated with lameness.

TREATMENT

Lesions affecting individual animals should be treated topically. If necessary, the claw should be trimmed to a normal shape and necrotic tissue and pockets pared. After cleaning and drying, the lesion should be sprayed with an aerosol containing a solution of oxytetracycline hydrochloride.[47] Bandaging is not necessary. Topical treatment has not resulted in detectable residual levels of oxytetracycline in blood or milk.[2] Consistently good results are achieved if the lesion is treated on at least one further occasion, depending on the severity of the case. After treat-

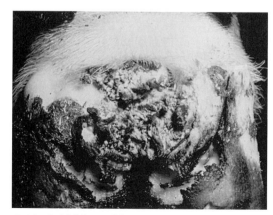

Figure 7–20. A highly proliferative lesion with horny papillae. (Photo courtesy of Carlo Maria Mortellaro, Milan, Italy.)

ment, the lameness typically is reduced within 24 hours and a normal gait can be expected after 2 to 3 days.

Herd outbreaks are best treated with a footbath. DD can be successfully controlled by a single passage through a foot bath containing 5 to 6 grams/liter of oxytetracycline or 150 grams Lincospectin, 0.75 to 1.5 grams/liter of water.[8] For optimum effect, the heels of the cows should be washed thoroughly before they enter the footbath. Repeat treatments may be needed after 4 to 6 weeks, depending on the extent of the environmental challenge.

The use (see p. 134) of copper sulfate, zinc sulfate, formalin, dimetridazole, or citric acid in footbaths has given poor to inconclusive results. These footbaths may, however, have a beneficial effect in reducing the prevalence of ID and may thus decrease the susceptibility to DD.

In general, parenteral antibiotics have not shown any effect on either the erosive or proliferative type of DD. For chronic lesions, the only effective treatment is complete resection of the proliferation under regional anesthesia. A topical antiseptic dressing and a compression bandage should be applied for several days after surgery.

CONTROL

General hygienic precautions and reduction of high-moisture conditions are mandatory. In herds with chronic infection, the symptoms may be masked for a while. Therefore, in order to control the disease, routine inspection of all animals should be carried out regularly. It is imperative not to spread infection between animals or between farms with poorly sterilized claw-trimming equipment or in other comparable ways. Unaffected animals introduced into an affected herd are particularly susceptible to infection. Disinfection and quarantine procedures should be used before animals are introduced to healthy herds. Vaccination has not been successful.

REFERENCES

 1. Andersson L, Törnqvist M: Toxic effects of ethylenediamine dihydroiodide treatment in Swedish calves. Vet Rec 113:215–216, 1983.
 2. Anfossi P, Roncada P, Tomasi L, et al: Indagine su una presenza di ossitetraciclina nel siero e nel latte di bovine trattate per via topica con una formulazione spray. (Oxytetracycline determination in serum and milk of cows topically treated with a spray formulation). Societa Italia di Buiatria (Italian Association for Buiatrics) 25:431–435, 1993.
 3. Arkins S: Lameness in dairy cows. Parts I & II. Irish Veterinary Journal 35:135–140, 163–170, 1981.
 4. Berg JN: "Foot rot complex" in cattle. Current Veterinary Therapy, Food Animal Practice. Philadelphia, WB Saunders, 1981, pp. 1104–1106.
 5. Berg JN, Maas JP, Paterson JA, et al: Efficacy of ethylenediamine dihydroiodide as an agent to prevent experimentally induced bovine foot rot. Am J Vet Res 45:1073–1078, 1984.
 6. Bergsten C, Pettersson B: The cleanliness of cows tied in stalls and the health of their hooves as influenced by the use of electric trainers. Prev Vet Med 13:229–238, 1992.
 7. Blowey RW: Interdigital causes of lameness. Proceedings of the 8th International Symposium on Disorders of the Ruminant Digit. Banff, Canada, 1994, pp 142–154.
 8. Blowey RW: Studies on the pathogenesis and control of digital dermatitis. Proceedings of the 8th International Symposium on Disorders of the Ruminant Digit. Banff, Canada, 1994, pp 168–173.
 9. Braun RK, Bates DB, Shearer JK, et al: Efficacy of amoxicillin trihydrate for the treatment of experimentally induced foot rot in cattle. Am J Vet Res 48:1751–1754, 1987.
10. Brizzi A: Bovine digital dermatitis. Proceedings of the 26th Annual Conference of the American Association of Bovine Practitioners, Albuquerque, NM, 27:33–37, 1993.
11. Cheli R, Mortellaro CM: La dermatite digitale del bovino. (Digital dermatitis in dairy cows.) Proceedings of the 8th International Meeting on Diseases of Cattle. Milan, Italy, 1974, pp 208–213.
12. Clark BL, Emery DL, Stewart DJ: Aetiology and prevention of interdigital necrobacillosis (foot abscess) in cattle. In Stewart DJ, Peterson JE, McKern NM, Emery DL (eds): Footrot in ruminants. Proceedings of the Workshop. Melbourne, Victoria, Australia, Commonwealth Scientific and Industrial Research Organisation (CSIRO), 1986, pp 275–279.
13. Clark BL, Stewart DJ, Emery DL, et al: Immunisation of cattle against interdigital dermatitis (footrot) with an autogenous Bacteroides nodosus vaccine. Aust Vet J 63:61–63, 1986.
14. David GP: Severe foul-in-the-foot in dairy cattle. Vet Rec 133:567–569, 1993.
15. Dehoux JP: Note clinique sur une epizootie de Phlegmons interdigites sur bétail N'Dama importé de Senegambia au Gabon, sur le ranch de la Ngounie. (Clinical note on an outbreak of foot rot in N'Dama cattle imported from Senegambia into Gabon.) Rev Elev Med Vet Pays Trop 42:509–510, 1989.
16. Egerton JR: Footrot of cattle, goats and deer. In Egerton JR, Yong WK, Riffkin GG (eds): Footrot and Foot Abscess of Ruminants. Boca Raton, FL, CRC Press, 1989, pp 47–56.
17. Egerton JR, Laing EA: Characteristics of Bacteroides nodosus isolated from cattle. Vet Microbiol 3:269–278, 1978.
18. Emery DL: Host responses to footrot and foot abscess. In Egerton JR, Yong WK, Riffkin GG (eds): Footrot and Foot Abscess of Ruminants. Boca Raton, FL, CRC Press, 1989, pp 141–153.
19. Emery DL, Vaughan JA, Clark BL, et al: Cultural characteristics and virulence of strains of Fusobacterium necrophorum isolated from the feet of cattle and sheep. Aust Vet J 62:43–46, 1985.
20. Espinasse J, Savey M, Thorley CM, et al: Colour Atlas on Disorders of Cattle and Sheep Digit—International Terminology. Maisons-Alfort, Editions du Point Vétérinaire, 1984.
21. Faye B, Lescourret F: Environmental factors associated with lameness in dairy cattle. Prev Vet Med 7:267–287, 1989.
22. Frankena K, Van Keulen KAS, Noordhuizen JP, et al: A cross-sectional study into prevalence and risk indicators of digital hemorrhages in female dairy calves. Prev Vet Med 14:1–12, 1992.
23. Gourreau JM, Scott DW, Rousseau JF: La dermatite digitée des bovins. (Digital dermatitis of cattle.) Le Point Vétérinaire 24:49–57, 1992.
24. Jubb TF, Malmo J: Lesions causing lameness requiring veterinary treatment in pasture-fed dairy cows in East Gippsland. Aust Vet J 68:21–24, 1991.
25. Kasari TR, Scanlan CM: Bovine contagious interdigital dermatitis: A review. Southwest Vet 38(2):33–36, 1987.
26. Kasari TR, Marquis H, Scanlan CM: Septic arthritis and osteomyelitis in a bovine digit: A mixed infection of Actimomyces pyogenes and Fusobacterium necrophorum. Cornell Vet 78:215–219, 1988.
27. Laing EA, Egerton JR: The occurrence, prevalence and transmission of Bacteroides nodosus infection in cattle. Res Vet Sci 24:300–304, 1978.
28. McLennan MW: Incidence of lameness requiring veterinary treatment in Queensland. Aust Vet J 65:144–147, 1988.
29. Monrad JA, Kassuku AA, Nansen P, Willeberg P: An epidemiological study of footrot in pastured cattle. Acta Vet Scand 24:403–417, 1983.

30. Mortellaro CM: Digital dermatitis. Proceedings of the 8th International Symposium on Disorders of the Ruminant Digit. Banff, Canada, 1994, pp 137–141.
31. Murphy PA, Hannan J, Monaghan M: A survey of lameness in beef cattle housed on slats and on straw. *In* Wierenga HK, Peterse DJ (eds): Cattle Housing Systems, Lameness and Behaviour. Dordrecht, Martinus Nijhoff, 1987, pp 67–72.
32. Peterse DJ: Lameness in cattle. Proceedings of the 14th World Congress on Diseases of Cattle. Dublin, Ireland, 1986, pp 1015–1023.
33. Plym Forshell L, Andersson L: Infektion med *Bacteroides nodosus* vid klövspaltdermatit hos ko. (*Bacteroides nodosus* infection in bovine interdigital dermatitis.) Sven Vet Tidn 33:551–553, 1981.
34. Read DH, Walker RL: Papillomatous digital dermatitis and associated lesions of dairy cattle in California: Pathologic findings. Proceedings of the 8th International Symposium on Disorders of the Ruminant Digit. Banff, Canada, 1994, pp 156–158.
35. Read DH, Walker RL: Papillomatous digital dermatitis and associated lesions of dairy cattle in California: Clinical characteristics. Proceedings of the 8th International Symposium on Disorders of the Ruminant Digit. Banff, Canada, 1994, pp 159–163.
36. Rowlands GJ, Russell AM, Williams LA: Effects of season, herd size, management system and veterinary practice on the lameness incidence in dairy cattle: Vet Rec 113:441–445, 1983.
37. Smith GR: Pathogenicity of *Fusobacterium necrophorum* biovar B. Res Vet Sci 52:260–261, 1992.
38. Smith GR, Wallace LM: Further observations on the weak immunogenicity of *Fusobacterium necrophorum*. Res Vet Sci 52:262–263, 1992.
39. Thorley CM, Calder HAMcL, Harrison WJ: Recognition in Great Britain of *Bacteroides nodosus* in foot lesions of cattle. Vet Rec 100:387, 1977.
40. Thysen I: Foot and leg disorders in dairy cattle in different housing systems. *In* Wierenga HK, Peterse DJ (eds). Cattle Housing Systems, Lameness and Behaviour. Dordrecht, Martinus Nijhoff, 1987, pp 166–178.
41. Törnqvist M: Evaluation of animal health in beef production in relation to housing and feeding systems: "The Götala husbandry project." Bovine Pract 26:57–58, 1991.
42. Toussaint Raven E, Haalstra RT, Peterse DJ: Cattle Footcare and Claw Trimming. Ipswich, UK: Farming Press, 1985.
43. Tranter WP, Morris RS: A case study of lameness in three dairy herds. N Z Vet J 39:88–96, 1991.
44. Vermunt JJ: Lesions and structural characteristics of dairy heifers in two management systems (M.V.Sc. thesis). Saskatoon, Saskatchewan, Canada, University of Saskatchewan, 1990.
45. Wilkinson FC, Egerton JR, Dickson J: Transmission of *Fusiformis nodosus* infection from cattle to sheep. Aust Vet J 46:382–384, 1970.
46. Williams LA, Rowlands GJ, Russell AM: Effect of wet weather on lameness in dairy cattle. Vet Rec 118:259–261, 1986.
47. Zemljic B: Current investigations into the cause of dermatitis digitalis in cattle. Proceedings of the 8th International Symposium on Disorders of the Ruminant Digit. Banff, Canada, 1994, pp 164–167.

Donald W. Collick *United Kingdom*

A. David Weaver

Paul R. Greenough *Canada*

8

Interdigital Space and Claw

Pododermatitis Circumscripta (Sole Ulcer)

Donald W. Collick

DEFINITION

A sole ulcer is a specific lesion located in the region of the sole-bulb junction, usually nearer the axial than the abaxial margin (region 4). Damage to the dermis is associated with a circumscribed zone of localized hemorrhage and necrosis (Fig. 8–1).

INCIDENCE

Sole ulcers commonly affect one or both lateral hind claws, predominantly in heavy, high-yielding dairy cattle kept under confined conditions.[2, 10, 24, 40, 47] In the forelimb, it more often involves the medial claw. Bulls are less frequently affected.

The condition is common in dairy herds worldwide,

although most reports have come from European countries. The incidence is higher in herds managed in loose housing systems or otherwise confined for long periods on concrete, particularly if conditions are moist as during the winter months. Cases tend to predominate in the late winter months and early spring. In 1977, a national United Kingdom survey of practitioner-treated lameness reported an annual incidence of 5.5%,[47] of which 12% showed sole ulcer lesions (1100 of 9178 cases).

In France, systematical examination of one hind foot of 4896 cows, a third of which were lame, revealed 5% affected with sole ulcers.[44] A 2½-year epidemiological study in the United Kingdom concluded in 1991[13] reported that sole ulceration accounted for 28% of a total 8645 primary diagnoses reported and ranked it as the most common lesion in the four regions studied.

The incidence of sole ulceration is increased when cows are fed high levels of concentrates[31] or high levels of dietary protein.[33] Grass silage high in dry matter, high in fiber, and low in crude protein were associated with less lameness.[13]

Friesian cattle are more susceptible to laminitis than other breeds of dairy cattle.[32, 39] Swedish Friesians are prone to sole hemorrhage and ulcers.[1] Russell[46] found that daughters of certain bulls had a higher incidence of sole ulcers and white line lesions.

Sole ulcers have been observed more frequently in animals kept in cubicles with concrete floors than straw yards.[47]

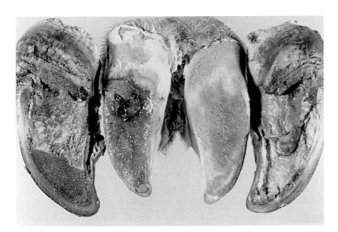

Figure 8–1. Exungulated claws of the pelvic limb showing widespread hemorrhage in the lateral claws, especially severe at the specific site for the sole ulcer (pododermatitis circumscripta). (Photo courtesy of P. Ossent.)

LITERATURE

Sole ulceration was first described accurately by Rusterholz.[48] Numerous theories about its etiology have subsequently been advanced. Today the condition is considered to be a sequel to laminitis,[32, 39, 40, 42] nutrition being an important factor.[43] Laminitis is considered in greater detail in Chapters 18, 19, and 20.

Heel erosion and interdigital dermatitis are considered to be predisposing or contributory causes of sole ulcers.[52]

Sole ulcers are associated with reduced fertility, particularly when diagnosed as the cause of lameness in the period 76 to 120 days after calving.[16] Service numbers, days to conception, and cull rates are increased.

ETIOLOGY AND PATHOGENESIS

Current opinion about the cause of sole ulcers favors the concept that subclinical laminitis damages horn-producing tissues, with the result that the sole horn is softened. This weakened state, probably exacerbated by the effects of the environment, such as prolonged standing in slurry, makes the sole vulnerable to the effects of trauma. Conditions that predispose to laminitis are discussed in Chapters 18, 19, and 20.

The lesion occurs immediately adjacent to the plantar process of the distal phalanx. This very specific site (region 4, see Fig. 1–2) suggests that anatomical and mechanical factors have a significant role. The majority of lesions occur in hind lateral claws. The outer hind claw is broader, and its distal phalanx is rougher than the inner, indicating that the forces affecting the claws are not equal.[41, 51] The mechanical forces of weight-bearing are discussed fully on pp. 123–124. It is not clear whether an exostosis is involved in the etiology, because secondary bone changes occur later in the healing process.[37] In cows that have flat soles, the area subjected to maximum pressure during weight-bearing is located at the sole ulcer site. Factors that flatten the sole and so increase the risk of sole ulcers include wear due to walking on hard surfaces or incorrect hoof trimming.

Toussaint Raven[51, 52] postulated that when the heel region of the lateral claw suffers an insult, hyperplasia of the keratogenic layer causes the horn to grow more rapidly. Therefore, the lateral claw in mature cows frequently bears more weight than the medial claw.[38] This process is favored if cows are maintained on concrete surfaces. Excessive periods of standing on hard surfaces lead to localized circulatory disturbance and ischemic changes. Lying is considered to be an important aspect of behavior in dairy cattle. In a herd with a high incidence of lameness, cows and heifers spent more time standing.[14]

Mechanical pressure on the corium, sandwiched between the sole and the plantar process of the distal phalanx, causes an ischemic necrosis of the corium. This necrosis leads to discoloration in the horn at the specific site because of poor-quality horn production and hemorrhage.[25] Impaired activity of the keratogenic layer of the corium caused by injury leads to

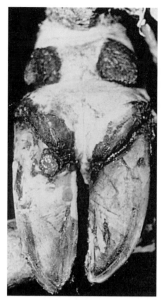

Figure 8–2. Classical case of sole ulcer at the sole-bulb junction of the lateral claw with protruding granulation tissue. The deep V-shaped grooves typical of heel erosion should be noted. Long toes and reduced heel height create a pressure point over the plantar process of the distal phalanx.

further local hemorrhage and necrosis. Erosion of the heel and interdigital dermatitis can complicate the disease process by increasing the breakdown of the already compromised horn, eroding through to the corium and disturbing claw balance (Figs. 8–2 and 8–3).

Repair of the lesion occurs from the periphery. Granulation tissue, which is easily damaged and bleeds, may protrude through the perforation in the sole.

CLINICAL SIGNS

The majority of cases occur in the lateral claw in one or both hind limbs. Bilateral lesions of differing

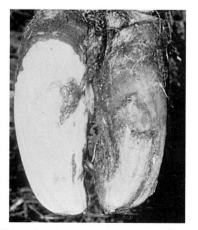

Figure 8–3. This sole ulcer was revealed beneath normal horn during the process of routine claw trimming.

severity are common, a high proportion of cases being associated with claw overgrowth.[13, 15, 53] The progress and severity of lameness are variable and often masked in bilateral cases, depending on the size of lesion and the extent of secondary infection. Because the lateral digit is usually involved, the limb is often held slightly abducted with weight-bearing on the unaffected medial digit. As the disease progresses, the hind toes may be rested on the edge of the heel stone in an attempt to relieve pressure on the heel-sole junction. On flat surfaces, an affected animal stands with its hind limbs camped back. Some cows may shake the affected foot frequently, and those with bilateral lesions may continually shift weight from limb to limb and lie down more often.

Grossly, the lesion varies from a soft, slightly discolored area, which may be painful under pressure, to an obvious circumscribed perforation. This is often the stage at which lameness becomes severe enough to be noticed. In later stages, granulation tissue protrudes through the sole defect (Fig. 8–4). Infection of the exposed corium may cause various degrees of separation of the sole.

Once the corium is exposed, infection can invade the deeper structures of the claw and travel proximally to involve the navicular bursa, resulting in necrosis of the flexor tendon and ligaments of the navicular bone (Fig. 8–5). Rupture of the flexor tendon leads to dorsal rotation (upward) of the toe (cocked toe) (Fig. 8–6). Infection involving the distal interphalangeal joint produces marked swelling and pain. In complicated cases, infection may even travel up the deep flexor tendon sheath.

DIAGNOSIS

The site and nature of the condition are characteristic. The area is often covered by a ledge of sole horn,

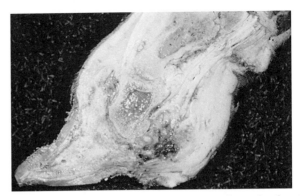

Figure 8–5. Cross section of a digit affected with a sole ulcer in which infection has invaded the deep tissues of the digit. The deep flexor tendon, its sheath, the navicular bursa, and the retroarticular space are all affected. (Photo courtesy of C. Bergsten, Sweden.)

which protrudes toward the interdigital space (Fig. 8–7), or the thickness of the heel horn may be excessive.[7] Paring the excess growth reveals hemorrhagic horn. This can indicate when the initial laminitic insult first occurred. Depending on the rate of wear, the new horn may take 3 months to reach the surface. In contrast, the wall at the abaxial groove grows at about 5 mm/month.[27] Further paring exposes the ulcer and separation of the sole around the periphery of the lesion.

Other causes of foot lameness, all of which are easily differentiated from sole ulceration by careful examination, include punctured sole, white line disease, bruised sole, and exposed corium due to extensive horn erosion or wear. Acute laminitis often produces a similar stance in a cow with bilateral sole ulcer.

TREATMENT

The therapeutic claw-trimming procedure is described in Chapter 9 (see pp. 129–133). Protruding granulation tissue at the sole ulcer site may be resected at sole level, but this is not essential.

Local anesthesia facilitates the treatment of more

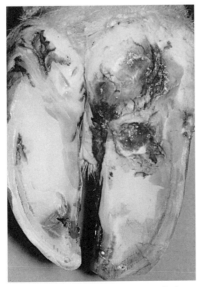

Figure 8–4. The heel has been completely eroded, and as a result, weight-bearing has been transferred to the typical sole ulcer site.

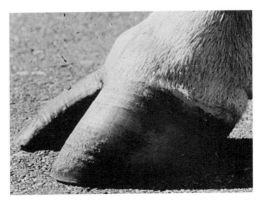

Figure 8–6. A typical cocked-up toe that is indicative of pathological avulsion of the insertion of the deep flexor tendon into the distal phalanx.

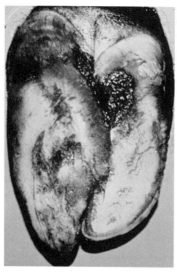

Figure 8–7. Displaced sole horn causing abnormal pressure over the typical site. The horn covers a typical sole ulcer, which is revealed after paring. (Photo courtesy of R. Blowey, United Kingdom.)

painful lesions. Paring the diseased claw as described in simple cases forces the inner claw to act as a functional block while the ulcer heals. In more complicated cases, application of a wooden or rubber block to the unaffected medial claw removes all weight-bearing from the ulcer region and is an ideal treatment. Claw blocks should be kept on for a *maximum* of 6 weeks.

Topical application of copper sulfate or other astringent dressings or the use of actual cautery to control granulation tissue is contraindicated because it retards new horn development. Bandages should not be applied because they result in continued weight-bearing at the ulcer site. Furthermore, covering the lesion causes it to remain moist and promotes maceration and bacterial infection. In the opinion of the author, the most rapid method of resolving a lesion is to rest the affected digit.

Many ulcers never fully resolve. Cows can continue to have a chronic low-grade lameness, needing corrective foot trimming two to four times yearly for the rest of their productive lives. The author believes that if an ulcer is found in the lateral claw of one hind limb, it is mandatory that the contralateral digits be examined and that both hind limbs be pared and balanced. Sole ulcers are commonly bilateral and are usually associated with claw overgrowth and weight-bearing imbalance between claws.

If the lesion is purulent, parenteral broad-spectrum antibiotic therapy is advisable for a minimum of 3 days. Currently favored are tylosin, oxytetracycline, and lincomycin. Application of a foot poultice may also help. Radical surgery is required in cases of deep sepsis (see Chapter 16).

PREVENTION AND CONTROL

Because the occurrence of sole ulcers is believed to be intimately related to subclinical laminitis, the presence of this condition should be investigated and appropriate control measures instituted (see Chapters 19 and 20).

White Line Disease at the Heel

Donald W. Collick

DEFINITION

White line disease is characterized by disintegration of the fibrous junction between the sole and wall and its penetration by debris. The abaxial white line immediately distal to the heel bulb junction of the lateral hind claw is commonly affected (region 3).

INCIDENCE

White line disease is a commonly observed lesion and has frequently been reported as a major cause of lameness, particularly where cattle are housed and fed concentrates. Several United Kingdom reports cite the condition as responsible for between 18% and 35% of lameness.[13, 19, 47] French workers[44] identified 20% of cows affected, and in Quebec[10] 12% were affected. Two Australian studies[28, 35] found the condition to be less common, although in New Zealand[54] pasture-fed cattle, an incidence of 39% was reported in three herds.

ETIOLOGY AND PATHOGENESIS

The white line is only as deep as the contiguous sole. Even in a normal claw, it is usually delineated by dirt and grit that have become embedded in the soft horn. At this stage, lameness may be present as a result of simple pressure on the corium. Unless dislodged or removed, foreign bodies eventually penetrate the sensitive laminae and initiate a septic laminitis/coriitis.[20] If a purulent abscess becomes established, pressure and inflammation cause lameness. As the abscess enlarges, intraungular pressure causes pus to spread from the initial focus to underrun the wall or sole. Horn becomes separated from the keratogenic layer by purulent material. Dependent on the origin site, pus takes one or more of several routes:

- Discharge at the coronary band, leaving a sinus (Fig. 8–8)

- Emergence at the skin-horn junction at the heel

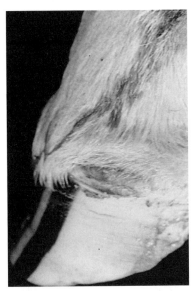

Figure 8–8. A discharge of purulent material from the skin-horn junction usually indicates that a tract of infection has ascended beneath the wall from a lesion in the white line.

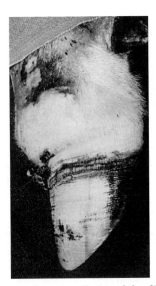

Figure 8–10. In cases of septic arthritis of the distal interphalangeal joint, the region above the skin-horn junction becomes edematous and tender.

- Penetration to the navicular bursa, producing a septic arthritis of the distal interphalangeal joint (Figs. 8–9 and 8–10). In 14 (18.3%) of 76 cows referred for digit amputation, the primary lesion had been white line disease[20]

The abaxial border of the sole is the area of first impact in locomotion, and it absorbs maximum pressure during midstance.[49] Compression of the structures inside the claw, especially at the digital cushion, then results in abaxial expansion and transfer of forces to the wall. This gives rise to mechanical stress and a potential separation of the white line.[4] In pedobarometric studies,[18, 49] high-pressure values were usually recorded in the heel area, abaxial walls, and toes. It has been suggested[53] that weight-bearing by the lateral claw varies more widely with successive movement of the body, whereas loads on the medial claw are more even.

Hard surfaces, soft horn as a result of wet condi-

tions, claw deformities, and laminitis all have been associated with white line disease.[20, 25]

Breakdown of the white line may be related to subclinical laminitis (see Chapter 18). Hemorrhage into the white line may reduce its quality and strength, thereby reducing its integrity. Transmission electron microscopic studies of ultrathin sections of the white line have confirmed the breakdown in horn quality and hemorrhage.[30] Significant sole hemorrhage became apparent about 10 weeks after calving, the period required for the white line and sole horn to grow from the basal layer to the ground surface.

Long distances walked to pasture, wet weather during early lactation, unsuitable materials in track construction, and impatient herding[9, 12] allegedly increase the incidence of the condition.[54]

CLINICAL SIGNS

The lateral claw of the hind digits is usually involved. White line disease frequently involves both hind limbs. If bilateral, the disease may remain unnoticed until lameness is more pronounced in one limb than the other. Because the outer hind claw is affected, the limb is abducted, allowing more weight to be borne by the inner digit. White line separation without complications is frequently seen at claw trimming.

In early uncomplicated cases, claw examination reveals little heat or pain on percussion. In severe cases, the claw is hot and percussion of the wall in the affected area is resented. Coronary sinus formation or separation of heel horn at the heel bulbs may be seen in advanced cases.

Spread of infection to the navicular bursa is accompanied by heel swelling and increased lameness. Further spread of sepsis can involve the distal interpha-

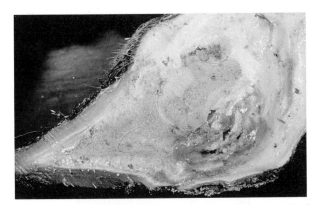

Figure 8–9. Cross section of a digit showing a typical retroarticular infection involving the distal interphalangeal joint, distal sesamoid, and deep flexor tendon. The infection originated at the white line. (Photo courtesy of C. Bergsten, Sweden.)

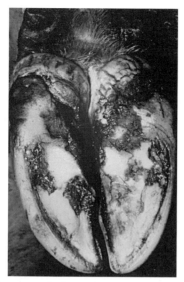

Figure 8–11. An unpared sole in which small stones can be observed embedded in the white line.

langeal joint and can cause erosion of the flexor process of the distal phalanx and necrosis of the deep flexor tendon. Involvement of the deep flexor tendon sheath is uncommon.

DIAGNOSIS

Separation of the wall from the sole is often obvious, but claw examination involves careful paring to expose and excavate any small black areas in the white line that could mask the site of an abscess (Figs. 8–11 and 8–12). In the author's experience, penetration in the toe and axial white line is easily missed. Hoof testers are helpful in locating regions of pain. The original lesion may be partially covered by new horn

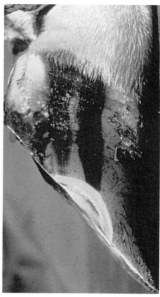

Figure 8–13. A smooth elliptical segment of the abaxial wall can be removed to provide a self-cleansing surface to enable a white line lesion to drain freely.

growth. Involvement of deeper tissues is shown by a painful swelling at the heel and sinus formation. The diagnosis may be confused with lesions such as punctured sole, bruised sole, sole ulcer, and fracture of the distal phalanx.

TREATMENT

Drainage is effected by removing foreign bodies and necrotic debris and creating an opening sufficient to allow the continued flow of pus. It is recommended that both claws be pared and balanced initially. Many small white line defects are removed in this procedure, and the significant lesions become obvious.

The sole should be thinned on either side of the lesion, and heel height reduced. Removal of an ellip-

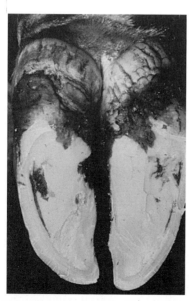

Figure 8–12. The same sole shown in Figure 8–11. After paring, damage to the white line can be seen. The black areas should be carefully explored with a hoof knife.

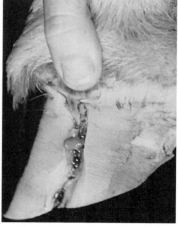

Figure 8–14. A lesion in the white line should be followed throughout its length. In this case, the tract passes the distal interphalangeal joint, from which pus is oozing.

tical segment of the wall adjacent to the lesion aids free drainage by providing a self-cleansing abaxial opening (Fig. 8–13). Opinions on the need to apply a dressing to the exposed corium are divided. An increasing number of veterinarians (including the author) now consider that new horn forms more rapidly in the absence of a dressing. There is a danger that a dressing will physically cause the exposed corium to remain weight-bearing and impede drainage. In a trial to evaluate bandaging in various digital horn diseases,[57] cows with unbandaged feet were significantly less lame 1 week after treatment, but no significant difference was observed at 1 month. A block on the sound claw promotes healing and is recommended for serious cases.

Lesions in the axial white line and toe region often develop a painful protrusion of granulation tissue, which is associated with movement of the sole and side wall caused by destabilization from the defect. This may also indicate that initial paring was insufficient. Resection of the granulation tissue followed by claw blocking should be sufficient to ensure recovery.

Abscessation with sinus formation to the coronary band requires the removal of the abaxial wall throughout the length of the defect (Fig. 8–14). This procedure may be painful, and local anesthesia is required. A plug of necrotic debris is often found in the tract. A sinus located near the bulb usually signals involvement of deeper structures for which resection or amputation may be needed (see Chapter 16). Antibiotic therapy (tetracycline, tylosin, or lincomycin) for 4 to 5 days may be required.

PREVENTION AND CONTROL

It is important to minimize wet and unhygienic conditions. Trim the claws regularly to prevent overgrowth, but avoid trimming when animals must walk long distances. Improve walkways to pasture, gateways, and areas of congestion. Repair or replace damaged or broken concrete surfaces. Allow cows to move at their own pace without bunching. An astringent footbath can be used to harden horn (see Chapter 9).

White Line Disease at the Toe (Toe Ulcer)

Paul R. Greenough

DEFINITION

A hemorrhage or separation of the white line in the toe region (region 1) is considered to be white line disease at the toe.

INCIDENCE

The incidence is sporadic and may be associated with subclinical laminitis.

ETIOLOGY AND PATHOGENESIS

In one study,[26] this phenomenon was thought to be associated with congestion of the circumferential artery in the toe region after sudden introduction to high-energy feed. The increased intraungular pressure was believed to cause depression of the distal phalanx (Fig. 8–15) and rupture of the white line in region 1. During this study, it was noted that each animal that had a dropped sole or rotated digit also had a ridge (the reaction ridge) extending around the wall (Fig. 8–16). The ridge was similar in location to

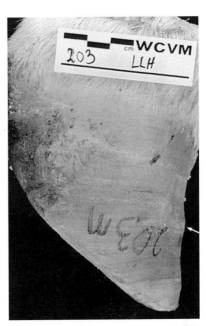

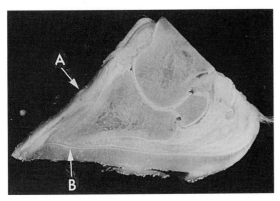

Figure 8–15. Cross section of a digit showing the early stages of digital rotation (B) (sunken sole). Note the reaction ridge at point A.

Figure 8–16. A reaction ridge (arrow) is a slight buildup of horn on the wall extending more or less parallel to the coronary band.

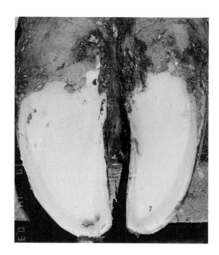

Figure 8–17. A typical early toe ulcer in a recently calved heifer.

Figure 8–18. An advanced toe ulcer in which the tip of the distal phalanx has started to penetrate the sole. (Photo courtesy of K. Mortensen, Denmark.)

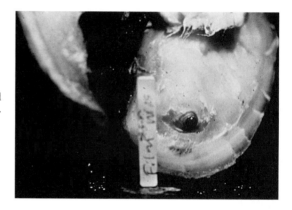

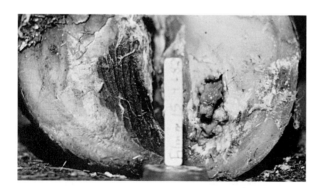

Figure 8–19. A toe ulcer in which the corium has become infected and necrotic. (Photo courtesy of K. Mortensen, Denmark.)

a hardship groove and was displaced distally in a similar manner. The distance from the skin-horn junction to the ridge divided by an appropriate monthly growth rate would indicate the time of the insult. Osteomyelitis of the distal phalanx has been observed[6] in complicated cases of white line disease in the toe region (region 1).

CLINICAL SIGNS

In many cases, the white line in region 1 may only be stained with serum or blood (Fig. 8–17). In more advanced cases, penetration of the sole may take place, with associated infection (Figs. 8–18 and 8–19).

TREATMENT AND CONTROL

Insufficient experience with this phenomenon has generated no reports on treatment; however, it seems rational to provide protection with a methyl methacrylate covering. Control of subclinical laminitis is likely to ameliorate this condition.

Vertical Fissure (Sand Crack)

Paul R. Greenough

DEFINITION

Commonly referred to as a sand crack, a vertical fissure originates as a vertical separation of the periople and horn of the coronary band and extends distally for a variable distance.

LITERATURE

The veterinary literature contains little on the etiology of sand cracks. In one study,[13] it ranked first as the condition causing considerable pain in dairy cows, although the incidence was extremely low. By contrast, in another study,[56] the incidence was found to be extremely high in beef cattle and 2.7% of the animals observed were lame.

INCIDENCE

The incidence of vertical fissure in dairy cows is low; in one study, only 38 of 6901 animals had primary lesions.[13] The incidence could be higher, because the condition may not cause lameness in a dairy cow. The lesion is often obscured by dried manure. In western Canada, the incidence of sand cracks in beef cattle averages 37.2%,[55] with an individual herd variation of 20.5% to 64.3%. The number of cows affected within each farm was markedly different within the same region and did not appear to be related to area or soil moisture content. One western Canadian study[23] reported a 22.7% prevalence of sand cracks in pastured beef cows.

Of 1191 sand cracks recorded in one study,[55] 85.6% were observed in the front lateral claw. These results agree with the 80.6% found in a second investigation.[23] In this last mentioned study, 62% of the affected animals had one sand crack, 29% had two, 5.4% had three, and 3.4% had four or five.

According to Goonewardene and Hand,[23] beef cows with sand cracks were 1.5 years older and were 43 kg heavier and fatter than cows that showed no lesions. They suggested that overconditioning of older breeding cows resulting in higher body weight can increase the risk of sand cracks. Lameness becomes an economic problem when the incidence of sand cracks is high and otherwise productive animals are culled.

ETIOLOGY AND PATHOGENESIS

The lesion commences as one or more fine fissures extending distally across the perioplic corium and the coronary band. Considerable disruption of the structure of the corium occurs beneath the lesion. The fissure may extend distally to the bearing surface on the dorsal wall. The larger cracks usually have ragged edges and may have accumulations of horn on one or both borders. Natural resolution is rare.

The cause of vertical fissures is unknown. There has been speculation about the significance or relative importance of several possible contributory factors including trauma, dehydration, laminitis, and trace element deficiencies.

Historically, it was believed that the disease was caused by factors that dehydrate the claw, such as low humidity and loss of the stratum externum. The term *sand crack* is found in 18th century books on farriery, where it is associated with mechanical damage to the claw.

The high incidence in the lateral foreclaw suggests a possible anatomical component of the etiology. The lateral foreclaws have a significantly larger area of ground contact than the medial claws. The forelimb carries more than half of the body mass.[49] The inclination of the forepastern (which may be heritable[26]) and toe angle is steeper than that of the hind claws. The lesions occur near the center of the dorsal wall of the claw, which is directly over the non-resilient

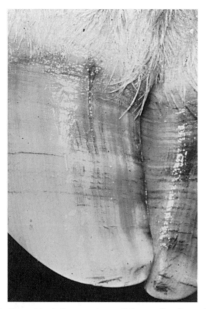

Figure 8–20. A vertical fissure type 1 is confined to the coronary band. This type of lesion is commonly obscured by mud. If it is located abaxial to the extensor process of the distal phalanx, the dorsal pouch of the distal interphalangeal joint is vulnerable to infection. Digital pressure along the coronary band is recommended if the seat of digital lameness is not obvious.

extensor process of the distal phalanx. Because these features are found equally in both affected and non-affected animals, they serve to explain the location of these lesions but are not a predisposing cause.

Sand cracks in beef cattle can occur with several different abnormalities of the claw wall surface. Some changes are reminiscent of chronic laminitis, but other affected claws have distinct stress grooves

(hardship groove, see p. 111). These observations, combined with the consistent finding that the condition is more prevalent in overconditioned beef animals, strongly indicate an underlying nutritional factor.

The role of trace elements in the etiology of claw diseases is not known. Copper and zinc can affect both skin and hair in cattle on a deficient diet. They are essential elements for the growth of good-quality claw horn. The picture can be complicated by low levels of selenium or high levels of molybdenum. The soil pH, the presence of sulfate in drinking water and pasture, or forage legumes also affect the equation. Empirical evidence, based on the sale of large quantities of trace element supplements, suggests they have beneficial results. Supplements should be formulated strategically to meet individual circumstances.

DIAGNOSIS

Sand cracks usually occur on the dorsal surface of a claw where the distal interphalangeal joint is protected by the extensor process. The lesion rarely occurs over the abaxial border of the extensor process, where the dorsal joint pouch is quite superficial. An infected sand crack at this location presents a very high risk of joint infection.

A vertical fissure is categorized as being one of several types:

Type 1. Limited to the coronary band (Fig. 8–20)

Type 2. Skin-horn junction to middle of the claw (Fig. 8–21)

Type 3. Skin-horn junction to distal wall (Fig. 8–22)

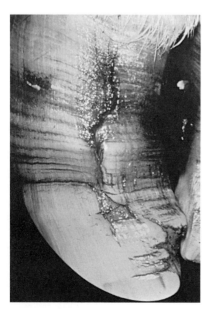

Figure 8–21. A vertical fissure type 2 extends from the skin-horn junction to the middle of the wall. These cracks are frequently associated with deep horizontal fissures. In this case, the horn between the horizontal groove and the skin-horn junction is of poor quality.

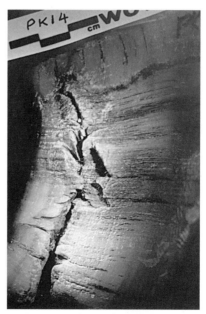

Figure 8–22. A vertical fissure type 3 extends from the skin-horn junction to the bearing surface of the wall.

Type 4. Middle of claw to distal wall

These types probably represent stages in the evolution of a vertical fissure. A type 4 lesion is probably resolving. Lesions are classified in severity from 1 to 3. A type 1 lesion has no separation of the fissure edges. A type 3 lesion is marked by a wide gap with ragged edges, and the corium may be exposed.

Fissures are easy to observe, with the exception of type 1, in which mud often obscures the lesion to the extent that it can lead to failure to make a diagnosis. Palpation along the coronary band is essential when examining the digit. Type 1 sand cracks are most likely to become infected and result in a painful abscess below the horn. Very few of the large fissures cause lameness. However, if the seat of lameness can be traced to a claw with a sand crack, hoof testers should be applied to each edge of the crack throughout its length.

TREATMENT

Most sand cracks in beef cattle are benign and require no treatment. Some type 1 fissures become infected. In these cases, a small wedge of horn should be removed from either edge of the fissure to facilitate drainage. Anesthesia usually is not required for this procedure because the tissue that is removed is already detached. However, the wound should be dressed with an astringent/bacteriostat and pressure applied to reduce granulation tissue production. A very small gauze dressing may be held in place by a 2.5-cm adhesive bandage applied around the coronary band.

Cosmetic treatment using staples and methyl methacrylate to stabilize the fissure may be attempted, but it is doubtful if any intervention will resolve the lesion. If lameness can be traced to the limb in which a large (type 3) sand crack is present, it is wise to trim the edges of the fissure to remove debris and foreign bodies from its depth. To minimize movement of a large fissure during weight-bearing, the axial portion of the toe should be removed.

The possibly beneficial effect of biotin on claw horn quality has attracted much attention. Although the rumen synthesizes adequate quantities of this vitamin, biotin demand increases during periods of stress, and the blood levels for biotin found in lame cows are lower than in normal animals.

CONTROL

The control of vertical fissures is of major concern only in beef herds with a high incidence (more than 35% of adults affected). Although successful control measures have not been reported, some recommendations may be made:

- Estimate the body condition score, particularly in the spring. Above average weight may predispose to fissures. Some producers feel obliged to "flush" their stock before the breeding season, despite their excellent condition.

- Examine the claws of at least half of the mature animals. If a hardship groove is present, measure its distance from the horn-skin junction on the dorsal surface of the claw. Because the claw *at this point* grows at 2.5 mm/month, calculate the approximate date of the insult and determine any management changes at that time.

- Investigate the potential role of trace elements.[5]

Horizontal Grooves and Fissures

Paul R. Greenough

DEFINITION

A horizontal groove (known in lay terms as a *hardship groove*) is a depression of varying depth extending parallel to the rugae around the axial and abaxial walls of the claw. A horizontal fissure (known in lay terms as a *thimble*) is a complete breach of the wall of the claw in a plane parallel to the rugae.

INCIDENCE AND LITERATURE

Westra[56] reports that 0.8% of the beef cattle that he examined had horizontal fissures. In another study,[10] 2.05% of 245 lame cows examined had horizontal fissures.

ETIOLOGY AND PATHOGENESIS

Horizontal Groove. A horizontal (hardship) groove is indicative of stress such as a sudden nutritional change. For example, the weaning groove in beef calves forms when the animals are subjected to a number of stresses, including transportation, market, dehorning, vaccination, and the different ration of the feedlot.

Grooves are usually painless. They are important to clinicians as a temporal indicator of stress. In beef cattle, the dorsal claw wall normally grows at a rate of 2.5 mm/month but grows faster in winter and in intensively fed cattle. Dairy cows may generate wall horn at the heel at a rate of 5 to 6 mm/month. This phenomenon is an excellent tool for calculating the date of an insult. The distance from the skin-horn

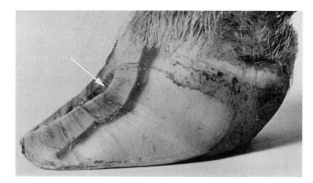

Figure 8–23. A buckled toe (arrow). A series of minor stresses cause a fault line, at which the dorsal wall of the claw bends and becomes concave.

Figure 8–24. A thimble is produced from a very deep horizontal groove that partially breaks when the groove has been displaced by growth to a point more than halfway along the dorsal wall. The thimble causes considerable pain when the attached fragment moves during locomotion. (Photo courtesy of K. Mortensen, Denmark.)

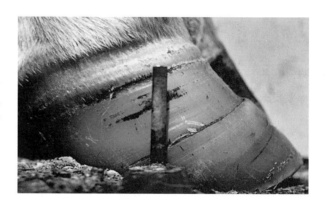

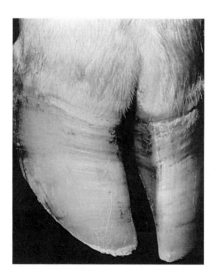

Figure 8–25. The claw of a young beef bull 3 months after weaning. The distal horn was produced before weaning and indicates that management and nutrition before weaning were good. The horn closest to the coronary band reflects the animal's inability to adapt to intensive feeding during a 3-month period.

Figure 8–26. The claws of a beef steer with good-quality horn distal to the hardship groove. This indicates favorable preweaning conditions. The length and quality of the proximal band of the claw horn are suggestive of a very inadequate growing ration.

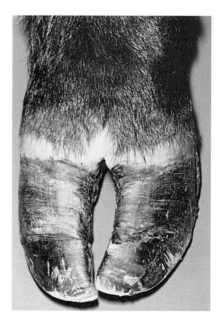

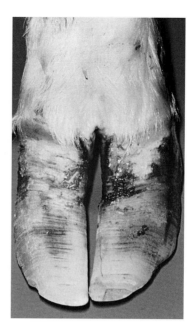

Figure 8–27. The claw of a steer fed barley and straw. The horn distal to the groove is of defective quality, indicating relatively poor nutrition before weaning. This type of appearance is most commonly observed in a beef calf suckling a poorly milking cow, a cow with a three-quarter udder, or a heifer. The horn closest to the coronary band is also poor and reflects the quality of nutrition during the finishing period.

junction to the groove is measured, and the resultant figure is divided by the appropriate monthly growth rate.

As a groove moves distally, it becomes a fault line. Bearing pressure exerted on the apex of the toe may cause the claw to bend (buckling of the claw) at the fault line, causing concavity of the dorsal wall (Fig. 8–23). The toe eventually fractures at the fault; a so-called broken toe results.

Horizontal Fissures (Thimbles). Horizontal fissures are uncommon and are caused by a serious systemic insult as a result of which horn production at the coronary band ceases altogether for a short time. When horn growth resumes, the fissure moves distally until the distal portion of the claw is only loosely attached. At this stage, the condition is extremely painful because the distal section of the claw is hinged at the fissure, which causes the underlying sensitive tissues to be traumatized. This mobile distal section of horn is often called a *thimble* (Fig. 8–24). Horizontal fissures result from any serious febrile disease. They are a characteristic clinical sign of foot-and-mouth disease. Horizontal fissures usually affect all eight claws similarly.

CLINICAL SIGNS

A hardship groove often marks a time at which nutritional changes have taken place. In a beef calf, the horn produced distal to the groove represents the period when the calf was with the cow. The quality of the horn may reflect the milking capacity of the dam. The quality of the horn proximal to the groove reflects the ability of the animal to adapt to its new environment or changed nutrition (Figs. 8–25, 8–26, and 8–27).

At the acute thimbling stage, an affected animal is in pain whenever it bears weight. When standing, it moves agitatedly. It may lie down for prolonged periods. The presence of the fissures is obvious on inspection.

TREATMENT

Pain from a thimble can be relieved by removing the section of the toe distal to the fissure, thus reducing movement of the loose wall during locomotion. Because the procedure is extremely painful, it is advisable to administer a regional nerve block. The horn is removed with shears or an electric cutter.

CONTROL

Horizontal fissures are uncommon and warrant no special control measures.

Traumatic Injuries to the Sole

Donald W. Collick

DEFINITION

The horn and corium of the sole can be damaged by wear or a foreign body. A foreign body may be a sharp stone, a piece of glass, a nail, a fragment of metal, the sharp roots of a cast molar tooth,[7] or any other sharp material capable of penetrating the sole or heel.

INCIDENCE

Penetration of the sole by a foreign body is usually sporadic and is primarily dependent on the condition of the roadways or the accidental presence of materials that can penetrate the sole. In one study,[45] 3.6% of the cases of lameness in 5854 cows examined was caused by a foreign body in the sole, and another 10.7% of the animals had a punctured sole with pus. Another study[10] found that 8.6% of 245 lame cows had septic pododermatitis. Eddy and Scott[19] reported that 20.4% of 1256 lame cows had a pricked sole and 4.8% had a foreign body.

Generalized bruising of the sole can occur if the sole is worn thin or has been subjected to excessive paring. Eddy and Scott[19] found that 1.2% of their lameness cases involved an overworn sole. In another study,[13] 12.7% of the cases resulted from bruising of the sole.

PATHOGENESIS

Localized pressure from a foreign body embedded in the sole but not penetrating through it causes pain and damages the sensitive tissues. If the condition is not rapidly relieved, focal necrosis may occur, and pain increases as an abscess develops.

The distal interphalangeal joint is not directly vulnerable to foreign bodies, although nails have been known to penetrate through the axial groove and enter the joint.

Predisposing factors for solar penetration include the following:

- Conditions that soften the horn or sole; excessive moisture or laminitis
- Excessively worn soles from walking long distances or the abrasive effect of newly laid concrete
- Foreign body risk: sharp aggregate in roadways and gateways and around water troughs[9, 22]
- Driving animals too forcefully along rough roads or tracks[9, 12]

CLINICAL SIGNS

A foreign body that penetrates the sole usually causes lameness that increases in intensity owing to rapid accumulation of pus. The onset of lameness is usually rapid and the pain intense if the penetration occurs in region 5, because the infection is trapped between the arch of the distal phalanx and the sole. In this case, the pain can only be compared with that of fracture of the distal phalanx. In very acute cases involving the lateral claw, the animal abducts the limb; if the medial foreclaw is involved, the limbs may be crossed. The animal may become recumbent and anorexic, erroneously presenting a clinical picture suggestive of a systemic disease.

Beneath the bulb, the horn is flexible and the digital cushion resilient. Therefore, penetration of the sole in region 6 produces a less acute lameness. In these cases, pus often escapes at the skin-horn junction of the bulb, where separation of the sole can be observed (Fig. 8–28).

Generalized bruising occurs when the sole is abnormally thin. The sole depresses easily under thumb pressure, and dark clots of blood are visible through the sole (Fig. 8–29). The blood observed in cases of subclinical laminitis stains the sole pink, and the sole is relatively resilient. Blood and serum from the damaged tissues separate the keratogenic layers from the sole, and a new sole develops. In some cases, if the wear has made the horn extremely fragile, the sole is repeatedly traumatized until the corium is exposed, damaged, infected, or eroded. This condition affects all claws similarly; therefore, the gait is abnormal, although a specific limb lameness may not be identified.

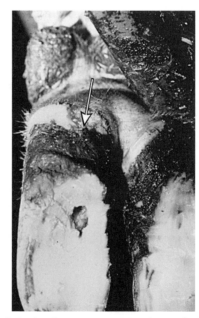

Figure 8–28. Infection from a penetrating foreign body in the heel region causes the sole to separate from the keratogenic layers. The skin-bulb junction (arrow) is no longer attached.

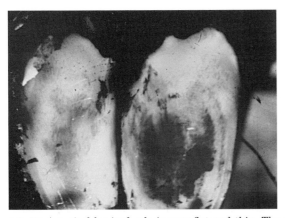

Figure 8–29. A typical bruised sole is very flat and thin. The sole depresses easily on pressure and causes the animal pain. Dark blue-black blood clots are usually visible through the horn of the sole.

DIAGNOSIS/DIFFERENTIAL DIAGNOSIS

Wash and dry, dry brush, or clean the sole with sawdust or shavings. Using the back (blunt) edge of a search knife, carefully scrape across the sole to remove or locate any remaining foreign bodies (stones) that would blunt the knife. Remove a thin slice of sole to reveal a clean surface. Often all that remains is a black tract or blemish. Each mark in the sole should be explored. Hoof testers may aid diagnosis by pinpointing areas of localized sensitivity.

Diagnosis may be confused by acute lameness caused by distal phalangeal fracture, white line disease, interdigital phlegmon, and horizontal and vertical horn fissures.

TREATMENT

A subsolar abscess should be opened with a fine-pointed hoof knife. The hook on the tip of the knife should be sharpened with a fine chain saw file. Each blemish in the surface of the sole should be explored by rotating the tip of the knife to produce a conical incision. Once pus has been released, further exposure of the lesion is usually contraindicated because the larger the opening the more prone it is to contamination. Intraungular pressure usually seals the opening quite rapidly, making an external dressing unnecessary. Intramammary antibiotics may be injected into the opening. Resolution is usually un-

eventful. Extensive undermining of the sole should be pared away.

Cattle with extensively bruised soles should be confined for 1 month in a deeply bedded loose box or straw yard. If the remaining sole is damaged, a protective device such as a plastic shoe (shoof) or boot may be applied.

If the sole is completely absent, the animal may have to be slaughtered on humane grounds. In some cases, an attempt may be made to salvage such an animal by applying a prosthetic sole (see Chapter 9).

At the site of penetration, an osteomyelitis of the distal phalanx may occasionally develop. If this fails to resolve even after local curettage, drainage, and prolonged use of antibiotics, claw amputation needs to be considered.

CONTROL

Control measures are aimed at avoiding the precipitating factors. In the United Kingdom, many tracks were designed to allow machinery access to pasture. Consideration needs to be given to the construction of tracks specifically for cattle.[22] Such tracks require good drainage, a firm non-abrasive base, a soft surface, and an adequate maintenance program. Similarly, gateways and areas around drinking troughs require attention.

Concrete surfaces must be kept free of loose stone material, which may be carried there by machinery or cattle, with regular cleaning or brushing. Construction material must be kept away from stock walk areas. Chalk bedding base material should be flint free.

When new concrete is being prepared, smooth stone should be used in the aggregate. It should be tamped mechanically to ensure that the stone is sufficiently covered by "fines." Before use, smooth out the surface with a slurry scraper and power clean. The initial surface is extremely abrasive to the sole, making the claw more vulnerable to penetration.

Newly surfaced public roads, because of the size of the surface chips, sometimes pose a special hazard and can result in a herd outbreak of lameness due to solar penetration from walking four times daily over such material.[24]

Trimming inevitably reduces sole thickness and must be avoided when animals have to walk long distances to pasture. Sufficient sole thickness must be left to allow for greater protection (>5 mm), or conversely, trim at "drying off," when cattle have a rest period from walking tracks.

Traumatic Exungulation

Paul R. Greenough

DEFINITION

Traumatic exungulation is defined as loss of the entire horny claw.

PATHOGENESIS

An affected animal usually has accidentally caught its limb in some object such as a gate, fence, or farmyard equipment and torn off the claw in its struggling. It also occurs as a severe complication of fescue foot when cattle are transported or subjected to conditions where their movements are uncontrolled. It is occasionally encountered in lateral hind claws of very heavy bulls with relatively small claws.

TREATMENT

In some instances, the claw may not have become completely detached (Fig. 8–30). Regional anesthesia should be administered. The space between the capsule and claw should be examined for debris, which should be removed by a jet of water under moderate pressure. If the area can be cleansed, the claw should not be removed because it provides ideal protection for the germinal layers to produce a new claw. Topical antibiotics may be applied; then the entire digit should be enclosed in a fiberglass cast for several weeks unless signs of increasing discomfort are seen. On removal of the cast, the affected claw will usually have become detached, and healing will have taken place. Casting should be repeated because generation of adequate horn protection by the coronary band requires several months.

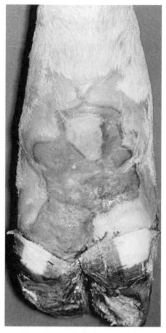

Figure 8–30. This animal caught its extremity in a gate, causing a serious skin defect. The claws were partially torn away. Treatment consisted of enclosing the digits in a cast for 1 month while a new horn capsule replaced the old one, which eventually dropped off.

If the claw capsule has been completely detached, secondary damage to the digital structures is usually severe. If adequate viable tissue (75% of the corium) is visible, the claw should be dressed with antibiotic-impregnated petroleum jelly gauze and bandaged. A wooden or rubber block must be applied to the sound claw. A methyl methacrylate prosthesis can be applied (see p. 137).

Heel Horn Erosion

Donald W. Collick

DEFINITION

Heel horn erosion is defined as irregular loss of bulbar horn in the form of multiple pitlike depressions or deep oblique grooves.

LITERATURE AND INCIDENCE

Heel horn erosion (slurry heel, erosio ungulae) is a benign condition of older animals exposed to an unhygienic moist environment. Very few mature dairy cows that are intensively managed do not have some erosive lesions in their heels. However, the condition can predispose the heel region to complications that do cause lameness. In one study,[13] 6.5% of the diagnoses made involved heel horn erosion; in another,[10] 11.84%. The majority of the lesions occurred in the first 6 months of the year (winter and spring). In a French survey[44] conducted during the winter housing period, heel horn erosion was the most common lesion found (55%), but in only 11% of those cases was it the primary cause of lameness. In a study of 17 United States herds,[21] the condition was found in 44% of animals in first lactation and 69% of animals in later lactations.

ETIOLOGY AND PATHOGENESIS

Toussaint Raven[53] considered that *Bacteroides nodosus*, which is allegedly the cause of interdigital dermatitis, is also involved in the etiology of heel horn erosion. *B. nodosus* is the predominant and often only bacterial invader of skin and cornified epithelium of the claw. The pili of *B. nodosus* help maintain the commensalism of the bacterium, while its proteases damage the horn. In chronic infections, the epidermal infection spreads from the interdigital skin to the bulbs of the heel, resulting in pits in the bulbar epidermis (Fig. 8–31). The pits eventually coalesce to form linear black fissures of varying depth in the bulbar epidermis and, if severely involved, the heel horn (Fig. 8–32). The fissures always course posteriorly in an axial to abaxial direction.[29]

High concentrations of cattle increase the likelihood of heel horn erosion owing to high levels of pathogens in the environment. Warm, humid conditions favor its development. After destruction of the heel horn, a compensatory proliferation of horn can occur in the sole region directly anterior to erosion. This wedge of abnormal horn causes pressure on the corium (contusion), which becomes inflamed and painful. The balance of the claw is disturbed (see Chapter 9). The heel, denuded of horn, then becomes vulnerable to secondary infection.

Observation of experimentally produced laminitis in beef steers[26] revealed episodes of hemorrhage producing layering of hemorrhages in the sole. Each layer was observed to end in a groove identical to that in heel horn erosion (Fig. 8–33).

CLINICAL SIGNS

Lameness is not a clinical sign of uncomplicated heel horn erosion; therefore, the presence of the condition

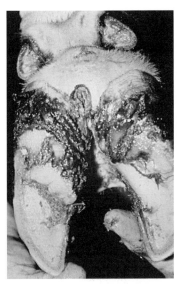

Figure 8–32. Typical heel erosion showing easily recognizable ridges. In this case, evidence of a concurrent interdigital dermatitis is present, affecting the interdigital skin between the bulbs.

is not known until the digit is elevated and examined. The lesions vary widely from light grooving to deep V-shaped channels running diagonally across the heel. Loss of horn tends to be greatest in the axial part of the heels. Long-term chronic advanced cases are marked by an extremely ragged and fragmented heel horn.

The heel horn fissuring may conceal other lesions such as sole ulcers and white line disease near the abaxial wall and sole junction. Necrotic laminitis occasionally occurs if the heel horn has completely separated from the corium. Although all four feet can be affected, the hind feet, especially the lateral claws, tend to be more frequently involved.

Sequelae to chronic extensive heel erosion include sole ulcer, sole abscess, white line disease, and complete heel loss (Fig. 8–34).

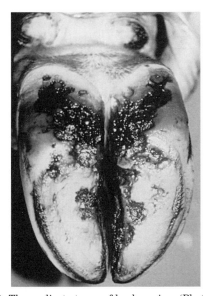

Figure 8–31. The earliest stages of heel erosion. (Photo courtesy of Roger Blowey, United Kingdom.)

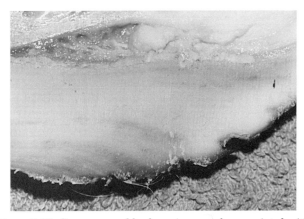

Figure 8–33. Some cases of heel erosion may be associated with subclinical laminitis. In this cross section of the heel, layers of blood in the sole end at the heel grooves are typical of heel erosion.

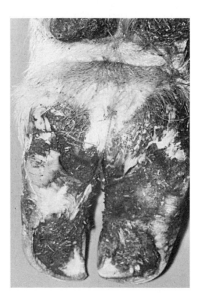

Figure 8–34. Complete heel loss is one sequela of severe heel erosion. In this case, the balance of the digit is seriously disturbed.

DIAGNOSIS/DIFFERENTIAL DIAGNOSIS

Heel erosions have a very characteristic appearance, but this may be confused with the sequelae of a sole abscess deep to the horn, caudal to the sole-heel junction. In such cases, pus causes the heel to separate from the underlying corium as a single flap of heel horn. Heel erosion is commonly present when another lesion is the actual cause of lameness—for example, sole ulceration.

TREATMENT

Pare excess horn to obliterate deep grooves in uncomplicated heel horn erosions. If a steep wedge of horn has accumulated on the sole slightly anterior to the heel, this should be shaped with a hoof knife to slope toward the abaxial wall (Fig. 8–35). Both hooves should be equally high for correct weight-bearing.

In addition to paring, clean and dress with an astringent or antibacterial spray. Keep affected animals on clean bedding for several days while the exposed horn hardens.

CONTROL

Attention to hygiene and reduction of slurry are important control measures. Regularly trimming the claws of dairy cows twice yearly is very helpful, but trimming itself has been shown to be a high-risk factor.[21] Cows that had their claws trimmed in the period from July to December and that calved from March to October were more likely to develop heel erosion.

Weekly footbaths (3% to 5% formalin) during the winter months, commencing in the late fall, harden the claw horn and limit the progression of heel horn erosion.[3, 17, 50]

The use of lime in cubicles to reduce the incidence of mastitis has been suggested,[6] and it may also decrease heel erosion. Provision of cubicles of sufficient length, allowing cows to stand up in their cubicle rather than with their back feet in the gutter, may also help. A period of summer grazing allows the heels to recover and to form again.

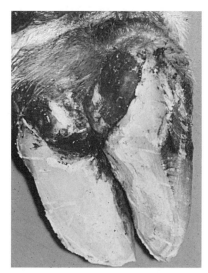

Figure 8–35. The buildup of horn in the heel region may result in a ridge of horn that presses on the sensitive tissues to cause pain. To correct this, the horn should be sloped to the abaxial wall, which must be lowered to an appropriate depth. Failure to do this results in abnormal pressure placed on the region of the digital cushion.

Interdigital Hyperplasia

Donald W. Collick

DEFINITION

Interdigital hyperplasia (hyperplasia interdigitalis) is a proliferative reaction of the interdigital skin or subcutaneous tissue to form a firm mass, which occupies part or all of the interdigital space. It has been variously referred to as *corns, interdigital granuloma, limax, fibroma, tyloma,* and *wart.*

INCIDENCE

The condition is usually sporadic but is common in certain breeds such as the Hereford. Cirlan[11] quotes 80% of affected bulls as having interdigital skin hyperplasia in their antecedents. Dairy cattle surveys[13, 44, 47] indicate an incidence of approximately 4% in examined lame cattle. Enevoldsen and colleagues[21] recorded a frequency of less than 1% in first lactation, rising to nearly 6% in later lactations. Rowlands and associates[45] show a significant decrease in incidence in the summer and a greater incidence associated with winter cubicle housing.

ETIOLOGY/PATHOGENESIS

Interdigital skin hyperplasia is caused by chronic irritation or dermatitis in the interdigital region. This may result from protracted mild interdigital dermatitis and heel erosion or may be a chronic sequela of interdigital phlegmon.[8, 21, 53] Irritation by slurry may aid these effects. A high incidence of the condition has been observed where slurry is removed from free stalls by automatic scrapers. Claws are often drier, but the movement of the scrapers tends to coat the claws with a layer of slurry, which eventually builds up to encase the whole claw.

The lesion is a protuberance of skin in the interdigital space (Fig. 8–36). When large, it appears to originate from the middle of the space and is frequently in the dorsal half of the cleft. Vaughan and Osman, cited by Greenough and colleagues,[24] found that the lesion generally started at the axial aspect of the lateral digit, rarely on the medial digit. Szalay, also quoted by Greenough and associates,[24] histologically found a subacute or chronic inflammatory process, with hyperkeratosis, parakeratosis, and superimposed secondary damage (wounds, pressure necrosis, splitting of the keratinized layer, and local infection). Both epidermal and dermal tissue may have a combined thickness of about four times normal (i.e., 16 mm compared with 4 mm).

Skin hyperkeratinization starting in the dorsal interdigital region with hyperplasia has been observed as early as age 8 to 12 months.[8]

Interdigital hyperplasia forms between the two digits as a pseudotumorous fibrous mass, covered in hyperkeratinized epidermis, barely sensitive to pain. Advanced cases present more proliferative centers with desquamation of epidermis and ulcerative necrotic lesions, caused by trauma and the large size of the lesion. The highly vascularized fibrous tissue contained granulomas, some of which involved hair follicles. A superficial caseous purulent exudate is often present. Microbial cultures from the granulomas grew mixed fungi or actinomycetes. *B. nodosus* was isolated in about half the lesions.

Considerable confusion surrounds the possible role of inheritance.[14] Stretching of the distal interphalangeal ligament is implicated in the etiology of this condition. This results in excessive spreading of the distal phalanges, which in turn stretches the interdigital skin. *Splay toes* (German *Spreizklauen*) is related to interdigital hyperplasia. It involves abnormal separation of the claws at the toes and excessively wide and folded interdigital skin. Affected bulls are rejected for breeding.

In older animals, skin hyperplasia arises as a lesion secondary to chronic infection or localized irritation in the area.

CLINICAL SIGNS

Interdigital skin hyperplasia is more common in the hind limbs than the forelimbs and may be unilateral or bilateral. A bilateral or quadrilateral lesion is suspicious of a primary inherited condition, particularly if observed in an animal younger than 2 years.

The degree of lameness depends on the size and situation of the lesion, the degree of infection, and stress placed on the affected digit. Simple small lesions producing no mechanical interference cause lit-

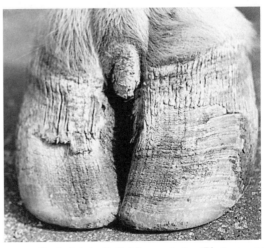

Figure 8–36. Typical interdigital hyperplasia. (Photo courtesy of Vet Medicine VFU, Orthopedic Clinic, Brno, Czech Republic.)

tle or no lameness. Many moderate-sized lesions (1 to 2 cm wide, 2 cm deep) may persist for years without resulting in lameness. Larger lesions with infection, ulceration, and necrosis result in more severe lameness. In untreated cases, infection and necrosis may eventually extend deeper. Surfaces in contact with the axial wall are often moist and exudative owing to slight pressure necrosis, and they have the typical odor. The distal surface is particularly likely to become traumatized by impact with the ground.

TREATMENT

In simple cases, treatment may be unnecessary, but the digits should be trimmed and balanced with special attention to the axial walls, to allow more space for the lesion.[8, 53] Modeling or dishing of the sole in the middle third to produce a concavity extending to the axial border allows improved self-cleaning. Systemic antibiotics plus thorough cleansing and topical antibacterial spray aid control of secondary infection. Application of local caustic agents (silver nitrate, copper sulfate) is appropriate to treat small lesions. Larger lesions, especially those associated with clinical lameness, require resection.

Invasive therapy includes knife surgery, electrocautery, or cryosurgery.[55]

- Administer a sedative (xylazine or acepromazine) and restrain in lateral recumbency or in a crush in the paring stance.

- Administer local analgesia by intravenous regional anesthesia, nerve block, or local infiltration.

- Cleanse the area thoroughly and disinfect it. Apply a tourniquet. Use a retractor or an assistant to separate the digits.

- Grasp the protruding mass with Allis tissue forceps or Backhaus towel forceps.

- Remove the entire mass in a wedge-shaped pattern by making two longitudinal incisions, leaving a small margin of skin by the axial coronary band. Remove any protruding interdigital fat with blunt scissors, avoiding the distal cruciate ligaments.

- Apply a topical antibacterial powder (e.g., oxytetracycline).

- Wire the toes together through drill holes to prevent separation of the two claws. Bandage the two claws together tightly (wiring toes together may not be necessary when using a tight elastic bandage). The bandage may be further protected by placing a polythene bag over the extremity and covering it with a second elastic bandage. Change the dressing in 5 days.

- Systemic antibiotics should not be necessary.

The lesion heals in about 3 weeks.

As an alternative to knife surgery, an electrocautery knife may be used with the advantage of reduced intraoperative and postoperative hemorrhage.

Cryosurgery may also be used to remove the hyperplastic skin.[36] Applying a tourniquet keeps the heat of the arterial blood out of the fibromatous tissue, improving the efficiency of cryosurgical treatment. The cryospray needle is placed in the middle of the growth, passing through in a longitudinal direction. Freezing is continued until the whole growth is visibly frozen (5 minutes). The needle is withdrawn, and a flexible mandrin is inserted and left in the channel during a 10- to 15-minute thawing period. A second freezing cycle is carried out similarly. Remove the tourniquet 15 minutes after the second freezing process. The cryosurgically treated lesion is sloughed after about 2 weeks, and a wound filled with granulation tissue appears.

An open cryoprobe spray system may be used, in which case the lesion may require some initial debulking.

PREVENTION

Simple isolated cases in adult cows due to secondary factors respond well to surgical treatment. When genetic studies have not been performed, an attempt must be made to establish the inheritance of the condition. Affected animals shown to have a genetic defect should not be used for breeding purposes.

Attention to foot hygiene may prevent the early development of secondary infections in existing lesions. To avoid the buildup of crusted slurry firmly dried on the claws, the times and frequency of automatic scraping have been changed, with good effect, from eight to four times daily—twice while the cattle are milked and at midday and midnight, when the cows tend to be resting.

Traumatic Injuries to the Interdigital Space

A. David Weaver

DEFINITION

Damage to the interdigital space can be caused by materials similar to those traumatizing the sole (see p. 114).

INCIDENCE

The diagnosis of interdigital foreign body accounted for 2.2% of the lesions causing lameness in British dairy cows.[47] Lesions were equally distributed between fore and hind limbs. This incidence is low compared with punctured sole and pus (9.2%, 80% being in hind claws), white line abscess (13.8%, 85%, respectively), and foul in the foot (or interdigital phlegmon, 14.7%, 75%).

ETIOLOGY

During weight-bearing, the dorsal aspect of the interdigital space opens as the skin stretches while the palmar/plantar section remains relatively closed and may even be compressed by the digital cushion. The interdigital space is considerably farther from the ground dorsally (5 cm) than between the heels (3 cm). The thickness of the interdigital skin averages approximately 4 mm.

Conformation plays a part in that a decreased fetlock angle (dropped, overextended fetlock) tends to bring the palmar/plantar interdigital space closer to the ground and potentially make it more liable to trauma. The same circumstances result from a low heel, which may be either congenital or acquired after heel horn erosion.

The interdigital space is considered to be self-cleansing as a result of regular changes in its shape. When the claws are lifted, the space becomes constricted from side to side, and momentarily impacted material tends to be squeezed out. At pasture, movement of grass stems also cleans the space.

Foreign bodies may lacerate or even puncture the surface skin. With lacerations, there is a greater chance that the foreign body will remain in the interdigital space. Also, the narrowness of the volar interdigital space between the heels means that a self-retaining action is more likely, especially if irregular objects such as stones become impacted.

CLINICAL SIGNS

The onset of lameness is usually sudden, but the degree (lameness score) variable. Sometimes the animal, usually a cow, shakes the limb when the foreign body (e.g., twig, stone) is still lodged. When only mild

trauma has resulted, the condition often resolves spontaneously.

Careful visual inspection and palpation of the interdigital space are essential in all cases of suspected digital lameness.

DIFFERENTIAL DIAGNOSIS

The clinical signs may be similar to those of other common interdigital disease such as ulceration, dermatitis, and phlegmon. Infectious diseases (foot-and-mouth disease, bovine virus diarrhea/mucosal disease [BVD/MD] complex) must always be borne in mind, especially when several animals become lame (see Table 7–1).

TREATMENT AND CONTROL

Any foreign body should be removed, and deep perforations should be explored for any residual foreign body then irrigated with a dilute organic iodide solution (e.g., 0.5% povidone-iodine [Betadine]). Any partly detached tissue should be resected. Cattle that have localized swelling and cellulitis should be given systemic antibiotics (see p. 93).

Cows with interdigital trauma should have limited exercise on dry bedding (e.g., straw yard) for a week to provide optimal healing conditions. Those that fail to respond within 48 hours (reduced lameness and swelling) should undergo a second careful examination.

REFERENCES

1. Andersson L, Lundstrom K: The influence of breed, age, body weight and season on digital disease and hoof size in dairy cows. Zentralbl Veterinaermed A28:141–151, 1981.
2. Arkins S: Lameness in dairy cows. Part II. Ir Vet J 35:163–170, 1981.
3. Arkins S, Hannan J, Sherington J: Effect of formalin footbathing on foot disease and claw quality in dairy cows. Vet Rec 118:580–583, 1986.
4. Baggott DG, Russell AM: Lameness in cattle. Br Vet J 137:113–132, 1981.
5. Blood DC, Radostits OM, Henderson JA: Veterinary Medicine, 6th ed. London, England, Baillière Tindall, 1983.
6. Blowey RW: Diseases of the bovine digit. Part 2: Hoofcare and factors influencing the incidence of lameness. In Pract 14:118–124, 1992.
7. Blowey RW: Cattle lameness and hoofcare. Ipswich, England: Farming Press, 1993, p 75.
8. Bolte S, Decun M, Igna C, et al: Aetiopathogenesis of interdigital lesions in cattle. Proceedings of the 6th International Symposium on Diseases of the Ruminant Digit. Liverpool, UK, 1990, pp 255–257.
9. Chesterton RN, Pfeiffer DU, Morris RS, Tanner CM: Environmental and behavior factors affecting the prevalance of foot lameness in New Zealand dairy herds on case control study. N Z Vet J 37:131–142, 1989.

10. Choquette-Levy L, Baril J, Levy M, St-Pierre H: A study of foot disease of dairy cattle in Quebec. Can Vet J 26:278–281, 1985.
11. Cirlan M: Risk factors for pododermatitis in bulls for AI. Proceedings of the 6th International Symposium on Diseases of the Ruminant Digit. Liverpool, UK, 1990, pp 262–268.
12. Clackson DA, Ward WR: The effect of farm tracks and attendants patience on the incidence of summer lameness in dairy cows. Proc BCVA 1991, pp 425–434.
13. Clarkson MJ, Downham DY, Faull WB, et al: An epidemiological study to determine the risk factors of lameness in dairy cows. (University of Liverpool, Faculty of Veterinary Science, CSA 1379), 1993.
14. Colam-Ainsworth P, Lunn GA, Thomas RC, Eddy RG: Behavior of cows in cubicles and its possible relationship with laminitis in replacement heifers. Vet Rec 125:573–575, 1989.
15. Collick DW: Applied techniques for diagnosis of lameness. Proceedings of the 6th International Symposium on Diseases of the Ruminant Digit. Liverpool, UK, 1990, pp 103–106.
16. Collick DW, Ward WR, Dobson H: Associations between types of lameness and fertility. Vet Rec 125:103–106, 1989.
17. Davies RC: Effects of regular formalin footbaths on the incidence of foot lameness in dairy cattle. Vet Rec 111:394, 1982.
18. Distl O, Mair A: Pedobarometric forces at the sole/floor interface. Proceedings of the 6th International Symposium on Diseases of the Ruminant Digit. Liverpool, UK, 1990.
19. Eddy RG, Scott CP: Some observations on the incidence of lameness in dairy cattle in Somerset. Vet Rec 106:140–144, 1980.
20. Edwards GB: White line disease of the foot in cattle. Vet Annu 20:227–232, 1980.
21. Enevoldsen C, Grohn YT, Thysen I: Heel erosion and other interdigital disorders in dairy cows: Association with season, cow characteristics, disease and production. J Dairy Sci 74:1299–1309, 1991.
22. Faull WB, Hughes JW: A study of walking surfaces and their association with cow lameness. Cattle Pract 1(4):344–359, 1993.
23. Goonewardene LA, Hand RK: A study of hoof cracks in grazing cows—association with age, weight and fatness. Can J Anim Sci 75:25–29, 1995.
24. Greenough PR, MacCallum FJ, Weaver AD: Lameness in cattle, 2nd ed. Bristol, UK, John Wright & Sons, 1981.
25. Greenough PR, Vermunt JJ: Evaluation of subclinical laminitis and associated lesions in dairy cattle. Proceedings of the 6th International Symposium of diseases of the Ruminant Digit. Liverpool, UK, 1990, pp 45–54.
26. Greenough PR, Vermunt JJ, McKinnon JJ, et al: Laminitis-like changes in the claws of feedlot cattle. Can Vet J 31:202–208, 1991.
27. Hahn MV, McDaniel BT, Wilk JC: Rates of hoof growth and wear in Holstein cattle. J Dairy Sci 69:2148–2156, 1986.
28. Jubb TF, Malmo J: Lesions causing lameness requiring veterinary treatment in pasture-fed dairy cows in E. Gippsland. Aust Vet J 61:21–24, 1991.
29. Kasari TR, Scanlon CM: Bovine contagious interdigital dermatitis: A review. Southwest Vet 38(2):33–36, 1987.
30. Kempson SA, Logue DW: Ultrastructural observations of hoof horn from dairy cows. Changes in the white line during first lactation. Vet Rec 132:524–527, 1993.
31. Livesey CT, Flemming FL: Nutritional influences in laminitis, sole ulcer and bruised sole in Friesian cows. Vet Rec 114:510–512, 1994.
32. Maclean CW: The long term effects of laminitis in dairy cows. Vet Rec 89:34–37, 1971.
33. Manson FJ, Leaver JD: The influence of concentrate amount on the locomotion and clinical lameness in dairy cattle. Anim Prod 47:185–190, 1988.
34. McDaniel BT, Wilk JC: Breeding to reduce lameness in dairy cattle. Proceedings of the 6th International Symposium on Disorders of the Ruminant Digit. Liverpool, UK, 1990, pp 64–65.
35. McLennan MW: Incidence of lameness requiring veterinary treatment in Queensland. Aust Vet J 65:171–176, 1988.
36. Menzel A: Cryosurgical treatment of interdigital fibromas under field conditions. Supplementary Paper to the 6th International Symposium on Diseases of the Ruminant Digit. Liverpool. Proc BCVA 1990, pp 98–102.
37. Moldovan M, Bolte S, Igna C: Radiological research on phalangeal changes in pododermatitis circumscripta in cattle. Proceedings of the 6th International Symposium on Diseases of the Ruminant Digit. Liverpool, UK, 1990, pp 269–275.
38. Murray RD, Singh SS, Ward WR: Pathophysiology of lameness in dairy cattle. Cattle Pract 1,4:322–331, 1993.
39. Nilsson SA: Clinical, morphological and experimental studies of laminitis in cattle. Acta Vet Scand 41(Suppl 1):9–304, 1963.
40. Nilsson SA: Recent opinions about the cause of sole ulceration of the hoof of cattle. Nord Veterinaermed 18:241–252, 1966.
41. Ossent P, Peterse DJ, Schamhardt HC: Distribution of load between the lateral and medial hoof of the bovine hind limb. J Vet Med Ser A 34:296–300, 1987.
42. Peterse DJ: Assessment of the bovine hoof on the appearance of sole lesions (PhD Thesis). Utrecht, Netherlands, Rijksuniversiteit, 1980.
43. Peterse DJ, Vuuren AM Van, Ossent P: The effect of daily concentrate increase on the incidence of sole lesions in dairy cattle. Proceedings of the 6th International Symposium on Disorders of the Ruminant Digit. Dublin, Ireland, 1986, pp 39–46.
44. Philipot J, Pluvinage P, Cimarosti I, Luquet F: On indicators of laminitis and heelhorn erosion in dairy cattle: a research based on the observation of digital lesions, in the course of an ecopathological survey. Proceedings of the 6th International Symposium on Diseases of the Ruminant Digit. Liverpool, UK, 1990, pp 184–198.
45. Rowlands GJ, Russell AM, Williams LA: Effects of season, herd size, management system and veterinary practice on the lameness incidence in dairy cattle. Vet Rec 113:441–445, 1983.
46. Russell AM: Influence of sire on lameness in cows. Proc British Cattle Veterinary Association 213–220, 1986–87.
47. Russell AM, Rowlands GJ, Shaw SR, Weaver AD: Survey of lameness in British dairy cattle. Vet Rec 111:155–160, 1982.
48. Rusterholz A: The specific traumatic sole ulcer of claws in cattle. Schweiz Arch Tierheilk 62:421–466, 1920.
49. Scott GB: Lameness and pregnancy in Friesian dairy cows. Br Vet J 144:273–281, 1988.
50. Sumner J, Davies RC: Footbaths on dairy farms in England and Wales. Vet Rec 114:88, 1984.
51. Toussaint Raven E: Determination of weight-bearing by the bovine foot. Neth J Vet Sci 5:99–103, 1973.
52. Toussaint Raven E: Lameness in cattle and footcare. Neth J Vet Sci 5:105–111, 1973.
53. Toussaint Raven E: Cattle foot care and claw trimming. Ipswich, UK, Farming Press, 1989.
54. Tranter WP, Morris RS: A case study of lameness in three dairy herds. N Z Vet J 39:88–96, 1991.
55. Weaver AD: Bovine Surgery and Lameness. Oxford, UK, Blackwell Scientific Publications, 1986, pp 199–200.
56. Westra R: Hoof problems in cattle—is there a relationship with trace mineral levels? Proceedings of the 2nd Western Nutrition Conference. Edmonton, Alberta, Canada, 1981, pp 114–132.
57. White EM, Glickman LT, Embree C, et al: A randomised trial for evaluation of bandaging sole abscesses in cattle. J Vet Med Assoc 178:375–377, 1981.

9

Claw Care

FUNCTIONAL CLAW TRIMMING

The objective of functional claw trimming is to restore the normal shape of the claw and the angle of the toe and thereby the position of the limbs in the standing animal.[23] The normal function of the limb is thus restored.

Under normal conditions, horn wear is balanced by horn production. Claw wear is reduced if cattle are confined on non-abrasive surfaces (e.g., straw yards) or if the climate is very dry, in which case the horn becomes extremely hard. Horn production is greater on abrasive wet surfaces and slatted floors. Animals on a heavily concentrated diet produce horn more rapidly than those that are less well nourished.[11] The rate of claw horn production may be variable in beef cattle owing to age, the season, and the quality of nutrition.

Annual preventive claw trimming may increase the functional life of the herd by one lactation. The explanation may be that artificially removing horn from the sole stimulates the natural compensatory reaction of growth, balancing wear. The new horn may be stronger than that removed. On the other hand, not all reports on the value of claw trimming are positive.[4, 20] An incorrect technique is likely to produce negative results (i.e., cause lameness).

NORMAL CLAW

The length of the dorsal wall of the claw is measured along the dorsal border from the apex of the toe to the distal border of the coronary band (see Chapters 6 and 14). In Holstein cows, average length is about 7.5 cm, with some variation according to frame size and body weight. Claw lengths normally differ slightly between breeds.

The angle of the claw is about 45°.

The apical region of a normal sole is about 5 to 7 mm thick. The prebulbar region is approximately 50% to 100% thicker. The horn of the bulbar bearing surface is more flexible than other regions of the sole.

The ground surface of the wall is flat from toe to heel. However, weight normally is not only borne on the wall but also on a zone of the sole about 2 to 3 cm wide adjacent to the wall. In addition, both the toe region of the sole and the prebulbar and bulb regions are weight-bearing areas.

More lameness-producing lesions occur in the lateral hind claw[4] than in any other claw of dairy cows. In the hind limb, the posterior region of the abaxial wall touches the ground first during locomotion. This region and the adjacent ground surface bear the first impact of locomotion. The bulb horn is soft and flexible and, together with the digital cushion, absorbs the forces transmitted during locomotion and weight-bearing.[12, 14–16, 22]

The medial hind claw is narrower than the lateral. The ground surface of the medial claw has considerable slope from its abaxial to axial borders, whereas the lateral claw tends to be flatter and has more ground contact, giving it greater stability. On soft bedding (sand, straw, or pasture), both claws bear weight equally (Fig. 9–1). On hard surfaces, such as concrete, the lateral claw bears more than 50% (even as much as 70%) of the weight.[12, 22]

STABILITY OF CLAWS

A stable claw has an even distribution of weight-bearing (Fig. 9–2). This minimizes the effect of trauma and makes a major contribution to claw health.

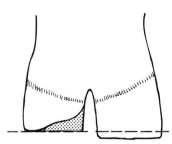

Figure 9–1. The medial claw is narrower than the lateral claw and slopes upward toward the interdigital space. On concrete, the lateral claw tends to grow thicker and gradually bear more weight. (From Toussaint-Raven E, Haalstra RT, Peterse DJ: Cattle Foot Care and Claw Trimming. Ipswich, UK, Farming Press, 1985.)

123

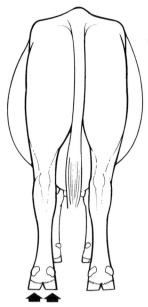

Figure 9–2. When the claws bear weight equally, the limbs are held in correct alignment. (From Toussaint-Raven E, Haalstra RT, Peterse DJ: Cattle Foot Care and Claw Trimming. Ipswich, UK, Farming Press, 1985.)

Weight-shifting on concrete surfaces is mainly a function of the lateral claw. In modern dairy units, cows spend much time walking on concrete. This causes claw stability to deteriorate gradually because increased loading of the lateral claw causes it to wear more rapidly than the medial. A compensatory reaction of increased horn production should result in a natural balance. However, growth of the lateral claw tends to be greater than wear. The outer claws then slowly but gradually increase in thickness beneath the bulb.

When the sole dries out, it tends to flake away, giving the false impression that the wall is growing more rapidly.[23]

Claw stability is optimal with the limb axis perpendicular to the ground surface of the sole. Weight-bearing should be equally distributed between the medial and lateral claws. The objective of claw trimming, therefore, is to create a balance between weight borne by the toe and heel and between the claws.

If the stability of a claw is lost, a cow may slip or may exert more pressure on one area of the sole than another.

Overgrowth of the lateral claw may also result from *laminitis* or *interdigital dermatitis* and sometimes from *digital dermatitis*. A bilateral aberration of hind limb gait around calving time suggests the presence of *pododermatitis circumscripta* (ulcers) or *laminitis*.

In summary, overgrowth of horn is a result of environmental factors exacerbated by predisposing disease factors. Functional claw trimming restores equal weight-bearing between the two claws. This does not mean that claw trimming replaces other appropriate disease control measures but that it is an essential component of any lameness control program.

EVALUATING THE CLAW BEFORE TRIMMING

The three basic types of claw abnormalities are discussed next.

Long Claws

A long claw is one that exceeds 7.5 cm (dorsal wall length). Weight-bearing on a long claw is shifted back onto the prebulbar region of the sole and the flexor process of the distal phalanx (Fig. 9–3).

Some long claws have a concave dorsal surface (buckled toe). Closer examination reveals that it is bent slightly at each of a series of horizontal grooves. This phenomenon is probably a result of a laminitis-like process. In these cases, the angle of the toe is significantly less than 45°.

Overburdened Lateral Claws

In an overburdened claw, the sole thickness at the toe is correct but the depth of the heel (usually a lateral hind claw) is greater than normal (Fig. 9–4). When horn builds up beneath the bulb of the lateral hind claw, its shock-absorbing function is reduced and trauma is inflicted on the corium. This contusion causes pain, which in turn leads to an even greater accumulation of sole horn. A base-wide or cow-hocked posture is adopted in these cases (Fig. 9–5). The animal is then likely to become lame. This process is often bilateral, in which case lameness may not be noticed, although the animal walks stiffly and carefully.

Short Claws

If a claw is too short, the thickness of the anterior sole (apex) usually is dangerously thin and should

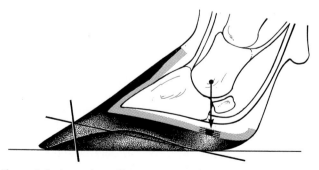

Figure 9–3. As a claw elongates, it is tipped backward, causing more weight to be shifted onto the prebulbar area. Strain is placed on the flexor system as the pastern is overflexed. (From Toussaint-Raven E, Haalstra RT, Peterse DJ: Cattle Foot Care and Claw Trimming. Ipswich, UK, Farming Press, 1985.)

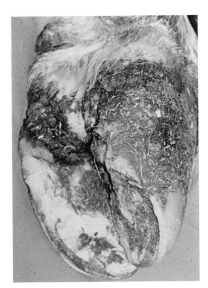

Figure 9–4. An overburdened lateral claw, associated with a cow-hock stance.

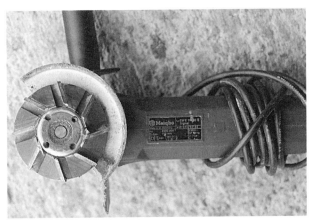

Figure 9–6. An angle grinder fitted with a convex eight-bladed disk. An additional guard has been added because this can be a dangerous instrument to use.

never be trimmed. If the lateral claw is overburdened, the medial claw should not be trimmed at all. The posterior region of the lateral claw should be reduced as much as possible, but it is often impossible to level the bulbs.

EQUIPMENT

Many different types of restraining devices and claw-cutting equipment are available. Each operator has personal preferences. This section offers only an overview of the instrumentation.

Some trimmers use gloves to protect their hands from rope burns and from trauma due to operating a metal retaining device. If gloves are used, they should be considered as a potential vector for spreading infection from one farm to another.

CLAW-TRIMMING INSTRUMENTS

Motorized Disk Cutter (Angle Grinder)

Motorized disk cutters have gained favor with many professional claw trimmers because they can be fast and effective and virtually eliminate the need for a hoof knife, pincers, and rasp. In inexperienced hands, however, they are extremely dangerous to both the operator and the animal (Figs. 9–6 to 9–8). Safety precautions may necessitate that the operator wear protective goggles. Sanding disks are not recommended because they generate considerable heat.

Hoof Pincers (Nippers, Claw Cutters)

Double-action pincers must be used while standing behind the cow. Restraint must therefore be ex-

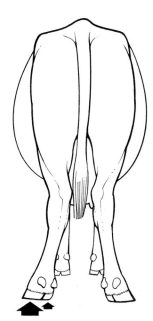

Figure 9–5. When horn builds up on the lateral claw, the hocks are forced inward. (From Toussaint-Raven E, Haalstra RT, Peterse DJ: Cattle Foot Care and Claw Trimming. Ipswich, UK, Farming Press, 1985.)

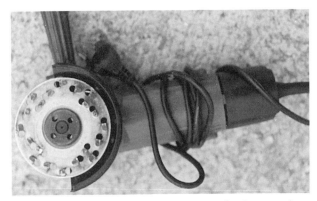

Figure 9–7. A flat, perforated disk is more popular for general use.

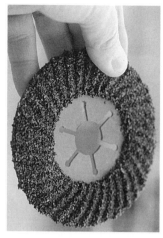

Figure 9–8. Some operators prefer an abrasive disk.

Figure 9–9. A fine-bladed hoof knife manufactured from the highest-quality steel. This type of knife is ideal for the exploration of lesions.

tremely effective, or there is considerable risk that the instrument will be driven into the operator if the cow kicks. Furthermore, this instrument is the least accurate of the pincers because the blades are flat and the jaws are large, making the instrument difficult to manipulate.

Single-Action Pincers

Preferred by most workers, single-action pincers are used to remove claw wall at the bearing surface and to reduce the length of the dorsal wall. For cutting the abaxial wall, the jaws of the pincers are placed at right angles to the sole. For reducing the length of the dorsal wall, the pincers are held at 90° to the sole. The quality of the pincers varies with the quality of the steel, and their efficiency is usually relative to their cost.

Shears

Shears are long-handled instruments of two types. In one, the blades resemble tree branch–cutting shears; in the other, blades are short and square and operate like scissors. The ends of the handles should be directed to the side of the operator, because if the animal kicks the blades, the handles are driven forcibly backward.

Hoof Knives

Both left- and right-handed hoof knives should be available, preferably in two sets. The quality of the knife usually is related to its price. The highest-quality steel accepts the sharpest edge. Particularly good-quality knives are produced by a number of reputable European manufacturers (Fig. 9–9).

Because the hard (or coarse) work can usually be performed with an electric disk cutter or pincers, a hoof knife is used for delicate work and for shaping

the sole to a smooth surface. It is also used for removing loose, irregular sole horn and exploring fissures.

Trimming should proceed from heel to toe, with the blade held at an angle to the direction of the cut. The cut should be made in a sweeping action slightly across the sole in an axial-to-abaxial direction. Two hands may occasionally need to be used. It is often easy for a beginner to remove more horn from the central sole than from the toe, and the central sole thus becomes dangerously thin and dished in an anteroposterior plane. The easiest way to control the knife is to pull from toe to heel on one claw and from heel to toe on the other.

Some workers prefer a Swiss knife, sometimes called a *treen knife*. This knife is shaped as a 3-cm-diameter metal band. Its lower border is sharpened to an edge, and a handle is attached to the upper border. The knife is used as a gouge, which is most effective on the center of the sole. In unskilled hands, this knife can render the sole too concave.

The once popular Allgäu is not used in the Dutch method of claw trimming. However, it may be useful in the removal of thimbles. Similarly, rasps including the Surform plane have largely been replaced by disk cutters.

MAINTENANCE OF INSTRUMENTS FOR CLAW CARE

Claw care is unpopular with both farmers and veterinarians for several reasons, including difficulty with restraint and lack of skill or knowledge of the correct principles. Even when these skills have been acquired, it is surprising that so many operators struggle on with blunt, rusty, or unsuitable (usually the cheapest) instruments. They should be cleaned *and disinfected* after use. Oil should be applied to moving parts, and they should be stored in a suitable container. Veterinarians should take every precaution to avoid spreading infection from one farm to another.

Appropriate storage avoids accidental misuse by other individuals, who may use the instrument as nail pullers or wire cutters. Sharpening and alignment of pincers should be carried out by professionals. Hoof knives must be sharpened by the individual user.

New Hoof Knife

When a hoof knife is purchased, its blade may have a cutting edge that is convex. If so, the convexity

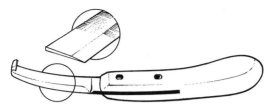

Figure 9–10. A hoof knife is sharpened on the curved side only. The cutting edge must be flat, not rounded.

must be flattened. The quickest method is to use a bench grinder with a 36-grit disk. After a flat surface has been established, it should be polished with a standard 120-grit abrasive disk. After many years of manual sharpening, a blade may also be reconditioned in the same way.

Manual Sharpening (Whetting)

Manual sharpening is appropriate if the blades are used only occasionally. *Oil stones* are used with whetting oil and are usually made of carborundum. Ideally they have two sides, one fine grain and the other rough grain. *Whetstones*, used extensively in North America, are manufactured from various grades of naturally occurring rock. They measure approximately 7 cm long and 2 cm wide. The stones are wedge-shaped across their width, and some may be lubricated with water. A coarse followed by a fine stone should be used.

Technique

The stone is first applied to the concave (bow) side of the blade (Fig. 9–10). The stone must be maintained at an angle of 30° throughout the entire procedure (Fig. 9–11). The tip of the blade should be held firmly to a stable surface, and the stone stroked with a rotating action from shaft to hook with significant pressure. A common error is stroking the blade like a bow on the strings of a violin. Such an action produces a convex cutting edge that is not sharp. When the sharpening process is complete, a burr may have been created on the flat, convex side of the blade. If so, the flat surface of the stone should be stroked several times along this side of the blade

(Fig. 9–12). The backside of the knife must remain absolutely flat; otherwise, it becomes uncontrollable by the user.

Hook

At each sharpening, a chain saw file should be applied to the convexity of the hook. Stroking should commence 0.5 cm from the hook, and the file should be rotated by the fingers as it is pushed through the hook. When this procedure has been completed, the surface should be polished with fine emery paper (360 grit), which for convenience can be wrapped around a small piece of hard board (approximately 0.3 cm thick).

Selection of at least one knife with a small hook permits a veterinarian to create an instrument capable of delicate exploration with a minimum of destruction to normal horn. A knife with such a hook should be used only for therapeutic or diagnostic procedures and never for routine trimming.

Mechanical Sharpening

Mechanical sharpening is preferable for hoof knives in constant use. The procedure takes less time and effort.

Electric Bench Grinder. An electric bench grinder (2899 to 3000 rpm) should have one rubber-backed 120-grit wheel and a second cloth or felt polishing wheel. The wheels should rotate away from the operator; otherwise, the blade (hook) may catch and cause personal injury. The concave edge is first sharpened with the abrasive disk and then polished on the felt disk to which an abrasive paste has been applied.

Dremel Tool. Originally designed as a hobby tool, this hand-operated unit can be fitted with various types of small sharpening, grinding, and polishing heads. Its advantages are portability, precision, and the compact size of the grinding and polishing surfaces. The instrument can also be used for other claw-related tasks such as cutting the wall (e.g., trimming vertical fissures) or methyl methacrylate.

RESTRAINING EQUIPMENT

Many different types of equipment are manufactured worldwide to facilitate the examination of bovine

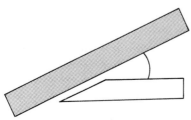

Figure 9–11. When a stone is applied to a cutting edge, it must be held at a constant angle of 30°. Rocking the stone across the blade results in a rounded cutting edge that lacks sharpness.

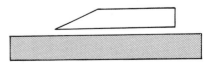

Figure 9–12. If a burr forms on the flat surface of the knife after sharpening, it should be removed with a few strokes of the stone.

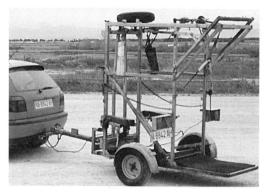

Figure 9–13. A lightweight mobile chute that is very popular in Europe.

claws and for trimming. This section includes two examples of mobile equipment. Manual elevation of the limb is described in Chapter 2, and although these methods are appropriate for an isolated single examination or therapy, they are impracticable for routine claw care. A mobile crush or tipping-table should be available for large herds, and the joint purchase of such equipment by producer groups is recommended as a cost-effective protocol for the control of lameness through regular claw trimming.

Mobile Walk-in Crush

A good example of this system is manufactured in the Netherlands (Figs. 9–13 and 9–14). This model can be towed by a light car and maneuvered into place by one person. It is ideal for dairy cows that are being regularly handled because it causes them less distress than some other systems.

The cow is led into the crush and restrained in a head gate. The hind limbs are elevated either with a manual crank or with the electric or hydraulic systems of more expensive models. The animal has restricted movement in all directions, and the operator can work from the side.

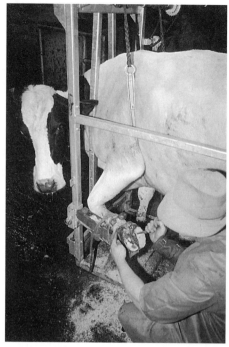

Figure 9–15. The mobile chute has a support to which the forelimb can be attached.

The forelimbs can be managed by using a belly band and forelimb support (Fig. 9–15).

Tipping-Table

Tipping-tables (Fig. 9–16) are the system of choice for the restraint of beef cattle, particularly heavy bulls. This equipment is also used for dairy cattle, although it should not be used with animals that are heavily pregnant. An animal is brought to the vertically positioned table, its head is tied, and belly bands are applied. The table is then moved to the

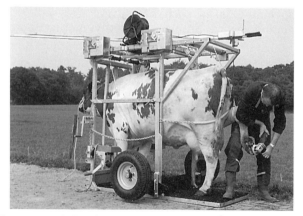

Figure 9–14. A Dutch chute can be motorized to facilitate ease of use.

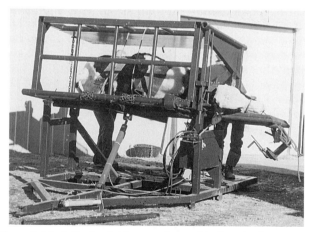

Figure 9–16. A tipping-table, seen here with the wheels removed, is also mobile. The animal enters a chute, its head is secured, and belly bands are applied. A motorized hydraulic ram operates the table. The extremities are secured for examination and treatment by means of wheel and pulleys. (Photo courtesy of High-Hogs Farm and Ranch Equipment Ltd, Calgary.)

horizontal position by means of an electric or gasoline-driven hydraulic ram. The animal's digits are tied by rope or soft nylon bands that are tightened by means of a ratchet pulley. Care should be taken to avoid overextension of the shoulder, which may result in radial paralysis (see p. 207).

Stationary Crush

Many makes and types of permanent facilities are found on beef ranches in North America. They are primarily installed for the purpose of examination, treatment, surgical procedures, and pregnancy diagnosis. Being the only such facility available on the farm, they may be used for the examination of hind feet, but they are generally unsafe for trimming the claws of a herd.

Larger dairy units also may have permanent treatment facilities. If large numbers of animals have to be processed for claw care, many of the features of the mobile Dutch unit should be incorporated.

TECHNIQUE OF FUNCTIONAL CLAW TRIMMING

The following technique is sometimes termed the *Dutch standard*. The method is divided for convenience into the three steps of routine trimming and two additional steps if lesions are present in the sole. The claws should be cleaned and evaluated for length and angle of the toe. Some fractious animals may require sedation (see p. 47).

ROUTINE TRIMMING

Step One

The length of the dorsal wall of the *medial* claw is 7.5 cm, measured from the apex to the coronary band. The wall should be reduced to approximately

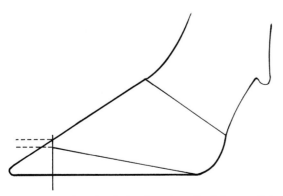

Figure 9-17. The length of the dorsal wall of the medial claw should be reduced to approximately 7.5 cm, leaving 5 to 7 mm thickness at the tip. (From Toussaint-Raven E, Haalstra RT, Peterse DJ: Cattle Foot Care and Claw Trimming. Ipswich, UK, Farming Press, 1985.)

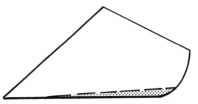

Figure 9-18. If the outer claw is damaged, make this claw lower toward the heel to transfer more weight to the sound claw. (From Toussaint-Raven E, Haalstra RT, Peterse DJ: Cattle Foot Care and Claw Trimming. Ipswich, UK, Farming Press, 1985.)

this length by making a vertical cut with hoof cutters (dumping) (Fig. 9-17).

The tip of the toe has to be left 5 to 7 mm thick. The posterior region of the sole should not be trimmed at this stage. The sole has to be flat—that is, the wall and sole must be at the same level. The toe angle should now be approximately normal.

Step Two

The *lateral claw* is next reduced to the same length as the medial claw. This may not be possible if the dorsal wall of the medial claw is less than 7.5 cm, in which case the lateral claw should be maintained at 7.5 cm. The sole is then trimmed, if possible, to the same level as that of the medial claw. If the heel of the lateral claw is significantly deeper than that of the medial claw, an attempt should be made to equalize the heel depth (Fig. 9-18). However, in some cases this is not possible. The sole in the bulbar region should have some resilience, but no flexibility should be detected in the apical region. The bearing surface of the lateral claw must also be left flat and at the same level as the medial claw.

Iatrogenic sole ulcers can develop if too much horn is removed from the posterior region of the sole. When animals are to walk on abrasive surfaces such as new concrete, rough concrete, or stony roadways, an increased thickness of the claws should be allowed.

It is not unusual for sole horn to grow across into the axial space, forming a ridge that should be removed to restore the normal contour.

Step Three

The central region of the sole is shaped to slope toward the axial border (Figs. 9-19 to 9-24).

THERAPEUTIC TRIMMING

The term *therapeutic* here emphasizes the philosophy that treating a lesion alone is inappropriate. A lesion often develops because the claws are not stable and balanced. Thus, steps 1 to 3 should always precede the treatment of a lesion.

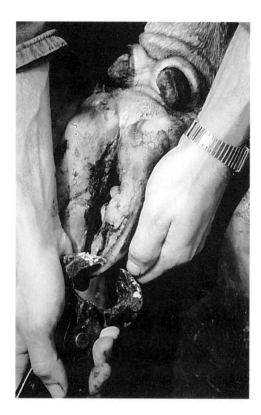

Figure 9–19. The toe of the medial claw is cut back with hoof cutters.

Figure 9–20. The cut end of the toe enables the sole thickness to be seen.

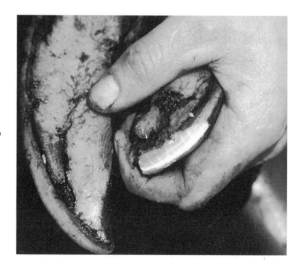

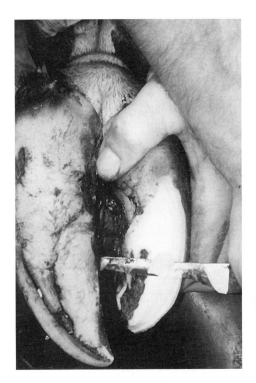

Figure 9–21. The sole is pared down.

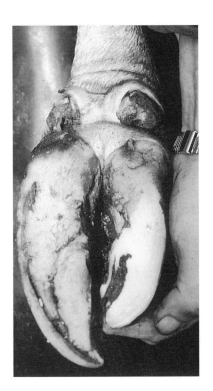

Figure 9–22. The medial claw has been shaped as a pattern for the lateral claw.

Step Four

Assuming that the lesion is located in the lateral hind claw, the thickness of the sole in the apical region should not be reduced but horn should be removed from the posterior two thirds (Fig. 9–25). The aim is to transfer as much weight-bearing as possible to the medial claw. If impossible, apply a block to the medial claw.

In the case of a toe lesion, blocking of the medial claw is necessary.

Infrequently, a lesion may be encountered in a medial claw, in which case the procedure should be reversed.

Step Five

Remove loose horn and thin out hard ridges, sparing the posterior aspect of the medial claw as much as possible.

Now check the claws of the contralateral limb.

Post-trimming Hemorrhage and Lameness

Hoof cutters or a knife may occasionally penetrate to the corium, and hemorrhage may occur. The bleeding normally ceases spontaneously. If the wound is an open cut, a topical dressing with a bacteriostatic pow-

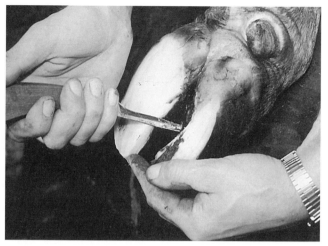

Figure 9–24. The final step creates a slight concavity in the sole facing the axial border.

der should be applied and held in place with a very light elastic bandage. The same treatment is used if a purulent fistula is opened. If the wound, usually made by cutters, is a penetrating slit, removing the overlying horn may be wise.

Clients should be advised to contact the operator if the animal becomes lame within 10 days of its claws being trimmed. Lameness is caused most frequently by removal of too much horn from the sole of the claw, in which case a lift (block) may have to be applied to the sound digit.

FREQUENCY OF CLAW TRIMMING

The frequency of claw trimming is once or twice each year, depending on conditions in the herd. Other variables also apply:

- Summer-pastured cows are more likely to require claw trimming during the early housing period.

- It is preferable to trim the claws when cows are not heavily pregnant or during peak lactation.

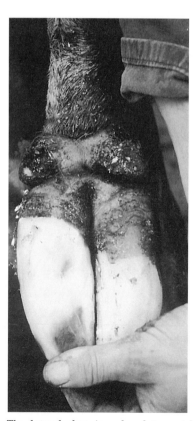

Figure 9–23. The lateral claw is reduced to match the medial counterpart as nearly as possible.

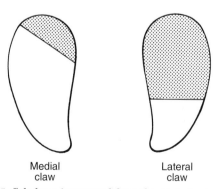

Medial claw   Lateral claw

Figure 9–25. Sole horn is removed from the posterior two thirds of the sole of a lateral claw to transfer weight-bearing to the medial claw. (From Toussaint-Raven E, Haalstra RT, Peterse DJ: Cattle Foot Care and Claw Trimming. Ipswich, UK, Farming Press, 1985.)

- Hind claws usually require more attention than foreclaws.

- The trimming procedure should not be conducted in association with the milking parlor, lest milk letdown be compromised by association.

- Problem cows inevitably require more attention (e.g., three to four times annually).

LESIONS ENCOUNTERED DURING CLAW TRIMMING

The main sole lesions are *pododermatitis circumscripta* (sole ulcer, see p. 101), *white line disease* (see p. 104), *toe ulcer* (see p. 107), *double sole* (see p. 286), and *sole trauma*.[10] The general aim of therapy is to remove pressure from the lesion.

Sole Ulcer. The horn around the circumference of the lesion should be thinned, sloped, and freed from hard or ragged edges. This area should react to light thumb pressure. A lesion is further relieved of mechanical pressure if horn is removed from the posterior region of the affected sole (i.e., the last two thirds of the weight-bearing surface of the sole). The anterior third of the sole, the toe region, should not be lowered, because this is the weight-bearing area.

In selected cases, a block or shoe may be applied to the healthy claw for 4 to 6 weeks. However, a block can overburden a healthy claw and should be removed immediately if lameness occurs. A block can be a good curative measure in exceptional cases.

Bruising. Depending on its severity, bruising should be treated by removing any overburdening of the posterior region of the claw (Fig. 9–26). The operator should attempt to transfer weight-bearing to the toe region. The sole should remain resistant to digital pressure. Rarely the sole becomes very thin owing to road wear. Blood is visible through the horn. The horn reacts to pressure, and the animal experiences

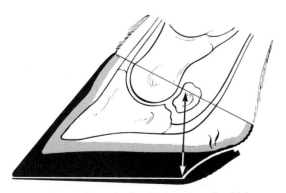

Figure 9–26. Excess horn in the heel region should be removed particularly if underrunning or heel erosion is present. Care should be taken to slope the region to distribute weight-bearing over a wide area. (From Toussaint-Raven E, Haalstra RT, Peterse DJ: Cattle Foot Care and Claw Trimming. Ipswich, UK, Farming Press, 1985.)

pain. In these extreme cases, the animal should be allowed to rest on soft bedding for at least 4 weeks.

Sole Trauma. Cuts or blemishes may be encountered in any part of the sole. Each should be explored thoroughly with a hoof knife, but the greatest care should be taken not to remove more horn than is absolutely necessary. Any tract should be opened up so that the sides of the channel, made smooth and sloping, provide a self-cleaning surface.

CLAWS OF THE FORELIMB

The claws of the forelimb have fewer problems than those of the hind limb. Lesions are found most commonly in the forelimb medial claw. In particular, hooking (overlapping of the toe over the adjacent lateral toe) of the medial claw is encountered quite frequently. The clinical importance of this phenomenon is uncertain. *Laminitis* and *interdigital dermatitis* increase the growth of the medial claw in much the same way as occurs in the lateral hind claw. The foreclaws are trimmed the same way as the hind claws, with the exception that the role of the medial and lateral claws is reversed. The length of the foreclaws is slightly longer than the length of the hind claws.

FOOTBATHS

Footbaths are used routinely as a measure directed toward the control of infectious diseases of the digital and interdigital skin.[1, 6, 7, 21, 22] In one study, it was found that the use of a 1% formalin footbath decreased the incidence of lameness by 5.3%, whereas an untreated group showed an increase of 9.6%.[7]

A footbath is not a substitute for attentive hygiene but assists in control of the environmental bacterial burden. Farmers should not overlook the use of a footbath for dry cows. The bath may also be used for replacement stock and bulls, depending on the system of management.

CONTROL

Interdigital dermatitis responds to formalin footbathing, commencing in the early winter and continuing throughout the housing period (see p. 134). Some clinicians advocate footbaths for the control of *interdigital phlegmon*. The effectiveness of this practice is uncertain, although it is believed that the cleansing bactericidal action reduces the level of the interdigital bacterial burden. *Laminitis*, being a multifactorial disease, does not respond directly to footbathing.

TREATMENT

In *digital dermatitis*, the footbath is currently the most recommended vehicle for therapeutic herd medication. Topical applications are also popular for treating individual animals.

PRODUCTS USED IN FOOTBATHS[5, 17]

Formalin

A solution of 3% to 5% formalin is made up from the generic chemical product, which is usually marketed at a concentration of 40% by volume. If a commercial product is used, label instructions should be followed. Inhalation of formalin fumes is harmful to the health of both animals and humans.[9]

- Use the bath twice daily on 3 consecutive days.
- Repeat every 3 or 4 weeks (depending on the infection level on the farm).
- *Do not* use formalin on open lesions.
- Replace the fluid when contaminated with mud and manure. Replacement means draining *and* cleaning the footbath before using fresh fluid.
- Formalin is ineffective at temperatures less than 13°C.
- After a footbath, allow the cows to walk or stand for 5 to 30 minutes on a clean floor to permit excess fluid to drain. If the animals are immediately allowed onto bedding, it will become contaminated with formalin, and the teats may be blistered after the animal lies down.

Formalin is an irritant chemical. Concentrations exceeding 5% or used for more than 3 consecutive days can cause skin blistering. An early sign is erection of the hairs over an erythematous coronet. Formalin is poorly biodegradable, and its release into natural waterways or ground water may contravene local statutes.

In addition to being bactericidal, formalin has been found to harden claw horn.[13]

The bath should be sited in a well-ventilated area. Cows should never use a formalin bath before entering the milking parlor because the milk may become tainted.

For *ad hoc* treatment of individual cows, a knapsack sprayer is useful and inexpensive.

Formalin has two major advantages:

- It is the least expensive footbath solution.
- It retains its effectiveness longer in the presence of organic matter (manure) than do other products.

Solutions should be renewed after every 500 to 800 uses (e.g., 100 cows could pass through eight times before renewal). In one study, it was found that in a 360-liter footbath containing a 2.2% solution of formaldehyde, no bacterial growth occurred until it had been used by 330 cows.[8]

Copper Sulfate and Zinc Sulfate

Copper sulfate[17] and zinc sulfate[19] are more expensive and slightly less effective than formalin. Fur-thermore, they combine with manure and thereby rapidly lose potency, making solutions ineffective when very contaminated.

Antibiotics

Veterinarians are prescribing antibiotics for use in footbaths for the treatment of *digital dermatitis*. This form of treatment is expensive, and it is generally advocated that only a *minimal-fluid footbath*[26] be used (see Fig. 9–27). Various products are currently in use. A typical regimen for use might be as follows:

- Use antibiotics for 2 consecutive days and repeat after 3 to 5 days.
- Use formalin 10 days after the last antibiotic footbath.
- Continue regular formalin footbaths.
- Antibiotic footbaths must not be used more than twice a year in order to prevent increasing the resistance of the causal organism. Antibiotics should be used only to treat *digital dermatitis* or for individual animal therapy (see p. 99).

FOOTBATH SYSTEMS

Walk-Through Footbaths

Walk-through footbath systems must be located near to the parlor exit in order to keep fumes out of the parlor. The fumes are an irritant to the workers, may excite the cows, and may contaminate the milk.

Permanent System

Walk-through footbaths are valuable adjuncts for the maintenance of hygiene in loose housing systems, where foot bathing should be repeated at frequent intervals.

The footbath may be a permanent construction created as a concrete trough in a convenient passageway. The approach should be funneled if necessary to manage cattle entering the footbath. The facility should be under cover to avoid dilution with rainwater. The optimal dimensions are as follows:

- Length, 3 meters minimum
- Width, 1 meter minimum; the walls may be sloped inward toward the base
- Depth, 0.15 meter (10 to 12 cm depth of liquid)

Permanent installations require a drain running into a 10-cm pipe and appropriate access for correction of a blockage. The floor of the footbath should be grooved to prevent slipping. An ideal system includes a washing trough or power water spray that removes mud and manure *before* the cows enter the milking parlor.

In climates that are so cold that a liquid footbath is impractical, a covered passage may be used for the cattle to walk through slaked lime. The material should be spread to a depth of about 10 cm.

Portable System

Portable fiberglass footbaths are now available. Some have inverted lips to minimize loss of fluid due to splashing. A minimal-solution footbath is also available (Fig. 9–27). This bath is constructed of very durable plastic, and the bottom is lined with foam plastic and covered by a tough, impermeable membrane. As an animal bears weight on the membrane, the resulting depression causes the liquid to swirl around the digits.[26] The bath needs about 10 to 15 liters, compared with 125 to 200 liters in a traditional footbath. It is claimed that about 4 liters must be added for each 25 cows passing through.

Stand-In Footbath

If animals need to be treated individually, a portable footbath may be used if all four extremities need exposure to the therapeutic agent. If only one foot requires treatment, it is often more practical to use a rubberized horse-feeding bowl (metal buckets usually are not tolerated by cattle) that is about 0.75 to 1.0 meter in diameter and 24 cm deep. Liquids should be slightly above ambient temperature. Quiet cattle accept individual treatment in this way.

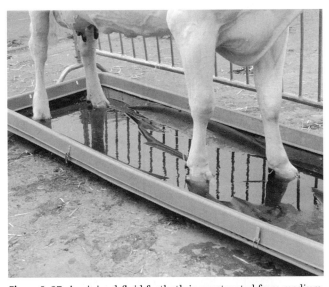

Figure 9–27. A minimal-fluid footbath is constructed from medium-density polyethylene. It measures 3000 × 838 × 150 mm (118 × 33 × 6 inches) and contains a plastic-encased foam rubber pad that is 55 mm deep. A sheet of butyl is extended over the pad and sides of the tray and held in place by a polyethylene rim, which is attached by catches. About 15 liters of fluid is used. The bath is topped up every 20 to 25 cows with 4 liters of solution. (Photo Courtesy of G&E Stable & Son, Little Urswick, Ulverston, Cumbria. Patent pending.)

DEALING WITH CLAW DEFORMITIES

Some abnormal claw shapes have traditionally been described in picturesque terms. Very few objective studies have been conducted.

NORMAL OVERGROWTH

Definition

A claw in which horn production has exceeded wear is said to have normal overgrowth.

Etiology

Beef cattle fed a high-energy diet frequently have overgrown claws.[9] Therefore, culling young bulls with overgrown claws after periods of intensive feeding may be inappropriate. On the other hand, workers in Colorado believe that claw horn production in some breeding lines of beef cattle may be abnormally high.[3]

The soles of cattle kept on concrete surfaces wear selectively, as already described under Stability of Claws (see p. 123).

Clinical Signs

The claw length is much increased in animals with normal overgrowth. The dorsal surface is often concave. An abnormal increase in the horn thickness is evident beneath each bulb. The claw width is unaltered, and twisting of the claw is minimal.

Treatment

Normal overgrowth is treated by functional claw trimming.

CORKSCREW CLAW

Definition

A corkscrew claw is a claw in which the abaxial wall, usually of the lateral hind claw, grows beneath the distal phalanx and displaces the sole dorsally, giving the claw a twisted, corkscrewlike appearance (Figs. 9–28 and 9–29).

Incidence and Etiology

Most descriptions of corkscrew claw are about 30 years old and were contributed by workers in Belgium and the Netherlands.[2, 23–25] In one study from the United Kingdom during that period, approximately 3% of mature Holstein cows were found to have a corkscrew claw.[11]

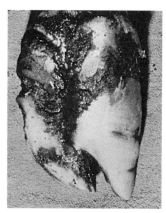

Figure 9–28. The wall of a corkscrew claw grows so rapidly that it displaces the sole axially and dorsally. This rind of horn wall is exceptionally hard.

Corkscrew claws are usually bilateral and not obvious before 3 years of age. Bulls rarely have a severe corkscrew claw, but lines of cows with corkscrews have been traced back to a single bull. For this reason, many workers believe that it is unwise to select young bulls for breeding if they have any abnormal degree of concavity in the lateral hind claw.

Pathogenesis

The middle phalanx is twisted so that its proximal and distal surfaces are out of alignment by as much as 11°.[2] The distal phalanx is abnormally narrow and long. Whether these abnormalities are cause or effect is not known. In addition, exostosis formation occurs on the abaxial border of the joint, suggesting a possible reaction to strain on the collateral ligament of the coffin joint. Exostosis formation may be severe enough to cause ankylosis of the joint.

Isolated cases of corkscrew claw can occur in any digit as a result of trauma or septic arthritis of the coffin joint.

Clinical Signs

The condition is easily recognized. Affected animals tend to hold their limbs camped back. Their ability to forage is often sufficiently limited to cause loss in bodily condition. The animal ultimately has to be culled for low production.

Treatment

Therapeutic claw trimming can be difficult to perform because it is very difficult to judge the thickness of the toe. The claw should first be shortened in stages. The first cut may be made on the dorsal border of the claw at a point 10.0 cm from the coronary band. If the cut end shows no sign of hemorrhage, shortening should continue by removing 0.5 cm at a time until traces of blood are observed. It should be noted that one feature of the condition is molding of the distal phalanx into an elongated narrow shape. This makes it difficult to cut the claw without causing hemorrhage. It is usually essential to trim such claws three to five times each year to keep them in shape.

The next step is to cut back the exceptionally hard wall with pincers or shears, but a skilled operator often finds an angle grinder easier to use. After the hard wall has been removed from beneath the distal phalanx, the sole may be shaped with a hoof knife.

Once established, however, this condition is irreversible. If the tendency to curl is noted early in life, regular claw trimming at intervals of 3 months can

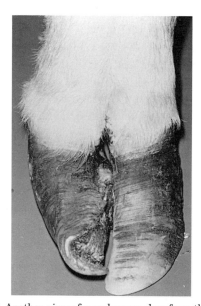

Figure 9–29. Another view of a corkscrew claw from the dorsal aspect.

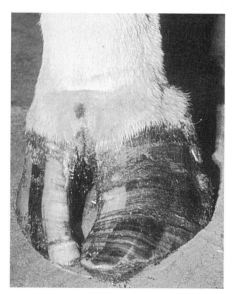

Figure 9–30. A slipper foot affecting only the lateral claw. The claw is flatter and wider than normal. The obvious ridging is probably associated with chronic laminitis.

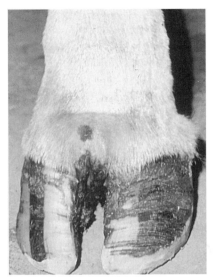

Figure 9–31. The same claw shown in Figure 9–30 after it has been trimmed.

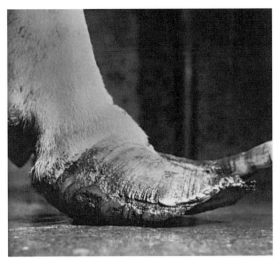

Figure 9–32. A slipper foot showing the Persian slipper characteristic.

prolong the useful life of an animal. Even though such an animal may have very high production, its progeny should not be retained for breeding purposes.

SLIPPER FOOT

Definition

Most workers agree that a slipper foot is an indication of chronic laminitis. The claw is characteristically long, the toe square, the width increased up to 50%, and the normal convexity of the dorsal wall flattened. The claw is heavily rippled or rough and appears dull. A marked concavity in the dorsal wall evokes comparison with a Persian slipper (Figs. 9–30 to 9–32).

Etiology

There is no objective evidence that slipper foot is a result of either acute or subclinical laminitis. The histopathology of chronic laminitis is described in Chapter 18.

Treatment

Therapeutic claw trimming is contraindicated in all but the mildest cases. It is rarely possible to restore normal weight distribution, because horn of the entire claw has softened, causing the wall to collapse. The wall frequently is partially detached from the sole.

BEAK CLAW

In a beak claw, named after the psittacine beak, the bearing surface is entirely convex. The animal's stance is extremely unstable. The significance of beak claw may not be appreciated until an affected animal is 6 months old. The condition is congenital, and the animal should be eliminated from the herd as soon as possible.

Methyl Methacrylate and Claw Prosthetics

Paul R. Greenough   *Canada*

First used to manufacture human dentures, methyl methacrylate (MM) has many purposes in veterinary practice, from the reconstruction of the beak of a Toucan to the repair of hoof defects in horses.

MM is supplied for veterinary use as a premix consisting of two parts. The first is a fully polymerized powder mixed with a catalyst. The second is the unpolymerized product in liquid form. When the liquid is mixed with the powder, the catalyst causes the liquid to cure, with the generation of considerable heat. Therefore, an operator should always wear disposable gloves when mixing and applying MM. After the polymerization phase and the time of maximum heat generation, the puttylike mixture may be molded with gloved hands that have been immersed in water. The product is manufactured by several companies and is variable in both cost and suitability.

Cured MM is extremely abrasion resistant, has

considerable tensile strength, and yet has some degree of flexibility. Its use is limited only by personal ingenuity.

ADHESIVE

The most common use of MM is to fix a wooden block to the sole of a claw. The sole should be prepared by creating a surface free of loose or flaked horn. The surface is thoroughly dried; a small domestic hair dryer is suitable. The sole should be rasped to roughen the surface, or the sole and the distal 2 cm of the abaxial wall may be lightly scored with a hoof knife. The objective is to increase the surface area for contact with MM. The bonding surface of the claw is lightly painted with the liquid, which is allowed to dry. The MM is mixed, and when it has the consistency of butter it is quickly applied to the surface. The wooden block is then pressed firmly into the MM covering the sole. The MM that squeezes out should be molded over the wall and sides of the block. Final molding is facilitated by putting a little water on the surface to reduce the stickiness. The block should not project beyond the toe, otherwise repeated trauma may cause its premature loss.

PROTECTION

MM may be usefully applied to the bearing surface of any part of a fiberglass cast that contacts the ground (see p. 259). Fiberglass, although strong and water resistant, has poor resistance to abrasion.

OTHER INDICATIONS

- MM may be applied directly over a worn (and bruised) sole. The thickness of layer should be 1.0 to 1.5 cm, depending on body weight (Figs. 9–33 and 9–34).

- In pathological fracture of the distal phalanx complicated by osteomyelitis, the toe may be amputated to remove the sequestrum. The toe may occasionally be broken off, accidentally exposing the corium. In either case, the exposed tissue should be dressed with gauze impregnated with petroleum jelly containing an antibiotic. Once a regenerative process has commenced (after 3 to 4 days), with the appearance of granulation tissue, the defective area can be protected with MM (Figs. 9–35 and 9–36). The curing process must be slowed down by running cold water over the MM to dissipate heat.

- A complete claw can be created to protect tissue exposed during traumatic exungulation of a single claw. A wooden block is applied to the sound claw. The prosthesis is built in stages using the sound claw and pastern as the foundation. Fiberglass can provide a platform from which MM can be molded around the defective claw (see p. 116).

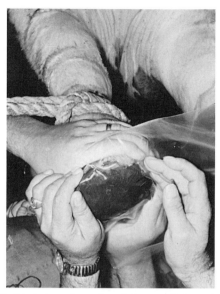

Figure 9–33. Methyl methacrylate being applied to the sole of a claw. The material, because of its sticky qualities, is best molded through plastic.

- *Immobilization of claw movements.* Movement of a diseased digit is undesirable either because healing is retarded or infection is actively moved around fascial planes. MM can be applied to minimize the movement of one claw relative to the other. For example, toes can be wired together as reinforcement for a bridge of MM (Fig. 9–37). This technique is useful in aiding healing after surgical treatment of a retroarticular abscess or for stabilizing a claw as a phase in arthrodesis.

- *Repairing articular fractures of the distal phalanx.* A bridge is used to maintain a claw in forced flexion

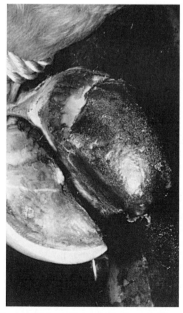

Figure 9–34. The methyl methacrylate forms a tough covering for a fragile or damaged sole.

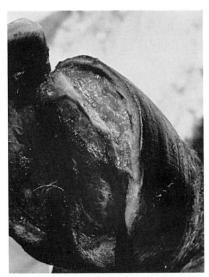

Figure 9–35. In this case, the toe of the claw and distal phalanx were fractured and the bone exposed. Covering the wound with petroleum jelly/penicillin gauze and a bandage for 4 days allowed sufficient time for granulation tissue to cover the bone. Methyl methacrylate can be applied directly to the lesion, provided it is allowed to cure slowly.

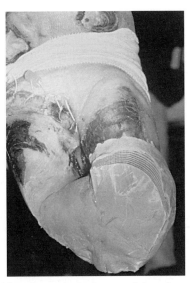

Figure 9–37. After the navicular bone and deep flexor tendon were resected, a block (lift) was applied to the sound claw. A bridge was created to envelop the affected claw. Arthrodesis was effected in the distal interphalangeal joint, and recovery was uneventful.

to eliminate movement and so permit the healing of a distal phalangeal intra-articular fracture. However, application of a block to the sound claw is usually an adequate method of resting the fractured phalanx.

PROTECTING THE CLAW

The digits of most cows are exposed continuously to slurry, mud, straw, and abrasive materials. Good

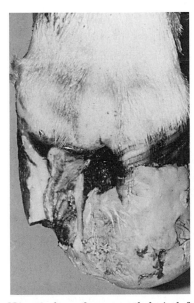

Figure 9–36. Necrotic bone from a pathological fracture of the distal phalanx was removed by amputating the dorsal surface of the claw. A lift was applied to the sound claw, and a bridge was created to envelop the damaged claw. A new claw grew beneath the prosthesis.

postsurgical healing is difficult under such conditions owing to contamination. Simple protective measures are often required to ensure the successful resolution of such cases. Covering the digital region, however, has the major disadvantage of permitting moisture to collect under the protective cover, creating an atmosphere that is deleterious to healing.

BANDAGES

A bandage may be used to provide complete protection for the digital region or can be applied to one claw. The use of bandages, however, should be strictly limited to postsurgical applications and even then applied for as short a period as possible. Bandages have potential disadvantages[27]:

- They are bulky, and if applied over a sole lesion, undesirable pressure may inhibit healing.
- Used alone, a cotton bandage absorbs moisture, which may carry infection to the lesion. Therefore, a waterproof external covering such as a plastic freezer bag (or portion of a plastic fertilizer bag) must be applied. Both plastic and cotton bandages are easily worn away; thus, they in turn must be protected with a tough adhesive bandage.

Readers are advised to consult Chapters 7 and 8 for advice about the treatment of lesions of the digital region.

Technique of Application

A bandage 5 to 10 cm in width is wound around the pastern (between the bulbs and dewclaws) several times. The bandage must be wrapped around the abaxial claw of one digit, across the soles of the two

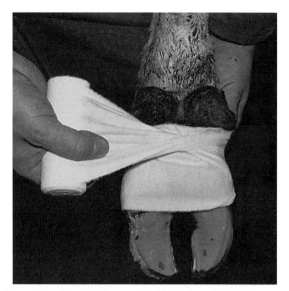

Figure 9–38. The bandage is firmly fixed around the pastern.

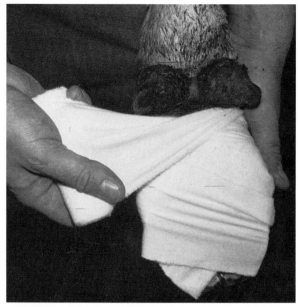

Figure 9–40. Successive turns of the bandage completely envelop the claws.

claws, back around the opposite abaxial wall, and once more around the pastern. The procedure is repeated several times. The objective of this method is to ensure that the two claws are bound closely together to prevent movement that may retard healing of interdigital lesions (Figs. 9–38 to 9–43). Bandaging between the claws is strictly contraindicated in the management of interdigital lesions because this practice separates the claws and tends to open the lesion. Wiring the toes together or applying an MM bridge (discussed earlier) aids healing of interdigital trauma.

BOOTS

A boot, usually of rubberlike material and canvas, can be used to protect the entire digital region. It provides complete but clumsy protection for any topi-

cal dressing that may be applied to a lesion or wound in an animal that can be confined to a small area (box, stall). A boot is not suitable for an animal required to walk any distance, because the sharp edges of the claw can eventually penetrate the material. A boot must be disinfected between each use.

A boot can also be used to soak the digits for preoperative cleaning or exposure to medication.

OTHER DEVICES

Shoof

A shoof is constructed of extremely durable plastic material. It is a slipper into which both claws are

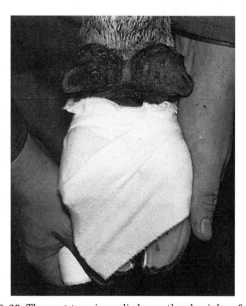

Figure 9–39. The next turn is applied over the abaxial surface, and the claws are pulled closely together.

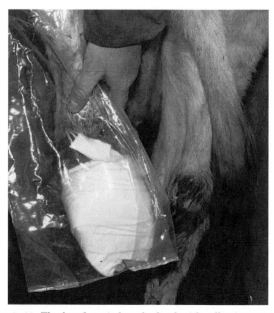

Figure 9–41. The bandage is loosely fixed with adhesive tape, and the foot is covered with a plastic bag.

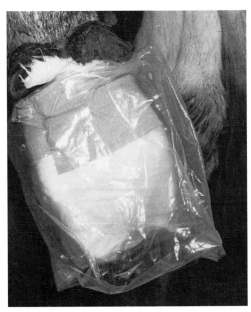

Figure 9–42. The bag is fixed with an adhesive bandage passed around the pastern. The bag is then folded back over the foot to provide a second layer of protection.

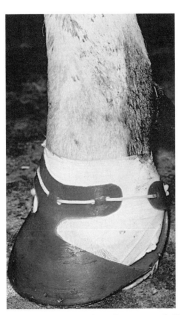

Figure 9–44. A shoof is a lace-on shoe that is available in a number of sizes and configurations.

inserted, and it is held in place by a strap laced around the pastern. Several sizes and models are available. Some incorporate a lift beneath a sound claw. A thin bandage is supplied by the manufacturer for the purpose of providing a tight fit. The shoof *must* be fitted with the limb extended; otherwise, the laces will be too loose in the standing position (Fig. 9–44).

Cowslip

A cowslip is similar to a thimble, shaped exactly to the conformation of a normal claw.[18] Adhesive mate-

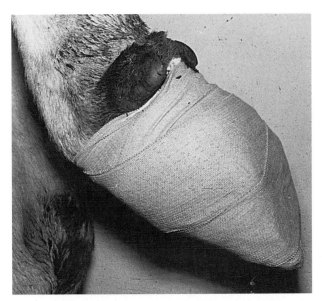

Figure 9–43. The digits are completely enclosed in an elastic bandage covering. Bandages are recommended for only 2 or 3 postoperative days.

rial (a rapidly polymerizing form of MM) is mixed and poured into the cowslip, which is applied over the cleaned and trimmed claw. The large contact area of MM between the cowslip and the horn considerably reduces the chance of failure to adhere. This is a good system for either elevating a sound claw (the prime use) or occasionally providing protection for an extensively damaged sole. A disadvantage is that the cowslip elongates the sole and disturbs the balance of the claw; therefore, it is very unwise to use this device for a prolonged period. It is best removed using a hammer and chisel.

Wooden Blocks and Composite Shoes (Lifts)

Wooden blocks have been in use ever since MM became commercially available. However, the high price of MM has stimulated the production of rubber or composite blocks. The surface to which a rubber block is applied must be quite flat in order for it to seat correctly. It is applied with not less than four pony nails, preferably five. The shoeing technique is easily learned. As in horses, the major hazard is possible misdirection of a nail through the white line and into sensitive laminae. The width of the wall and white line is narrower in cattle than in horses, making precision imperative. In some countries, a wood shoe is secured by three steel screws to a metal shoe that has first been nailed to the sole (modified Wiessner shoe). The wood wears away; the metal shoe may be reused.

Claw Hardeners

Liquids available for painting on the claws reputedly improve the durability of claw horn. These substances conserve horn moisture and make the external surface of the sole resistant to abrasion.

REFERENCES

1. Arkins S, Hannan J, Sherington J: Effects of formalin footbathing on foot disease and claw quality in dairy cows. Vet Rec 118:580–583, 1986.
2. Bouckaert J, Oyaert W, Deloddere E: The corkscrew claw. Vlaams Diergeneeskd Tijdschr 27:149, 1958.
3. Brinks J: Hoof health is inherited. Cattleman Sept:86–88, 1984.
4. Clarkson MJ, Downham DT, Faull WB, et al: An epidemiological study to determine the risk factors of lameness in dairy cows. (Ref; University of Liverpool, Veterinary Faculty, CSA 1370) Final report. 1993.
5. Cornelisse JL: Some observations on the disinfection of ruminant claws. Proceedings of the 3rd International Symposium on Disorders of the Ruminant Digit. Vienna, Austria, 1980, pp 137–138.
6. Cornelisse JL, Peterse DJ, Toussaint Raven E: Formalin foot baths in the prevention of interdigital dermatitis. Tijdschr Diergeneeskd 107:835–840, 1982.
7. Davies RC: Effects of regular formalin footbaths on the incidence of foot lameness in dairy herds. Vet Rec 111:394, 1982.
8. David EA: Personal communication, 1975, Agriculture Development and Advisory Service, Ministry of Agriculture, Trescoyd, Wales.
9. Epstein E, Maibach HI: Formaldehyde allergy: Incidence and patch test problems. Arch Dermatol 94:186–190, 1966.
10. Greenough PR: Observations on lameness in cattle. Fellowship of Royal College of Veterinary Surgeons, London, UK, Thesis, 1962.
11. Greenough PR, Vermunt JJ, McKinnon JJ, et al: Laminitis-like changes in the claws of feedlot cattle. Can Vet J 31:202–208, 1990.
12. Ossent P, Peterse DJ, Schamhardt HC: Distribution of load between the lateral and medial hoof of the bovine hind limb. J Vet Med Ser A 34:296–300, 1987.
13. Pietzsch W, Schauer W: The water content of bovine digital horn under different conditions of husbandry and the effect of copper sulphate and formalin on the hardness of horn (thesis). Berlin, Dept. of Animal Production and Veterinary Medicine, Humboldt University, 1970.
14. Scott GB: Variation in load distribution under the hooves of Friesian heifers. In Wierenga HK, Peterse DJ (eds): Cattle Housing Systems, Lameness and Behaviour. Boston, Martinus Nijhoff, 1987, pp 29–36.
15. Scott GB: Studies of the gait of Friesian heifer cattle. Vet Rec 123:245–248, 1988.
16. Scott GB: Changes in limb loading with lameness for a number of Friesian cattle. Br Vet J 145:28–38, 1989.
17. Serieys F: Comparison of eight disinfectants for cattle footbaths. Proceedings of the 4th International Symposium on Disorders of the Ruminant Digit. Paris, France, 1982.
18. Shearer JK, Elliot JB: Preliminary observations on the application of cowslips as adjunct to treatment of lameness in dairy cows. Proceedings of the 7th International Symposium on Disorders of the Ruminant Digit. Banff, Canada, 1994, p 71.
19. Skerman TM, Moorhouse SR, Green RS: Further investigations of zinc sulphate footbathing for the prevention and treatment of bovine foot rot. N Z Vet J 31:100–102, 1983.
20. Stanek CH, Thonhauser M-M, Schroder G: Does the claw trimming procedure affect milk yield and milk quality factors. Proceedings of the 8th International Symposium on Disorders of the Ruminant Digit. Banff, Canada, 1994, p 306.
21. Sumner J, Davies RC: Footbaths on dairy farms in England and Wales. Vet Rec 114:88, 1984.
22. Toussaint-Raven E: Determination of weight-bearing by the bovine foot. Neth J Vet Sci 5:99–103, 1973.
23. Toussaint-Raven E, Haalstra RT, Peterse DJ: Cattle Foot Care and Claw Trimming. Ipswich, UK, Farming Press, 1985.
24. Van Schaik P: A gradually increasing defect in black and white cattle. Tijdschr Diergeneeskd 70:908, 1952.
25. Van Schaik P: Defects of the hind hooves and hind limbs of Dutch Friesian cattle. Tijdschr Diergeneeskd 81:624, 1956.
26. Ward WR: The minimal solution footbath—an aid to treatment of digital dermatitis. Proceedings of the 8th International Symposium on Disorders of the Ruminant Digit. Banff, Canada, 1994, pp 184–185.
27. White EM, Glickman LT, Embree C, et al: A randomised trial for evaluation of bandaging sole abscesses in cattle. J Vet Med Assoc 178:375–377, 1981.

Conditions Affecting Other Skeletal Structures

Marion Smart *Canada*
Nadia F. Cymbaluk

10

Role of Nutritional Supplements in Bovine Lameness— Review of Nutritional Toxicities

The impact of mineral (macromineral and micromineral) deficiencies on the integrity of claw horn, bone, and muscle is complex. Livestock breeding, feeding, and management are becoming more sophisticated through advances in biotechnology and animal husbandry but are constrained by environmental and animal welfare issues. The complexity of these interactions and issues no longer permits veterinarians to investigate nutritional problems in isolation. An excessive or deficient mineral intake often complicates these interactions. As a result, veterinarians must be able to identify and correct often subtle nutritional imbalances. Nutritional consultants and local agricultural specialists are a valuable and necessary resource required for nutritional evaluation. Several methods are used to establish published nutritional requirements. The most common are

- Factorial modeling[1]

- An expert committee's review of the appropriate literature[31, 32]

The factorial method uses experimental data to determine maintenance requirements for each production group by evaluating the amount of nutrients absorbed, used, stored, and excreted. Because many of the conclusions drawn by both methods are based on controlled nutritional research conducted in a temperature-neutral environment, they do not always reflect real farm conditions. Chronically fistulated and cannulated cattle are often used. If these animals have a chronic low-grade infection, the results of the trial may reflect a response to this infection and not to the nutrients studied. Chronic infections can significantly alter trace mineral metabolism.

Published macromineral and micromineral requirements are of value only as a starting point in ration evaluation and formulation. Values for minimum requirements must be adjusted for specific environmental, dietary, and animal factors (Table 10–

1). The importance that a veterinarian or nutritionist gives to these factors depend on his or her experience in formulating supplements. An on-site evaluation of the producer's nutritional and management practices is essential.

The primary objective of this chapter is to review those nutrients related to lameness in cattle. The role that these nutrients have in reproduction, stress, and the immune response must also be considered, because lameness may be only a symptom of a more complex problem.

IMPACT OF SOILS ON NUTRIENT INTAKE

Soils play a significant part in the nutrient status of crops grown for feed or used as pasture. Soils vary in their mineral content depending on the origin of the parent rock, soil type and pH, level and type of fertilization, climatic conditions, content of organic

TABLE 10–1. KEY ENVIRONMENTAL, DIETARY, AND ANIMAL FACTORS THAT ALTER PUBLISHED NUTRITIONAL REQUIREMENTS OF CATTLE

Environmental factors	Climate/season/precipitation/soil type
	Housing/shelter/pasture management
	Feed bunk management
Dietary factors	Water quality/availability
	Feedstuffs (fresh or dry)/actual analysis/weight/process method
	Interactions/digestibility/ bioavailability/chemical structure and solubility
	Growing/harvesting conditions/ method of preservation/plant genetics
Animal factors	Breed/age/body condition/welfare
	Production status/metabolic state
	Disease/stress/tissue reserves
	Compensatory growth

material, and microbial population. None of these factors acts alone, and all can be significantly altered by farming practices.

Soil conditions can affect the availability of minerals to plants. Sandy soils low in organic matter tend to be low in copper and sometimes selenium. Peat soils are marginal in copper. Molybdenum is high in forages grown on soils originating from shale. Acid soils favor plants' uptake of molybdenum but not copper. Selenium is low in forages and grains grown in the gray luvisolic soil zones. Plant genetics (bioengineering), species, and rate and stage of growth can alter the uptake of minerals by a plant.

Fertilization can change the nutrient uptake of plants. Nitrogen fertilizers depress the uptake of copper, cobalt, molybdenum, and manganese. Lime applied to pastures to increase soil pH tends to reduce the availability of copper, cobalt, zinc, and manganese and to increase the availability of molybdenum. This effect depends on the degree of change in soil pH produced by the lime. Molybdenum fertilizer used to enhance nitrogen-fixing bacteria on legume roots can cause a secondary copper deficiency. Superphosphate fertilizers can reduce the selenium content of young clover pastures.

NUTRIENTS AND THEIR ROLE IN CLAW INTEGRITY

The exact role of minerals in the pathogenesis of claw diseases is unknown. As a result, the rationale for the often excessive mineral supplementation of cattle diets is poorly based. Inappropriate mineral supplementation can create interactions and imbalances that can exacerbate a deficiency or create a toxicity. The clinical effects of a marginal mineral intake are difficult to evaluate and diagnose unless supplementation yields an obvious clinical or production response. Nutrient interaction alters not only

intestinal absorption but also the bioavailability* of the mineral within body tissues.[33]

Although supplemental macrominerals and microminerals are available to cattle, *ad libitum* intakes depend on the animals' preferences, their access to the minerals, and the palatability and form of the supplement. For example, block mineral is consumed 10% less than the same mineral in loose form. The formulation of commercial mineral supplements assumes that all animals consume a minimum amount (Table 10–2). Because many factors influence voluntary mineral intake, one cannot assume that free-choice access to minerals ensures adequate intake. If minerals are available by free choice, an individual animal's intake may be greater or less than requirements.

As illustrated in Table 10–2, mineral and salt intakes can be modified by diet, water quality, and location of the supplement. On pasture, supplemental salt and minerals should be located in an area where cattle spend a large portion of the day. Systemic (injectable) forms, oral boluses, and chelated minerals (Table 10–3) have been developed to circumvent problems associated with voluntary intake and interactions.[9]

STRESS, NUTRITION, AND THE CLAW

Stress in animals originates from powerful external stimuli that may be psychological or physical. Disruption of the body's homeostasis may alter the nutritional requirements for the periods of stress and recovery. This catabolic state results in metabolic changes that use the nutrients in tissue reserves. Intensive animal management practices generate stress in different ways depending on the group and types of cattle. Stress can be categorized as follows:

Sensory Stress (Short-term Pain and Discomfort). At weaning, beef calves are removed from their dams, perhaps castrated, dehorned, and vaccinated. Then they are transported, sold, and relocated to groups in conditions of relative confinement. Confrontations to establish a hierarchical order are stressful and can impair disease resistance and performance.

Emotional/Physical Stress. In late pregnancy, dairy heifers are removed from their peer group and confronted by mature dominant cows. They suddenly get less exercise, walk on concrete surfaces, and face a new management regimen that changes their diet and nutrient intake. Another stress for first-calf heifers is parturition (Fig. 10–1). The temporary decline

TABLE 10–2. CONVENTIONAL VS. ACTUAL FREE-CHOICE SALT AND MINERAL INTAKE (GRAMS/HEAD/DAY) OF BEEF COWS UNDER DIFFERENT DIETARY AND MANAGEMENT CONDITIONS

	Conventional*	Hay§	Silage§	TDS>2000†	Pen Location‡
Salt	45	—	—	11	35–75
Mineral	60–80	14–17	25–28	9–11	—

*Commercial salt and mineral supplements are usually formulated to this level of individual intake.

†Total dissolved solids in the drinking water.

‡The intake of 35 grams was by a group of pregnant beef cows penned in a quiet area. The intake of 75 grams was by a group of pregnant beef cows penned near an area of high activity on the same farm.

§Ho SK, Hidiroglou M, Wauthy JM, et al: Effects of chelated trace mineral supplement on the copper and iron status of wintering pregnant beef cattle fed hay or grass silage. Can J Animal Sci 57:727–734, 1977.

*Bioavailability is the amount of a dietary nutrient available for metabolism after dietary, intestinal, and systemic interactions are considered. Mineral available as indicated on the label of a mineral supplement only reflects the actual amount in the supplement. For example, the actual copper in a mineral may be 0.3% (3000 mg/kg), but the bioavailability may be only 3%, or 90 mg.

TABLE 10–3. EXAMPLES OF THE TYPES OF TRACE MINERAL SUPPLEMENTS AVAILABLE FOR CATTLE

Supplement	Type	Example	Applications/Limitations
Chelate	1. Inorganic	Cu EDTA	Forms a stable bond with mineral
			Oral form not readily available
	2. Organic*		
	a. Metal amino acid chelate†	Cu amino acid chelate†	Conflicting results about benefits in scientific literature
	b. Metal amino acid complex‡	Cu amino acid complex‡	Bypass rumen degradation and dietary interactions
	c. Metal proteinate§	Cu proteinate§	Expensive but less is required
	d. Metal polysaccharide complex	Cu polysaccharide complex	Stable in processed feeds
	e. Metal-specific amino acid complex	Cu lysine	Amino acid content variable except in e.
Systemic (injectable)	Subcutaneous injection	Cu EDTA	Not approved in all countries
			Vary in toxicity, bioavailability
		Cu oxquinoline sulfonate	Occasional severe local reactions
			Individual treatment
			Protects for 3 months
		Cu glycinate	Ideal for pasture cattle
			Transfers to fetus independently of dam's status
		Cu methionate	Decline in efficacy with repeated use
			Bypass dietary interactions
Oral	Free choice	Trace mineral fortified salt or mineral	Individual intake variable
			Interactions a problem
			Be aware of factors that influence intake and availability
	Mix in ration		Interactions a problem
			Uniform mixing to ensure adequate intake
	Bolus	Slow-release soluble glass	Not approved in all countries
			Erratic rumen breakdown in some cases
			Individual protection up to 7 months
		Copper oxide needles	Bypass rumen interactions
			Retained in abomasum
			Individual protection
			Slow release over time
		Slow-release bolus (selenium)	As for other bolus products

*An *in vitro* study of organic chelates and complexes found that between a pH of 2 and 5 all products were soluble at low concentrations. This mimics the conditions in the abomasum and upper intestines. The authors conclude that these chelates are not absorbed or metabolized any differently than the inorganic sources. Inorganic chelates have a low solubility and are not available.[9]

†*Chelate*—a chemical reaction of a soluble metal salt with amino acids (1 mole metal to 1 to 3 moles amino acid).

‡*Complex*—complexing of soluble metal salt amino acid or polysaccharide solutions (polysaccharide coats metal).

§*Proteinate*—chelation of a soluble salt with amino acids or partially hydrolyzed protein.

in plasma zinc level related to stressful calving may disrupt nutrient delivery to the claws and briefly compromise horn integrity.

Nutritional Stress. Beef or dairy cows turned out on young lush pastures in the spring encounter a dramatic change in their diet from their winter feed. The quality of fiber changes, and protein solubility increases. Moreover, the nutrient profiles of the pastures can change significantly as they mature and respond to environmental stresses related to extremes of precipitation, wind, and temperature. The nutritional picture is further complicated by the types of plant species, amount of fertilization (commercial or manure), age of pasture, length of the grazing period, and pasture management.

Disease Stress. Disease alters the nutrient balance in the body (Table 10–4 and Fig. 10–2). Nutrients and tissue reserves are used to assist the immune system and the body to control and eliminate offending pathogens. In response to a viral or bacterial infection, serum iron is shunted into the reticuloendothelial system, away from the pathogen that requires iron. Table 10–5 illustrates the changes that occurred in plasma zinc and iron levels after beef calves were experimentally infected with infectious bovine respiratory (IBR) virus and then with *Pasteurella haemolytica* to simulate the pathogenesis of shipping fever. In response to the IBR aerosol, plasma iron level dropped significantly and plasma zinc level fell slightly. A marked decline in plasma zinc level occurred the day after the *P. haemolytica* aerosol and 1 day before death. In this experimental model, plasma iron level was more responsive to a viral infection and zinc to a secondary bacterial infection. This nutrient shift, as in emotional and physical stress, may temporarily deprive the claws of nutrients essential for normal horn growth (see pp. 111–113).

Strategic supplementation of appropriate nutrients

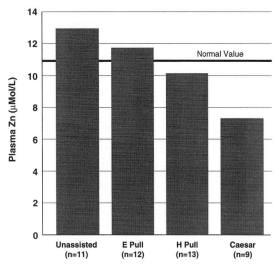

Figure 10–1. Heifer plasma zinc concentrations related to calving ease. E Pull, easy pull (by hand); H Pull, hard pull (use of traction); Caesar, cesarean section. (From Termuende Farm, Lanigan, Saskatchewan, Canada.)

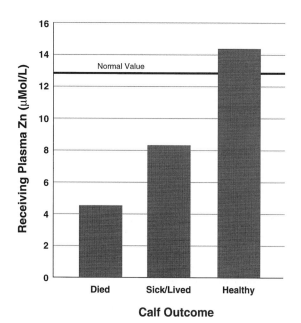

Figure 10–2. Plasma zinc concentration on the day the calves came into the feedlot. Final outcome of the calves evaluated at the end of the feeding period. (From Alberta, Canada, feedlot.)

may address the nutrient requirements of stress, *but* a supplement formulated to meet these needs may create an imbalance if fed to non-stressed cattle.

TRACE MINERALS, SULFUR, AND BIOTIN

Dietary copper and zinc deficiencies can produce skin and hair lesions related to their role in the maturation of keratin. These minerals are essential for growth of good-quality claw horn. The effect of marginal intakes of these nutrients on horn development is controversial and poorly understood. Although these two microminerals are "popular players," other trace minerals (cobalt, selenium, molybdenum, manganese) and sulfur may have less obvious but important roles in the production of healthy claw horn.

COPPER

Copper deficiency can result from an inadequate dietary intake (primary) or from complex dietary (mo-lybdenum/sulfur)[27] or systemic interactions (secondary).

The normal level of copper in plasma is 12.6 to 18.9 μmol/L. Plasma concentrations fluctuate with season, breed, age, and the metabolic or disease state and may not be a reliable indicator of the true copper status. If a clinical copper problem is suspected and the only diagnostic tool available is plasma concentration, then at least 15% to 20% of the affected group must be sampled. Liver copper concentration (normal 1.4 to 8.3 μmol/gram of dry matter [DM]) is a more reliable measure of copper status. These data can be obtained by biopsy[47] or by liver samples taken at slaughter. Determination of plasma levels of ceruloplasmin and amine oxidase and measurement of erythrocyte superoxide dismutase are indirect methods used to evaluate copper status.

An adequate concentration of copper in the diet is

TABLE 10–4. RESPONSE IN TISSUES OF IRON, ZINC, COPPER, AND MANGANESE TO ACUTE INFECTION AND STRESS

	Iron		Zinc		Copper		Manganese	
	Infection	*Stress*	*Infection*	*Stress*	*Infection*	*Stress*	*Infection*	*Stress*
Blood	⇓	↓	⇓	↓	⇑	↔	↓	↔
Liver	↑	↑	⇑	↑	↓	↔	↔	↔
Absorption	↓	↔	↓	↔	↔	↔	?	?
Excretion	↔	↔	↓	?	↔	↔	?	?
Requirement:								
During	↓	↓	↔	↔	↔	↔	?	?
After	↑	↑	↑	↑	↑	↑	?	?

From Klasing KC: Nutrition and Metabolism of Trace Minerals During Stress. Fresno, California Animal Nutrition Conference, 1983.
⇓, major decrease; ↓, measurable decrease; ⇑, major increase; ↑, measurable increase; ↔, variable; ?, not known.

TABLE 10–5. THE EFFECT OF EXPERIMENTAL INFECTIOUS BOVINE RESPIRATORY (IBR) VIRUS AND SECONDARY *PASTEURELLA HAEMOLYTICA* ON PLASMA COPPER, ZINC, AND IRON CONCENTRATIONS (μmol/liter) OF BEEF CALVES

Treatment	Day 1	Day 4 (IBR*)	Day 8 (P. haemolytica*)	Day 9	Day 10
Plasma copper	11.1	13	12.7	13	
Plasma zinc	17.9	14.4	11.2	4.5	Died
Plasma iron	20.3	19.9	9.4	7	

*Active pathogens administered intranasally by an aerosol.

10 mg/kg dietary (DM) intake. This is a baseline value that must be adjusted if interactions are suspected. Dietary copper concentrations of up to 80 mg/kg of DM can be fed to improve the copper status of the group but not as a long-term solution. Once improvement is seen, the copper intake should be adjusted to a maintenance level (approximately 20 mg/kg of DM) to avoid long-term toxicity in cows and perhaps acute toxicity in perinatal calves. The maintenance concentration of copper in the diet should accommodate nutrient interactions, age, stage of pregnancy, and production group.

ZINC

Claw horn quality was improved by supplementation with zinc proteinate. In Scotland, fattening cattle with infectious pododermatitis responded to oral zinc therapy without the use of parenteral antibiotics, suggesting a zinc deficiency. Brazele found a reduced incidence of foot rot (interdigital phlegmon) in animals given zinc methionate supplementation.[8] Zinc supplementation may reduce the prevalence and severity of digital disease. Zinc-treated animals had an increase in serum carotene and zinc levels, and the vitamin A content of the liver was increased.[16] Zinc deficiency can produce a secondary vitamin A deficiency because the lack of zinc reduces retinol-binding protein, resulting in a failure of vitamin A release from the liver. In adult cattle, zinc deficiency causes parakeratosis starting above the bulbs of the heels. This progresses up the leg to the udder and may eventually involve the head. Affected cattle become thin and lame and are susceptible to infections. An inherited form of zinc deficiency is reported in Friesian cattle (lethal trait A-46). The affected calves are unthrifty and develop parakeratosis, lameness, joint swelling, and abnormal claw and horn growth. These calves are susceptible to infection as their immune system is compromised. They respond to oral zinc sulfate but quickly suffer relapse if treatment is stopped.

Normal plasma zinc concentrations are 11 to 14 μmol/liter, and normal liver concentrations are 15 to 18 μmol/grams of DM. Plasma zinc concentration may not be a reliable index of zinc status as values decline with stress and acute bacterial infections.

Serum alkaline phosphatase can be used as an indirect measure of zinc status.

The published zinc requirements are 40 to 50 mg/kg of dietary DM.[2, 3] This concentration is adjusted to account for those factors that alter zinc requirements. Dietary zinc concentrations exceeding 2000 mg/kg of DM cause a secondary copper deficiency by interfering with the intestinal absorption of copper.

COBALT

Soils with cobalt concentrations less than 0.25 mg/kg of DM are likely to lead to marginally deficient pastures. Cobalt requirements are 0.1 to 0.2 mg/kg of diet DM. Cobalt is essential for the production of vitamin B_{12} by rumen microorganisms. The primary feature of cobalt deficiency is chronic wasting related to impaired protein and energy metabolism. Lameness is a consequence of a chronic deficiency.

SULFUR

Sulfur is a macromineral (requirement in the diet is 0.30% of dietary DM) important in the synthesis of methionine and cysteine, two amino acids required in the maintenance of horn quality.

BIOTIN

Some reports indicate that biotin improves the integrity of the claw horn in cattle. The metabolic role of biotin is in carbohydrate and lipid metabolism.[15] Biotin is unstable in oxidizing conditions; thus, processing of feedstuffs can result in substantial losses. The bioavailability of biotin in most feeds is low.

The developed rumen is considered capable of synthesizing adequate quantities of biotin. Recent evidence suggests that ruminal synthesis of biotin is not significant.[18] The demand for biotin increases during periods of stress, and the blood levels found in lame cows are lower than normal.

A PRACTICAL APPROACH TO EVALUATING THE STATUS OF TRACE MINERALS

Evaluation of dietary trace mineral status must be part of any investigation into a herd lameness problem. The trace mineral content of the forage/pasture component of the diet varies from field to field and year to year. This variation is related to time of year, fertilization practices, plant species, grazing density, forage management, and a host of environmental factors. The trace mineral content of grains grown in the problem area is more constant from year to year.

Feed-testing laboratories often have summaries of the nutrient content of feedstuffs grown in their service area. Depending on the level of client service provided, the professional people associated with these laboratories can be a valuable resource.

Appropriate ration and supplement formulation must be based on a detailed history of the problem, gained from an on-farm evaluation of the overall management of cattle, feed mixing, and the feed bunk. For a complete dietary evaluation, a veterinarian should

- Examine the pasture to determine the plant species, stage of maturity, condition (e.g., overgrazed), and application rate and type of fertilization.

- Take multiple pasture clips of the plants grazed over the season to identify nutrient changes and potential problems. A single clip of pasture plants and a nutrient analysis are of limited value, because skeletal and claw changes occur over time.

- Determine the availability, source, and quality of *all* water supplies (optimal DM consumption is dependent on adequate water intake).

- Take appropriate feed/pasture and water (Table 10–6) samples for nutrient analysis. For dry forages, core sample 10% to 20% of representative bales with a forage probe. For silage, take 10 grab samples from the face of the pit or as the silage is discharged from the silo. Question whether these samples are representative of all forages/silage that are to be fed over the entire feed period, because all forages/silage are not harvested at the same time or from the same fields. A sudden drop in the quality and palatability of silage, not considered in the initial formulation, can alter the forage-to-concentrate ratio and lead to an acute production decline, indigestion, and acute laminitis. Forage/silage quality can be appraised visually and by smelling samples.

- Attempt to solve or treat any obvious problems before receiving the formal feed analysis.

- Once the feed analysis is available, convert all results to 100% DM (most feed-testing facilities can do this). This brings all the feeds to an equal base.

- Determine the present nutrient intake from the

TABLE 10–6. A SUMMARY OF ACCEPTABLE WATER QUALITY FOR CATTLE*

Element	Maximum Safe Level (mg/liter)	Significance
pH	Minimum 5, maximum 9	Palatability problems pH >9 may cause a mild metabolic alkalosis and is a potential risk factor for milk fever
Hardness	180	Very hard water No obvious health problems in cattle Hard on equipment
Total dissolved solids (TDS)	7000–10000	Impact on animal production depends on salt composition Sodium chloride is tolerated at higher concentrations than sodium sulfate Can alter the dietary cation anion balance [(Na + K) − (Cl + S)]
Magnesium (Mg)	800	May be laxative when cattle are first introduced to the water
Sodium (Na)	800	See TDS
Calcium (Ca)	1000–2000	If the diet is also high in Ca, may predispose high-risk cows to milk fever
Iron (Fe)	300	Along with high Mn, reduces water palatability >1500 reduces dietary Cu availability
Sulfates (SO_4)	900	Found in deep wells and in surface water associated with alkaline soils Interacts with copper alone or with molybdenum (thiomolybdate) to decrease Cu bioavailability Decreases Se, Fe, and Mn availability Associated with feedlot and pasture polioencephalomalasia (thiamine deficiency)
Nitrates (NO_3)	100	Additive with dietary nitrates Converted in rumen to nitrates that produce methemoglobin Surface water and shallow well should be monitored because nitrate comes from surface contamination
Zinc (Zn)	25	—
Copper (Cu)	1	30% of sheep's daily requirements
Selenium (Se)	0.1	10-fold margin of safety
Chlorides (Cl)	1000	>250 causes corrosion of plumbing
Mercury (Hg)	0.01	—
Lead (Pb)	0.1	—
Fluoride	3	At this concentration may cause mild mottling of teeth

*These values are guidelines and may vary with local conditions. An adequate and palatable water supply is essential in maintaining optimal dry matter intake in each production group of cattle.

TABLE 10–7. THE INFLUENCE OF FORAGE QUALITY ON VOLUNTARY DRY MATTER INTAKE*

Forage/ Pasture Quality	Voluntary DM Intake as % BW	Crude Protein % DM		TDN % DM	% DM Digestibility†	Examples	
		Grass	Legume			Forage	Pasture
Excellent	Up to 3	15	21	63	75	Legume prebloom	Vegetative
Good	2.5	11	16	52	65	Legume midbloom	50–70% bloom
Mature	1.5–2.0	8	12	50	60	Legume full bloom	Full bloom
Poor	0.5–1.0	4	7	44	50	Legume late bloom	Late bloom
						Rice or wheat straw	Mature

*Mold or spoilage can decrease dry matter (DM) intake 0.5% or more.
†Dependent on degree of weathering, environmental conditions during growth, and the degree of spoilage. These numbers are to illustrate the decline of digestibility with maturity.
 DM, dry matter; BW, body weight; TDN, total digestible nutrients.

feed intake data collected on the farm visit (all feeds should have been weighed and individual consumptions calculated). For pastures and some forages, individual intake may be difficult to determine but can be calculated on the basis of the voluntary intake of forages/pastures of different quality (Table 10–7).

- Compare the calculated results with adjusted published requirements.

- Formulate a new diet or supplement to correct any existing nutritional imbalances. The *actual* trace mineral content and the *bioavailability* of the mineral are important considerations (Table 10–8). A number of computer-assisted ration evaluation/formulation programs are available. They all come

with a warning that "a sound nutritional background is required to successfully use the program." If these programs are used, always check that the input data are in the correct form (DM or as fed), make sure the correct requirements and adjustments are chosen, and evaluate the results starting with the DM intake, then in turn consider the macronutrients, minerals, trace minerals, and vitamins.

- Advise the client of the changes required. The dietary changes should be not only in the weights of the feeds to be fed but also in terms understood by the producer (e.g., number of coffee tins per cow, number of buckets per pen). Clients should be educated to use actual weights and a weigh scale

TABLE 10–8. EXAMPLES OF COMMONLY USED TRACE MINERAL SUPPLEMENTS, THE ACTUAL MINERAL PERCENT AND BIOAVAILABILITY, AND SOME FACTORS THAT INFLUENCE BIOAVAILABILITY

Supplement	Actual % of Trace Mineral*	Bioavailability
Copper (Cu)		
1. Inorganic		Altered by purity (reagent grade vs. feed grade)
Cu sulfate	25.6	Processing to remove impurities can increase or decrease bioavailability
Cu carbonate	53	Experimentally induced interactions may not replicate field situations
Cu oxide	75	For high-molybdenum diets, the availability of proteinate is greater than
2. Organic		sulfate
Cu proteinate	Supplied by manufacturer	
Cu lysine	5 or 10	
Manganese (Mn)		
1. Inorganic		Mn methionine complex most available
Mn sulfate	25	Mn oxide least available and depends on the source and purity, a high-
Mn oxide	60	dioxide content decreases bioavailability
2. Organic		
Mn methionine complex	8 or 16	
Zinc (Zn)		
1. Inorganic		Inorganic sources may not be equal in bioavailability
Zn sulfate	36	Bioavailability increases with increased purity
Zn oxide	73	Organic sources are similar to ZnO, but metabolism may be different
2. Organic		Organic sources alter rumen microorganisms by increasing protozoa;
Zn methionine	4, 10, or 20	they also increase the uptake of vitamin A and beta-carotene
Zn lysine	10	

*Percentages may vary. Regulations require that the minimum percentage of trace minerals be specified on the label.

rather than measure by pail units. For some clients, this transition is not practical.

- Obtain direct (plasma, blood, hair, liver) or indirect (enzymes) measures of the affected animals' nutritional status. These values may not be necessary for the diagnosis of the problem but can be used as a baseline to monitor the group's early response to treatment.

NUTRITION, THE GROWTH PLATE, AND BONE METABOLISM

The growth/repair pattern of bone and the growth plate are altered by nutritional factors that impair

- Cell differentiation and multiplication
- The formation and maturation of the intercellular substance
- The mineralization of this organic matrix
- Capillary penetration (angiogenesis) of the mineralized organic matrix

Nutrition has an important role at all four levels,[44] particularly during the active growth phase of a calf's skeleton. A fetus or calf whose growth is temporarily arrested by disease or malnutrition may go through a period of compensatory growth associated with increased nutritional requirements. Growth arrest lines are often evident in the diaphysis on radiographs.

In a young adult, 3% to 5% of the total skeletal tissue is remodeling at one time. Mechanical load bearing requires adequate amounts of functional bone.[39] Nutritional alteration of bone quality can lead to skeletal deformities, fractures, or growth retardation.

GROWTH PLATE (Fig. 10–3)

The primary growth plate is responsible for longitudinal bone growth.[23] The secondary growth plate (ossification center) is responsible for endochondral ossification of the epiphyses (see p. 229).[36]

BONE METABOLISM

In bone metabolism, nutrients are essential for normal enzyme activity, as free radical scavengers, and in hormonal regulation. Normal bone growth, turnover, and repair can proceed only if the following components have matured in an orderly fashion: collagen and mucopolysaccharide synthesis and calcification.

COLLAGEN

Collagen is rich in glycine, proline, and lysine. Collagen maturation takes place rapidly, and once the

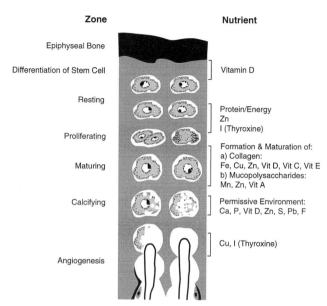

Figure 10–3. Nutrients essential for normal maturation of the growth plate at the different zones of maturity.

collagen cross-linkages are stabilized, mineralization proceeds. Intracellularly, collagen synthesis begins with the uptake and hydroxylation of proline. Vitamin D, vitamin C, iron, and zinc are important at this level. Extracellularly, the cross-linkages of the polypeptide chains of immature collagen to mature collagen are dependent on vitamin E, copper, and zinc.

MUCOPOLYSACCHARIDE

Mucopolysaccharide forms the extracellular interfibrous component (proteoglycans) in which maturing collagen fibers are embedded. Manganese is essential for the synthesis of chondroitin sulfate A, an important component. Decreased uptake of sulfate is reported in zinc-deficient rats. Zinc, through alkaline phosphatase, is involved in matrix formation. Poor control of matrix calcification is attributed to a decrease in sulfate groups.

CALCIFICATION (MINERALIZATION)

Calcification begins once a mature organic extracellular matrix is formed. Three zones are present in the mature mineralized matrix. The interior zone has the lowest rate of ion turnover and is the site of strontium, radium, and lead sequestration. Because of the low turnover rate, it is difficult to treat and determine a withdrawal period for cattle with chronic lead poisoning. Fluoride incorporation results in a very stable crystal (see Fluoride Toxicity, p. 157).

A decline in bone mineralization or matrix formation results in *osteopenia*, which is defined as decreased bone density. This can be *osteoporosis*, a loss of bone matrix and mineral, or *osteomalacia*, a decrease in bone mineral but not matrix.

CLINICAL IMPLICATIONS OF ALTERED BONE METABOLISM

In a calf, the most obvious skeletal lesions are asymmetrical enlargement of the physis of the distal ulna/radius, femur, metatarsus, metacarpus, and costochondral junctions. Varus or valgus deformities may develop at the carpus/tarsus and fetlock. Spontaneous fractures occur in the long bones and vertebral bodies, resulting in severe lameness or recumbency. Neurological signs (posterior paralysis) signal damage to the spinal cord. If articular cartilage is involved, distention of the synovial joint can occur. Histologically, a widening of and irregularities in the growth plate are observed. Islands of poorly mineralized cartilage are evident in the metaphysis, and microfractures of primary trabeculae occur. Other histopathological changes are specific for the cause of the skeletal lesions.

In mature cattle, osteopenia results in lameness and spontaneous fractures. Because of the low bone turnover rate, the skeletal changes follow a decline in production, body condition, and reproduction.

MACROMINERALS

Although each mineral is next considered individually, metabolic bone disease is seldom associated with a deficiency or excess of a single nutrient. A veterinarian who focuses on a single nutrient without thoroughly evaluating the problem can be misled and may implement inappropriate treatments.

CALCIUM

Calcium deficiency in a calf results in a failure of adequate mineralization of the zone of hypertrophying cartilage and a failure of the bone matrix. Lysine, arginine, lactose, and vitamin D increase calcium absorption. Oxalates, phytates, fiber, and saturated fats can impair calcium absorption; these are not significant if the rumen is functional. Diets that increase the abomasal pH can decrease calcium absorption. A high dietary intake of phosphorus in association with a low dietary calcium intake causes hyperparathyroidism.[11] A low-magnesium diet fed to dry dairy cows reduces the rate of calcium mobilization at parturition.

In an adult, efficiency of intestinal absorption declines with age. A chronic dietary deficit is compensated by increased bone resorption.[43] Stimulation of the resorptive remodeling units causes cortical thinning and porosis. Highly acidic diets (milk fever prevention) produce a larger pool of exchangeable calcium by bone resorption. If these diets are misused and cause a chronic metabolic acidosis, osteoporosis may develop.[40]

A chronic excess of dietary calcium (alfalfa hay) in bulls leads to hypercalcitonism (C-cell hyperplasia or neoplasia), arrested bone resorption, and osteopetrosis, in an attempt to regulate serum calcium.[29] The primary lesion is osteophyte formation in T11–L1 vertebrae. These osteophytes can fuse the vertebrae and fracture, resulting in pain, reluctance to move, ataxia, and posterior paralysis if the spinal cord is damaged.

Because milk is considered adequate in calcium for a preruminant calf, published requirements vary. Ten to 20 grams/day is considered adequate.[1] If a calf is fed milk at 10% of its body weight (BW) (a conventional standard), the calf's intake of calcium and phosphorus is deficient based on a milk content of 1.05 grams of calcium and 0.55 grams of phosphorus per liter. This deficit can be corrected if milk is fed at 20% BW (three equal feedings versus two per day) or by early introduction of a balanced creep ration. The finishing ration of feedlot cattle should have a calcium content of 0.5% to 0.8%. Maintenance requirements for adult cattle are 24 to 50 grams/day; lactational requirements are calculated according to the average daily milk production (1.02 gram of calcium per liter of milk). For maximum milk yield and fertility, a calcium-to-phosphorus ratio of 1.4:1 is ideal. Cattle can tolerate a ratio of 8:1 if lactating and if the phosphorus requirements are met. This ratio should be avoided in mature dry cows because it may predispose them to milk fever.

PHOSPHORUS

In cattle, phosphorus depletion occurs primarily with an inadequate dietary intake. The forage/pasture component of the diet is often deficient. The grains and oilseed meals are high. The efficiency of phosphorus absorption is altered by age, the source of phosphorus, vitamin D status, rumen and intestinal pH, other minerals, and dietary fat.[30] Ruminants recycle large amounts of inorganic phosphorus through the saliva; therefore, the calcium-to-phosphorus ratio of the ingesta presented for absorption is altered.[57]

A secondary phosphorus deficiency can be caused by ingestion of an excess of aluminum,[14] iron, beryllium, calcium, magnesium, strontium, and molybdenum.[41] Highly leached acid soils and alkaline soils are associated with phosphorus deficiency.[41]

Long-term (2 years) dietary intake of less than 6 grams of phosphorus per day produces clinical signs in mature cattle, of weight loss, reduced feed intake, reluctance to move, abnormal stance, and spontaneous bone fractures (osteoporosis) of ribs, vertebrae, and the pelvis.[45] Before skeletal changes are clinically evident, the early signs of phosphorus deficiency are infertility and pica (depraved appetite). In New Zealand, osteodystrophy related to a phosphorus deficiency is described in yearling Angus steers grazing a winter pasture of swedes *(Brassica napus)*.[51] Postpartum downer cows that fail to respond to calcium supplementation yet are bright and alert are often hypophosphatemic.

Rib bone density and mineral content per unit volume of bone are sensitive indicators of dietary phosphorus intake.[55] Serial biopsy specimens taken from the 9th to 12th ribs can be used to monitor changes in calcium and phosphorus concentrations related to dietary intake.[6]

The dietary requirement for a milk-fed preruminant calf is 8 to 11 grams/day, for optimal gain.[1] For feedlot cattle, the dietary requirement is between 0.3% and 0.5% of dietary intake. For adults, the maintenance requirements are 17 to 25 grams/day, with an additional requirement of 10 grams when pregnant. Lactational requirements are based on the level of production (0.55 grams of phosphorus per liter of milk). Care should be taken to balance the dietary intake of phosphorus with that required for maintenance, growth, and lactation. This reduces fecal excretion of phosphorus and lessens environmental pollution.[30]

TRACE MINERALS

Determination of dietary trace mineral status should be part of any nutritional evaluation in which herd lameness is a problem. The risk factors involved apply primarily to the forage/pasture component of the diet, particularly if the pastures are intensively managed (mismanaged) or in areas known to be deficient or marginally deficient in one or more of the minerals.

COPPER

Copper acting through the enzyme lysyl oxidase is responsible for the formation of cross-linkages in collagen and elastin. Abnormal collagen leads to osteoporosis and spontaneous fractures in adults. In calves, copper deficiency results in defective mineralization of abnormal collagen in the immature growth plate. Clinically, enlargement of the distal tarsal and carpal epiphyseal plates (epiphysitis) occurs.[48] Affected calves are unthrifty and may have a dry, faded hair coat (depends on initial pigmentation), diarrhea, and a limited response to the treatment of lice and coccidiosis.

Lameness due to copper deficiency is associated with microfractures in the primary trabeculae. Microscopically, focal widening of the growth plate consists of tongues of uncalcified cartilage with delayed or impaired provisional calcification in the presence of active osteoblast.

ZINC

Alkaline phosphatase, a zinc-dependent enzyme, has a role in bone metabolism through extracellular matrix secretion and collagen and mucopolysaccharide synthesis. Zinc is an activator and constituent of numerous enzyme systems involved in nucleic acid metabolism, protein synthesis, and carbohydrate metabolism. An excess of zinc or vitamin A has been suspected in cases of congenital skeletal abnormalities.[34]

MOLYBDENUM

Molybdenum interacts with sulfur to impair dietary and systemic availability of copper. Molybdenum levels in soils of shale origin vary between 10 and 100 mg/kg of soil DM. Levels exceeding 3 mg/kg of dietary DM are toxic if the sulfur intake is high (>0.45% total dry diet) and the copper status low (<7 mg/kg of dietary DM). The concentration of molybdenum in plants varies with the season and is highest in spring and fall. The concentration of molybdenum in legumes is higher than in grasses. Molybdenum is considered to be a conditioning agent for copper, as are zinc, iron, lead, and calcium carbonate. The critical ratio of copper to molybdenum in the diet is considered to be 4:1. The impact of molybdenum on bone integrity is through a secondary copper deficiency.

MANGANESE

Manganese is required for normal fetal skeletal and inner ear development. Manganese deficiency results in failure of chondrocyte maturation, inhibition of chondroitin sulfate synthesis, and decrease in mucopolysaccharides. A manganese deficiency in a fetus can result in contracted tendons, impaired inner ear development, and other abnormalities related to chondrogenesis. Skeletal abnormalities occur in a neonate when the dam's dietary intake of manganese is less than 17 mg/kg of DM.[1]

Manganese status of cattle is difficult to determine because tissue reserves are minimal. Hair analysis (deficient <14 mg/kg of hair DM) has been used to evaluate the manganese status in neonatal calves. A detailed analysis of a cow's ration during pregnancy is the most reliable indicator of manganese status. Most diets are formulated to contain 40 to 80 mg of manganese per kilogram of DM.[21]

IODINE

Depletion of thyroid iodine stores decreases the production of thyroxine, which influences cartilage growth and endochondral ossification. In a deficiency, differentiation of chondrocytes is impaired and vascular penetration (angiogenesis) of cartilage is depressed. The iodine status of a dairy herd can be monitored by an analysis of bulk milk samples (>12 µg/liter is considered normal). The iodine requirement for maintenance is 0.12 mg/kg of dietary DM, for pregnancy and lactation 0.80 mg/kg of DM, and 1.20 mg/kg of DM if goitrogens are present.

IRON

Rations should contain 25 to 30 mg of soluble iron per kilogram of dietary DM. Ground water should not be overlooked as a source of iron. Ferrous iron along with other nutrients is required in early collagen production (proline → proline protocollagen). Excessive iron in the diet (>1500 mg/kg of dietary DM) can decrease copper availability and create a secondary copper deficiency.

VITAMINS

VITAMIN D (RICKETS)

Vitamin D (vitamin D_3) metabolism interacts with that of calcium, phosphorus, calcitonin, and parathyroid hormone to regulate blood calcium levels closely.[3] A decrease in extracellular calcium concentration stimulates parathyroid hormone secretion, which in turn stimulates renal production of vitamin D_3. Vitamin D_3 enhances the intestinal absorption of calcium by production of a D_3-dependent calcium-binding protein in the enterocyte. Vitamin D_3 recruits bone marrow stem cells for new bone formation and remodeling.[49]

Seasonal and geographical variations in ultraviolet activation of provitamin D occur in the skin.[20] In northern climates, ultraviolet activation is minimal from October to March. Thus, supplementation of diets during this period may be necessary. The level of vitamin D supplementation is generally not adjusted from published requirements. A calf receives vitamin D from milk for the first 10 days. If calcium and phosphorus are adequate in the calf's diet, vitamin D requirement is small (7 IU/kg of BW per day or 0.175 μg/kg of BW per day).

VITAMIN A

Vitamin A is involved with the synthesis of specific glycoproteins that control cellular differentiation. Although not directly linked to lameness, vitamin A does have a role in bone metabolism. If vitamin A is deficient, sulfur uptake is diminished in the formation of chondroitin sulfate. Thus, cartilage cells do not follow the normal pattern of growth, maturation, and degeneration. Vitamin A in excess may impair the ability of periosteal progenitor cells to differentiate into osteoclast, and subperiosteal reabsorption of bone thus fails.

A calf's initial source of vitamin A is colostrum. The requirement for a preruminant is approximately 47 IU/kg of BW. Thirty times the requirement is the safe upper limit, and 100 times the requirements can cause skeletal lesions. For mature cattle, published requirements are used in ration evaluation and formulation.

VITAMIN K

Vitamin K,[53] through its role as a cofactor for the formation of carboxyglutamate residues in protein may have an effect on bone metabolism. Osteoblasts produce three carboxyglutamate-containing proteins: osteocalcin, matrix carboxyglutamate protein, and protein S. Their specific function in bone metabolism at this time is speculative. The most significant one is osteocalcin, which has a regulatory role in mineralization and remodeling of bone tissue. Serum osteocalcin is used as a marker for osteoblast activity and bone formation in humans and animals because it correlates with bone formation. In humans, a poor vitamin K status has been associated with an increased risk for osteoporosis.

NUTRIENT DEFICIENCIES RELATED TO MUSCLE INTEGRITY

NUTRITIONAL MYOPATHY

Nutritional myopathies occur as a result of selenium or vitamin E deficiency. The clinical signs and response to therapy depend on the age of the animal, the muscle groups affected, and the identification of dietary and environmental stressors that increase the oxidative load or impair selenium and vitamin E availability (Table 10–9).

PATHOGENESIS

Both selenium and vitamin E protect the cell from free radical injury. Free radicals are generated during normal cell metabolism, and their production is accelerated in an animal under stress.[37] Selenium functions in the cytosol through glutathione peroxidase (GSH-Px). Lipid-soluble vitamin E prevents lipid peroxidation of the polyunsaturated fatty acids in cell and organelle membranes.[38] If one or both of these systems are compromised in striated muscle, an intracellular cascade of events occurs. Initially, uncontrolled free radicals cause intracellular membrane damage; as a result, an increased net flux of calcium occurs. This results in an excessive uptake of calcium by the mitochondria. As a consequence, initial functional damage then structural damage occur to the mitochondria. This impairs the energy metabolism of the cell. The next step is an elevated cytoplasmic concentration of calcium, which causes hypercontraction of muscles and eventually cell necrosis and hyalinization. In the muscle cell, the contractile elements are most vulnerable. If the sarcolemmal sheath remains intact, regeneration can occur with no scarring. Aerobic muscle fibers are

TABLE 10–9. ENVIRONMENTAL, DIETARY, AND ANIMAL FACTORS THAT IMPACT ON SELENIUM/VITAMIN E AVAILABILITY

	Selenium	Vitamin E (Alpha-Tocopherol)
Environmental factors	Decrease Se: Gray luvisolic soils Acidic soils with high iron oxides; Se availability to plant 4% Heavy fertilization/heavy rainfall/lush growth High soil Se General: Alkaline soils 40% Se availability to plants	Decrease vitamin E: 60% loss if cut forage lies in the field 4 days Weathered forage
	Sudden inclement weather Stressful transportation of deficient or marginally deficient cattle	
Dietary factors	Replace Se-rich plant proteins with a non-protein nitrogen source Dietary antagonists: 3 gm Zn/kg DM 5 gm Fe and S/kg DM 100 mg Ca/kg DM 500 mg Cu/kg DM	Method of ration processing (large round bales) Trace minerals in supplement Hay has less than silage High-moisture grains preserved with propionic acid
	Increase oxidative load (involves both Se and vitamin E): High C18:3 fatty acids High dietary polyunsaturated fatty acids Rancid fats Lipids in early lush pastures Cupric or ferric ion in supplement High dietary vitamin A Mycotoxins	
Animal factors	Rumen environment influences Se bioavailability as most rumen Se is insoluble	
	Sudden unaccustomed exercise Age, vitamin E/Se status	

affected first. Mineralization of the degenerating myofibrils can occur within 6 to 8 hours.

CLINICAL SIGNS

Perinatal (White Muscle Disease)

Affected calves may be stillborn or weak. If the skeletal muscles are involved, the calf is stiff and sore and its affected muscles are painful and firm. Dyspnea and abdominal breathing are noted if the intercostal muscles and the diaphragm are involved (can be misdiagnosed as pneumonia). If the tongue is involved, a calf is unable to suck. Sudden death can occur if the myocardium is involved.

Young Adults (Myoglobinuria)

An acute azoturia syndrome was diagnosed in calves transported to a feedlot and was related to a selenium-deficient diet from the place of origin. The muscles primarily involved were the back and thigh.[12] In one feedlot study, the sentinel case was recumbent and had diarrhea. Subclinical myopathy was diagnosed in the group based on elevated serum creatine phosphokinase and aspartate amino transferase con-

centrations, and a myopathy was noted in biopsy specimens.[48] This myopathy was related to a low vitamin E concentration in the high-moisture corn component of the ration.

Mature (Recumbency)

A milk fever–like syndrome has been described; affected cows did not respond to conventional milk fever therapy. The researchers attribute the problem to the stress of repeated dietary changes, a digestive upset, and low selenium and vitamin E intake.[19] In one case report, pregnant Chianina heifers experienced abortion and periparturient recumbency. This was associated with a combined vitamin E/selenium deficiency, rapid growth, and the stress of pregnancy and calving.[24]

CLINICAL PATHOLOGY

The plasma activity of several enzymes of muscle origin is used as a diagnostic tool and to monitor the response to treatment.[4] The concentrations in the plasma vary in relation to the severity of the muscle damage and the plasma half-life of the enzyme. Plasma activity of creatine kinase, a muscle-dependent enzyme, is significantly correlated with microscopic damage of the muscle and is a useful tool for monitoring recovery and identifying animals that are affected subclinically.[2]

Other enzymes used to assess muscle injury are not muscle specific. These are aspartate aminotransferase, lactate dehydrogenase,[4] alanine aminotransferase, and pyruvate kinase.

Plasma selenium concentrations are used as a measurement of selenium status (normal 0.05 to 0.4 µg/mL). Normal liver selenium concentrations are 0.35 mg/kg of DM. Erythrocyte GSH-Px (normal >30 IU/liter) is a stable measure of selenium status, which depends on the availability of selenium during erythropoiesis.[28] A calf's plasma selenium concentrations at birth are significantly correlated with that of its dam at parturition.[22] Plasma or serum tocopherol concentrations (normal >4 µg/mL) are not always useful indicators of vitamin E status, because the body has limited stores. The liver is the principal site of vitamin E storage. These stores and circulating tocopherol concentrations vary in relation to the season of the year, physiological state, breed, and dietary intake.[13] Plasma concentrations are low in calves despite their dams' status.[22]

TREATMENT AND SUPPLEMENTATION

Selenium

Dietary selenium requirements are 0.1 to 0.1 ⌣ ⌣ of DM for all ages of cattle.

In areas where selenium deficiency is a problem, the cow herd should receive a year-round supplement. If this is not possible, the cows should receive a supplement during the last 3 months of pregnancy to build up fetal reserves. The amount of selenium in commercial mineral supplements fed free choice or in a mixed ration is government regulated but is at a level that should be adequate for preventing white muscle disease. The selenium content of commercial supplements is under review in the United States. Sustained-release oral boluses slowly release selenium into the rumen for a specified period. Their advantage is that the amount of selenium available for an individual animal is known. Systemic (injectable) supplements are used in the prevention and treatment of white muscle disease. The bottle dose and instructions should be followed carefully to avoid toxicity (lethal dose 1 to 2 mg/kg of BW). Selenium and vitamin E are slowly released for 14 to 18 days. No matter what method of supplementation is used, multiple sources can result in acute or chronic selenium toxicity.

Vitamin E

In supplementation trials, the bioavailability of vitamin E is poor. This in part may be related to individual animals' response, vitamin degradation by rumen microorganisms associated with high-grain diets, the form of the supplement,[35] and the level of unsaturated fat in the diet. Unesterified tocopherol improves plasma alpha-tocopherol levels better than an equivalent amount of tocopherol acetate.[13] Thus, if a high oxidative load exists, published requirements must be adjusted. An adequate dietary vitamin E intake is 100 mg of alpha-tocopherol per kilogram of dietary DM (1 IU vitamin E = 1 mg alpha-tocopherol). If unsaturated fats are added to the ration, increase vitamin E at 2 mg/g of added fat. This may be important in early lactation and for calves fed milk replacer, when additional fat may be added to the diet.

TOXICITIES

IONOPHORE TOXICITY

Ionophore antibiotics are used in cattle feeds to improve feed efficiency and as a coccidiostat. Toxicosis occurs with improper mixing, accidental contamination, or formulation of rations. The ionophore most commonly associated with toxicity is monensin sodium. The LD_{50} for cattle is 21.9 mg/kg of BW.[42] The newer ionophores have a higher LD_{50}. Monensin toxicity results in edema, hemorrhage, and coagulation necrosis of cardiac and skeletal muscle. Clinical signs are anorexia, depression, dyspnea, and a stiff gait.

FLUORIDE TOXICITY

Acute fluoride toxicity occurs if the dietary intake reaches 100 mg/kg of DM. Long-term exposure to fluorine (>50 mg/kg of DM) can result in periosteal hyperostosis, compactness of bone tissue, and osteoporotic changes.[25] Teeth lesions seen are mottling, hypoplasia, and abrasions of permanent incisors.[45] Fluoride can pass the placental barrier and result in a five- to eightfold increase in a calf's skeletal fluoride concentrations.[50] The toxicity of fluoride depends on the chemical composition and water solubility. Calcium fluoride is the least toxic, and sodium fluoride the most.[54] Undernutrition accentuates the toxic affects.

In chronic fluorosis, cattle are lame and have difficulty eating and drinking. A drop in milk production occurs, as well as a loss of body condition. Fracture of the distal phalanx (P3) may occur.[54]

Fluorosis occurs in cattle grazing on contaminated pastures (plants have a limited capacity to take up fluoride) or drinking polluted water (>35 mg/liter). Raw rock phosphate supplementation was a source of fluoride. Historically, bone meal supplements have been a source. Mineral supplements must now contain a fluoride-to-phosphorus ratio of 1:100. Pollution comes from industrial plants. An outbreak of fluorosis in cattle occurred after a volcanic eruption in the southern Andes. The eruption resulted in fluoride contamination of the forage.[5] Fluorosis is enzootic in parts of India, Australia, and Africa. Aluminium salts are used to decrease intestinal absorption of fluoride.

MYCOTOXINS

ERGOTISM

Description

Claviceps purpurea is a natural fungal inhabitant of soils. Under high-moisture conditions, this fungus infects the ovary of the plant during development of the flower stage, resulting in ergot bodies in the mature seed. The fungal elements or sclerotia are slightly larger than the original whole seed, oblong, and black to deep purple. Immature ergot, the honey-dew stage (honey colored), contains less toxin than the darker sclerotium. Cattle become affected after consuming mature contaminated grass, hay, or concentrate feed.[17] Rations containing 0.6% or more of ergot are potentially toxic.

If infected grains are milled, the toxic principles involved, ergotamine and ergonovine, can be identified by laboratory evaluation. Forty alkaloids have been identified. Although rye is considered the main grain infected, ergotism occurs in association with triticale, wheat, barley, oats, wild grasses, tall fescue, and crested wheat grass.

Pathogenesis

The toxins cause arterial spasm, endothelial degeneration, and dry gangrene. The sequence of events following the ingestion of ergot varies.[10] The fungus grows more rapidly in wet, warm seasons. Cold temperatures accelerate the development of skin necrosis. The larger the amount consumed or the younger the animal consuming the toxin, the more dramatic (acute form) may be the clinical signs, which may include nervous excitement.

Clinical Signs

Lameness, first occurring in the hind limbs, is a consistent finding with ergot toxicity. Necrosis of the tip of the tail and ears and of the distal limbs occurs later.[56]

If consumption of ergot takes place for 7 to 10 days, a chronic form of ergotism occurs.[10] The clinical signs of the chronic form of ergotism appear from 3 to 6 weeks after the first ingestion of the toxin. One of the early signs of chronic ergotism is lameness, an indicator of a wide range of diseases and not specific to ergot poisoning. During early painful phases, the body temperature rises, the respiratory rate increases, and the animal becomes dull and declines to eat and drink. At the same time when the lameness appears, the skin over the distal extremities might feel cold and clammy. This could be easily overlooked. Within a week of the onset of lameness, an indented line appears at the limit of the normal skin. Distal to this point, the skin progressively dries out and darkens in color (a change that may not be noticed in black-pigmented animals). The skin is insensitive at this stage owing to nerve death.

As the dry gangrene progresses, the skin and claws separate from the tissues beneath. The dry skin forms a casing around the structures beneath, protecting them and preventing examination of the deeper structures. As long as this casing remains intact, affected animals experience no pain. As the protective casing breaks down, a bed of granulation tissue is exposed.

FESCUE FOOT

Definition

Fescue foot is a syndrome of peripheral dry gangrene (similar to ergotism) manifested primarily in hindquarter lameness. The offending mycotoxins are produced by the fungus *Epichloe typhina* or *Acremonium coenophialum (Sphacelia typhina)*, found in tall fescue grass, hay, or seed. The endophyte fungus (invisible to the naked eye) within the grass alters the plant's metabolism to produce the toxin. The alkaloids isolated from tall fescue grass are pyrrolizidine, *N*-formyl loline, and ergot-like. The toxicosis primarily affects cattle in the southeastern and midwestern states of the United States, where tall fescue *(Festuca arundinacea Schreb)* is the major grass variety, covering more than 35 million acres (= 14 million hectares).[26] High environmental temperatures can increase an animal's sensitivity.

Pathogenesis

The mycotoxin reduces prolactin secretion.[7] Vasoconstrictor agents in the mycotoxin produce marked peripheral vasoconstriction by direct stimulation of the adrenergic nerves supplying arteriolar smooth muscle.

Clinical Signs

Affected cattle are lame as a result of a dry gangrene of the distal limbs (hind limbs first). The cattle lose weight, develop fat necrosis, and are agalactic. Signs usually develop in some stock within a short period (10 to 21 days) after turnout into a contaminated fescue pasture in fall. A period of frost tends to contribute to an increased incidence.

Signs of fescue foot are seen in fattening steers and heifers in the fall and winter, although cases can occur year-round. Cattle are alert but lose weight and develop a hind leg lameness, often preceded by a period of paddling or weight shifting. The back is slightly arched. Knuckling of a hind pastern may be an initial sign.

Erythema and swelling of the coronary region are associated with progressive lameness, poor appetite, and depression. Severely affected animals develop skin necrosis and dry gangrene from the pastern distally. The skin is hard and cold and may slough. Sometimes one or both horny claws are shed (exungulation), usually when the animal is forced to move fast or awkwardly (e.g., transport to or movement in a sale barn or cattle market). Necrosis of the ear tips or tail switch is often observed.

Differential Diagnosis

Differential diagnoses include ergotism (which can coexist), selenium toxicosis, frostbite, foot rot (phlegmona interdigitalis), and simple trauma.

Diagnostic Tests

The endophyte is readily seen under the microscope in infected feed or plant stems but not in the leaf. Serum prolactin levels are elevated in steers on endophyte-infected pastures.[26] Quantitative laboratory tests, including enzyme-linked immunosorbent assay, are available to measure and monitor the fungal concentration in plant tissue.

Treatment and Prevention

The entire group should be removed from the affected pasture, or if fed contaminated hay, an alternative roughage should be found. If cattle must be maintained on the same land, supplementary endophyte-free hay and, if economical, concentrates should be fed. Problem pastures can be reseeded with certified endophyte-free fescue strains or seeded with a legume to dilute the fescue component. Fungicides are unsuccessful in control. High-risk pastures can sometimes be grazed more safely by adult breeding stock.

OTHER TOXIC PLANTS CAUSING LAMENESS

TOXIC SHRUBS AND PLANTS

Certain well-defined geographical areas have major problems of developmental diseases that result when the dam or offspring ingests toxic plants. Examples in the United States include lupinosis (crooked calf disease), *Cassia* species toxicity, and others. Many signs are not associated with the locomotor system, but the two examples just mentioned are briefly discussed next.

Lupinosis

Crooked calf disease is induced in a variable proportion of calves (as many as 30%) born to dams that ingested specific toxic lupine plants primarily in the period of days 40 to 70 of gestation. The condition is reported from varied regions, primarily the United States. Toxic species include *Lupinus caudatus, Lupinus sericeus,* and *Lupinus laxiflorus.* Anagyrine, a quinolizidine alkaloid isolated from the plant, is the likely toxic agent.

Calves are born with severe skeletal deformities including limb malformations, especially in the forelimbs. Abnormalities include flexure contraction and arthrogryposis, resulting from disordered joint growth, and shortening and rotation of long bones. Other skeletal deformities include torticollis, scoliosis, and skull deformities including cleft palate. Calves are born alive but suffer severe growth retardation. Minor degrees of deformity may occur but tend to be recognized easily because of the grazing history and concomitant severe cases.

Control, which is often difficult, depends on grazing management, which involves making sure that pregnant cows avoid dangerous pastures during the susceptible period.

Cassia *Species Toxicity*

Various *Cassia* plant species (e.g., *Cassia occidentalis,* or coffee senna; and *Cassia obtusifolia,* or sickle pod senna) that flourish in sandy southern areas of the United States have regularly caused severe illness and death as a result of skeletal myopathy and less pronounced myocardial lesions. The first signs, after diarrhea, include weakness and a swaying and stumbling gait. Some affected animals are already recumbent at the first examination. Affected stock tend to be yearlings, in contrast to the younger calves suffering vitamin E–selenium myopathy.

A prominent clinical sign is myoglobinuria following muscle degeneration, as well as elevated levels of muscle enzymes. Moderate pallor of major skeletal muscle groups is observed at autopsy.

Careful differential diagnosis is vital because treatment of *Cassia* toxicity with vitamin E or selenium potentiates the toxicity.

Control, as in lupinosis, is by appropriate pasture management and is outside the scope of this text.

Selenosis

Selenosis (alkali disease) has been reported in cattle when the long-term dietary intake of selenium (as selenoamino acids or inorganic selenium compounds) was greater than 5 mg/kg of dietary DM.[52]

Certain plants, termed alkali accumulators, grow on seleniferous soils and can accumulate selenium in excess of 1000 ppm. They are unpalatable to livestock, and cattle are poisoned only when good forage is scarce. Chronic selenium poisoning is characterized by signs of stiffness, lameness, claw malformations, and hair loss, as well as emaciation due to reduced feed intake and mobility. The claw horn is occasionally shed but more frequently develops multiple horizontal fissures.[28]

REFERENCES

1. Agricultural Research Council: The Nutrient Requirements of Ruminant Livestock. Wallingford, UK, Commonwealth Agricultural Bureau, 1980.
2. Allen WM, Bradley R, Berrett S, et al: Degenerative myopathy with myoglobinuria in yearling cattle. Br Vet J 131:292–308, 1975.
3. Allen TA, Weingand K: The vitamin D (calciferol) endocrine system. Comp Cont Ed 7:482–488, 1985.
4. Anderson PH, Berrett S, Patterson DSP: The significance of elevated plasma creatine phosphokinase in muscle damage of cattle. J Comp Pathol 86:531–538, 1976.
5. Araya O, Wittwer F, Villa A, et al: Bovine fluorosis following volcanic activity in the southern Andes. Vet Rec 126:641–642, 1990.
6. Beighle DE, Boyazoglu PA, Hemken RW: Use of bovine rib bone in serial sampling for mineral analysis. J Dairy Sci 76:1047–1052, 1993.
7. Bernard JK, Chestnut AB, Erickson BH, et al: Effects of prepartum consumption of endophyte-infected tall fescue on serum prolactin and subsequent milk production of Holstein cows. J Dairy Sci 76:1928–1933, 1993.
8. Brazele F: Zinc methionine appears to improve hoof condition of grazing beef cattle. Feedstuffs 64:10, 1992.
9. Brown TF, Zeringue LK: Laboratory evaluation of solubility and structural integrity of complexed and chelated trace mineral supplements. J Dairy Sci 77:181–187, 1994.
10. Burfingen PJ: Ergotism. J Am Vet Med Assoc 163:1288–1290, 1973.
11. Calvo MS: Dietary phosphorus, calcium—metabolism and bone. J Nutr 123:1627–1633, 1993.
12. Chalmers GA, Decaire M, Zacher CJ, Barrett MW: Myopathy and myoglobinuria in feedlot cattle. Can Vet J 20:105–108, 1979.
13. Charmley E, Hidiroglou N, Ochoa L, et al: Plasma and hepatic-tocopherol in cattle following oral or intramuscular supplementation. J Dairy Sci 75:804–810, 1992.
14. Crowe NA, Neathery MW, Miller WJ, et al: Influence of high dietary aluminum on performance and phosphorus bioavailability in dairy calves. J Dairy Sci 73:808–818, 1990.
15. Dakshinamurti K, Chauhan J: Regulations of biotin enzymes. Annu Rev Nutr 8:211–233, 1988.
16. Dembinski Z, Wieckowski W: Bull Vet Inst Pulaway 30–31(1–4):104–112, 1987/1988.
17. Fraser CM: The Merck Veterinary Manual, 7th ed. Rahway, NJ, Merck & Co, 1991, pp 1684–1685.
18. Frigg M, Hartmann D, Straub OC: Biotin kenetics in serum of cattle after intravenous and oral dosing. Int J Vit Nutr Res 64:36–40, 1994.
19. Gitter M, Bradley R: Nutritional myodegeneration in dairy cows. Vet Rec 103:24–26, 1978.
20. Henry HL, Norman AW: Vitamin D: Metabolism and biological actions. Annu Rev Nutr 4:493–520, 1984.
21. Henry R, Ammerman CB, Littell RC: Relative bioavailability of manganese methionine complex and inorganic sources for ruminants. J Dairy Sci 75:3473–3478, 1992.
22. Hidiroglou M, Batra TR, Roy GL: Changes in plasma alpha-tocopherol and selenium of gestating cows fed hay or silage. J Dairy Sci 77:190–195, 1994.
23. Hill MA, Ruth GR, Van Sickle DC, et al: Histochemical morphologic features of growth cartilages in long bones of pigs of various ages. Am J Vet Res 48:1477–1484, 1987.
24. Hutchinson LJ, Scholz RW, Drake TR: Nutritional myodegeneration in a group of Chianina heifers. J Am Vet Med Assoc 181:581–584, 1982.
25. Kapoor V, Prasad T, Bhatia KC: Effect of dietary fluorine on histological changes in calves. Fluoride 26:105–110, 1993.
26. Kerr LA: Fescue toxicosis. In Howard J (ed): Current Veterinary Therapy. Food Animal Practice. Philadelphia, WB Saunders, 1993, pp 370–371.
27. Kincaid RL, Blauwiekel RM, Cron R, et al: Supplementation of copper as copper sulphate or copper proteinate for grazing cattle fed forages containing molybdenum. J Dairy Sci 69:160–163, 1986.
28. Koller LD, Exon JH: The two faces of selenium—deficiency and toxicity—are similar in animals and man. Can J Vet Res 50:297–306, 1986.
29. Krook L, Lutwak L, McEntee K, et al: Nutritional hypercalcitoninism in bulls. Cornell Vet 61:625–639, 1971.
30. Morse D, Head HH, Wilcox CJ, et al: Effects of concentration of dietary phosphorus on amount and route of excretion. J Dairy Sci 75:3039–3048, 1992.
31. National Research Council: Nutrient Requirements of Beef Cattle, 7th ed. Washington, DC, National Academy of Sciences, 1984.
32. National Research Council: Nutrient Requirements of Dairy Cattle, 6th ed. Washington, DC, National Academy of Sciences, 1989.
33. Nelson J: Bioavailability of trace mineral ingredients. Proceedings of the 6th Western Nutritional Conference. Winnipeg, Manitoba, 1985, pp 60–72.
34. Orr JP, McKenzie GC: Unusual skeletal deformities in calves in a Saskatchewan beef herd. Can Vet J 22:121–125, 1981.
35. Pehrson B, Hakkarainen J, Tornqist M, et al: Effect of vitamin E supplementation on weight gain, immune competence, and disease incidence in barley-fed beef cattle. J Dairy Sci 74:1054–1059, 1991.
36. Poole AR: The growth plate: Cellular physiology, cartilage assembly and mineralization. In Hall BK, Newman SA (eds): Cartilage: Molecular Aspects. Boca Raton, FL, CRC Press, 1992, pp 179–211.
37. Rice D, Kennedy S: Vitamin E: Functions and effects of deficiency. Br Vet J 144:482–496, 1988.
38. Rice DA, Kennedy S: Assessment of vitamin E, selenium and polyunsaturated fatty acid interactions in the aetiology of disease in the bovine. Proc Nutr Soc 47:177–184, 1988.
39. Rodan GA: Introduction to bone biology. Bone 13:S3–S6, 1992.
40. Romo GA, Kellems RO, Powell K, et al: Some blood minerals and hormones in cows fed variable mineral levels and ionic balance. J Dairy Sci 74:3068–3077, 1991.
41. Schryver HF, Hintz HF: Handbook series in Nutrition and Food. In Richeigh M (ed): Nutritional Disorders, vol II, Section E. Effect of Nutrient Deficiencies in Animals. Boca Raton, FL, CRC Press, 1978.
42. Schweitzer D, Kimberling C, Spraker T, et al: Accidental monensin sodium intoxication of feedlot cattle. J Am Vet Med Assoc 184:1273–1276, 1984.
43. Scott D, McLean AF: Control of mineral absorption in ruminants. Proc Nutr Soc 40:257–266, 1981.
44. Seyedin SM, Rosen DM: Cartilage growth and differentiation factors. In Hall BK, Newman SA (eds): Cartilage: Molecular Aspects. Boca Raton, FL, CRC Press, 1992, pp 131–151.
45. Shupe JL, Butcher JE, Call JW, et al: Clinical signs and bone changes associated with phosphorus deficiency in beef cattle. Am J Vet Res 49:1629–1636, 1988.
46. Shupe JL, Christofferson PV, Olson AE, et al: Relationship of cheek tooth abrasion to fluorine induced permanent incisor lesions in livestock. Am J Vet Res 48:1498–1503, 1987.
47. Smart ME, Northcote MJ: Liver biopsies in cattle. Comp Cont Ed Pract Vet 7:S327–S332, 1985.
48. Smith DL, Palmer ST, Hulland TJ, et al: A nutritional myopathy enzootic in a group of yearling beef cattle. Can Vet J 26:385–390, 1985.
49. Suda T, Shinki T, Takahashi N: The role of vitamin D in bone and intestinal cell differentiation. Annu Rev Nutr 10:195–211, 1990.
50. Suttie JW, Clay AB, Shearer TR: Dental fluorosis in bovine temporary teeth. Am J Vet Res 46:404–408, 1985.

51. Thompson KG, Cook TG: Rickets in yearling steers wintered on a swede (*Brassica napus*) crop. N Z Vet J 35:11–13, 1987.
52. Traub-Dargatz JL, Knight AP, Hamar DW: Selenium toxicity in horses. Comp Cont Ed 8:771–776, 1986.
53. Vermeer C, Jie G-S, Knapen MHJ: Role of vitamin K in bone metabolism. Annu Rev Nutr 15:1–22, 1995.
54. Wheeler SW, Fell LR: Fluorides in cattle nutrition. Nutr Abs Rev 53:741–761, 1983.
55. Williams SN, Lawrence LA, McDowell LZR, et al: Dietary phosphorus concentrations related to breaking load and chemical properties in heifers. J Dairy Sci 73:1100–1106, 1990.
56. Woods AJ, Jones JB, Mantle PG: An outbreak of gangrenous ergotism in cattle. Vet Rec 78:742–749, 1966.
57. Yano F, Yano H, Breves G: Calcium and phosphorus metabolism in ruminants. Physiological aspects of digestion and metabolism in ruminants. Proceedings of the 7th International Symposium on Ruminant Physiology. San Diego, CA, Academic Press, 1991, pp 277–291.

A. David Weaver   *United Kingdom*

11

Joint Conditions

This chapter discusses the anatomy, pathobiology, clinical signs, and diagnosis of diarthrodial joint diseases and includes brief descriptions of their treatment. It concentrates on diarthrodial joints, because other types (fibrous, synostoses, as between the tibia and fibula or cartilaginous joints comprising synchondroses and symphyses) rarely have clinical problems.

The typical diarthrodial joint comprises two or more bones covered with hyaline cartilage, connected by a joint capsule that is lined by the synovial membrane, and supporting ligaments (e.g., collateral, cranial cruciate). The stifle additionally has paired menisci; the hip joint has an accessory fibrocartilaginous rim over the dorsal edge of the acetabulum.

ARTICULAR CARTILAGE

Articular cartilage is hyaline and translucent owing to its high water content (about 70% in mature cartilage, greater in neonatal). Cartilage (dry matter basis) contains about 50% collagen, 35% proteoglycan, 10% glycoproteins (protease inhibitors, lysozyme, fibronectin, and chondronectin), minerals (3%), lipids (1%), and chondrocytes.

The significance of the composition of articular cartilage in the context of bovine joint disease is that major pathological conditions (infectious or septic arthritis, degenerative joint disease [DJD], osteochondrosis) derive in part from degradation of matrix proteoglycans by proteolytic enzymes. Chondrocytes themselves may be an important source of such enzyme activity in horses.[7] This may also be true of cattle.

Articular cartilage is arbitrarily subdivided into four zones, the more superficial unmineralized zones (I to III) being separated from the mineralized zone IV by a conspicuous tidemark or blue line. Chondrocytes in the articular cartilage become progressively more numerous, smaller, and elongated toward the surface. Collagen fibers rarely extend parallel to the cartilaginous surface, being tangential or oblique in a decussating pattern. Mechanical strength of the articular cartilage is enhanced by this complex meshwork.

Articular cartilage tends to be thicker over areas of maximal pressure, as in the middle of convex surfaces (e.g., proximal humeral head) and the periphery of concave surfaces (e.g., acetabulum).

Synovial grooves (fossae synoviales) are normal irregular depressions, usually bilaterally symmetrical, on the surface of certain joints (e.g., carpal, tarsal). Their dimensions vary from 1 to 2 cm long to 2 to 9 mm wide. These depressions develop in early postnatal life. They have distinct borders and a relatively smooth surface and appear bluish pink because the subchondral capillary bed lies beneath their surface. They are most apparent in the carpal and tarsal joints. Their morphology has been reviewed.[29] Their appearance should not be confused with early degenerative change. Their function is disputed but is thought to involve joint lubrication.

JOINT CAPSULE

The joint capsule forms a sleeve that encloses the articular structures. Ligaments act with the joint capsule to maintain the correct location of bone ends and restrict movement to various degrees depending on their thickness and strength.

The joint capsule has three layers, an outermost fibrous structure, a thin connecting lamina propria, and the synovial membrane.

The blood supply to the joint capsule ramifies in the fibrous outer layer to supply smaller branches to the subsynovial and synovial membrane. Lymphatics and nerves accompany these vessels into the joint capsule. The articular cartilage has no nerve supply. The pain of arthritis originates in the well-innervated joint capsule.

The innermost layer of the joint capsule, the synovial membrane, is critically involved in the production and turnover of synovia through the inner lining intima. This layer is smooth, only a few cells thick, and is very well vascularized.

The synovial membrane is of particular interest from the physiological and pathological viewpoints. The intima consists of both type A phagocytic and type B secretory or fibroblastic cells. The former are more numerous and more superficial and act as macrophages. Type B cells produce hyaluronic acid. Other types of cells are intermediate between types A and B, and it is possible that types A and B are different functional stages of the same cell.

The synovial membrane is permeable in either direction to small molecules, which are removed by capillaries and lymphatics. Phagocytes remove particulate matter, which is deposited in the subintimal layer. If the amount of debris is great, as in disease processes such as DJD, capsular fibrosis may be stimulated. This fibrosis in turn can contribute to swelling and stiffness of joint movement.

SYNOVIAL FLUID

Synovia, a plasma ultrafiltrate, is a clear, viscid, colorless or pale yellow, nonclotting fluid. It contains most molecules that are present in plasma, but large protein molecules are lacking. Mononuclear cells account for about 90% of the total (synoviocytes, monocytes, lymphocytes), the remaining 10% being polymorphonuclear leukocytes. The protein content is about 1.5 grams/liter.

Synovia is viscid owing to hyaluronan, which is synthesized within the cell on the plasma membrane of synoviocytes and chondrocytes. The viscosity, which results from the overlap of the large hyaluronan molecules, has three major biomechanical properties: it functions as a boundary lubricant, absorbs some of the energy produced by joint movement, and aids in strain resistance. A second significant function of synovia is to supply nutrients to articular cartilage by diffusion from subchondral vessels and from the cartilage itself.

SYNOVIAL FLUID PATHOBIOLOGY

Synovia may easily be collected (arthrocentesis) from normal joints (e.g., tibiotarsal) in cattle (see p. 228, Fig. 14–13, for sites and technique) and is placed in a sterile glass tube (for bacterial culture), a heparinized tube (for cell count and general examination), or a sodium fluoride tube (for glucose estimation).

Table 11–1 lists some characteristics of normal and abnormal synovial fluid. The abnormal states are septic, suspected septic, aseptic, degenerative osteoarthritis, and hydrops. The major potential changes are in color and turbidity, clotting property, total leukocyte count and proportion (percentage) of polymorphonuclear neutrophils, total protein, and the nature of the mucin precipitate.

The volume and appearance of synovial fluid vary among different bovine joints of the same animal. Exercise tends to increase the volume, and inactivity to decrease it. Older cattle often tend to have a more yellow synovia. Blood in synovial fluid renders it pink if fresh (e.g., iatrogenic arthrocentesis) and amber if old. Any turbidity is pathological and represents cellular debris. Floccules may result from the presence of degenerated cartilage.

Viscosity may be simply and semiquantitatively estimated by observing one drop falling from a syringe hub. The normal length of "string" before separation is at least 2 cm. A reduction is due to synovial dilution (e.g., by effusion into a joint, as in hydrarthrosis or inflammation), severe synovitis (decreased production and poor polymerization of hyaluronic acid by synovial lining cells), or hyaluronic acid degradation by bacterial hyaluronidase.

The mucin clot test is similarly easily performed by adding a few drops of synovia (0.5 mL) to about 3 mL of 2% acetic acid solution and gently shaking the mixture. The normal effect is a tight, ropey clot. An abnormal result is a loose clot and particles floating free in the surrounding solution, an effect due to similar changes in synovia as reduced viscosity. EDTA may decrease the mucin clot quality.

In the category of suspected septic, the presence of bacteria on a Gram-stained smear does not necessarily indicate a current infection. Particularly if most cells are phagocytosed, it may rather be evidence of a past infection, which may nevertheless still be active. *Actinomyces pyogenes* is by far the most common isolate in septic arthritis in mature cattle, followed by streptococci and staphylococci in a mixed culture.

SYNOVITIS

Synovitis involves infiltration of inflammatory cells into the synovial membrane, vascular proliferation

TABLE 11–1. CHARACTERISTICS OF NORMAL AND ABNORMAL SYNOVIAL FLUID

	Appearance	Clot	Leukocytes/μL Total	Leukocytes/μL %	Protein (g/dL)	Mucin Precipitate
Normal	Clear	−	<250	<10	<1.8	Tight, ropy
Septic	Very turbid	+	100,000	95	>4.0	Flakes
Suspect septic	Very turbid	+	50,000	90	>4.0	Flakes
Aseptic	Slightly turbid	+ or −	3,000	Variable	2–4	Normal or slightly abnormal
Degenerative osteoarthritis	Clear or slightly turbid	−	<250	<15	<2	Normal or slightly abnormal
Hydrops	Clear or slightly turbid	−	<350	<10	<2	Normal

Modified from Kersjes AW: Over Synovia et Synovitis. Utrecht, Netherlands, Proefschrift, 1963.

and both hyperplasia and hypertrophy of the lining cells, and fibrosis. It may be divided into primary (or type 1 traumatic arthritis) and secondary (type 2 traumatic arthritis) synovitis.

Primary synovitis or inflammation of a synovial membrane is uncommon. It does not initially result in gross damage to the articular cartilage or supporting structures.

Secondary synovitis results from trauma to or degeneration of the articular cartilage or subchondral bone. The etiology is multiple: DJD, articular malformation or maldevelopment, intra-articular fracture (e.g., Salter-Harris type), or ligamentous instability or rupture (e.g., cranial cruciate). Hard and soft tissue disease usually occur at the same time.

Fibrin clots are the major gross feature of the inflammatory exudate resulting from primary or secondary synovitis. Fibrin is deposited on both the cartilage and synovial villi, disrupting their function and contributing to permanent damage and maintenance of an inflammatory cycle. Removal of such fibrin (see p. 168) is an important step in therapy of joint inflammation.

Synovitis results in the release of histamine and 5-hydroxytryptamine and activation of the kinin, complement, and clotting system (Fig. 11–1). Metabolites of arachidonic acid develop in cell membranes and are powerful endogenous mediators of inflammation.

Synoviocytes and oxygen free radicals (produced by neutrophils and macrophages) are responsible for the formation of lysosomal enzymes. These enzymes degrade hyaluronan in the synovia and interstitium.

Other major effects of synovitis include hypertrophy and hyperplasia of the synovium and increased pain perception mediated by prostaglandins of the I and E series (see Fig. 11–1).

SPECIFIC CONSIDERATIONS IN EXAMINATION FOR JOINT DISEASE

Stance. Clinicians may be misled by a stance suggestive of a joint problem—namely, reduced weight-bearing and apparent prominence of a large joint such as the shoulder or stifle. All cases should have the possibility of a claw lameness excluded.

Muscle Atrophy. Localized muscle atrophy is a nonspecific sign and may reflect a nerve lesion resulting in disuse atrophy. A specific paralysis should be excluded in all cases of unilateral atrophy. Atrophy also tends to throw related joint areas into prominence. The suspected prominent joint should be contrasted with the contralateral joint.

Palpation of Suspected Joint. The prominence of bony landmarks should be contrasted, as should any swelling and fluctuation possibly involving the joint capsule and an increased synovial fluid volume. Heat may sometimes be appreciated in the overlying skin.

Manipulation. Digital pressure on a joint may be resented (possible septic arthritis). Flexion and extension should be practiced with great care, be-

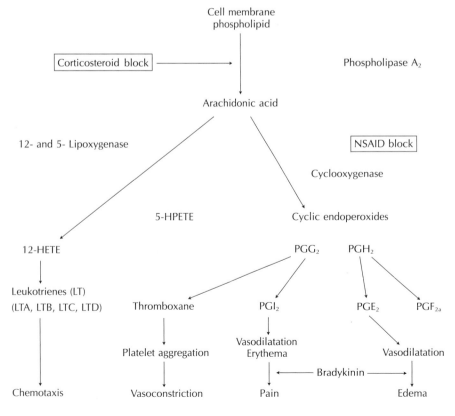

Figure 11–1. Arachidonic acid cascade. NSAIDs, nonsteroidal anti-inflammatory drugs; BW 755C, a lipoxygenase and cyclo-oxygenase blocker; 5-HPETE, 5-hydropero-oxyeicosatetraenoic acid; 12-HETE, 12-hydroxyeicosatetraenoic acid; SRS-A, slow-reacting substance of anaphylaxis; PG, prostaglandin. (Modified from Todhunter and Lust: Synovial joint anatomy, biology, and pathobiology. *In* Auer J [ed]: Equine Surgery. Philadelphia, WB Saunders, 1992.)

cause pain may be pronounced. Crepitus (a grating sound) may be evinced. It is due to bone, exposed as a result of cartilaginous erosion or loss, rubbing on bone. In some instances, fractured bone ends are the cause of crepitus. In others, periarticular new bone surfaces grate against each other. False-positive findings can confuse a clinician when sound is transmitted from a more distal site. An example is the click appreciated when, with the hand on the stifle area, the claws intermittently contact the ground as the cow is gently rocked in a transverse plane.

Rectal Palpation. Rectal palpation is essential in any case in which joint disease may be located in the pelvic area (coxofemoral joint or sacroiliac region). The symmetry of the pelvis can be assessed (including the region of the obturator foramen). The animal may be rocked gently from side to side with one hand in the rectum and the other, palm flat, over the greater femoral trochanter. If doubt remains, the patient may, if its temperament allows, be walked slowly while continuing this examination. The major abnormality to be detected, apart from asymmetry, is crepitus originating proximally. Again, one should beware of false-positive findings.

SPECIAL TECHNIQUES

Radiology

Routine radiographs, using a minimum of two views, have frequently been of great value in differential diagnosis of joint diseases in cattle. Technical difficulties are greater than in small animals. Economics are often a limiting factor. In the forelimb, the shoulder and elbow, because of their size and proximity to the trunk, and in the hind limb the coxofemoral joint and pelvis can present difficulties in positioning and in exposure factors. Pelvic radiographs in the ventrodorsal projection may require deep sedation or general anesthesia (see pp. 47–48). An atlas of bovine radiology includes many excellent examples of joint diseases.[1] As in other species, it is essential to take appropriate safety measures to avoid exposure to radiation, particularly to the primary beam. The nature of the species and surroundings may mitigate against effective control of potential radiation hazards when compared with the more routine use of such facilities in small animal and equine practice. Whenever possible, grids and, in proximal limb joints (shoulder, hip, stifle), rare earth screens are advisable to improve quality and reduce the exposure time and radiation hazard (see pp. 24, 32).

Conditions in which radiographs are of particular value in establishing the differential diagnosis and the progress of a lesion include septic physitis, fractures (for deciding on the optimal methods of fixation), physeal separation, dislocations, and septic arthritides.

Septic arthritis in its early stages (up to day 7 after infection) may not lead to suspicious radiographic changes, except some soft tissue swelling. Later, a slight widening of the joint space reflects an increased volume of synovial fluid. Lack of definition of the joint surfaces reflects early damage to the subchondral bone. Free air is occasionally evident in the joint space (see p. 38). Later radiographic stages involve intracapsular and extracapsular periosteal reaction, subchondral sclerosis, exostosis formation, osteomyelitis and bone destruction in smaller limb bones (carpal, tarsal, proximal sesamoidean pathological fractures), and dislocations (see Fig. 3–12). In advanced stages of septic arthritis, osteolysis is more advanced, the new bone is denser and has clearer borders, and pathological fractures can occasionally be seen.

Ultrasonography

A real-time linear scanner (e.g., 7.5 mHz) with video images recorded on tape has been developed as a useful and, after purchase of the equipment, economical method of assessing both joint disease and soft tissue damage (e.g., tendons, tendon sheaths) in cattle.[15] Examination involves recording in both the sagittal and transverse planes of the bovine limb. The transducer is applied to the limb after skin clipping, cleaning, and application of a high-viscosity coupling gel. Manual or chemical restraint should be sufficient to permit safe skin contact of the transducer.

Arthroscopy

Rapid advances in the field of diagnostic and surgical arthroscopy in horses have not been matched by similar applications in cattle. The reasons are the different nature of lesions (the high incidence of chip fractures in the equine carpus has no parallel in cattle) and economical and management considerations (see p. 252 for some criteria).

Specialized clinics can successfully use this technique for the confirmatory diagnosis and treatment of septic arthritis of larger limb joints such as the stifle, tarsus, carpus, and fetlock.[18] Apart from use as a diagnostic aid, intra-articular cartilaginous and subchondral bone may be curetted, and accurate, efficient joint irrigation is facilitated.

Punch Biopsy

Punch biopsy of the synovial membrane is seldom indicated, having been superseded by arthroscopy. It may avoid the more traumatic diagnostic arthrotomy of open surgery and removal of a wedge of a suspected abnormal joint. The preferred instrument is a Tru-Cut assembly 4½ inches (10.8 cm) long (Travenol Labs, Deerfield, IL). The maximum sample size is 2 cm × 1 to 2 mm. This instrument is delicate and is very likely to bend if the animal moves. The subject should be tranquilized before infiltration of local anesthetic solution subcutaneously and along the proposed tract. Strict skin asepsis is mandatory. A small 0.5- to 1-cm skin incision is made over the site. The assembly is relatively atraumatic, and several samples may be taken from one entry port.

Another punch biopsy instrument that is stronger and that delivers a large specimen (diameter 3 mm) is the Polley-Bickel assembly. It is manipulated in a similar manner.

Biopsy material may be cultured, being placed in a suitable growth medium and later streaked on agar plates. Another specimen may be prepared for histopathology. To maintain orientation, the specimen should initially be pinned onto a flat surface before immersion into fixative.

Complications of bovine punch biopsy include mild hemarthrosis, septic arthritis (due to inadequate aseptic precautions), breakage of the instrument resulting from a patient's unexpected movement, and inadequate sample size.

INFECTIOUS ARTHRITIS

Infectious arthritis is caused by bacteria, mycoplasmas, viruses, fungi, or rickettsiae and may be limited to one joint or, as part of a systemic infection, may produce pathological changes in several joints (polyarthritis) and other tissues (e.g., lungs, brain).[3, 21]

Common causes of infectious arthritis include *Streptococcus* spp. and *Escherichia coli* in young animals and *A. pyogenes, Salmonella* spp., *Mycoplasma bovis,* and *Haemophilus somnus* at any age.[10, 21]

Infectious arthritis may be primary, resulting from direct penetration of the joint by a foreign body. Involvement of a joint by extension of cellulitis and necrosis from a decubital lesion (e.g., lateral aspect of hock, dorsum of carpus) is also primary. Secondary arthritis results from spread of pathogens from an adjacent localized focus (Fig. 11–2). Tertiary infectious arthritis follows systemic, usually hematogenous spread and is typically represented by "joint ill" or neonatal polyarthritis (discussed later).

Infectious arthritis, whether primary, secondary, or tertiary, starts with an inflammatory process in the capillary walls of the interstitial tissue of the synovial membrane and results in a synovitis (see p. 163). In cattle, the natural development after introduction of infection is a purulent arthritis (septic, pyogenic, or suppurative).

The following sections first consider an infectious (bacterial) arthritis in calves, joint ill or neonatal polyarthritis. This is followed by (1) septic arthritis of older cattle; (2) an unusual and poorly defined condition, Lyme borreliosis arthritis; (3) DJD; and (4) osteochondrosis and osteochondritis dissecans.

JOINT ILL (NEONATAL POLYARTHRITIS)

Joint ill in calves is a tertiary hematogenous septic arthritis, often affecting several joints in neonates or

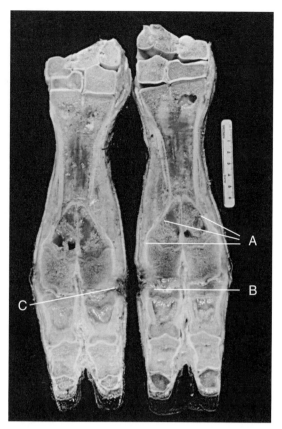

Figure 11–2. Bilateral open fractures of the metacarpus and spread of osteomyelitis to the fetlock joint in a 7-week-old Angus calf. Longitudinal section of one forelimb showing the fracture site (A) and the septic fetlock joint (B). Skin necrosis (C) resulted from severe traction on the obstetrical chains. Secondary septic arthritis.

very young (<4 weeks old) calves and almost always originating from an umbilical focus.

Incidence

Joint ill is a major nontraumatic cause of acquired joint disease. National figures for incidence have not been compiled. Dairy calves are more susceptible than beef calves. The incidence is higher in an unhygienic environment, where immediate postnatal disinfection of the umbilicus (e.g., by organic iodide) is not practiced, and where calves are immune compromised owing to inadequate colostral intake in the first few hours of life. Small, weak calves that remain recumbent for some hours, apart from failing to take colostrum, are also more likely to contaminate the abdominal skin of the umbilical region. Some premises may have a dangerously high and persistent level of potential pathogens in the calving area, leading to an increasing incidence. Surprisingly, the majority of calves with umbilical abscessation do not develop joint ill.

Etiology and Pathogenesis

Of the three tubular structures composing the umbilical remnant (umbilical vein, artery, and urachus), contamination and infection are most likely to develop in the flaccid and thin-walled vein. The other structures have a smaller lumen and, with more elastic tissue in the wall, tend to retract into the abdominal cavity after rupture of the umbilical cord. Any one of the three may be secondarily involved in infection through contiguous spread. Abscessation may initially be limited to the extra-abdominal remnant but tends to spread rapidly as an omphalophlebitis toward the liver and into the systemic circulation. *Streptococcus* spp. are probably the most common infectious agents. Somewhat less frequently, *E. coli, A. pyogenes,* and *Staphylococcus* spp. are isolated. *Salmonella* spp. are involved in a specific syndrome, affecting the metaphysis of slightly older calves and likely to spread to the joint cavity.

The route of hematogenous spread is either through metaphyseal or epiphyseal vessels or through the capillaries supplying the joint capsule, into the subsynovial layer and synovial membrane of one or more major joints (hock, carpus, stifle).

From the metaphysis, hematogenous organisms tend to be held up as sludge in end-arterioles adjacent to the growth plate. Organisms can then track along the line of least resistance through both the adjacent cortex at the physeal margin and the attachment of the joint capsule.

Spread from adjacent soft tissue injury, such as decubital lesions on the carpi of a calf unable to stand, into the bloodstream or directly into an adjacent joint capsule seems to be relatively less common. Another variation—a penetrating wound into a joint—is rare in calves and more common in adult cattle, in which a different monoarticular infection arises. Open fractures of the metacarpus resulting from excessive traction on calving chains can later result in septic arthritis, again through the pathway of cortex–metaphysis–margin of articular capsule–joint.

A sporadic cause of neonatal bovine polyarthritis is *Chlamydia psittaci*, serotype 2, which also causes encephalitis and conjunctivitis and is preceded by a severe bloody or watery enteritis. Joints are infected in a secondary chlamydemia.

In summary, the common form of infectious arthritis in younger cattle is septic, polyarticular, and hematogenous, and in neonates it originates from a primary umbilical focus.

Clinical Signs

Lameness develops suddenly and is severe. Systemic signs include joint effusion, pain, and usually fever, lassitude, and even recumbency. Joint swelling may not be appreciated in the initial 24 hours, but careful palpation including flexion of major weight-bearing joints may reveal heat and pain. Joint swelling develops within 24 hours of the establishment of infection. Despite involvement of several joints, the condition is rarely bilaterally symmetrical. The swelling is due to both an increased volume of synovia and periarticular edema. Pain on forced flexion and extension results from stimulation of nerve endings in the fibrous layer of the joint capsule. A limited range of movement follows later from capsular fibrosis and persisting edema.

Because visible signs of umbilical infection are inconsistent in joint ill, the umbilical area should be palpated deeply to detect possible involvement of the abdominal cavity adjacent to the umbilicus.

The intra-articular reaction is initially serofibrinous and later purulent. The synovial villi become hyperemic and edematous at the fibrinous stage. In the purulent phase, the exudate, containing large numbers of neutrophils (see Table 11–1), loses its normal viscosity and becomes cloudy. Ulceration of the articular cartilage occurs, with possible development of pannus. The articular cartilage is slowly destroyed by neutrophilic enzymes, bacterial lipopolysaccharides, and cytokines produced by macrophages (interleukin-1 and tumor necrosis factor).[21] Degenerative changes, which are most severe in major weight-bearing areas, include cartilaginous cleft formation and erosion. These changes permit organisms to attack the deeper mineralized layer (zone 4) of cartilage or even the subchondral bone. They may also undermine the peripheral cartilage. The result in either case is development of osteomyelitis.

Streptococcal polyarthritis may be associated with simultaneous development of meningitis, iridocyclitis, obvious nervous signs, and probable recumbency, possibly with convulsions.

In neonatal chlamydial polyarthritis, the joint capsule is the most severely damaged structure. Calves may be weak at birth and develop joint swelling at 2 to 3 days. Both subcutaneous and periarticular tissues are edematous. Joints contain turbid gray-yellow fluid and fibrin. Calves die 2 to 14 days after the development of signs.[21]

Radiographic changes 24 hours after the onset are limited to soft tissue swelling. Some days later, the subtle changes may include signs of subchondral osteolytic erosion (blurring of the normal bone outline), an associated widened joint space, early periosteal new bone formation, and occasionally gas formation within the joint capsule or joint space. Later still, a sclerotic zone may surround the advancing osteolytic lesion.[1] A helpful aid to interpretation is a radiograph of the contralateral joint.

These radiographic changes in bone and cartilage may be delayed in some slowly progressive cases and may first appear 2 to 3 weeks after infection; hence, radiology has a limited role in the diagnosis and management of joint ill of calves. The disease process in these cases may be due to limited multiplication of the invading organisms and their confinement to a small region of the joint.

Arthrocentesis of the suspected joint at the earliest stages of an infectious (septic) arthritis reveals an increased volume of abnormal synovia. The fluid is cloudy, turbid, and gray, yellow, or serosanguineous.

It has a low viscosity and poor mucin clot, and it clots on standing.

Typical features from synovial analysis in joint ill further include a very elevated total protein content (>4.0 grams/dL), total leukocyte count in the range of 50,000 to 100,000 cells/μL, and >90% neutrophilia. Samples may prove to be negative on bacterial culture, despite the presence of organisms on a straight Gram stain.

Diagnosis

A sudden onset of lameness in a neonatal calf that was normal and standing shortly after birth should arouse suspicion of joint ill. If joint swelling is apparent, the condition is at least 24 hours old. In the absence of joint swelling, all major limb joints should be flexed and extended to assess the pain response, and compared with the contralateral limb.

A recumbent neonate that was normal at birth may have a case of calfhood meningitis with an associated infectious arthritis. Calves may be slightly febrile, with tachycardia and a poor volume pulse resulting from dehydration.

The presence of purulent synovial fluid is diagnostic. In calves with a clinical course of 2 weeks or more, radiographic changes may also be diagnostic.

On early diagnostic arthroscopy, the appearance of the villi (fibrin deposition, hyperemia, edema) may suggest an inflammatory process. Superficial fibrillation and erosion of articular cartilage can be detected.

Treatment

Even if the diagnosis of joint ill is initially tentative, a course of systemic antibiotics should be started as a precautionary measure. Most drugs given systemically achieve therapeutic tissue levels in synovial membrane and synovia (see pp. 68–69). Suitable drugs include the beta-lactam penicillins (e.g., procaine penicillin G, 22,000 IU/kg IM BID; ampicillin trihydrate, 20 mg/kg IM BID), third-generation cephalosporins (ceftiofur, 1 mg/kg IM once a day), tetracyclines (oxytetracycline hydrochloride, 11 mg/kg IV BID), or potentiated sulphonamides (trimethoprim/sulfa, 30 mg/kg IV BID).

Systemic antibiotic therapy should be continued for 10 to 30 days even if an initial improvement is noted. Results of sensitivity testing of synovia taken at arthrocentesis during the initial examination and before any antimicrobial therapy may necessitate a change of drug.

Analgesic therapy should supplement antibiotics. The aim is not only to reduce pain but to encourage the calf to stand and (if appropriate, e.g., beef cattle) to nurse to increase the frequency of feeding and to avoid additional problems of recumbency.

Early consideration should be given to the possible value of joint irrigation, preferably a through-and-

through system with two wide-bore (e.g., 14-gauge) needles placed at opposite sides of the affected joint. Warmed polyionic solution (e.g., lactated Ringer's) should be flushed through to remove fibrin (early stages) or purulent fluid that is both free floating and attached to deformed villi.

Limited reports suggest that arthroscopic management is advantageous if facilities exist. Arthroscopic examination and surgery of neonatal septic arthritis in two calves (10 days old with right carpal and right femoropatellar involvement; 7 days old with left carpal infection) resulted in rapid improvement after drainage, debridement of diseased synovial membrane and articular cartilage with rongeurs, and joint lavage.[18] The advantages claimed for this approach were the excellent exposure with minimal surgical trauma (compared with arthrotomy) and the possibility of large-volume lavage, permitting the removal of large amounts of deposited fibrin. The reduced postoperative management costs partially offset the high expense of the procedure, which is likely to be limited to valuable stock.

Arthrotomy is not often advisable in advanced severe septic arthritis, because this major surgery necessitates prolonged postoperative therapy as the wound heals slowly. One possible modality, however, is open surgery with the aim of joint arthrodesis. This technique involves curettage of all the articular surfaces and postoperative joint immobilization (see Chapter 16 for details of techniques for carpal and fetlock joints).

Prognosis

Cases of joint ill treated early have a favorable prognosis, provided complications such as rapid spread to several other joints or meningitis do not develop. The prognosis is guarded when multiple joints are affected and treatment is delayed.

SEPTIC ARTHRITIS IN OLDER CATTLE

In older cattle, septic arthritis tends to be monoarticular. It may be primary or secondary, rarely tertiary. The most common location of a septic (secondary) arthritis is the distal interphalangeal joint (see p. 250). Trauma often predisposes to infectious arthritis of the tarsus or carpus (see p. 166). As in joint ill, large weight-bearing joints are more frequently involved. Specific infectious agents include the common organisms involved in joint ill as well as *Mycobacterium mycoides* or *bovis*, *Brucella* spp., and *H. somnus*.

Etiology and Pathogenesis

A primary origin is direct traumatic penetration of a joint (e.g., carpus, fetlock) by a wood or metal stake, barbed wire, or corrugated iron. Such wounds tend to be grossly contaminated. Their treatment is discussed elsewhere (see pp. 182–184). Another common route of infection is by contiguous secondary spread, for example, from a septic peritarsitis or tenosynovitis.

In addition to the specific microbiological agents and syndromes just mentioned, a tertiary infection in adult cattle may involve spread from suppurative mastitis, chronic (e.g., hepatic) abscessation, and septic metritis. One of the foregoing foci sometimes first involves the heart in septic endocarditis or myocarditis. Sudden deterioration in some recumbent cattle (downer cow syndrome) with severe joint sepsis is sometimes at autopsy demonstrated to have been due to acute inflammatory lesions of the heart, almost certainly associated with pyemic spread.

Septic arthritis occasionally arises from iatrogenic infection such as nonsterile arthrocentesis.

Two specific septic arthritides affect cattle. An acute suppurative gonitis has been reported in the United Kingdom and United States. It is characterized by severe lameness and synovitis and radiographic signs of articular erosions on the lateral tibial plateau.[4, 16, 30] In these reports, *Brucella abortus* vaccination was considered the cause of the lameness.

Group outbreaks of arthritis that has involved one or more hind limb joints in calves and feedlot cattle, often with systemic signs of pneumonia, can be due to *Mycoplasma agalactiae* var. *bovis* and *Mycoplasma bovigenitalium*. The respiratory signs of a cuffing pneumonia and alveolitis in calves may be overshadowed by the stiffness and lameness caused by arthritis, which develops in 5% to 10% of the susceptible stock.[10] Lameness may shift from one leg to another. The joints are warm to the touch and distended, and the synovia (arthrocentesis) appears cloudy. Culture of *Mycoplasma* requires special techniques and is most successful in early stages of infection.

Clinical Signs

The severe systemic response occurring in calves as a result of a joint infection is less consistent in older cattle. Nevertheless, most cases of monoarticular sepsis show marked lameness, pain and heat on palpation and gentle manipulation, and swelling due to increased synovial fluid volume and thickening of the soft tissues. The hock, stifle, and carpus are most frequently involved. Further signs indicative of a systemic disease include mild pyrexia, a reduced appetite, weight loss, and increased periods of recumbency.

Arthrocentesis and synovial fluid examination are helpful (see Table 11–1). Organisms usually are very difficult to culture from synovia. Tulleners[24] found no growth on aerobic or anaerobic culture of synovia taken from 14 female Holsteins aged 2 months to 2 years, despite physical features characteristic of joint sepsis. It is helpful if synovial samples are immediately inoculated into a diphasic culture bottle with sodium polyanethanolsulfonate to enhance recovery

of the organism.[28] Arthroscopic examination of joints may be easier than in neonates, if economic factors permit this approach.

Radiographic features of early septic arthritis are disappointingly few, being limited to soft tissue swelling and joint distention, as in neonatal polyarthritis. Radiographically, narrowing of the joint space resulting from destruction of articular cartilage and later, further widening due to destruction of subchondral bone can be visualized. Other radiographic signs include periosteal proliferation, exostosis formation, and possibly later osteomyelitis and ankylosis.[1]

Septic arthritis tends to be rapidly progressive, resulting in severe lameness, considerable pain, and increased periods of recumbency and anorexia.

Diagnosis

Differential diagnosis of septic (monoarticular) arthritis includes chronic hydrarthrosis, soft tissue swelling with periarticular abscessation, epiphysitis (usually bilaterally symmetrical), fractures involving joints, and dislocations. The last two categories, however, are often associated with crepitus. Diagnosis usually rests on positive findings on arthrocentesis and radiography.

Treatment

Treatment follows much the same principles as for neonatal joint disease. Early aggressive systemic and local therapy is essential for recovery. Systemic antibiotics (see p. 62, Table 5–3) should be given for a minimum of 2 weeks. Joint irrigation via a through-and-through system or so-called distention irrigation is recommended. Suitable solutions include polyionic solutions or physiological saline, possibly incorporating 0.1% povidone-iodine solution. This irrigation is thought to remove the lysozymes that destroy articular cartilage.

Failure of response may be due to selection of the incorrect antimicrobial agent, an inadequate intra-articular drug concentration, or the presence of excessive joint exudate and fibrin. In other cases, treatment has been initiated too late, and severe cartilaginous erosion has left subchondral bone exposed for the development of osteomyelitis. *Mycoplasma* arthritis responds only slowly to systemic therapy. Initiation of treatment for septic or infectious arthritis 1 week after the onset of disease leads to a poor prognosis for normal joint function.

Early treatment minimizes the deterioration in articular cartilage and development of pannus. Intra-articular medication is not recommended. Systemic antibiotic administration achieves adequate bactericidal/bacteriostatic levels in the synovia and avoids the risk of a chemical synovitis.

Radical arthrotomy has been successful in the treatment of septic arthritis in some of the more distal limb joints, such as the fetlock (see Chapter

16). In the past 10 years, however, the trend has been toward surgical procedures undertaken during arthroscopy (see p. 238).

Analgesic and anti-inflammatory drugs are useful supplementary therapy for infectious and septic arthritis. Suitable drugs include[22]

Phenylbutazone (initial dose 9 mg/kg PO, then 4.5 mg/kg every 48 hours)

Aspirin (100 mg/kg PO BID)

Flunixin meglumine (11 mg/kg IM BID)

Further details of indications, dosage regimens, and contraindications are given in Chapter 5 (see pp. 61, 68).

Prognosis

The prognosis is usually poor and is always guarded, even when therapy is promptly instigated.

LYME BORRELIOSIS ARTHRITIS

Borrelia burgdorferi is a spirochete transmitted by ticks (e.g., *Ixodes* spp.). It may occasionally cause abortion and arthritis in cattle. The organism has been isolated from blood, urine, colostrum, and synovial fluid of cows in North America.[6] The significance of this organism in clinical lameness of cattle is not clear because of the limited number of investigations.

Pathogenesis

The mechanism of infection may be twofold, first by direct effects of the spirochete in producing a lipopolysaccharide having pyrogenic activity and a cell wall peptidoglycan, and second by immune complex formation suggestive of an immune-mediated disease.

Clinical Signs

The organs involved at autopsy of an affected cow included joint synovia and cartilage, kidneys, lymph nodes, heart, liver, lungs, and udder.[6] The signs in one report[5] included mild lameness with swollen pastern and fetlock joints as well as erythema, swelling, and increased sensitivity of the udder and distal parts of the hind legs. Necropsy findings include thickening of the joint capsule and lymphoplasmacytic inclusions in a proliferative synovial membrane.

Diagnosis

Diagnosis of Lyme borreliosis depends on recognition of the clinical signs of sudden onset of lameness in one or more legs, possible fever and joint swelling, and later weight loss and arthritis, together with positive serology (indirect fluorescent antibody test, enzyme-linked immunosorbent assay, Western blot, polymerase chain reaction).

Treatment and Prevention

No information is yet available on the effectiveness of antibiotics against this spirochete. No vaccine is currently available. Prevention is based on tick control and strict sanitary measures.

DEGENERATIVE JOINT DISEASE

Definition

DJD is a chronic progressive, noninfectious, and initially noninflammatory disease characterized by primary degeneration of articular cartilage. Synonyms include degenerative arthritis, osteoarthrosis, osteoarthritis, and degenerative arthropathy.[11, 21]

Etiology

DJD is classified as primary or secondary. Secondary DJD results from known nutritional, traumatic, developmental, or other causes, leading to injury to joint cartilage or subchondral bone. Secondary DJD is, for example, an almost inevitable result of cranial cruciate rupture in the stifle joint. The primary DJD, of unknown cause, has a specific progressive cause starting with softening and fibrillation of articular cartilage, which then ulcerates to expose subchondral bone. This bone is eventually eburnated. Simultaneously, the joint is remodeled by the osteophyte formation at the joint margin at the attachment of the joint capsule, thickening of the lamina propria of the capsule, chronic villous proliferation, low-grade synovitis, and the accumulation of debris in the synovial fluid. In the end-stage joint, the differentiation between a primary inflammatory disease and DJD may be impossible.

The precise cause of osteophyte proliferation, which, together with capsular fibrosis, is responsible for joint enlargement, remains unknown.[21] Suggested explanations include synovial membrane stretching at its point of insertion, vascular-mediated effects at the marginal transitional zone of cartilage where it merges with the synovial membrane, inflammation of the synovial membrane, or a remodeling component of the degenerative process associated with changes in the structure of cartilage.

The metabolic, biochemical, and gross changes that occur in articular cartilage in DJD do so faster and more profoundly in infectious arthritis (see p. 166). The proteoglycan content of articular cartilage is decreased, and the water content is increased, leading to a decreased tensile strength of the collagen fibers when subjected to mechanical load-bearing pressure.

Matrix loss, physical compression, and both fragmentation and ulceration lead to a progressive thinning of cartilage.[21]

In cattle, an example of secondary DJD is chronic hip dysplasia, a sex-limited developmental malformation believed to be inherited through recessive genes[11, 27] (see p. 173). Another example reported to be inherited is DJD of the stifle in Holsteins and Jersey cows.[14]

Incidence

The incidence is higher in older cattle of both sexes. The major weight-bearing joints are involved in heavier animals (e.g., stifle and hock joints of breeding bulls). Hip joint involvement is also common. In the forelimb, the carpus has been investigated: An osteoarthritis deformans occurs in younger Simmental cattle (Switzerland) and in Japanese Black beef cattle.[11, 23] The incidence of DJD in proximal limb joints has been little investigated owing to problems of loss of carcass value after boning-out procedures in the abattoir.

Clinical Signs

A chronic lameness of slow onset is characteristic of DJD. In mild cases, a stud bull may have moderate lameness for years. It may be unwilling to mount cows but may be used for electroejaculation. Bulls with DJD in beef herds and working under range conditions tend to lack libido and lose weight because of difficulty in foraging. In other cases, cows and bulls experience rapid weight loss after the onset of severe pain and lameness. Muscle wasting is most marked over the hindquarters. Many mature cattle have bilateral DJD, although one limb tends to be more clinically affected.

Joint swelling is not often an obvious feature, although muscle atrophy tends to increase the prominence of the stifle. Cattle may walk slowly and stiffly and have a tendency to drag the claws. Palpation of the stifle or hock may reveal diffuse swelling due to chronic fibrosis. An increased volume of synovia and resulting joint puffiness are unusual.

Crepitus can easily be elicited in advanced cases. For the hip, the limb should be abducted and circumrotated. Rectal examination during gentle rocking of the animal from left to right and when walking slowly ahead may reveal crepitus. For the stifle, on the other hand, abduction and attempted rotation of the tibial plateau on the femoral condyle, by inward and outward movement of the tuber calcanei as well as flexion and extension, are vital steps to elicit abnormal sounds.

Degenerative coxitis comprised more than 50% of one series of cases of hip joint disease.[27] The average age was 8 years (range 2 to 17). In most cases, lesions were bilateral but rarely were symmetrical. The course of disease was 6 months to 6 years. No animal

made a complete recovery, although one 3-year-old (beef) bull improved for 2 years, only to relapse suddenly. The signs of degenerative coxitis included dragging of the limbs due to poor hip flexion, progressively severe atrophy of the hindquarters, localized crepitus, and in some cases evidence on rectal palpation of new bone formation on the obturator foramen and acetabular rim.[27] Osseous bulla formation has been seen in severe degenerative coxitis. The bulla develops at the cranial margin of the obturator foramen and adjacent to the caudal end of the acetabular notch, which is occupied by fat and the origin of the ligament of the head of the femur.[11]

The hock may show incongruities on visual examination. Bone proliferation tends to be in a similar position to equine spavin, being located distally and dorsomedially. Many such osseous proliferations in these distal tarsal joints, which normally have little movement, have no clinical significance because the animal never shows lameness. DJD rarely involves the tibial tarsal joint.

Synovial fluid in DJD may be pale and may contain debris such as cartilage and damaged villi. The total leukocyte and red blood cell counts are slightly elevated. Protein level is in the normal range. Viscosity is slightly decreased. Results of microbiological culture are negative.

Radiography in the early stages may fail to reveal changes. Massive periarticular osteophyte proliferation is apparent in chronic DJD.[1] In a typically severely affected stifle, as much as a 2-cm width of new bone may be evident at the caudal edge of the tibial plateau and around the femoropatellar joint capsule. Calcification of the joint capsule (osteochondroma formation) may be seen. Cavitation of the medial or, less commonly, lateral femoral condyle can sometimes be appreciated. The tibial eminence may be displaced dorsally after rupture of the cranial cruciate ligament (CrCL).[1, 2] Free-floating bone particles (joint mice) may be evident in either the femorotibial or femoropatellar joints.

Pathology

Gross pathology of chronic coxitis includes severe thickening of the joint capsule with areas of ossification, hyperplastic synovial villus proliferation, loss of the ligament of the head of the femur in some cases, and eburnation both of much of the acetabulum—especially dorsally, where pressure from weight-bearing is maximal—and also of the femoral head.[21] Peripheral exostosis is seen at the attachment of joint capsule to bone and over the region dorsal to the acetabulum and femoral neck. Severe cases have considerable remodeling of the acetabulum, which becomes shallow. Chip fractures of new bone can sometimes be seen around the joint margin and may explain sudden episodes of increased lameness.

Diagnosis

DJD is usually well advanced when chronic lameness draws the owner's attention to the cow or bull. Most bilateral cases tend to have the signs masked more than in unilateral involvement. Joint swelling is non-diagnostic. Arthrocentesis may be performed as a confirmatory step, and at the same time an opportunity may be taken to inject 10 to 20 mL of plain 2% lidocaine hydrochloride solution into the suspected joint. A reduction in the degree of lameness confirms the suspected site. In most cases, such a step is unnecessary because crepitus and evidence of discomfort can be localized by palpation and manipulation.

Differential diagnosis includes septic arthritis that has a sudden onset and rapid course and three conditions seen in young cattle—namely, rickets, osteoporosis, and nutritional osteoarthropathy due to a selenium and vitamin E deficiency.

Treatment

Only palliative treatment is possible. Possible drugs include phenylbutazone, aspirin, and corticosteroids (see p. 68). Dimethyl sulfoxide (DMSO) has been used with little success.[22] Cattle with DJD should, on welfare grounds, be confined to a limited area and have easy access to high-quality feed to slow the anticipated weight loss.

OSTEOCHONDROSIS AND OSTEOCHONDRITIS DISSECANS

Osteochondrosis involves an abnormality of physeal or epiphyseal growth cartilage. Its synonym is dyschondroplasia. Osteochondritis dissecans (OCD) is a manifestation of osteochondrosis in which a portion of articular cartilage splits as a result of fissure formation in an area of dysplastic subarticular cartilage to form a flap, which may separate entirely.[21]

Incidence and Pathogenesis

Osteochondrosis is less common in cattle than in pigs, horses, or dogs and frequently is of no clinical significan̪ e., does not result in lameness). OCD is also uncol. rarely groups, in t... the st... ho... and shoulder jo... In both young cattle and bulls, osteochondrosis may be manifested by subchondral bone cyst formation in either the tibial or femoral condyle.[2] Epiphysitis is a form of osteochondrosis encountered in United States feedlot cattle.[12] Others[9] describe radiographic features of an osteochondrosis-like lesion as a subchondral osteolytic form in the tarsal bones of 1- to 3-year-old bulls of fast-growing breeds. These foci, which appear in the pressure-bearing surfaces in young animals, disappear during bone maturation. Nevertheless, the articular surface fails to grow normally and predisposes the joint to DJD.[1]

The basic pathogenesis of osteochondrosis remains debatable.[21, 26] Retained growth cartilage is a hallmark of the condition. This results in disruption of ossification. The factors leading to the retained growth cartilage may include abnormal chondrocyte formation or structure, or abnormal matrix production or abnormal vasculature, the latter leading to inadequate chondrocyte nutrition. The result is areas of focal cartilaginous weakness on which shearing forces can act to produce cartilaginous flaps, some of which may break off, forming free-floating fragments and exposing subchondral bone (OCD). Another end process is the effect of compression forces acting on these flaps to produce areas of infolding, resorption, and the development of subchondral cystic lesions. A combination of ongoing ossification and continued infolding can then result in subchondral bone cyst formation. In horses, OCD lesions tend to develop in areas subjected to considerable shear forces, whereas bone cysts develop at points under substantial continuous and compressive loading.[26] Comparative studies in cattle are lacking.

Etiological factors have not been elucidated. Equine osteochondrosis has been variously related to a rapid growth rate stimulated by a high energy intake; deficiency of copper, zinc, and to a lesser extent calcium and phosphorus; as well as a postulated genetic predisposition. Trauma may act as a secondary etiological factor.[26]

It sometimes appears that OCD lesions are bilaterally symmetrical. They may quickly develop into DJD, when the joint capsule becomes thickened and the synovial volume increases. One such case has been illustrated.[11] In other instances, OCD is suggested by the development of a serous tarsitis involving all parts of this compound joint and provoking caudal extension of the limbs in an attempt to reduce discomfort.[11]

Clinical Signs

Generally, osteochondrosis is a pathological lesion unassociated with lameness unless it progresses to become OCD. At this latter time, an inflammatory response develops as a result of the release of tissue debris into synovial fluid. Synovial effusion, often accompanied by mild lameness, results.

Subchondral bone cysts, considered to be a mani-stifle lameness in Canada.ˀ Fifteen of 18 animals had no other abnormality to account for the lameness. Their ages ranged from 6 to 18 months. The lesion was usually (15/18) located in the lateral tibial condyle. Synovial fluid analysis ($n = 11$) revealed an elevated leukocyte count with a predominance of mature neutrophils and macrophages (6 cases) or degenerative neutrophilia (5 cases). Bacteria were isolated only in 1 of the 18 cases.

The most frequent sites of osteochondrosis lesions include the tarsus, especially the distal surface of the central tarsal and opposing metatarsal articular surface.[23] This report details erosive ("ulceric") lesions in all joints from the carpus and tarsus distally. Severe (70% of animals) or moderate (15% to 16%) lesions were very common. The incidence of lameness was not stated because the study involved 41 3- to 6-year-old Japanese Black steers at a slaughterhouse. The significance of these lesions remains doubtful, because these steers were not fast-growing cattle but husbandry usually involved strict confinement and limited movement.

Some cases of OCD doubtless show signs when secondary degenerative processes supervene (DJD). Exacerbations of a mild, slight lameness may be attributed to additional joint trauma and a flare-up in synovial fluid production, causing a suddenly increased joint swelling (Fig. 11–3).

If warranted economically, suspicious joints may undergo radiography, but changes confined to cartilaginous erosion may be difficult to appreciate. Carpal bones with osteochondrosis may have changes in the trabecular pattern and irregularity of the joint surface revealed when an intensifying screen and mammographic-type film are used.[1] Suspicious radiographic evidence of osteochondrosis is the presence of a free calcified body within the joint (joint mouse).

Today, after radiographic screening, investigation in valuable stock can include arthroscopy, which is easily used in joints with an extensive joint capsule such as the femoropatellar, scapulohumeral, and radiocarpal. Vision is more restricted in conventional approaches to the femorotibial, intertarsal, tarsometatarsal, and carpal joints.

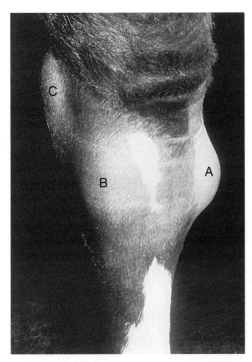

Figure 11–3. Suspected osteochondrosis dissecans of the left hock joint of a yearling steer (view from cranial). Note joint distention laterally (A), craniomedially (B), and caudomedially (C). The steer was slightly lame.

Diagnosis

Differential diagnosis of osteochondrosis includes DJD, chip fractures, and early low-grade septic arthritis, as well as recent trauma. Diagnosis depends on a history of chronic mild lameness, joint swelling, confirmatory synovial fluid analysis (sterile on culture, white blood cell population of macrophages and degenerating neutrophils), radiography (to rule out chip fractures), and possibly arthroscopy. In doubtful cases, consideration may be given to intra-articular anesthesia (see p. 226).

Treatment

OCD lesions resulting in lameness should initially be treated by strict confinement on soft bedding and, in fattening steers, by a more restricted calorie intake. The aim is to permit the lesion(s) to heal. Corticosteroids and antibiotics are contraindicated. Nonsteroidal anti-inflammatory preparations may be helpful (see p. 64 for dosage). If improvement is not seen with 1 to 2 weeks, consideration may be given to curettage of the lesion(s) via arthroscopy or arthrotomy, using surgical procedures as practiced in horses. In the Canadian study,[9] three of four cattle given stall confinement became functional and six of seven treated with systemic antibiotics (ampicillin, penicillin, kanamycin, or tetracycline) likewise recovered.

HIP DYSPLASIA

Hip dysplasia is an inherited bilateral malformation of the hip joint largely confined to beef breeds, principally Hereford and Aberdeen Angus but also reported in Galloway, Charolais, and Beef Shorthorn.[11, 27]

Incidence and Pathogenesis

Hip dysplasia occurs sporadically and has a low incidence, being reported mostly from Australia, the United Kingdom, and North America. Male cattle are usually affected, occasionally (Herefords) as neonates but commonly at 3 to 6 months.

The prime pathological lesion is a shallow acetabulum (primary acetabular dysplasia) and resulting incongruity of the coxofemoral (hip) joint. Severe cases inevitably develop a secondary DJD.

Inheritance is considered to be recessive and sex limited, with a higher penetrance in males than in females, as determined by pedigree studies in Hereford cattle in the United Kingdom.

Clinical Signs

The condition is occasionally suspected in a neonate that has difficulty rising, weak hindquarters, and hind limb lameness. More commonly, the onset is insidious at 3 to 6 months old and affects fast-growing male calves, which develop a slight swaying gait in the hindquarters. Other cases develop a mild unilateral lameness. Localized muscle atrophy of the hindquarters may be seen, or the history may involve a reduced rate of weight gain. Crepitus may be detected on manual or, in older cases, on rectal palpation. Abduction and flexion of the hip may accentuate the severity of crepitus. More severe cases may have a subluxation, demonstrated by placing the palm of the hand over the greater femoral trochanter and pushing the hindquarters laterally to transfer weight-bearing to the opposite leg. At this time, the trochanter moves inward and downward, reflecting the movement of the femoral head back into the acetabulum.[11] This movement may be accompanied by an audible click (Ortolani sign). Manipulation of the affected joint occasionally causes resentment and pain.

The availability of powerful radiographic equipment permits confirmation of the clinical diagnosis. The technique should be limited to a maximum of three exposures because the skin dose of radiation in the middle of the primary beam is considerable (140 to 155 rad) and is close to the scrotum, as the animal is radiographed in dorsal recumbency under deep sedation or general anesthesia and with the hind limbs extended caudally. The stifles are rotated slightly inward. The scrotum should be surrounded by 1-mm-thick lead sheeting.

Radiographic changes in bovine hip dysplasia include shallowness of the acetabulum. The acetabular margin and femoral neck may have exostoses. Gross coxofemoral subluxation may be evident.[11]

Advanced cases may have severe changes in one hip, leading to increased weight-bearing by the opposite dysplastic hip, which may demonstrate subluxation. As in chronic osteoarthritis of senility, bouts of more severe lameness may be reported because, it is proposed, chip fractures occur in the periarticular new bone, releasing more debris into the joint capsule and resulting also in further damage to and hemorrhage in the dense fibrocartilage dorsal to the acetabular rim.

Pathology

Gross pathological changes in dysplastic joints include confirmation of acetabular shallowness, severe cartilaginous loss especially in the dorsal half of the ~abulum (Fig. 11–4) and the dorsal surface of the ~al head (Fig. 11–5), dorsal displacement of the fibr~ ~inous rim dorsal to the acetabulum, and proliferat~ ~ses around the acetabulum and along the femor~ ~ an intact ligament of the head of the femur (teres or round ligament), but it later ruptures. Chronic changes resemble those of any degenerative osteoarthropathy. Minor degrees of arthritis such as cartilaginous erosion, suggestive of a subclinical

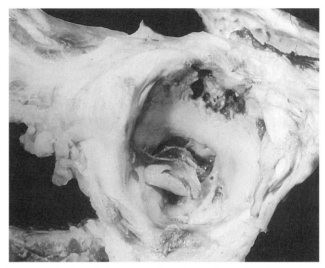

Figure 11–4. Acetabulum (R) of an 8-month-old Aberdeen Angus bull with hip dysplasia, showing severe cartilage loss and bone erosion dorsally over the region of maximum pressure.

OCD, may be noted in other major weight-bearing joints (stifle, hock, shoulder, elbow).

Diagnosis

A unilateral or bilateral progressive lameness in the hip joint of young, fast-growing beef bulls, accompanied by crepitus or subluxation of one or both joints, is strongly suggestive of hip dysplasia. Mineral imbalance and more generalized joint disease should be ruled out. Radiographic examination can confirm the clinical suspicion.

Treatment

No treatment is possible. Investigation should concentrate on related stock and analysis of suspected

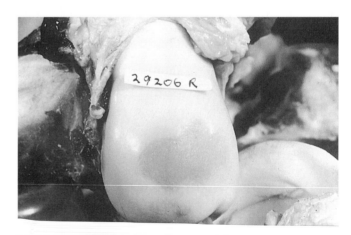
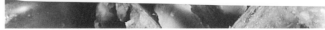

Figure 11–5. Femoral head of an 11-month-old Hereford bull with hip dysplasia, showing an extensive area of cartilaginous loss but no exposure of bone.

families. Hip dysplasia is a breeding unsoundness. The program introduced in the United Kingdom to control the condition, based on diagnostic pathology of cases suspected by the Society's veterinarian and notification of positive findings to the owner as well as the breeder of sire and dam, has successfully controlled the problem in the United Kingdom.

LUXATIONS AND SUBLUXATIONS

SACROILIAC LUXATION AND SUBLUXATION

Introduction and Etiology

Partial separation of synarthrodial joint surfaces is termed *subluxation,* which is more common than complete separation, or *luxation.* These conditions are generally associated with parturition, occurring soon after dystocia and rarely prepartum. Predisposing factors include physiological relaxation of pelvic ligaments due to hormonal effects at the time of parturition, overexertion in rising after parturition, and, rarely, excessive road work in advanced pregnancy.

Clinical Signs

Clinical signs include mild ataxia and weakness in the hindquarters (subluxation) or severe posterior paresis and recumbency (luxation). The lumbar spine and sacrum appear dropped or depressed relative to the abnormally prominent sacral tuberosities of the ilium. As a cow walks forward the tuber coxae rock back and forth as the hindquarters move independently of the spine. Crepitus may be detected on gentle lateral rocking of the hindquarters or during slow forward movement. Deep palpation over the sacroiliac joint may be resented. Rectal palpation may reveal a reduced dorsoventral diameter of the pelvic inlet due to ventral and caudal displacement of the sacral promontory. Recent acute cases may have a detectable edematous or fluid-filled (blood) swelling ventral to the spine. An initial subluxation sometimes slowly develops into luxation.

Diagnosis

Diagnosis depends on the history, gross appearance, detection of crepitus and pain, and rectal palpation. It is easier if the animal remains standing. Differential diagnosis includes an acute phase of an ankylosing spondylopathy, degenerative osteoarthritis of one or both hips or stifle joints, progressive hind limb paralysis, pelvic fractures, mild obturator damage, spinal lymphosarcoma, and spinal fracture.

Management

Rest is essential. Patients, usually adult cows, should be put onto straw bedding in a yard or box. Low-level analgesics may be given for some days (see p. 64). If subluxation or luxation develops prepartum, fetal delivery may require assistance or a cesarean section may be indicated. Cases of subluxation have a favorable prognosis, but cattle with a complete luxation have a guarded to poor outlook, and attentive nursing is essential to avoid both decubital injuries and mastitis. Animals that remain alert and eat well may be nursed for 10 to 14 days. Increasing dullness, weight loss, and failure at attempts to stand should be grounds for slaughter. Cows that recover after a complete sacroiliac luxation should not be bred owing to the narrowed pelvic inlet, making dystocia inevitable.

COXOFEMORAL (HIP) LUXATION

Introduction and Clinical Signs

Coxofemoral luxation is commonly seen in dairy cattle,[27] usually traumatic in origin and often related to postpartum events. A typical history involves a cow that, after dystocia, develops a bilateral obturator paralysis, goes down with both hind legs abducted, and either immediately or as a result of struggling to stand develops a unilateral coxofemoral luxation. Bilateral cases are rare. Cases also occur in younger animals, even in neonates after injudicious traction in dystocia. Jersey cows may be predisposed to this condition, and in these animals it may be related to a lack of supporting muscle mass.

The common direction of abnormal movement of the femoral head is dorsal and cranial, the head lying along the lateral aspect of the ilial shaft. The animal is usually unable to bear weight on this leg, which is rotated so that both stifle and digits are directed outward. The external pelvic landmarks are abnormal, the greater trochanter on the affected side also being dorsal and cranial to its normal position. Crepitus ("bone on bone") and localized pain may be elicited on rotational manipulation of the leg.

The less frequent directions of luxation of the femoral head (Fig. 11–6) are directly ventral, as well as caudoventral into the obturator foramen.[11] These positions have a significantly poorer prognosis, because other musculoskeletal and neurological injuries may also be present and replacement is more awkward. The animal is often recumbent. Manipulation of the limb with the hand placed over the greater trochanter should again be performed. Rectal palpation is mandatory. A distinct impression of a hard, bony mass moving in and out of the obturator foramen on abduction and adduction of the limb by an assistant is diagnostic of a caudoventral luxation.

Clinics with radiographic facilities should consider ventrodorsal radiography to confirm the diagnosis and the direction of luxation and to rule out additional trauma.

Differential Diagnoses

The major differential diagnoses are pelvic fracture, proximal femoral fracture, separation of the proximal

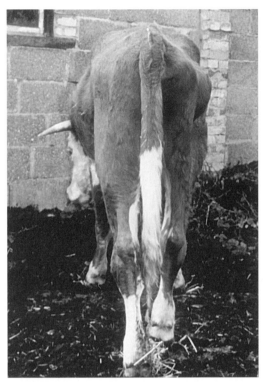

Figure 11–6. Right hip dislocation in a Hereford cow (chronic). Note the muscle atrophy and the more ventral position of greater femoral trochanter.

femoral epiphysis (see p. 272), fracture of the femoral neck, sacroiliac luxation, and acute septic arthritis of the hip or stifle joints.

Treatment

Animals with a hip dislocation remain severely lame and lose weight, and their milk yield declines drastically. Successful nonsurgical reduction is related to the interval since the trauma and using the appropriate manipulative procedures under sedation or general anesthesia.[13] Few animals with a hip luxation of more than 48 hours' duration can successfully undergo reduction by manipulation. Outcome in one series was statistically related to several factors[13]: the ability to stand (85% vs. 11%); age less than 3 years (81% vs. 23%); cranial as opposed to caudal direction of dislocation (82% vs. 31%); a duration of dislocation less than 12 hours (56% vs. 8%); occurrence during estrus and nonestrus (77% vs. 30%), and body weight less than 400 kg (63% vs. 30%). Younger, smaller animals with a cranial dislocation of short duration therefore warrant a more favorable prognosis.

MANIPULATIVE REDUCTION OF DORSOCRANIAL LUXATION

The approach to reduction of dorsocranial dislocation by manipulation is made under deep sedation or, if facilities permit, general anesthesia. The hindquarters are fixed by a rope passed round the inguinal region over the back and secured to a firm object (tree, post). A rope is fixed to the fetlock of the dislocated limb with the cow in lateral recumbency.

The limb is circumducted with maximal abduction to attempt to break down and disperse blood and edematous fluid that may have gathered around the joint. A pulley block system is fixed to the rope, and traction is exerted in the direction of a line passing through the femoral head and acetabulum. This direction is caudal. A block of wood may be placed medial to the stifle to act as a fulcrum when, during traction, inward rotational movement is attempted on the limb. At this time, the limb may be forcibly rotated by outward traction on the point of the hock. The rotation is aided by simultaneously pushing the stifle medially. The fulcrum assists by tending to elevate the femoral head off the ilial surface.

If successful reposition follows, indicated by a "clunk," traction must immediately cease; otherwise, the femoral head may be pulled over the acetabulum and into the obturator foramen. Successful reduction usually is immediately confirmed by an absence of crepitus on circumrotation. Check that the radiograms are confirmatory. Postoperative care is most important.

After reduction, the cow should be maintained in a recumbent position for 24 hours on a soft, clean straw bed with the hind limbs hobbled above the hock or fetlocks to reduce the risk of immediate recurrence of the dislocation on standing. This period also permits a little periarticular support to develop as a result of edematous swelling.

Attempts at closed reduction of caudal and ventral luxations usually fail because of an inability to direct traction in an appropriate direction. Should, exceptionally, reduction be achieved, these cattle often remain recumbent.

SURGERY

Reports from a United States veterinary school[25] show that open reduction can have a high success rate under good operating conditions (general anesthesia, strict aseptic surgery, equipment). In this referred series, in which many animals were immature and the etiology was traumatic but unrelated to parturition, a craniodorsal approach was adopted and 95% of cases underwent successful reduction. In open reduction, debris can be removed from the acetabulum and the surgeon can visually ascertain definite reduction. In this series,[25] craniodorsal luxations had a better long-term outlook (75%) than ventral cases (33%). The most common complication was reluxation.

Femoral head and neck resection has been carried out in cattle with chronic hip dislocation, but results have been poor as a result of continuing lameness and consequent unthriftiness.[27]

Prognosis

Chronic cases of hip dislocation tend to develop a pseudarthrosis as new bone formation occurs on the ilium around the pressure point of the femoral head. Continuing severe lameness and weight loss can be expected.

In conclusion, coxofemoral luxation in adult cows is a severe debilitating injury with a poor prognosis unless skillful and often prolonged manipulation can be undertaken in the first 12 to 24 hours or unless facilities exist for open surgical reduction if manipulation fails. The risk of recurrence after manipulative reduction is considerable. Left untreated, most cows deteriorate rapidly. In younger stock, the success rate for closed reduction is higher and the prognosis is correspondingly better.

FEMOROTIBIAL INSTABILITY

Rupture or partial rupture of the cruciate ligaments, primarily the cranial, is a common cause of femorotibial subluxation or instability.[2, 11] Trauma is invariably the cause. The complexity of this joint is reflected in the presence of intra-articular ligaments and paired menisci. Trauma often involves damage to several joint components.

Complete luxation, on the other hand, is a rarity, involving massive damage including rupture of the collateral and cruciate ligaments. It cannot be effectively treated, because even if reduction is achieved under general anesthesia, joint damage will have been too severe to justify repair attempts. The major concern here is with subluxation.

Etiology

The traumatic etiology of subluxation can involve a twisting action of the limb while the claws remain firmly placed on the ground. The hindquarters are swung around during weight-bearing, as during estrus, either mounting another cow that moves or being mounted by a bull or cow. A similar injury is possible if a claw is caught in a hole or between bars of a gate carelessly left on the ground. Major damage to the collateral ligaments seems to be less common than cruciate injury, in which the CrCL appears to be at greater risk than the caudal cruciate ligament (CaCL). Many other forms of trauma doubtless occur but are unobserved. The immediate injury is a partial or complete rupture of the CrCL and usually associated injury to the menisci. Cruciate damage (CrCL) is commonly near the insertion onto the tibial crest. A portion of the crest may be torn off. The result is an ability of the tibial plateau on weight-bearing to move cranially relative to the femoral condyles, and caudally when the limb is raised from the ground. The movement may be 1 to 3 cm.

Pathology

Surveys of bovine hind limbs condemned for atrophy reveal severe chronic gonitis in many cases. Exami-

nation of intra-articular structures in such cattle has revealed partial or complete rupture of the CrCL to be the most common abnormality, together with medial meniscal injury and erosion of the opposing medial femoral condyle. The periarticular structures are often severely thickened owing to chronic fibrosis, which may represent an attempt by the animal to restabilize the joint.[11] Additional features in these chronic cases of stifle instability include peripheral osteophyte proliferation, especially over the caudal aspect of the tibial plateau surface. In some cases, portions of these osteophytic ledges later fracture off.

Clinical Features—Acute Care

Clinical examination reveals an animal that suddenly develops a mixed lameness (i.e., in both the weight-bearing and non–weight-bearing phase), when the stifle is maintained in flexion. The stifle is swollen, and in very early acute stages it may be edematous. Palpation is not resented. The joint instability may be visible as the animal walks. Abnormal movement of the stifle joint may be provoked by moving the point of the hock medially and laterally, attempting rotation of the tibial shaft and plateau. The other hand is kept over the patellar and collateral ligaments to detect joint crepitus. The leg may often be elevated easily to attempt both abduction and adduction. This manipulation also may reveal joint instability. Another movement is best performed by attempting to move the tibial plateau cranially over the femoral condyles ("drawer-forward" movement). The subject sometimes must be placed in lateral recumbency with the affected leg uppermost for this test. A further suggestive but nondiagnostic sign is a lack of tone in the stifle region.

Clinical Features—Chronic Case

Unilateral muscle atrophy may exaggerate still further the enlargement of the affected joint. A variable degree of lameness accompanies this chronic gonitis. Palpation reveals that the usual landmarks such as the patellar ligaments, tibial crest, and collateral ligaments are obscured by joint fibrosis. Heat is absent, and crepitus, from the movement of the eroded femoral trochlear surfaces on the tibia, may be elicited. Consistent clicking sounds sometimes result during joint flexion from a flipping movement of torn menisci (Fig. 11–7). Increased synovial volume in chronic cases is inconsistent, but some cows with a volume in excess of 80 mL may show obvious joint fluctuation on palpation. The drawer-forward sign may no longer be demonstrable.

Further Investigations

Swelling of the joint capsule may justify arthrocentesis to permit differentiation of an acute septic goni-

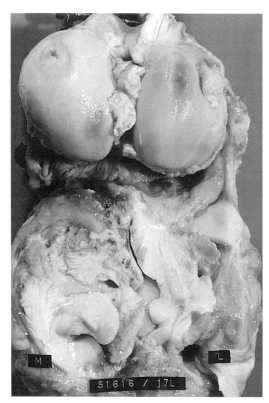

Figure 11–7. Necropsy specimen of a left stifle joint of an aged cow, showing severe chronic changes. Both femoral condyles have severe erosions, and the caudal horn of the medial meniscus has been ruptured and reflected forward. Severe periarticular fibrosis. Primary lesion was probably cranial cruciate rupture.

tis from an acute traumatic incident with possible hemarthrosis. Later synovial changes associated with cruciate rupture reflect the intra-articular damage (e.g., cartilaginous debris, synovial villous particles).

Arthroscopy of the femorotibial joint is hampered by its limited size, but examination may reveal CrCL damage, meniscal injury, and cartilaginous defects.

In radiography of the stifle joint in cattle,[1, 2] the lateral-medial view is more helpful for diagnosis of cruciate damage and requires a lower exposure than caudal-cranial projection, which often lacks detail owing to the superimposed depth of soft tissue (Fig. 11–8). The first feature is increased opacity due to excessive intra-articular fluid. Features suggestive of a CrCL rupture include cranial displacement of the tibial plateau: the intercondylar eminence is in the cranial third of the intercondylar fossa. Bone spicules visualized just proximal to the intercondylar tuberosity result from avulsion fracture and separation after severe traction at the insertion of the CrCL. The simultaneous existence of a CaCL rupture is unassociated with any specific radiographic features. On a caudocranial view, incongruity of the femorotibial surfaces is occasionally appreciated after meniscal damage or additional collateral ligamentous rupture.

Lateral-medial radiographs of chronic gonitis after rupture of the CrCL reveal increased opacity due

marked exostosis formation, in particular a calcified mass, which may measure 3×3 cm, at the caudal edge of the proximal tibial plateau. Some calcified areas on the tibial plateau may result from mineralization of the torn insertion of the CrCL or menisci.[1, 2] The drawer sign may not be evident on radiographs in chronic cases.

Differential diagnosis includes acute and chronic septic gonitis, simple collateral ligamentous injury, chronic osteoarthritis unassociated with ligamentous or meniscal damage, patellar fracture and fractures of the distal femur, and growth plate damage (including the proximal tibial plate, which is usually confined to young cattle).

Treatment

In acute cases, rest in a box or straw yard is essential. The aim is to avoid further injury and to permit development of a fibrotic reaction, which may help joint stabilization. Systemic phenylbutazone may be given in the acute early phase for 3 weeks, remembering the slow elimination rate, making injection or oral administration every second day advisable (see p. 64, Table 5–3).

Although several reports describe successful repair of a ruptured CrCL,[8, 17, 20] many have been experimental procedures in which the ligament was transected

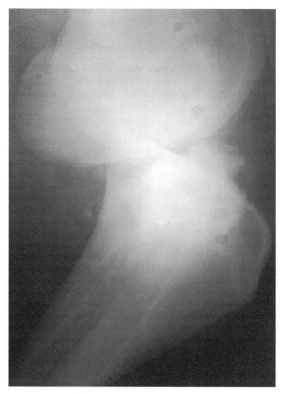

Figure 11–8. Lateral radiograph showing gross forward displacement of the tibial plateau relative to the femur. There is a severe periarticular soft tissue reaction and new bone formation or calcification of the joint capsule. The point of insertion of the cranial

and then, in the same surgical procedure, replaced by a fascial graft,[17] skin, or artificial prosthetic materials (e.g., carbon fiber). Such operations fail to account for the usual additional damage in clinical cases of cruciate rupture. Extra-articular plication of the dorsal retinaculum is a simple form of joint support[20] but, because of the considerable forces acting on the articulation, is rarely successful in clinical cases.[9] "Over-the-top" techniques using patellar ligamentous material have been successful.[8]

Prognosis

Because of accompanying damage in the menisci and articular surfaces of clinical cases, the prognosis is very guarded. Use of prosthetic ligaments continues to be a procedure limited to valuable stock of moderate weight that are treated in a referral clinic. Smaller breeds (e.g., Jersey) have a better but still guarded prognosis. Treatment of chronic cases can be only palliative.

INJURY TO MENISCI AND FEMOROTIBIAL COLLATERAL LIGAMENTS

Detachment of the medial meniscus has been reported[19] after injury to the medial collateral ligament in 50 cattle, predominantly dairy breeds, of all ages (1 month to 1 year) in Illinois. Reports from other centers are awaited.

Clinical Features

The injury is sudden and results in a shortened stride and swelling and pain over the damaged tissue. Manipulation of the distal limb medially causes an appreciable opening of the femorotibial joint medially. Caudocranial radiographs may reveal incongruity of the joint surfaces and spicules of subperiosteal bone from the origin and insertion of the ligament.

Laxity of the medial collateral ligament is apparent on varus stressing of the stifle. A separation between the medial meniscus and medial collateral ligament can usually be detected. This report[19] states that this ligament is normally securely attached to the medial border of the medial meniscus, which is also attached to the joint capsule. The anatomical relationship is disputed (see p. 228).

At arthrotomy in 34 cattle,[19] the medial meniscus was in all cases detached from its capsular attachment but not dislocated, resulting in a 1- to 3-cm-long cleft.

Treatment

Surgery has been undertaken (meniscopexy) in 34 cattle.[19] Twenty of 27 cattle with postoperative follow-up were either slightly or no longer lame. For economic reasons, 16 cattle did not undergo operation, and only 1 of the 11 cattle with follow-up after conservative management showed any improvement.[19]

Further reports on this medial meniscal and collateral ligamentous injury are lacking. Because 76% of the animals in this report were younger than 2 years, mounting activities during estrus are postulated as factors contributing to the lameness.

Because almost no reports describe other forms of collateral ligamentous stifle injury in cattle, unassociated with other pathology, it can be considered uncommon. Severe injury, such as rupture, to both collateral ligaments causes severe subluxation or luxation, invariably with damage to intra-articular structures, resulting in severe lameness. Such injuries cannot be successfully treated.

REFERENCES

1. Bargai U, Pharr JW, Morgan JP: Bovine radiology. Ames, IA, Iowa State Univ Press, 1989, pp 36–37, 82–86, 96.
2. Bartels JE: Femorotibial osteoarthrosis in the bull. 1. Clinical survey and radiologic interpretation. J Am Vet Radiol Soc 16:151–158, 1975.
3. Blood DC, Studdert VP: Baillière's Comprehensive Veterinary Dictionary. London, Baillière Tindall, 1988.
4. Bracewell CD, Corbell J: An association between arthritis and persistent serological reaction to *Brucella abortus* in cattle from apparently brucellosis-free herds. Vet Rec 106:99–101, 1979.
5. Burgess EC: Borreliosis in cattle. *In* Howard JL (ed): Current Veterinary Therapy. Food Animal Practice 2. Philadelphia, WB Saunders, 1993, pp 515–517.
6. Burgess EC, Gendron-Fitzpatrick A, Wright WO: Arthritis and systemic disease caused by *Borrelia burgdorferi* infection in a cow. J Am Vet Med Assoc 191:1468–1470, 1987.
7. Caron JP: Understanding the pathogenesis of equine arthritis. Br Vet J 148:369–370, 1992.
8. Crawford WH: A surgical technique for the intra-articular repair of cranial cruciate ligament injuries in cattle. Vet Surg 19:380–388, 1990.
9. Ducharme NG, Stanton ME, Ducharme GR: Stifle lameness in cattle at two veterinary teaching hospitals: A retrospective study of 42 cases. Can Vet J 26:212–217.
10. Frey ML: Mycoplasmosis in cattle. *In* Howard JL (ed): Current Veterinary Therapy: Food Animal Practice 3. Philadelphia, WB Saunders, 1993, p 455.
11. Greenough PR, MacCallum FJ, Weaver AD: Lameness in Cattle, 2nd ed. Bristol, United Kingdom, Wright Scientechnica, 1981, pp 295, 309–311.
12. Jensen R, Park RD, Lauerman LH, et al: Osteochondrosis in feedlot bulls. Vet Pathol 18:529–535, 1981.
13. Jubb TF, Malmo J, Brightling P, et al: Prognostic factors for recovery from coxofemoral luxation in cattle. Aust Vet J 66:354–358, 1989.
14. Kendrick JW, Sittmann K: Inherited osteoarthritis of dairy cattle. J Am Vet Med Assoc 149:17–21, 1966.
15. Kofler J, Edinger HK: Diagnostic ultrasound imaging of soft tissues in the bovine distal limb. Vet Radiol Ultrasound 36:246–252, 1995.
16. Madison JB, Tulleners EP, Ducharme NG, et al: Idiopathic gonitis in heifers: 34 cases (1976–1986). J Am Vet Med Assoc 194:273–277, 1989.
17. Moss EW, McCurnin DM, Ferguson TH: Experimental cranial cruciate replacement in cattle using a patellar ligament graft. Can Vet J 29:157–162, 1988.
18. Munroe GA, Cauvin ER: The use of arthroscopy in the treat-

ment of septic arthritis in two Highland calves. Br Vet J 150:439–449, 1994.

19. Nelson DR, Huhn JC, Kneller SK: Peripheral detachment of the medial meniscus with injury to the medial collateral ligament in 50 cattle. Vet Rec 127:59–66, 1990.

20. Nelson DR, Kosch DB: Surgical stabilisation of the stifle in cranial cruciate ligament injury in cattle. Vet Rec 111:259–262, 1982.

21. Palmer NC: Diseases of joints. *In* Pathology of Domestic Animals, vol 1, 4th ed. Jubb KVF, Kennedy PC, Palmer N (eds): San Diego, Academic Press, 1993, pp 138–145, 171.

22. Smith JA, Williams RJ, Knight AP: Drug therapy for arthritis in food-producing animals. Comp Cont Educ Pract Vet 11:87–93, 1989.

23. Taura Y, Sasaki N, Nishimura R, et al: Ulceric lesions of articular cartilages distal to carpal and tarsal joints in Japanese Black beef cattle. Jpn J Vet Sci 46:571–576, 1984.

24. Tulleners EP: Management of bovine orthopedic problems. Part II. Coxofemoral luxations, soft tissue problems, sepsis and miscellaneous skull problems. Comp Cont Educ Pract Vet 8:S117–S125. 1986.

25. Tulleners EP, Nunamaker DM, Richardson DW: Coxofemoral luxations in cattle: 22 cases (1980–1985). J Am Vet Med Assoc 191:569–574, 1987.

26. Watkins JP: Osteochondrosis. *In* Auer J (ed): Equine Surgery. Philadelphia, WB Saunders, 1992, pp 971–984.

27. Weaver AD: Hip lameness in cattle. Vet Rec 85:504–508, 1969.

28. Weaver AD: Lameness above the foot. *In* Andrews AH (ed): Bovine Medicine. Oxford, Blackwell Scientific, 1992, p 386.

29. Wegener KM, Heje NI, Aarestrup FM, et al: The morphology of synovial grooves (fossae synoviales) in joints of cattle of different age groups. J Vet Med Assoc 40:359–370, 1993.

30. Wyn Jones G, Baker JR, Johnson PM: A clinical and immunopathological study of *Brucella abortus* strain 19–induced arthritis in cattle. Vet Rec 107:5–9, 1980.

Jeremy Bailey   *Canada*

Christian Stanek   *Austria*

A. David Weaver   *United Kingdom*

12

Wounds, Tendons, Muscles, and Neoplasms

Wounds

Jeremy Bailey

Wounds in cattle result from blunt or sharp trauma, examples being bruising from doorways through which two cows attempt to pass simultaneously and accidents with farm machinery and equipment left in a yard or a corner of a field. Wounds may be closed or open, the latter being the major concern. Lacerations, incisions, stab and puncture wounds, and abrasions are different forms of injury.

Most injuries are minor, require minimal attention, and are easily treated by the stockperson. The minority, however, can present major problems because of their situation and extent, their proximity to joints or body cavities, and their early contamination by manure, soil, herbage, or other foreign material.

Predictably common sites of wounds resulting in lameness are the lower limb, from the carpus and hock distally. Falls through displaced or broken metal gratings covering slurry drainage channels, entanglement with discarded old corrugated metal sheets, and iatrogenic accidental damage to limbs from forks and shovels all are well-recognized patterns of injury (Figs. 12–1 and 12–2).

Although the biological principles of wound healing are introduced next, it should be recalled that in cattle, lameness control, economical considerations, and the available equipment and facilities are very important factors in assessing the most appropriate line of management.

Incorrect treatment and management of skin wounds and limb lacerations of cattle may reduce their soundness and productivity. A sound appreciation of the biology of wound healing is fundamental to an understanding of management strategies.

Wound healing can be divided into three stages:

1. The substrate phase (inflammatory, exudative, or lag phase). This phase is characterized by initial vasoconstriction followed by vasodilatation and

the damaged vessels and initiation of the coagulation cascade. The cellular or inflammatory response, starting about 12 hours later, is marked by the influx of large numbers of neutrophils and other cells that, through liberation of enzymes, have a vital role in breaking down devitalized tissue and removing bacteria. Wounds that are contaminated or infected or that involve much tissue trauma have both a prolonged inflammatory phase and an increased amount of exudate and discharge. Attempts at closing defects with marked contamination and a severe inflammatory response are likely to be unsuccessful.

2. The proliferative phase (fibroblastic phase). This commences when fibroblasts enter the wound and begin to produce collagen. In a wound that has been closed primarily, this process provides strength to the closure. This phase continues and overlaps considerably with the next phase.

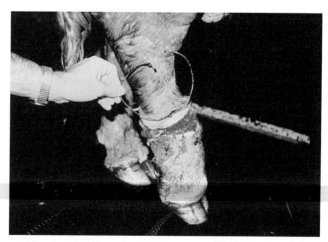

Figure 12–1. Extensive tissue damage resulting from a wire snar-

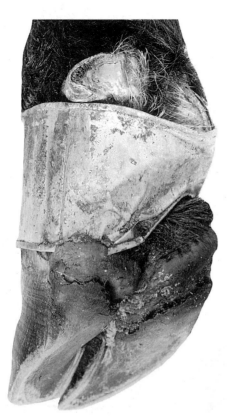

Figure 12–2. Portion of a tin can encircling the pastern of a steer.

3. Remodeling phase. Collagen synthesis and reorganization continue as the maturation or remodeling phase, which may persist for weeks or months.

In wounds in which closure is not an option, the proliferative stage still proceeds and eventually fills the defect with granulation tissue. Once soft tissue and skin defects are filled with granulation tissue, they become smaller after epithelialization and wound contraction. These two processes occur at an optimal rate in a healthy, even bed of granulation tissue. Both epithelialization and contraction are impeded by the development of excessive granulation tissue, the formation of hypermature or fibrous granulation tissue, and desiccation.

EVALUATION OF TRAUMATIC WOUNDS

Many systemic conditions, as well as economic considerations, can influence the ultimate method of wound management. Discussion here concentrates on factors related to the wound itself, many of which are interdependent. For example, a marked difference is seen between similarly contaminated wounds at 2 hours or 5 days old.

LOCATION OF THE INJURY

• Does the wound have effective gravitational drainage?

• Is it in close proximity to other important structures such as joints and tendon sheaths?

• If the wound is on the distal limb, is there sufficient skin to consider closure?

ELAPSED TIME SINCE INJURY

The degree of contamination of a wound and hence the probability of infection are related to the duration of the injury.

The so-called golden period is that time after which primary closure is probably contraindicated. This period is quoted as being 6 hours but is influenced by other factors such as the blood supply and the type of wound. Dogmatic adherence to specific time limits is inadvisable. A very fresh wound (<6 hours old) may be heavily contaminated but not yet infected. Organisms require time before they become established and replicate, and until this has occurred, contaminated wounds can in theory be converted to clean wounds and closure can be considered. The organisms in contaminated wounds more than 6 hours old have probably become established. Such wounds should be considered infected. Wounds more than 5 days old already have begun to form a bed of granulation tissue, which acts as a defense against any established organisms.

Determining the age of a wound also helps to make decisions about the viability of the adjacent tissue. Skin never regenerates, and because there is relatively little of it on the limbs, viable skin should not be debrided. The demarcation between viable and nonviable skin may not be very clear in the immediate post-trauma period. A delay in aggressive debridement for 24 to 48 hours may permit this distinction and may avoid the risk of removing potentially viable skin.

INFECTION

The risk of establishment of infection depends not only on the duration but also on the physical nature of the contaminating material—that is, infection-potentiating factors found in dirt, together with the quantity and virulence of the organisms, determine the risk that the infection will become established. The risk of infection is exacerbated by foreign bodies (including sequestra), excessive necrotic tissue, and impaired blood supply.

SIZE AND TYPE OF INJURY

The size of the wound is a major factor in deciding on any form of closure. Tension on sutures causes ischemia of the skin edges, leading to delayed healing and even wound dehiscence. The dimensions of the wound, the amount of skin loss, and the degree of swelling all are factors that must be considered.

The nature or type of wound is equally important. Clean lacerations (e.g., a knife cut) with no tissue loss and minimal tissue trauma lend themselves to primary closure.

At the other extreme are wounds that involve a lot of crushed and traumatized tissue with a high potential to become infected. Tissue damage, with its associated decreased blood supply, is one of the greatest potentiators of infection and prolongs the lag phase of wound healing.

Although the tissue damage of the traumatic insult is important, so too is the added insult of inappropriate wound management, rough tissue handling, and poor suture selection and application.

PUNCTURE WOUNDS

Puncture wounds, commonly encountered in food animal practice, can lead to devastating consequences if neglected. A penetrating object invariably introduces infection through a small aperture from which little or no drainage can occur. This enclosed environment is an ideal medium for organisms to replicate and for infection to develop readily. The lack of drainage results in accumulation of inflammatory and purulent exudate and formation of an abscess. The fluid may become walled off as it accumulates, or it may dissect towards and into more sensitive areas such

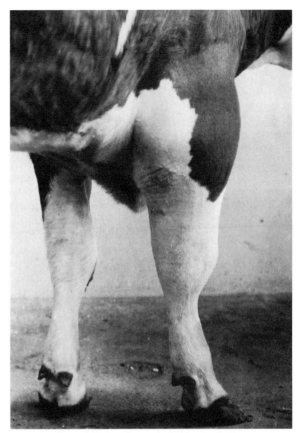

Figure 12–4. Infection of subcutaneous tissue following a puncture wound in the proximal region of the right forelimb has resulted in a massive phlegmon, subcutaneous cellulitis, and edema above the carpus and around the elbow. (Courtesy of Faculty of Veterinary Medicine VFU, Orthopedic Clinic, Brno, Czech Republic.)

as tendon sheaths and joints. Puncture wounds frequently affect the foot and axilla in cattle, and their early identification and treatment can prevent serious sequelae (Figs. 12–3 and 12–4). Adequate drainage should be a prime goal when dealing with puncture wounds. Systemic antibiotic therapy and local wound management, although important, are unlikely to prevent a fulminating infection and abscess formation if drainage is not established.

MANAGEMENT OF WOUNDS

The early management of a wound should be directed at containing the initial injury, preventing additional damage, and preparing the wound for the most appropriate type of repair. Adequate restraint, either physical or chemical, and local anesthesia establish suitable working conditions. Every wound is unique, and slight differences in treatment may change the overall result. These differences can be identified only if the unique characteristic of each wound is considered in the light of a sound understanding of the biology of wound healing.

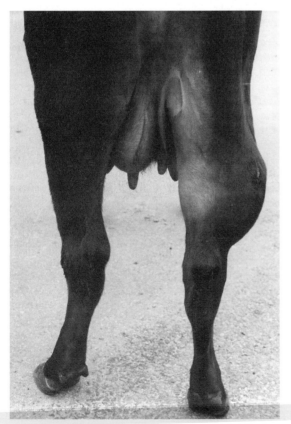

Figure 12–3. Abscess over the tibial region of the right hind limb resulting from a puncture wound. (Courtesy of Faculty of Veterinary Medicine VFU, Orthopedic Clinic, Brno, Czech Republic.)

CLEANSING

A wide area around the wound should initially be clipped and cleaned to minimize subsequent contamination from the surrounding skin and to facilitate surgical procedures. Protection of the wound bed during clipping using a water-soluble gel (e.g., K-Y Jelly, Johnson & Johnson) that can later be washed out is advised.

The wound should be thoroughly cleaned to reduce the level of contamination and bacteria. High-pressure lavage is more effective than low pressure for removing small particles and bacteria, and effective pressures can be obtained using a 35-mL syringe with a 19-gauge needle. High-pressure irrigation should avoid forcing the fluid between tissue planes, thereby posing the risk of driving contaminants deeper into the wound.

In the initial stages, the duration of hydrotherapy should be kept short to avoid waterlogging the tissue, as recognized by the development of a fairly characteristic grayish color.

In large animal practice, because of the nature of the wounds, the composition of the fluid is less important than the pressure or the volume. A 1% solution of a stock povidone-iodine preparation is readily available and practical, although some questions have been raised about its bactericidal properties.[22] A 0.05% solution of chlorhexidine diacetate has been shown to have better antibacterial activity without interfering with wound healing.[22] More concentrated solutions of these products either decrease the effectiveness of the product or increase tissue irritation.[28] The inclusion of antibiotics into irrigation solutions has also been shown to reduce the number of organisms in fresh wounds.[17] Economics usually dictate that antibiotic lavages should be used selectively and possibly as a final lavage. Some cases require physical scrubbing of the wound bed to remove the more adherent debris, but because this can increase tissue damage, it should not be overused.

In heavily contaminated wounds into which earth and manure have become impacted, some people have advocated the use of a mixture of equal parts of magnesium sulfate and glycerin. This material is packed into the wound and, because of its highly hygroscopic nature, is believed to be particularly useful in washing debris from fascial planes. Advocates of this method recommend that the mixture be used only for a maximum period of 2 hours.

DEBRIDEMENT

Removing dead and devitalized tissue decreases the rate of infection, shortens the lag phase, and helps prepare the wound for closure. Two practical methods can be used to debride a wound: either use sharp excision or allow time and the inflammatory phase to separate the nonviable tissue. Wet-to-dry dressings, recommended to aid in the removal of devitalized tissue[30] have practical limitations in large animal

practice. Sharp excision is quick and decisive and effectively shortens the lag phase, but which tissue needs removal may be difficult to determine. Clinical assessment based on capillary bleeding is usually adequate but can be misleading, particularly in the skin. If in doubt, debridement can be delayed for 24 to 48 hours, until the line of demarcation becomes more evident. Debridement of the skin margin should produce a smooth edge for improved apposition by sutures.

DRAINAGE

The drainage of serum, blood, inflammatory exudate, or pus from any wound remains a cornerstone of correct wound management. The accumulation of any such fluids is particularly devastating in closed wounds. Because open drains are not entirely without problems (providing a portal for retrograde infection), removal of fluids can be effected either by including closed drains or by gravity. Subcutaneous pockets involving one or more fascial planes must be identified and likewise drained. Seton drains are inexpensive yet effective. In some locations where wound configuration is such that gravity does not provide effective drainage, one must consider extension of the wound, establishing drainage portals or negative suction drains.

ANTIBIOTICS

The decision to use systemic antibiotics usually is easily made in acute wounds. The level of contamination and the nature of the wound are usually severe enough to justify their use. However, the decision to initiate parenteral antibiotic therapy depends on the evaluation of each individual situation. Systemic antibiotics are sometimes not required, as in more chronic wounds with a healthy bed of granulation tissue and adequate drainage. The choice of antibiotic drug should provide as broad a spectrum as possible (see pp. 62–63).

The use of topical antibiotics remains controversial. It is generally thought that topical antibiotics are useful only within the first few hours after injury.[28] Evidence shows that epithelialization in wounds treated topically with bacitracin/neomycin/polymyxin combination, silver sulfadiazine, or gentamicin solution proceeded at a faster rate than in untreated wounds.[31] Nitrofurazone, however, has been shown to slow epithelialization.[16] Petrolatum ointments also have a negative effect on some aspects of wound healing.[13] Care should always be used in selecting an appropriate medication. Ointments keep the wound environment moist, but the precise benefit has not been determined.

CLOSURE

Incorrect closure can result in early wound breakdown, abscess formation, poor cosmetic results, impaired function, prolonged treatment, and increased costs. The following methods can be used:

- *Primary closure* is used in sterile surgical incisions and can be applied to selected traumatic wounds that are very clean and have a healthy blood supply.

- *Delayed primary closure* of wounds may be preferable within the first 3 to 5 days before the onset of fibroplasia. Delayed closure follows treatment to reduce bacterial counts and to ensure that no devitalized tissue remains in the wound bed. In other words, wounds can be closed at any time after the contamination has been removed and the devitalized tissue debrided.

- *Secondary closure* applies to closing wounds after the formation of a bed of granulation tissue. It is useful in bovine lower limb wounds, which are often very contaminated. These wounds have a shortage of redundant skin to close over defects. The longer a wound is left before delayed or secondary closure, the more fibrotic is the surrounding skin. This decreased skin elasticity compounds the problem. In these cases or if the wound is too big to close, options are limited to treating it as an open wound or considering grafting or a skin mobilization procedure.

These options must also be considered in handling an extensive skin defect after removal of a neoplastic mass (e.g., melanocytoma) from the limb (e.g., hock, dorsal aspect of pastern), when primary closure is impossible. After a granulation tissue bed develops, a skin expansion technique or skin graft may be adopted.[1, 15]

The Skin Expansion Method

The skin expansion method is useful in closing larger wounds.[1] It entails undermining the surrounding skin and making several staggered rows of small stab incisions around the wound to expand the skin and to relieve the tension on the suture line (Fig. 12–5). Careful clinical judgment should determine how much of the surrounding skin can be undermined without compromising the blood supply. Clinical experience in lower limb injuries has shown that a 4- to 5-cm-wide margin of wound edge can safely be elevated. Stab incisions should be about 1.5 cm apart, with 2 cm between each row. A 10-mm stab incision is generally big enough to achieve the desired effect in fresh wounds, but older wounds need longer stab incisions to obtain the equivalent expansion. Postoperative support of the surgical site is very important, and plaster or fiberglass casts provide excellent support of the suture line and immobilization.

NONCLOSURE

When closure is not a viable option, the aim is to stimulate the processes of wound contraction and epithelialization, both of which are dependent on the presence of a healthy bed of granulation tissue. Management can be time consuming. Small limb wounds close if left completely alone, but the final result may not be as cosmetic as desired. To improve the cosmetic and possibly also the functional result, maintenance of an even, moist bed of granulation tissue is essential. Covering wounds with bandages maintains a moist environment, but increasing evidence suggests that bandaging open limb wounds promotes the formation of excessive granulation tissue.[2] Once a skin defect has filled with granulation tissue, the use of creams with very low levels of corticosteroids is very effective in controlling the formation of excessive granulation tissue (proud flesh) without inhibiting wound healing.[2] Many caustic products also control granulation tissue, but they also exert an equally caustic effect on the delicate migrating epithelial cells.

Casting the limb provides an effective physical barrier to prevent the formation of exuberant granulation tissue. It also effectively immobilizes the limb. Either plaster or fiberglass casts can be used, the latter being more expensive but having the distinct advantage of being resistant to water damage (see p. 259).

SKIN GRAFTING

The possible use of skin grafts in food animal practice is often overlooked. They have definite indications in lower limb wounds with extensive skin loss, especially when a good cosmetic result is sought.[15] Further details are published in an equine textbook.[4] Three types are commonly used in veterinary medicine: punch grafts (very similar to pinch or seed grafts), tunnel grafts, and sheet grafts. A sound understanding of basic graft biology is essential to ensure an acceptable success rate. Separation of the grafted skin from the recipient bed leads to failure. Accumulation of purulent fluid, blood, or serum at the graft-bed interface, movement of the grafted tis-

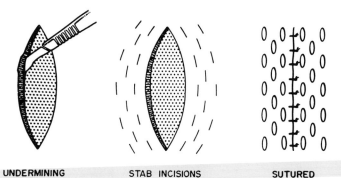

UNDERMINING   STAB INCISIONS   SUTURED

Figure 12–5. The mesh expansion method of wound closure showing the process of undermining, making stab incisions, and closing the wound.

sue, poor quality of the recipient bed, and poor collection techniques are common causes of failure of skin grafts. The donor site should be prepared as a sterile site, and the skin handled as atraumatically as possible. Although it is possible to graft to fresh wounds, it is customary to use a bed of granulation tissue as the recipient field. This should ideally be an even layer of fresh, highly vascular tissue that is level with the surrounding skin and free of any clefts or defects.

Sheet grafts require very exacting standards with very little room for error, and specialized equipment is required.[29] The technique is rarely used in cattle.

Tunnel grafts can be used in circumstances that are somewhat less than optimal and can easily be performed with minimal equipment.[14] Tunnel grafts have a high success rate but often poor cosmetic results. They do not require the same degree of immobilization as the other two techniques and thus can be used on areas where bandaging is difficult. The technique calls for a second surgical procedure to remove the roofs of the tunnels.

Punch or **pinch (seed) grafts** lie between these two extremes and are the most common technique. The success rate is moderately high, and a fairly pleasing cosmetic result can be obtained. Using disposable biopsy punches, punch grafts can readily be performed in cattle practice.

DEGLOVING INJURIES

In degloving injuries (Fig. 12–6), a large flap of skin is peeled back away from the underlying tissue. Lameness is uncommon unless the wound becomes severely infected and sepsis extends into muscles and tendons. These flaps can be large, and loss of this skin area can be potentially serious. It is often difficult to determine the integrity of the blood supply, which is influenced by the flap size, its width at the base, and the location. Debridement should be delayed until the line between the healthy and non-vascular tissues is well demarcated. Because skin cannot regenerate, all possible measures should be taken to preserve as much of the flap as possible. It should be returned to its normal position and held in place with stay sutures or bandages. Any tension on the flap is detrimental to an already tenuous blood supply. Drainage of any pockets formed in repositioning the flap should be established.

When the vascular integrity of the flap has been confirmed, immobilization is an excellent way to aid healing.

HEMATOMAS

Severe blunt trauma can result in vascular damage leading to the formation of large subcutaneous or intramuscular hematomas (Fig. 12–7). Differentiating hematomas from abscesses may be difficult without needle aspiration. Great caution should be taken to avoid inoculating an otherwise sterile hematoma

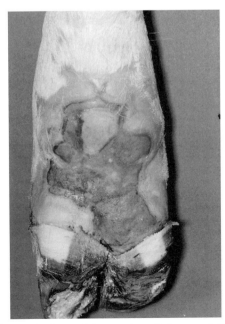

Figure 12–6. A degloving injury and partial exungulation caused when the animal struggled to release its limb from the rails of a gate.

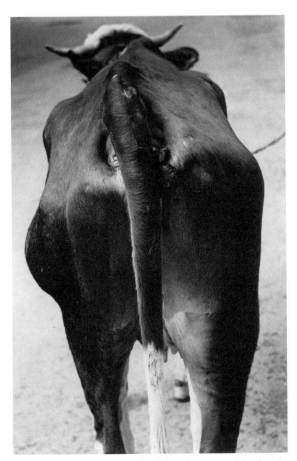

Figure 12–7. Hematoma over the left thigh caused by butting by another animal (Courtesy of Faculty of Veterinary Medicine VFU, Orthopedic Clinic, Brno, Czech Republic).

with organisms, thereby creating an abscess. If a diagnosis of a hematoma can be made on the basis of the history and clinical examination, it may be prudent to avoid taking such risks. Many hematomas spontaneously resolve eventually. A real danger of significant hemorrhage exists if a hematoma is lanced before the damaged vessel or vessels have had a chance to thrombose. Locating the offending vessel to control the bleeding or, depending on the location, applying sufficient pressure to minimize the blood loss may be difficult. It is therefore preferable to allow the hematoma to resolve on its own or to delay surgical drainage for at least 10 days.

INJURIES TO THE CLAW CAPSULE

Loss of the claw capsule may occur traumatically, as in a fracture of the toe, or may result from a surgical intervention. Severe lameness may result. In either case, with an intact blood supply, the hoof can re-form all of its components from the keratogenic dermal tissues. These wounds heal almost entirely by epithelialization but require more time than wounds on other parts of the body. Elsewhere, the defect first fills in with granulation tissue to allow the migration of germinal cells from the healthy surrounding corium. The same principles of treatment apply here as in skin lesions: careful assessment and debridement, cleaning, and preventing further contamination. To establish a bed of granulation tissue (even over exposed bone), gauze impregnated with antibiotic in petroleum jelly may be applied over the wound and held in place with a waterproof bandage. The germinal epithelium of the corium covers the deeper part of the defect and produces a layer of keratinized

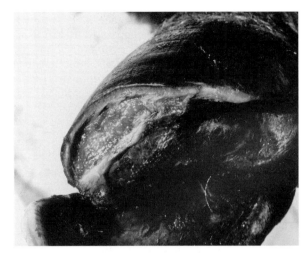

Figure 12–9. Granulation tissue is allowed to form under the protection of a bandage.

tissue, whereupon the remaining wall defect can be repaired with available acrylic materials (Figs. 12–8 to 12–10; see p. 137). Several such compounds generate heat, which can be dissipated by running cold water over the repair.

Injuries involving the coronary band are more serious. The hoof wall that grows down after the injury may be abnormal but may be quite functional. As with wall and sole defects, the germinal cells from the corium of the coronary band migrate over the defect. It is difficult to predict to what extent the hoof will be deformed, but experience has shown that even an abnormal-looking claw is better than no claw at all.

DISCUSSION

Medical management of skin wounds and injuries to deeper structures is discussed further in Chapter 16 (see pp. 248–254). Surgical management of a contam-

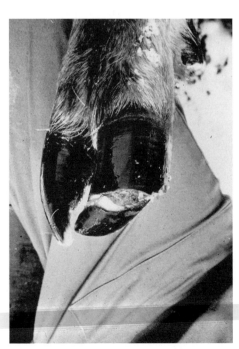

Figure 12–8. Fracture of the apex of a claw.

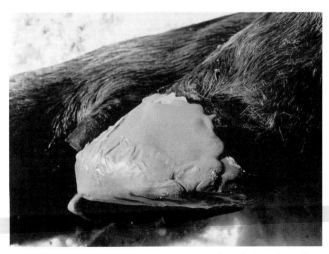

Figure 12–10. A semipermanent prosthesis of methyl methacrylate is applied over the tip.

inated wound has been covered (see p. 183), but the development of postoperative sepsis in a skin wound can be an equally difficult problem. The most common organism in this secondary infection is *Actinomyces pyogenes,* followed by streptococci, staphylococci, and *Proteus* and *Pseudomonas* spp.

Fortunately, rarely does a gas-forming organism (e.g., clostridia) complicate wound healing. The principles of adequate drainage, effective irrigation, and parenteral chemotherapy require intensive effort to avoid the development of systemic disease and irreparable damage to deeper vital structures.

Tendons and Tendon Sheaths

Christian Stanek

DIGITAL FLEXOR TENDON SHEATH

ANATOMICAL CONSIDERATIONS

The digital flexor tendon sheath (DFTS) is a synovial structure on the flexor aspect of the distal extremity, 16 cm long in adult cattle (see Chapter 14). The tendon sheaths of the third and the fourth digit are separated in the metacarpal region by an axial membrane. Communication with the fetlock, pastern, and distal interphalangeal joint is rare (<4%). The proximal limit of the DFTS is the distal third of the cannon bone, and it ends distally at the skin-horn border of the heel bulb. The distal recesses of the DFTS lie close to the palmar pouch of the distal interphalangeal joint and the navicular bursa. A thin synovial membrane separates these structures. Two flexor tendons, the superficial (SFT) and deep (DFT), are enclosed in this sheath. Proximally there are two separated compartments. The SFT forms a tendinous tube, enclosing the inner proximal compartment of the DFTS. The outer proximal compartment encloses the tendinous tube formed by the SFT concentrically. The inner compartment extends more proximally than the outer. Both compartments unite in the fetlock region. Puncture of the tendon sheath proximal to the accessory digits allows aspiration of synovial fluid from only one compartment, usually the outer. Pathological tendinous changes secondary to DFTS sheath infection can be quite different in this region. A vascularized mesotendon is limited to the proximal and the distal ends of the tendon sheath. The intervening structures have vessels passing mainly on the tendon surface or entering in a single vinculum in the fetlock region.[25] Blood supply should be taken into consideration when planning tendon sheath surgery, especially partial resection.

SEPTIC TENOSYNOVITIS OF THE DIGITAL FLEXOR TENDON SHEATH

Etiology

Septic tenosynovitis of the DFTS is either primary, caused by a penetrating wound (which is rarely iatrogenic), or secondary as a complication of a digital infection or spread of a local subcutaneous abscess.

In tie stalls, perforating fork wounds are seen, commonly on the pelvic limb above the dewclaw or in the pastern. Calves may have a metastatic infection of the DFTS, mainly caused by infection spreading into the tendon sheath from an infected fetlock joint or from a septic epiphysitis of the distal cannon bone. Metastatic infections in adult cattle are uncommon. Secondary septic tenosynovitis occurs as a sequel to a complicated digital infection, such as sole ulcer (pododermatitis circumscripta) (Fig. 12–11), white line infection, retroarticular abscess, or interdigital phlegmon. In complicated cases of pododermatitis circumscripta, the infection can extend into the tendon sheath as a result of deep flexor tendon necrosis (Fig. 12–12). In complicated sole ulcers, infections in the distal interphalangeal joint are generally more frequent than in the DFTS.[6]

Pathogenesis

The first stage is a marked fibrinous exudate (serofibrinous stage). Synovial fluid production and function are inhibited. Superficial venous thrombosis damages the vascular supply to the tendon sheath and related structures.

The next development is a purulent-necrotizing stage. Histological examination reveals the presence of leukocytes always associated with superficial ten-

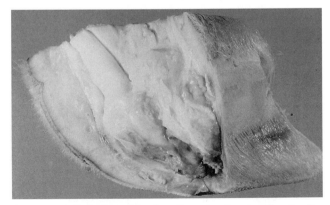

Figure 12–11. Infection of the deep flexor tendon sheath extending from a pododermatitis circumscripta lesion. The insertion of the deep flexor tendon into the distal phalanx can become necrotic and can avulse (horny capsule absent).

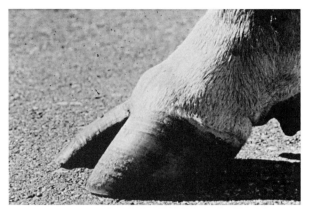

Figure 12–12. When the deep flexor tendon avulses from the distal phalanx, following necrosis resulting from septic tenosynovitis, the tip of the claw becomes overextended.

don necrosis.[25, 26] Adhesions later develop. Bacteriological isolates of adult animals are usually of *A. pyogenes*. Early stages of tendon sheath infection frequently have a negative result on bacteriological examination of the synovial fluid. The role of anaerobic bacteria is uncertain.

The various compartments may undergo different changes, especially in leukocyte count in the early stages of the infection. Advanced cases of distal interphalangeal infection may show alterations in DFTS synovia in the absence of infection of the tendon sheath itself. Increased fluid content within the tendon sheath should be evaluated,[10] but advanced cases may contain no fluid.

Clinical Signs

A mild to moderate lameness, usually of a hind limb, is present. Hyperflexion of the fetlock (knuckling) may occur. An edematous and phlegmonous swelling extends up the flexor surface of the midcannon region (Fig. 12–13). The dorsal aspect of the digit may be slightly swollen. Tendon sheath distention is palpable only in early stages. Rupture of the necrotic DFT results in upward tilting of the affected claw. Careful evaluation of the fetlock or distal interphalangeal joint may reveal the presence of pathological changes. The clinical symptoms of the joint infection predominate in most cases of combined distal joint sepsis and DFTS infection.

No diagnostic radiological changes are seen. Some cases have gas formation inside or adjacent to the tendon sheath. Ultrasonography may reveal enlargement of the peritendovaginal tissues, abscess formation, or tendon necrosis and pathological rupture.

Differential Diagnosis

The differential diagnosis includes localized phlegmon; septic arthritis of the distal interphalangeal, pastern, or fetlock joint; and other complicated digital infections.

Treatment

Medical Treatment. The precise stage of the infection has to be evaluated rationally. Local therapy must always be accompanied by parenteral antibiotics. In early cases, with no evidence of tendon or tendon sheath necrosis, repeated flushing of the tendon sheath with Ringer's solution plus an antibiotic or with a 0.1% povidone-iodine solution is recommended. Because part of the DFTS lies above the dewclaws, a second cannula can be inserted, directed distally, above the bulbs. This painful procedure should be performed using intravenous regional analgesia[27] with 10 megaunits of sodium benzyl penicillin added.

Surgical Treatment. Radical resection of the DFT and the SFT over the whole length of the DFTS is recommended for advanced cases.[34] This open exposure of all tendons permits the removal of necrotic tissue, including periarticular material (Fig. 12–14). Open wound drainage may prove useful.

The operation is performed best in a recumbent animal under sedation. A rubber tourniquet is applied around the proximal third of the metatarsus/metacarpus.[27] Intravenous regional analgesia is administered with 10 megaunits of sodium benzyl penicillin added. The site is clipped, shaved, and prepared for surgery. The flexor aspect of the affected digit is incised, starting 8 cm above the dewclaw in the sagittal plane of the accessory digit, circumscribing the dewclaw axially, then continuing distally to the skinhorn border of the bulb. Midline incisions between

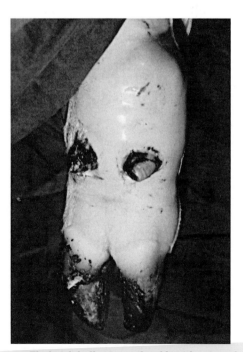

Figure 12–13. Fleckvieh bull, 10 months old, with a 2-week history of a small perforating wound above the dewclaw. Septic tenosynovitis of the lateral digital flexor tendon sheath is present despite vigorous antibiotic therapy. Note the marked swelling in the pastern area and above the accessory digits.

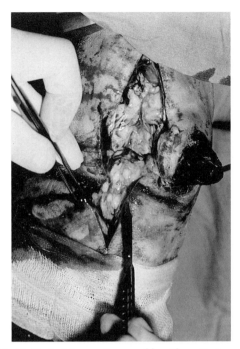

Figure 12–14. Fleckvieh cow, 6 years old, with septic tenosynovitis of the lateral digital flexor tendon sheath, which developed after pododermatitis circumscripta. Total resection of the deep and superficial tendons, which were embedded in a mass of multiple abscesses, was successful. Treatment with systemic antibiotics and lavage alone would have been inadequate.

the main digits should be avoided because of the risk of vascular injury. The subcutaneous tissue and annular ligaments are transected. The tendon sheath is opened along its entire length. The tendinous cord formed by the SFT and DFT is exposed, and the proximal extension of the DFTS is digitally explored. The SFT is then incised at its flexor aspect longitudinally, exposing the DFT, which is followed proximally to the division of the two branches to the medial and the lateral digit. The DFT is transected from axial to abaxial, carefully avoiding penetrating the soft tissue membrane dividing the tendon sheaths of the fourth and the third digit axially. The distal tendon stump is everted and, after dissecting the vinculum, is removed as far as possible from within the tendon sheath. In cattle with a complicated sole ulcer, the longitudinal incision is extended into the ulcer, exposing the tendon down to its insertion at the distal phalanx. The SFT is next transected proximally in an abaxial direction, carefully avoiding opening the DFTS on the other side. The accessory ligament of the interosseus medius muscle is transected, and the SFT is everted and dissected distally to its point of insertion, where special care should be taken not to open the distal interphalangeal joint. The peritendinous tissues of the DFTS are curetted to remove fibrous and necrotic material. A danger exists of opening the fetlock joint above the proximal sesamoid bones, as well as near the short distal sesamoidean ligaments. After thorough flushing, the wound is closed with interrupted sutures down to the level of the dewclaw, leaving the distal portion open

(Fig. 12–15). A gauze, rubber, or plastic (Penrose) drain should be inserted before wound closure. The sound contralateral claw is elevated by means of a wooden or rubber block (see pp. 137–141).

In cattle with localized pathological changes (e.g., perforating wounds of the fetlock region), partial distal resection of the tendon sheath is possible. Noninvolvement of the remaining portions of the tendon sheath can be confirmed by clinical, ultrasonographic, and intraoperative evaluation.[25, 26]

Bandage changes are recommended on postoperative days 3 and 6, thereafter at 4-day intervals. An average healing period of 42 days has been reported, with a success rate of 77%.[26] Infection of the contralateral digit is the most common complication. Because surgery is contraindicated, intensive medical therapy is the only option. The prognosis is poor. In cases with both infectious arthritis of the distal interphalangeal joint and infectious tenosynovitis, distal digital exarticulation is recommended, with partial or total tendon resection.

The postsurgical long-term results of the tendon and DFTS resection procedures show a mean survival period of 29.2 months under conventional (tie stall) conditions.[10]

TARSAL PERIARTHRITIS

Definition

Tarsal periarthritis is defined as chronic cellulitis of the epidermis, dermis, and subcutis of the lateral

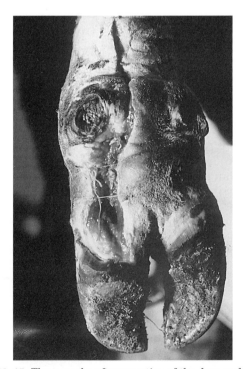

Figure 12–15. Three weeks after resection of the deep and superficial flexor tendons in a 5-year-old Brown Swiss cow. Open wound treatment was carried out. Two cutaneous sutures, visible distal to the dewclaws, were inserted to keep the wound edges in apposition without total closure.

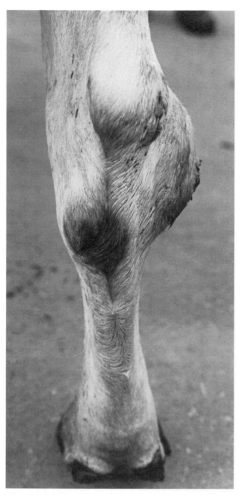

Figure 12–16. Purulent periarthritis with generalized involvement of extra-articular tissue (Courtesy of Faculty of Veterinary Medicine VFU, Orthopedic Clinic, Brno, Czech Republic.)

aspect of the hock joint (Fig. 12–16). Both limbs are involved to a variable extent.

Etiology and Pathogenesis

As a result of repeated trauma, an adventitious bursa forms on the lateral aspect of the hock joint. The swelling may become considerable (e.g., 20 × 20 × 12 cm deep). Predisposing factors are tie stalls lacking straw bedding or with sawdust bedding or short stalls or cubicles that force the animal to lie on the edge of the standing with its hocks rubbing on the curb. Cubicles in which cows find difficulty in standing, resulting in repeated scraping of the lateral aspect of the hock joint, also predispose to tarsal skin trauma and cellulitis. Fattening bulls kept on slatted floors are also affected. This chronic irritation first results in collection of blood and fibrin in a limited lateral subcutaneous position. A low-grade septic inflammation can develop later. Subsequent infection of the talocrural joint or the small distal tarsal joints is rare. Colonization of the bursa with *Brucella abortus,* reported previously,[7] does not appear to be

a problem today. Herds with multiple cases of tarsal cellulitis almost invariably have poor housing conditions, because the condition tends to respond when cattle are put to summer grazing.

Clinical Signs

The first sign is hairless, hyperkeratotic skin on the lateral distal tarsal region, as well as a localized soft swelling. A firm, thick-walled bursa then develops to various degrees, occasionally with minor signs of inflammation. The entry of infection does not cause major changes. Larger lesions may develop several interconnected pockets within the bursa, causing difficulties in the effectiveness of flushing this structure. Contusion results in a break in skin integrity, the entry of infection, and development of a chronic fistulous discharge of pus. This feature is uncommon. No systemic signs are noted unless septic infection extends elsewhere. Lameness is absent except in cases in which size causes mechanical impairment, such as might be the case if severe abscessation or inflammatory edema (phlegmon) is present. Advanced cases may occasionally show radiological changes such as periostitis and osteophytes on the lateral malleolus of the tibia, the centrotarsal bone, and the proximolateral aspect of the cannon bone. The soft tissue swelling is clearly visible, and a few cases have gas formation. Calcification of the bursal wall is rare. Ultrasonography is helpful in evaluating the internal structure.

Differential Diagnosis

The differential diagnosis includes perforating wounds, foreign body abscessation, localized phlegmon, septic tarsal arthritis, and serous tarsitis.

Treatment

Mild or moderate cases should, if possible, be put on to soft bedding (e.g., straw yard). Administration of antibiotics and corticosteroids often results in rapid improvement if not complete resolution of some cases.

When abscessation has occurred, the abscess cavity may be opened with a 5-cm vertical incision at the distal border. It should be irrigated (povidone-iodine) daily and possibly mildly curetted to remove infected granulation tissue. This wound should be kept open for further drainage and slow resolution.

Conservative treatment such as kaolin poultices and local hyperemic agents have little use. Bandages are difficult to maintain in position.

It is inadvisable to attempt radical surgery such as total resection of an infected bursa: the dissection plane is difficult to follow, the risk of entering the joint is high, and postoperative hemorrhage, skin necrosis, wound dehiscence, delayed healing, and eventual recurrence of the swelling are major disadvantages.

Prevention

Careful observation of a group problem reveals incorrect housing conditions (inadequate or poor bedding, incorrect stanchion or cubicle dimensions, bad position of rails) in most cases. Use of a straw yard resolves most such problems but may be economically difficult to justify.

PRECARPAL BURSITIS

Precarpal bursitis is a chronic inflammation of the subcutaneous adventitious bursa on the dorsal aspect of the carpal joint, occasionally with infection.

Etiology and Pathogenesis

Many features resemble tarsal cellulitis (see p. 190). It similarly results from chronic mechanical irritation, with the skin becoming thickened and hyperkeratotic. A distinct subcutaneous bursa develops. Predisposing factors are rough, hard floors without bedding, poor stanchion design that causes animals to creep backward to stand up, little or no bedding, and unhygienic conditions.

Clinical Signs

A hairless, hyperkeratotic skin initially develops with thick, firm subcutaneous tissue, followed by the formation of a subcutaneous bursa (Fig. 12–17). The size varies considerably. Carpal flexion is painful and reduced. The general condition of the animal is unaltered. Infection very rarely involves the joint. The bursal (or hygroma) contents resemble thin synovia. In the years 1970 to 1980, several publications reported the isolation of *B. abortus*, but its importance was unclear because the incidence was not significantly higher in animals with a positive agglutination titer than in animals in the same herd with a negative titer.[7]

Differential Diagnosis

The differential diagnosis includes septic carpitis, subcutaneous carpal abscessation (e.g., foreign body), and septic tenosynovitis.

Treatment

The condition should be treated only in animals that are in pain or that have infected lesions. Parenteral

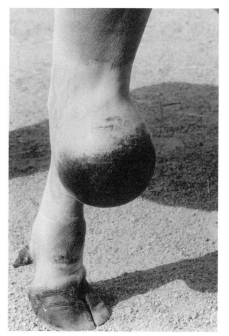

Figure 12–17. Severe case of bursitis precarpalis in a 7-year-old Brown Swiss cow. The bursa consisted of multiple cavities filled with 1.2 liters of pus containing *Actinomyces pyogenes.*

antibiotics should be limited to cases of acute infection. Appropriate treatment includes incision of a septic precarpal bursa at two or three points, especially at the most dependent point, careful limited curettage, and insertion of a plastic or latex (Penrose) drain (Fig. 12–18). The cavity should be repeatedly flushed. Surgical removal of the bursa should be

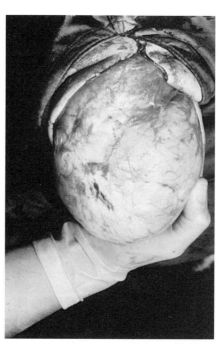

Figure 12–18. Total resection of an infected bursa in an advanced case of periarthritis tarsalis under intravenous regional anesthesia in a 5-year-old Fleckvieh cow.

avoided, as in tarsal cellulitis (see p. 190), because similar postoperative complications are most likely to develop.

SUBTENDINOUS (CALCANEAN) BURSITIS

Definition

Subtendinous (calcanean) bursitis is septic bursitis at the point of the hock (tuber calcanei with the bursa underlying the superficial flexor tendon). This condition is not synonymous with subcutaneous bursitis (Fig. 12–19).

Etiology and Pathogenesis

Septic inflammation of an adventitious subcutaneous bursa involves the subtendinous bursa beneath the superficial flexor tendon. Advanced cases also have osteomyelitis of the calcaneus. Cows are usually presented with severe changes. Dairy cows kept in tie stalls and loose stalls are affected, as are fattening bulls kept on slatted floors. No systemic disturbance is identified. The condition occurs mainly in animals tied in short stalls with sharp edges on the curb. Some cases result from fork wounds.

Clinical Signs

The clinical manifestation is an egglike bursa situated on the tip of the calcaneus (but actually lying beneath the flexor tendon), exhibiting signs of acute

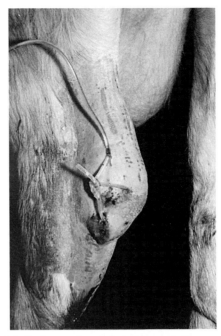

Figure 12–20. Drainage of an infected bursa calcanea subcutanea with a polyvinyl drain inserted in a proximodistal direction. Flushing was carried out two to three times daily.

infection. Complete tendon necrosis in this region is rare. The lesion is very painful, and a skin perforation is sometimes visible. Lameness is occasionally observed, as well as knuckling of the fetlock joint. In animals with a secondary osteomyelitis, osteolytic changes and a periosteal reaction are visible on radiography. In contrast, a subcutaneous bursitis is inconsequential except as a cosmetic blemish. The swelling is painless, and gait is not impaired. A bilateral presentation is possible.

Differential Diagnosis

The differential diagnosis includes traumatic aseptic subcutaneous bursitis, fracture of the calcaneus, other localized sepsis, and luxation of the superficial flexor tendon.

Treatment

Drainage is effected by means of a lateral incision followed by curettage and insertion of a drain (Fig. 12–20). The superficial flexor tendon should not be involved unless severe necrotic changes are present. Cases of osteomyelitis carry a guarded prognosis.

CELLULITIS OF THE LATERAL ASPECT OF THE STIFLE JOINT

Definition

Cellulitis of the lateral aspect of the stifle joint is a circumscript cellulitis, leading to subcutaneous pseu-

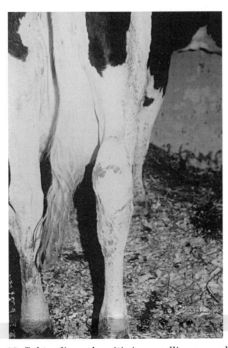

Figure 12–19. Subtendinous bursitis is a swelling around the tuber calcaneus.

dobursitis at the lateral aspect. If infected, necrosis and inflammation of the adjacent soft tissues may be present.

Etiology and Pathogenesis

Mechanical irritation can stimulate development of this lesion. It occurs mainly in older cows in tie stalls without bedding or with wood shavings. The partition separating one animal from another causes a contact irritation. Local infection is a secondary complication, with the condition worsening seriously within a few days. The lesion is allegedly the primary site for metastatic infection of liver, kidneys, and endocardium and for septic thrombophlebitis of the vena cava caudalis.

Clinical Signs

If the lesion is infected, cows usually are presented with systemic involvement (reduced appetite, pyrexia) and a large, hot, painful swelling. The whole stifle region sometimes is considerably enlarged and edematous. Gas is possibly palpable in the subcutaneous tissues. A moderate to severe swinging limb lameness is seen. Subsequent infection of the stifle joint is common. Diagnostic arthrocentesis of the joint is hazardous because of the severe surrounding infection. There may be a serious danger of abortion.

Treatment

The affected tissue should be incised distally to permit drainage and flushed with Ringer's or Betadine solution. Parenteral administration of high doses of antibiotic for several days is indicated.

Prognosis

The prognosis is guarded, with a long period of convalescence. A risk, in addition to abortion, is metastatic spread to internal organs. Exhaustion and recumbency are likely if the stifle joint is infected. The prognosis with involvement of the stifle joint is extremely poor, when euthanasia should be recommended.

Muscles and Neoplasms

A. David Weaver

MUSCLES

Several aspects of muscle disease related to lameness in cattle are discussed elsewhere in this text: muscle dystrophy (see Chapter 10, p. 155), double muscling and hypertrophy (see Chapter 6, p. 84), and adductor group rupture in the downer cow syndrome (see Chapter 13, p. 215).

This section considers some specific localized problems of muscle pathology resulting in lameness. Emphasis is placed on some examples of injuries, specifically rupture.

Injuries involve striated skeletal muscle, which comprises bundles of fibers each multinucleated and surrounded by a sarcolemmal membrane. Each muscle is attached proximally and distally to bone by fascia, aponeuroses, or tendons. The chemical energy for contraction of muscle comes from adenosine triphosphate (ATP). Muscle contains ATP and creatinine phosphate. The latter can aid resynthesis of ATP from adenosine diphosphate (ADP). Creatine phosphokinase catalyzes conversion of ADP to ATP and, found in high concentrations in skeletal muscle, is a useful indicator of the degree of muscle damage (e.g., in the downer cow syndrome—see p. 215).

Histological features of muscle rupture involve, in mild cases, sarcolemmal rupture, then hyaline and granular degeneration with an initial and transient neutrophil reaction.[9] Fibrin production can seriously interfere with regeneration. Any area of ischemic damage repairs badly. In considering a downer cow, a transient (pressure-induced) hypoxia, lasting a few hours only, results in coagulation of contractile proteins that are restored to normal by myoblast and myotube formation. Longer periods of hypoxia can result in irreversible changes in muscle fibers, explaining the need for frequent turning of a downer cow to the other side.

Apart from ischemia, local pressure from recumbency can lead to a compartment syndrome following increased fluid (blood, serum) within an osteofascial compartment of defined limits.

MUSCLE ATROPHY

Muscle atrophy is broadly considered to be a reduction in muscle size but more precisely a reduction in muscle fiber diameter or cross-sectional area. Pathological descriptions highlight a differential diminution of the type 1 and type 2 fibers.[9]

In relation to bovine lameness, muscle atrophy is important as a major sign of an underlying disease process.

Cachexia is associated with malnutrition and involves the entire body musculature. Such atrophy is gradual but tends to be prominent in the thigh muscles, leading to weakness rather than lameness.

Denervation atrophy, on the other hand, tends to affect a single region and is always associated with muscle weakness or paralysis. Proximal radial paralysis is a typical example (p. 207). Peripheral denervation leads to a rapid reduction of muscle volume (triceps group and extensors of the carpus and digits in this example).

Therefore, either generalized or localized muscle atrophy is an important parameter in considering both the duration and localization of a lesion causing lameness.

Localized muscle atrophy may not be a result of a so-called neurogenic atrophy. Further examples include disease atrophy after use of a limb cast or splint, chronic joint or tendon problems such as degenerative joint disease in a mature cow, or contracted flexor tendons in a neonatal calf.

SPECIFIC RUPTURES OF MUSCLE

Ventral Serrate Rupture

The ventral serrate muscle originates from the lateral thoracic wall and inserts onto the medial surface of the scapula, acting as the major component of the sling for the thorax between the forelimbs.

INCIDENCE

This rupture is sporadic in adult cows, especially Channel Island breeds (Jersey, Guernsey), and in young (6 to 18 months old) fattening cattle, among which several may be simultaneously affected (Fig. 12–21).

ETIOLOGY

In isolated adult cattle in which muscle paralysis or myositis is suggested but not demonstrated, it is most common in undernourished cattle in the Indian subcontinent. Nutritional muscular dystrophy or my-

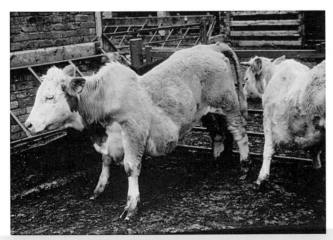

Figure 12–21. Rupture of the ventral serrate muscle in two fattening beef steers resulting from combined vitamin E and selenium deficiency ("flying scapula") (Courtesy V. I. Centre, Lincoln, M.A.F.F., England).

opathy can result in these signs in fattening animals (see p. 155).

CLINICAL SIGNS

One or both forelimbs may be affected. The onset is sudden, and stiffness or mild lameness is noted as the dorsal border of the scapula rides up some distance above the level of the cranial thoracic spine. In the non–weight-bearing phase, the scapula resumes its normal position. Pain is absent on palpation and abduction of the foreleg, and the disability may be classed as a mechanical lameness. Some cases are bilaterally symmetrical, with the chest then dropping between the shoulders.

In a closely related condition, the shoulder joint may be laterally displaced on weight-bearing ("loose shoulder," "Jersey shoulder"). The deformity is allegedly a result of partial rupture or reduced tone in the group of shoulder adductors (subscapularis, teres major, pectoral muscles), and in addition to its prevalence in Jersey cows is encountered in both thin dairy cows and grain-fed fattening steers and heifers. The lower limbs, compensating for the abducted shoulder, tend to be placed across the midline, incorrectly suggesting pain in the medial digit (e.g., fracture of medial distal phalanx or acute laminitis). The cause is not known. No nerve lesions have been demonstrated in either manifestation.

Necropsy reveals muscle rupture, serous infiltration, hematoma formation in early cases, and increased fibrous tissue.

DIAGNOSIS

The clinical signs are almost diagnostic in ventral serrate rupture. In lateral displacement of the shoulder, suprascapular paralysis (see p. 206) and fractures close to the shoulder joint should be excluded.

TREATMENT

Animals with recent signs should be confined to a well-bedded loose box for several weeks for spontaneous repair by fibrosis. More chronic cases remain unchanged or the animal deteriorates slowly, but few cows require emergency slaughter. Some Jersey cows adapt well to ventral serrate rupture and then remain in the herd for several lactations.

In fattening cattle, vitamin E and selenium injections should be given to the group to prevent the development of signs in other at-risk stock. Medical treatment fails to improve the clinical condition, and fattening cattle have a slow and uneconomical rate of weight gain.

Peroneus Tertius (Cranial Tibial) Rupture

The peroneus tertius and cranial tibial muscles are primary flexors of the hock and antagonists of the gastrocnemius.

INCIDENCE AND ETIOLOGY

Rupture occasionally occurs in the midbelly or at the proximal or distal tendon-muscle junction in mature cattle, usually in dairy breeds. It results from sudden trauma such as slips and falls, pulling the limb too high upward with a rope over a beam, and accidents in cattle chutes (crushes).

CLINICAL SIGNS

No abnormalities are apparent at rest, but locomotion is characteristic: the hock is abnormally extended while the stifle remains flexed, indicating a failure of the reciprocal apparatus. The limb is dragged, the claws scrape the ground, and the calcanean (Achilles) tendon is slack. The limb may be manually extended caudally so that the tibia and metatarsus are in a straight line while the stifle joint remains at 90° (Fig. 12–22).

Observation and palpation reveal painful, edematous, and hemorrhagic swelling in the cranial aspect of the gaskin over the tibial shaft in early cases. The swelling later becomes more localized and less painful.

DIAGNOSIS AND MANAGEMENT

The condition is easily recognized by the characteristic gait and site of the swelling, the location of which could initially be confused with a tibial fracture.

As in other conditions involving acute muscle trauma, plasma creatine phosphokinase levels are elevated in early stages.

Prolonged rest and confinement may resolve some cases in which rupture is in the muscle belly and fibrotic repair takes place. Cows with rupture and separation in the muscle tendon junction, muscle insertion or origin have a more guarded prognosis.

Adductor Muscle Group

The adductor group comprises the obturator, gracilis, pectineus, and adductor muscles, all of which originate from the pelvis (ilium, pubis) and from the sym-

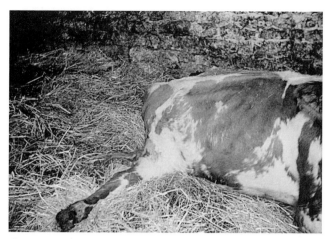

Figure 12–23. Cow recumbent after postparturient rupture of the adductor muscles. Note the typical positioning of the hind limb.

physeal and prepubic tendons to insert on the medial aspect of the femoral shaft (Figs. 12–23 and 12–24). The related nerve supply includes the obturator and sartorius.

CLINICAL SIGNS

The major abnormality is rupture of the bellies of several muscles, usually bilaterally, resulting from sudden marked abduction of the hind limbs (spread-eagling). In some cows, rupture occurs at its point of origin. This abduction may follow severe dystocia in cows of any age. Predisposed cows include younger animals with severe pelvic bruising and hemorrhage and older cows in poor condition with a large udder and overgrown claws, coupled with a slippery ground surface.

Examination (see p. 215) reveals skin abrasions in the medial aspect of the thigh and localized swelling due to intramuscular hemorrhage and early necrosis.

Diagnosis first depends on attempts to locate the site of muscle rupture, which is rapidly obscured by the developing swelling. Differential diagnosis includes spinal trauma, sacroiliac and coxofemoral lux-

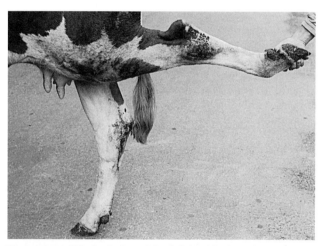

Figure 12–22. Manipulation of the left hind limb to demonstrate a position that can be produced in a case of peroneus tertius muscle rupture. The stifle is flexed, the hock is extended, and the gastrocnemius tendon is flaccid. (Courtesy of Faculty of Veterinary Medicine VFU, Orthopedic Clinic, Brno, Czech Republic.)

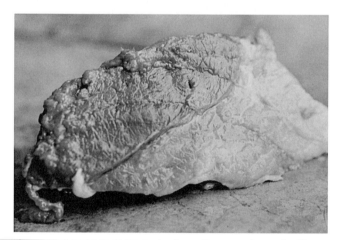

Figure 12–24. Adductor muscle from the cow shown in Figure 12–23. The lower muscle mass is pale and shows signs of ischemia.

ation, pelvic and femoral fractures, primary nerve damage, and muscle damage elsewhere (e.g., gluteal, gastrocnemius). All affected animals should undergo a careful rectal examination and general examination for signs of metabolic disease, because many have associated hypocalcemia and hypophosphatemia. Laboratory examination of levels of plasma or serum minerals and creatine phosphokinase may be undertaken.

TREATMENT

The course of disease depends on its severity, its unilateral or bilateral features, and supporting therapy. Management should primarily involve attentive nursing on soft bedding, appropriate mineral injections, and regular turning of the cow to avoid the development of both pressure sores on the lateral aspect of the dependent limb and compartment syndrome (see p. 215).

Gastrocnemius Rupture

The gastrocnemius muscle originates by two heads from the caudal femoral surface and inserts onto and just dorsal to the point of the hock (calcaneus) by two strong tendons.

Rupture can occur at three points:

1. In the muscle belly, some distance proximal to the point of the hock

2. At the muscle-tendon junction, about 8 to 12 cm proximal to the hock

3. At its insertion onto bone, more correctly termed avulsion

The incidence is low. It is usually unilateral. The typical case is seen in overweight, clumsy cows around the time of parturition. Older veterinary literature refers to several fattening animals of a group being simultaneously affected.[7] The common site is the muscle-tendon junction (number 2, listed earlier). Predisposing factors include prolonged recumbency (see p. 215), conformation (specifically excessive weight), mineral imbalance (calcium, phosphorus), bad flooring, and swampy pastures across which movement is excessively labored.

CLINICAL SIGNS

The hock is flexed, weight-bearing is reduced, and the point of the hock drops toward the ground, especially in walking. The fetlock may be flexed, initially suggesting a localized problem (Fig. 12–25 and 12–26). The typical case initially has a soft, warm, painless swelling containing blood and serous exudate and, later, edematous fluid. Several days later, the swelling is firm, larger, and somewhat painful. Animals with bilateral cases rapidly become recumbent, and early euthanasia on welfare grounds is usually indicated.

Type 3 cases may allegedly be lame for several days or weeks before the rupture, which is usually

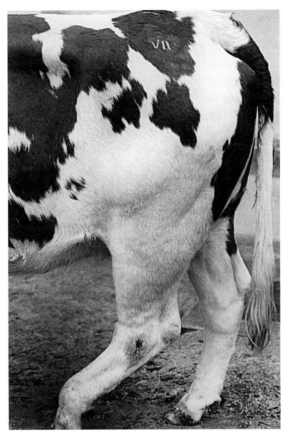

Figure 12–25. Partial rupture of the gastrocnemius muscle in a Friesian cow. Note swelling of the muscle, flexion of the fetlock, and reduced weight-bearing. (Courtesy of Faculty of Veterinary Medicine VFU, Orthopedic Clinic, Brno, Czech Republic.)

sudden. The distal gastrocnemius insertion separates, often with some bony spicules attached to the proximally retracted tendon. A diffuse, painful swelling develops around the point of the hock. In early cases, the area of separation can be palpated.

DIAGNOSIS

With the exception of the avulsion type 3, diagnosis is easy and based on the typical site and stance.

Although radiographic examination of the swelling is likely to be helpful only in diagnosis of type 3 cases, ultrasonography may be useful in differential diagnosis of hematoma, abscess, and seroma involving these soft tissues,[11] as well as defects in the continuity of muscle-tendinous structures. Both linear (7.5-mHz) and sector (5-mHz) scanning has been used in transverse and sagittal planes. This procedure is rapid, noninvasive, and harmless to both operator and patient. It will doubtless be extensively used as experience is gained in cattle clinics and on farms.

Differential diagnosis at the distal site (the third site mentioned earlier) includes calcanean bursitis (see p. 193), tarsal fracture (see p. 266), luxation of the superficial flexor tendon, and tarsal abscessation. In types 1 and 2 it includes discrete abscessation due to foreign bodies and hematoma formation, neither of which is likely to cause lameness.

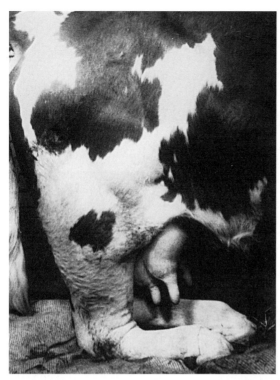

Figure 12–26. Bilateral complete rupture of the gastrocnemius muscle in a Friesian cow. Weight-bearing is primarily on the hock joints and metatarsi. (Courtesy of Faculty of Veterinary Medicine VFU, Orthopedic Clinic, Brno, Czech Republic.)

TREATMENT

An affected cow should be carefully moved a minimal distance to a well-bedded stall or loose box. It is important to avoid increasing the degree of damage. If the animal can stand, the preferred treatment includes support by a well-fitting Thomas splint to keep movement at the rupture site to a minimum. The inguinal padding of the splint must be kept in good condition to avert pressure necrosis. The device must be kept in place for a minimum of 6 weeks to permit healing of the partially ruptured muscle.

As an alternative to the splint device, yearling animals may have the hock immobilized for some weeks by drilling compression screws from the caudal surface of the calcaneus across the distal portion of the tibial shaft, with the tarsal joint in extension. Strict aseptic technique is essential. The wound is lightly bandaged for 1 week. After 6 weeks, the screws are removed and the patient is permitted gradually increased movement after a further week of strict confinement.

The prognosis is poor in complete rupture or avulsion of the tendon and is guarded in cases of muscle belly rupture.

Transection of the Gastrocnemius Tendon

Transection of the gastrocnemius tendon is discussed as a single specific entity rather than with wounds (see p. 181) or tendon sheath problems (see p. 188).

ETIOLOGY AND CLINICAL SIGNS

The lesion arises from severe trauma resulting in incomplete or complete transection and with accompanying contamination of the wound. The likelihood of simultaneous involvement of the superficial digital flexor tarsal sheath is slight. The signs are similar to rupture of the gastrocnemius muscle (see p. 197). The limb bears no weight, and when the animal is stimulated to walk, the hock drops markedly and the plantar aspect of the metatarsus may contact the ground.

TREATMENT

Every effort must be made to minimize the extent of contamination by immediately irrigating the wound with water and transporting the animal to dry surroundings, avoiding long distances that will increase the injury.

The treatment then follows the guidelines previously given (see p. 183) of preoperative systemic antibiosis, meticulous control of hemorrhage and debridement, and careful assessment of the possibility of suture coaptation of the transected tendon ends. This technique is usually limited to clean cuts with no loss of tissue. Surgery is performed on sedated recumbent patients under general anesthesia or epidural block. The preferred suture type, using stainless steel wire, monofilament nylon, or polydioxanone (PDS, Ethicon), is the locking loop or modified Kessler pattern, which provides close apposition and holding power that is superior to that of other simple interrupted tendon sutures.[12]

Other advantages of the locking loop include minimal disturbance of the extrinsic blood supply, little exposure of suture material, minimal damage to the epitendon, and adequate strength to prevent gap formation. These factors all promote tendon healing. Although important in equines, other perceived advantages such as a lack of peritendinous reaction and reduced fibrous tissue formation are unimportant in cattle.

Subcutaneous tissues and skin should be apposed over the tendon, and the area bandaged and placed in an appropriate splint to avoid overextension of the hock sufficient to cause immediate breakdown of the repair. Splintage should be maintained for several weeks, with weekly bandage changes.

In the healing process, fibroblasts and capillary buds from the surrounding connective tissue migrate and invade the wound. The fibroblasts synthesize collagen and mucopolysaccharides. The collagen polymerizes into fibrils, which are initially deposited in random fashion in and around the wound but later become longitudinally oriented parallel with the tendon fibers.

Infected wounds should be left open, and tendon sutures should not be placed. If splintage is adopted, there is a slight chance of repair by coaptation by new fibrous tissue, but it must be emphasized that most cases of complete transection carry a very poor prognosis.

CLOSTRIDIAL DISEASES OF MUSCLE

Lameness can be seen as a result of infection with

1. *Clostridium tetani*—tetanus

2. *Clostridium chauvoei*—blackleg

3. *Clostridium septicum* and others—malignant edema (gas gangrene)

This section briefly discusses the locomotor signs, gross pathology, and therapy. All these conditions may be prevented by appropriate vaccination programs. Standard textbooks cover other features in greater depth.

Tetanus

Generalized hypertonia, often with bouts of clonic muscle spasms, is the characteristic sign. Tetanus tends to be sporadic and predominantly occurs in younger stock. Slight stiffness is noted, rapidly worsening, and cattle prefer to stand still, sometimes adopting a rocking horse stance. If startled, the animal is likely to fall, keeping all limbs extended and being unable to rise.

Muscle enzyme levels are generally elevated. An infected wound is not often detected. Necropsy may not reveal any gross muscle pathology.

Differential diagnosis includes early hypomagnesemic tetany, bacterial meningitis, polioencephalomalacia, and polyarthritis.

Case management includes wound debridement and exposure to air (if detected), systemic and local penicillin G, tetanus antitoxin, tranquilization (acepromazine maleate), and attentive nursing.

Blackleg

A rapid onset of severe lameness is often missed because peracute cases are found dead. Most cases are encountered in 6- to 24-month-old stock. Lameness is more frequent in a hind leg, and muscle swelling of the gluteal region is then a feature. Foreleg lameness may be due to infection and swelling in the scapular region or brisket. The area is crepitant but painless on palpation. The skin may be discolored and colder than normal.

Incision into the swollen area releases rancid, thin, serosanguineous fluid. Muscle enzyme levels are elevated. Necropsy reveals discolored red and black necrotic muscle, serosanguineous fluid, and gas pockets and bubbles.

Differential diagnosis includes malignant edema (other clostridial spp.), bacillary hemoglobinuria, and, in afflicted animals found dead, lightning stroke and anthrax.

Therapy includes radical surgical exposure of affected tissue as well as drainage, systemic antibiotics, and supportive care.

Malignant Edema

Malignant edema develops after wound contamination (e.g., castration, vaccination) and causes severe local infection and systemic toxemia. Stiffness (resulting from scrotal infection) or hind leg lameness (from improper intramuscular injection, e.g., prostaglandins) are signs in some cattle. Local edema, swelling, and pain are apparent. Crepitus is not a consistent sign.

Necropsy features are similar to blackleg, and differential diagnosis may be difficult if no suspicious edematous wound is found.

Treatment is similar to blackleg (drainage, antibiotics), but the prognosis is poor owing to the severe systemic upset.

All three conditions are characterized by severe systemic signs. The disease is rapidly fatal, and intensive emergency treatment is essential for a realistic chance of recovery. Severely toxic, dehydrated, recumbent animals should be euthanized and necropsy performed at once.

Other muscular conditions in which stiffness of the hindquarters is observed include bacillary hemoglobinuria (*Clostridium haemolyticum*), postexertion azoturia (with muscle degeneration and myoglobinuria), and capture myopathy.

NEOPLASMS

This section considers some neoplasms of the skin and locomotor system that occasionally are associated with lameness. Lameness may be a simple mechanical impediment due to size and position, such as a large papilloma in the volar or plantar aspect of the pastern, preventing full flexion. Other neoplasms may cause pain, with the animal then being unwilling to flex or extend the limb. The incidence is low.

Benign tumors include papillomas and fibropapillomas,[7, 21, 23] melanocytoma,[5, 7, 19, 23, 32] schwannoma,[3] vascular hematoma (e.g., bovine cutaneous angiomatosis), and mast cell tumors.[8, 18, 21, 24] The last-named three forms are the basis of isolated reports only. Malignant tumors affecting the musculoskeletal system in cattle are rare. Reports include osteosarcoma,[7] malignant synovioma,[7, 20] and lymphosarcoma invading the spinal canal or, less commonly, appendicular joints.[7, 20, 21, 23, 33]

An extensive review (100 references) and 62 new cases have been published.[23] In this series, lymphosarcoma, fibropapilloma, and squamous cell carcinoma were the most common skin neoplasms. This review mentions lameness associated with a 25-mm-diameter fibroma on the right hind pastern and a 10-cm-diameter ulcerated fibrosarcoma on the coronary band region.

History

The history is usually of a slow-growing mass and correspondingly slow and insidious onset of lameness. Sudden onset of lameness is uncommon and then in association with neoplasia such as osteosarcoma with extension into soft tissues and major nerve trunks.

Clinical Examination

Observation and palpation should determine whether the lameness is purely mechanical interference or is due to pain. Neoplasms are rarely painful or warm to the touch, unlike localized subcutaneous abscesses.

Radiography and ultrasonography may be performed if bone structures could be involved (see p. 33). Needle, wedge, or excisional biopsy may be undertaken (see p. 165). Tissue may be examined grossly (e.g., melanoma confirmed as a solid black core) and a Gram stain smear performed to rule out bacterial infection. It may be justifiable in some cases to await a pathological diagnosis of the biopsy before proceeding with more extensive surgical resection.

Differential Diagnosis

Other conditions that may mimic neoplasms in cattle include slow-growing subcutaneous and localized periarticular abscesses, localized osteomyelitis of the diaphysis or metaphysis of long bones (e.g., metacarpus, metatarsus, tibia), especially of growing cattle (so-called Brodie abscess; see p. 246), spinal spondylosis or abscessation (differentiating spinal lymphosarcomatous infiltration), and digital dermatitis of the pastern.

Three neoplasms—melanocytoma, papilloma/fibropapilloma, and lymphosarcoma are briefly considered next.

MELANOCYTOMA (MELANOMA)

Melanocytic tumors (Fig. 12–27) account for 5% to 6% of tumors in surveys of bovine neoplasms. The skin is the common site. Black, red, and gray cattle have been affected most commonly. Although reported in older cattle, most cases develop in animals younger than 2 years. Neither site nor sex predilection has been established. Few melanocytomas invade deeper than the subcutis or metastasize. In one series[19] of 10 melanocytomas in young cattle, 4 occurred on the limbs (over the metacarpus, pastern, hock), causing some mechanical interference with locomotion but mostly of concern as a cause of disfigurement.

Most cases tend to be solitary gray to black masses, smooth surfaced, and ranging from 5 to 25 cm in diameter. Removal of such slow-growing masses should be undertaken as soon as practicable, because continuing infiltration of the subcutis results in involvement of adjacent tendon sheaths and joint capsules, leading to further gait impairment.

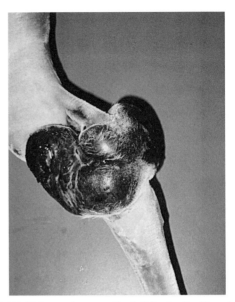

Figure 12–27. Melanocytoma on the left hock of a Charolais crossbred calf.

SURGERY OF MELANOCYTOMA

Most cases causing lameness are amenable to surgery under sedation (xylazine intravenously or intramuscularly) and intravenous regional analgesia distal to a tourniquet placed tightly around the proximal part of the affected limb (see p. 46).

After routine skin preparation for sterile surgery, *en bloc* resection of discrete masses should include a minimal 1-cm margin of apparently normal skin and subcutis. The lack of available skin on the limb usually makes it impossible to approximate the skin margins over the defect. Some residual small areas of black filamentous neoplastic tissues often are left adjacent to tendon sheaths but do not appear to result in subsequent regrowth. A firm occlusal dressing should be applied to prevent postoperative hemorrhage and the potential growth of excessive granulation tissue. After 3 to 4 days and a second dressing change, a paraffin tulle dressing or sheet of sterile equine amnion is a useful application to improve the rate of epithelialization over the defect. The prognosis is favorable, although residual scar tissue may present a cosmetic blemish.

Papilloma

Digital papillomatosis and its relationship to digital dermatitis are discussed in Chapter 7 (see p. 97).

One of the two types of lesions currently classified as digital dermatitis is a proliferative wartlike lesion (see Fig. 7–18). This papillomatous or verrucose type, characterized by a mass of hard fine tendrils, is histologically indistinguishable from a squamous papilloma.[23] Lameness was recorded in five Holstein cows with 3- to 6-cm-diameter verrucose lesions of interdigital fibropapillomatosis in hind limbs. Although papillomatosis caused by BPV1 and BPV2 usually regresses after 1 to 12 months, interdigital papilloma and papillomatosis caused by BPV3 and BPV5 rarely regresses spontaneously but responds well to surgical excision or cryotherapy. Histologic findings in these cows included an exophytic proliferation of epithelial and connective tissue without ballooning degeneration of keratinocytes or abnormal clumping of keratohyaline granules.[23] The precise cause remains obscure.

Nonfilamentous papillomas occasionally develop in the interdigital space or at the junction of the interdigital space and coronary band and are sometimes associated with skin hyperplasia manifested as a thickened fold of skin.[7] Larger masses are subject to pressure necrosis from expansion (interdigital space) and to external trauma, leading to intermittent hemorrhage and the development of an infected wound.

In terms of lameness, solitary papillomas or fibropapillomas on sites other than the distal extremity (pastern, interdigital space) are insignificant.

Papillomas extend peripherally, not into subcutaneous tissues, and do not metastasize. Surgery may be indicated in large masses (see p. 120), and healing may be slow as a result of contamination of the resulting wound. Radical (knife) excision, thermocautery (diathermy), and cryotherapy are the preferred surgical techniques. Recurrence at the same site is unlikely.

Lymphosarcoma

Lymphosarcoma is a sporadic condition, the adult form of which may cause lameness, commonly as a result of infiltration into the lumbar or sacral spinal cord or rarely into a peripheral joint such as the tarsus.[20, 33] Clinical signs may include a reluctance to rise, intermittent lameness, joint pain, and a shuffling or stilted gait. In spinal infiltration, the first sign may be knuckling of one or both hind fetlocks. Ataxia may be observed and crepitus may be appreciated.

In peripheral joints, the major pathology is in the articular cartilage, which becomes dull, pale, and eroded. The synovia undergoes degeneration and contains aggregates of neoplastic lymphocytes.

Lymphosarcomatous invasion of the lumbar spinal cord is usually an extension from the lumbar drainage nodes. The slow destruction of lumbar nerves results in a progressive posterior ataxia and paresis. Diagnosis is suggested on rectal palpation of irregular large sublumbar masses and possibly by other palpable foci of enlarged intrapelvic and intra-abdominal nodes.

Diagnosis of cases involving peripheral joint swelling depends on joint aspiration for demonstrating abnormal lymphocytes in the synovia and biopsy of the joint capsule.[20, 33] One case report[20] describes a 5- to 6-month-old Holstein heifer with a 3-week history of hind limb paresis and weakness, presenting with marked bilateral tibiotarsal joint distention. Arthrocentesis revealed a cloudy yellow fluid containing large numbers of small and large lymphocytes indicative of lymphosarcoma (bovine leukosis). Although a spinal tap revealed no abnormalities, at necropsy, gray ventral extradural masses were present throughout the spinal canal but were most prominent in the lumbar and sacral area, where they compressed nerve roots at lumbar 4 and 5.

After diagnosis, cattle should be culled as soon as possible, because spontaneous resolution, temporary remission, and successful therapy have not been recorded. Cases with disseminated lymphosarcoma are condemned for human consumption at meat inspection.

REFERENCES

1. Bailey JV, Jacobs KA: The mesh expansion method of suturing wounds on the legs of horses. Vet Surg 12:78–82, 1983.
2. Barber SM: Second intention wound healing in the horse. The effects of bandages and topical corticosteroids. Porceedings of the American Association of Equine Practitioners 107–116, 1989.
3. Canfield P: A light microscopic study of bovine peripheral nerve sheath tumors. Vet Pathol 15:283–291, 1978.
4. Caron JE: Skin grafting. In Auer J (ed): Equine Surgery. Philadelphia, WB Saunders, 1992, pp 256–272.
5. Gourreau JM, Scott DW, Charini JP: Les tumeurs mélaniques cutanées des bovins. Le Point Vét 26:55–62, 1994–1995.
6. Greenough PR, Ferguson JG: Alternatives to amputation. Vet Clin North Am Food Anim Pract 1:195–203, 1985.
7. Greenough PR, MacCallum FJ, Weaver AD: Lameness in Cattle, 2nd ed. Bristol, United Kingdom, Wright Scientechnica, 1981, pp 423–426.
8. Hill JE, Langheinrich KA, Kelley LC: Prevalence and location of mast cell tumors in slaughter cattle. Vet Pathol 28:449–450, 1991.
9. Holland TJ: Muscle and tendon. In Jubb KVJ, Kennedy PC, Palmer N (eds): Pathology of Domestic Animals, vol 1, 4th ed. San Diego, Academic Press, 1993, p 221.
10. Kofler J: Neue Möglichkeiten zur Diagnostik der septischen Tendovaginitis der Fesselbeugesehnenscheide des Rindes mittels Sonographie—Therapie und Langzeitergebnisse. Dtsch Tieraerztl Wochenschr 101:215–222, 1994.
11. Kofler J, Buchner A: Sonographische Differentialdiagnostik von Abszessen, Haematomen und Seromen beim Rind. Wien Tieraerztl Monatschr 82:159–166, 1995.
12. Krishnamurthy D: Tendons and ligaments. In Tyagi RPS, Singh J (eds): Bovine Surgery. Delhi, India, CBS Publishers, 1993, pp 304–309.
13. Lee AH, Swaim SF, Yang St, et al: The effects of petrolatum, polyethylene glycol, nitrofurazone, and a hydroactive dressing on open wound healing. J Am Anim Hosp Assoc 22:436–451, 1986.
14. Lees MJ, Andrews GC, Bailey JV, Fretz PB: Tunnel grafting of equine wounds. Comp Cont Ed Pract Vet 11:962–970, 1989.
15. Lees MJ, Fretz PB, Bailey JV, Jacobs KA: Principles of grafting. Comp Cont Ed Pract Vet 11:954–960, 1989.
16. Lesiewicz J, Goldsmith LA: Inhibition of rat skin ornithine decarboxylase by nitrofurazone. Arch Dermatol 116:1225–1226, 1980.
17. Lindsey D, Nava C, Marti M: Effectiveness of penicillin irrigate in control of infection in sutured lacerations. J Trauma 22:186, 1982.
18. McGavin MD, Leis TJ: Multiple cutaneous mastocytomas in a bull. Aust Vet J 44:20–22, 1968.
19. Miller MA, Weaver AD, Stogsdill PL, et al: Cutaneous melanocytomas in 10 young cattle. Vet Pathol 32:479–484, 1995.
20. Oliver-Espinosa O, Physick-Sheard PN, Wollenberg GK, Taylor J: Sporadic bovine leukosis associated with ataxia and tibiotarsal joint swelling: A case report. Can Vet J 35:777–779, 1994.

21. Palmer N: Bone and joints. *In* Jubb KVF, Kennedy PC, Palmer N (eds): Pathology of Domestic Animals, vol 1, 3rd ed. San Diego, Academic Press, 1993, pp 125–137, 181–182.

22. Sanchez IR, Swaim SF, Nusbaum KE, et al: Effects of chlorhexidine diacetate and povidone-iodine on wound healing in dogs. Vet Surg 17:291–295, 1988.

23. Scott DW, Anderson WI: Bovine cutaneous neoplasms: Literature review and retrospective analysis of 62 cases (1978–1990). Comp Cont Educ Pract Vet 14(10):1405–1418, 1992.

24. Shaw DP, Buoen LC, Weiss DJ: Multicentric mast cell tumor in a cow. Vet Pathol 28:450–452, 1991.

25. Stanek CH: Morphologische, funktionelle, chemische und klinische Untersuchungen zu den Erkrankungen der Fesselbeugesehnenscheide des Rindes. Wien Tieraerztl Monatschr 74:379–412, 1987.

26. Stanek CH: Morphologische, funktionelle, chemische und klinische Untersuchungen zu den Erkrankungen der Fesselbeugesehnenscheide des Rindes. Wien Tieraerztl Monatschr 75:14–29, 46–58, 84–102, 127–138, 170–180, 1988.

27. Stanek CH: Basis of intravenous regional antibiosis in digital surgery in cattle. Isr J Vet Med 49:53–58, 1994.

28. Stashak TS: Equine Wound Management. Philadelphia, Lea & Febiger, 1991, pp 24–27.

29. Swaim SF: Principles of mesh skin grafting. Comp Cont Ed Pract Vet 4:194–200, 1982.

30. Swaim SF: The physics, physiology and chemistry of bandaging open wounds. Comp Cont Ed Pract Vet 7:146–157, 1985.

31. Swaim SF, Lee AH: Topical wound medications: A review. J Am Vet Med Assoc 190:1588–1597, 1987.

32. Yager JA, Scott DW: Skin and appendages. *In* Jubb KVF, Kennedy PC, Palmer N (eds): Pathology of Domestic Animals, vol 1, 3rd ed. San Diego, Academic Press, 1993, pp 708–710, 719–721.

33. Van Pelt RW: Pathologic changes of joint disease associated with malignant lymphoma in cattle: Clinical, gross pathologic and histopathologic findings in cattle. Am J Vet Res 28:429–433, 1967.

34. Westhues M, Breuer D: Klauengelenks-resektionen und Sehnenresektion beim Klauengeschwür des Rindes. Nord Vet Med 16(Suppl 1):335–343, 1964.

Laura Smith-Maxie   *Canada*

13

Diseases of the Nervous System

Neurological problems, primarily of the peripheral nerves, can produce a gait problem that in the early stages may be difficult to distinguish from lameness of musculoskeletal origin. Once signs of general proprioceptive loss (knuckling of digits, dysmetria, spinal ataxia), paresis, neurogenic muscle atrophy, and even discrete sensory loss in parts of a limb are recognized, neurological gait problems are easier to diagnose. The emphasis in this chapter is on peripheral nerve diseases.

Several authoritative texts on the details of the neurological examination, special diagnostic techniques, and nervous diseases of the bovine species are available.[2, 14, 21, 23] Spinal column and spinal cord diseases discussed here are limited to those that tend to cause lameness in the early stages (e.g., spinal abscessation).

Most diseases of the brain can be ruled out on the basis of demeanor and behavioral disturbances, cranial nerve deficiencies, and signs of ataxias of vestibular or cerebellar origin. A few brain diseases are briefly discussed, because in the early stages, locomotor problems predominate and resemble musculoskeletal lameness.

EXAMINATION TECHNIQUES

PHYSICAL EXAMINATION

A thorough general physical examination is essential and may provide clues to the diagnosis of a neurological problem. Some examples follow:

- The fever and septicemia of *Haemophilus somnus* infection often cause a bilateral stiffness of gait just before hemorrhagic infarction of the brain or spinal cord.

- Limb deviations such as knuckling over of the fetlock or a dropped hock appearance, which tend to have neurological origins, must be distinguished from physical damage or congenital defects of the joints, muscles, or tendons.

- Rectal examination may detect internal lymphadenopathy suggestive of lymphosarcoma that has progressively infiltrated the spinal canal; this often results in cauda equina or spinal cord signs.[27]

- Thoracic and abdominal examination of unthrifty animals may support a diagnosis of abscesses that have also affected the spine.

- Progressive debilitation and gastrointestinal signs are also associated with the peripheral neuropathy of triorthocresyl (TOCP) phosphate poisoning.

- In newborn calves, abnormalities of the skull conformation and the eyes may occur in conjunction with congenital defects of the cerebral hemispheres such as hydrocephalus. It is important to realize that in ruminants, cerebral cortical diseases of a congenital or slowly progressive nature tend to cause a symmetrical or hemilateral gait disturbance that is often perceived as stiffness rather than paresis or conscious proprioceptive deficiency. Changes in mental status or visual deficiencies are helpful in the differential diagnosis but may become obvious only terminally if the problem is progressive. Hydrocephalus and brain abscessation are the most common examples.

GAIT AND POSTURE EXAMINATION

Careful observation of the gait of an ambulatory large animal is the most important examination procedure when attempting to identify neurological deficiencies and to differentiate neurological deficits from primary musculoskeletal disease. The weakness produced in the early stages of lower motor neuron (LMN) diseases, whether of the peripheral nerves, ventral root, or the neurons of the ventral horn of the spinal cord, often causes a stiff, short-strided movement of the affected limb(s). Until proprioceptive deficiencies or sensory loss is detectable, confirmation of neurological disease may be difficult.

Neurogenic atrophy of the affected muscles can take 5 to 10 days to develop. Diseases that irritate nerve roots and meninges, such as localized meningitis (often in association with vertebral/spinal cord abscessation and pathological vertebral fracture/collapse) or *Hypoderma bovis* migration, may cause stiffness. The initial differential diagnosis can include white muscle disease, arthritis, and tetanus.

General physical examination, laboratory tests, and ancillary diagnostic aids such as radiographs and arthrocentesis may be needed to make a diagnosis. Until a head tremor and truncal ataxia develop with progressive cerebellar disorders, the early signs of stiffness and mild hypermetria may be misdiagnosed as a primary disorder of the muscles or joints. A hereditary cerebellar disease that is subtle in its onset has been reported in young Holstein cattle.[36] Other insidious hereditary spinal diseases that may mimic primary musculoskeletal problems initially include bovine progressive degenerative myeloencephalopathy or Weaver syndrome of Brown Swiss cattle[31] and progressive ataxia or myelin disorder of Charolais cattle.[9, 21]

SPINAL REFLEX AND SENSORY EXAMINATION

If an animal is large and ambulatory, a complete spinal reflex examination is not possible unless it is cast into lateral recumbency. However, in combination with the gait evaluation and comparison of the various muscle groups that are prone to neurological problems, a practical assessment of reflex activity can be achieved. In any recumbent animal that is examined quickly after collapse, a complete reflex examination can be carried out to reveal specific nerve damage and diffuse or multifocal lower motor neuron deficits. If the animal becomes hypothermic or has been in prolonged recumbency resulting in muscle and nerve damage on the dependent side, identifying the primary problem is more difficult.

An animal being examined in lateral recumbency should later be turned onto the other side. Both upper limbs should be examined for evidence of injury that could impair the reflex test results (e.g., fracture, dislocation, extensive muscle damage, ankylosing arthritis, tendon contractures, and so on). Obvious muscle atrophy of any muscle groups should be noted at this time.

Passive Manipulation

Passive manipulation of each limb is performed by holding the claws and flexing and extending the limb several times. This allows assessment of general muscle tone and may reveal spasticity of upper motor neuron (UMN) diseases or may even detect the plastic rigidity of tetanus (often unbreakable extensor rigidity as opposed to the clasped-knife rigidity of UMN disease). In contrast, LMN disease often produces a remarkable flaccidity that is different from the normal muscle tone of a relaxed recumbent animal.

Flexor Reflexes

The flexor reflexes of both the pelvic and thoracic limbs must be tested carefully to assure the examiner that the animal can flex all joints completely. Application of sufficient stimulus to elicit full flexion is necessary. Superficial pinching or pinpricking of the skin of the lower extremity is rarely adequate. The use of hoof testers is appropriate. If no response occurs or if flexion of some or all of the joints is incomplete, a supramaximal stimulus in the form of an electric goad should be used. If this is not done, evidence of hypoflexia or areflexia of the limb is impossible to verify. With an animal that has adequate sensation in its distal extremities, a smooth flexor reflex of all joints is sometimes difficult to elicit before it kicks out in protest. These animals also tend to have considerable voluntary control, and the limb or its body may have to be repeatedly stimulated, during which time complete voluntary flexion may be observed. Pressing more gently on the bones of the phalanges sometimes produces a smoother complete flexor reflex.

In localizing lesions of the thoracolumbar spinal cord, it is important to be aware that pelvic limb reflexes will remain intact whenever the injury occurs between the *second thoracic (T2)* and *third lumbar (L3)* cord segments. A lesion in this section results in a *UMN paresis or paralysis,* which may cause spasticity of the hind leg reflexes. With a totally destructive UMN lesion of the thoracolumbar cord (T2 to L3), the limbs will react (involuntary flexion) to severe stimuli but there will be no voluntary movement or sensation to the body parts caudal to the level of the lesion. A severe but partial UMN lesion of the pelvic limbs usually causes loss of purposeful movement but preservation of some pain sensation distal to the lesion.

Damage to the mid to lower lumbar vertebrae affects the lower motor neurons of the lumbosacral cord segments that terminate within the first two sacral vertebrae in ruminants (Fig. 13–1). Lesions that are confined to the sacrum affect the cauda equina roots, which contribute to ischiadic nerve function, the pudendal nerve (voluntary control) and pelvic nerves (autonomic) that innervate the bladder, rectum, and perineum. Thus, bilateral LMN deficits of the back legs or perineum usually occur with spinal canal diseases of the lumbosacral area. Clinicians must always be alert to the possibility of the spinal form of rabies, which has a predilection for producing ascending hyporeflexia and analgesia of the perineum and pelvic limbs. In addition, bilateral damage to ischiadic and obturator branches can occur intrapelvically during difficult parturition in heifers and cows.

Patellar Reflex

The patellar reflex is the only *stretch* reflex that can be reliably elicited. This reflex must be tested with the animal in lateral recumbency. The limb is partially flexed, and the middle patellar tendon is tapped with a hammer or piece of metal piping that is of sufficient weight to stretch the tendon of a large

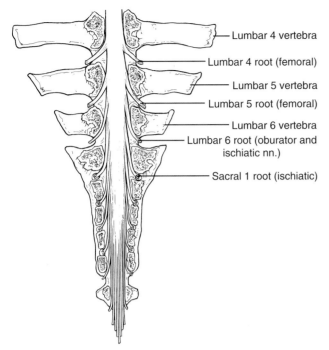

Figure 13–1. Dorsal view of the lumbosacral spinal cord and roots. Note the position of the spinal cord segments in relation to the exit of the nerve roots.

animal. A deficient or absent response indicates a lesion of either the femoral nerve or its root or more likely a lesion of the fourth and fifth lumbar cord segments. Except in the stretch injury of newborn calves, the femoral, unlike the ischiadic, nerve is much less susceptible to peripheral damage. The biceps and triceps reflex (tapping against a metal plexor held over the tendon is helpful) can be elicited by percussing the tendons just above the elbow. These tests are useful in assessing the musculocutaneous and radial nerves, respectively, but a negative or slight response is normal. A very brisk reflex may indicate hyperreflexia due to UMN damage (i.e., above the sixth cervical cord segment or white matter only of the lower cervical segments) (Fig. 13–2).

Perineal Reflex

The perineal reflex is assessed by stimulating the anal sphincter with forceps or a blunt pin and observing for contraction of the sphincter and clamping down of the tail. Lesions involving the last lumbar and sacral vertebrae may involve the sacral cord or cauda equina roots that supply the bladder and perineum. Sacral coccygeal injuries may affect only the caudal segments that control the tail. Severe tail stretch injuries can also occasionally involve sacral rootlets that affect rectal and bladder tone and control. Decreased tail tone also results from excessive traction applied to the tail when trying to assist a downer animal.

Sensory Testing

Conscious pain sensation is often determined in combination with the flexor and perineal reflex examination. A knowledge of the sensory distribution of the important nerves to the limbs is important to confirm specific nerve damage (Fig. 13–3). These are discussed under specific nerve deficits (palsies) that commonly affect the bovine species. Segmental testing for the level of a spinal lesion is usually valid only for severe lesions that significantly reduce sensation below the level of the lesion. Pinching the skin with a pair of hemostats, systematically progressing cranially on either side of the dorsal spinous processes, may define the vertebral level where conscious sensation becomes apparent or may detect a hypersensitive area that can result from nerve root or meningeal irritation. Loss of sensation to a body part indicates a severe injury that may be irreversible if improvement does not occur within 7 to 10 days after injury.

Postural and Attitudinal Reactions

The tests of hopping, righting, wheelbarrowing, hemihops, and proprioceptive positioning can be performed only in small calves. A modification for larger animals is described in several texts.[2, 14] The sway test, elevated head posture, tailing, circling, and blindfolding are maneuvers that may exacerbate subtle proprioceptive, motor weakness, cerebellar, and vestibular disease of cattle. For detecting peripheral nerve problems, ordinary gait examination and reflex and sensory testing of the affected limb are usually adequate.

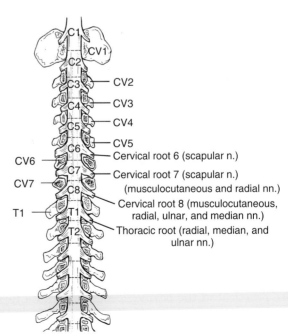

Figure 13–2. Dorsal view of the cervicothoracic cord segments and roots that contribute to the brachial plexus. CV, cervical vertebra.

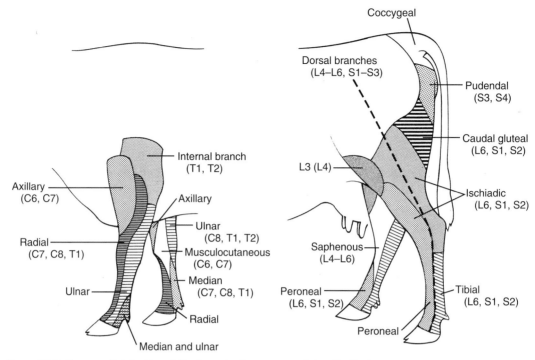

Figure 13–3. Sensory distribution of the important nerves supplying the limbs.

ANCILLARY DIAGNOSTIC AIDS

Electromyography (EMG) has been successfully applied to both small and farm animal neurology.[17, 21, 22, 30] It is most useful for detecting the denervation potentials that occur in muscles whenever the LMN unit is damaged, whether it be at the level of the ventral horn cells of the spinal cord, the ventral roots or motor axons carried in the peripheral nerve, the neuromuscular junction, or the muscle itself. Denervation potentials may not appear until a week after an injury and usually reach greatest activity by the third or fourth week. In mild or insidiously progressive conditions, such as diffuse degenerative neuropathy, EMG examination can detect the extent of LMN disease before it is clinically apparent. Active myositis can be detected on EMG examination, whereas degenerative muscle disorders such as white muscle disease usually yield negative results. With discrete peripheral nerve damage due to trauma, the EMG examination can be combined with a nerve conduction study; sequential examinations can assist in detecting recovery before it is clinically apparent. Estimates of time needed for recovery can be calculated on the basis of axonal regeneration at the rate of 1 to 4 mm/day.[14] This speciality area of neurology may be useful for valuable animals. Although such testing is best performed at a referral clinic, portable units are available for farm use.

Cerebrospinal fluid collection and examination is quite practical in the bovine species, even in a farm situation. In all recumbent animals in which the diagnosis is not obvious, it is one of the most useful tests to exclude the possibility of inflammatory spinal cord disease as well as the spinal form of lymphoma.

Details of the technique and interpretation of the analysis are well described.[14, 21]

Spinal myelography, valuable in calves, is an accurate diagnostic procedure for detecting space-occupying lesions encroaching on the spinal cord and for identifying spinal defects that produce stenotic lesions of the canal.[16, 21] Once an animal is anesthetized, lumbosacral injection of the dye is usually safe and easy and produces few side effects on recovery.[3] In adult animals, myelography is usually limited to the cervical area.

PERIPHERAL NERVE DISEASES

THORACIC LIMB

Suprascapular and radial nerve paralyses are the two most easily recognized and important neurological disabilities affecting the thoracic limb. It has been shown both clinically and experimentally that the gait and posture abnormality associated with the other major nerves of the brachial plexus (musculocutaneous, axillary, median and ulnar nerves) is relatively subtle, with minimal impairment in ambulation.[8, 14, 19, 21, 33] It is the neuroanatomical location and etiological factors that give rise to the common peripheral nerve syndromes encountered in cattle.

Suprascapular Paralysis

DEFINITION

Suprascapular paralysis is defined as paralysis of the supraspinatus and infraspinatus muscles of the scapula.

ANATOMY

The sixth and seventh cervical segments contribute to the formation of this purely motor nerve to the scapular muscles. It is vulnerable to injury by vertebral collapse at the C5–C7 vertebral articulations and may be stretched where the nerve crosses the cranial aspect of the neck of the scapula (Fig. 13–4).

CLINICAL SIGNS AND DIAGNOSIS

Depending on the cause of the problem, the lameness can be insidious or acute. Acute trauma to the prescapular area (such as violent struggling in a neck squeeze or a blow to the cervical-scapular area) may produce only the expected weight-bearing lameness initially. However, by 5 to 7 days after trauma, atrophy of the scapular muscles is often evident; irreversible damage to the nerve leaves only a scapula covered with skin within some weeks. The limb can be advanced actively but abducts on weight-bearing, causing the animal to circumduct the limb. This has been observed both naturally and experimentally.[19, 33] The stride may be shortened. Variations in the gait may depend on other concurrent muscle, nerve, and skeletal damage. Reflexes and sensation in the limb are normal if that is the only injury. Bilateral problems may be of peripheral origin, but a vertebral fracture or vertebral abscess in the lower cervical area may occasionally impinge on the nerve roots that contribute to the suprascapular nerve, before signs of spinal cord compression become obvious. Ra-

diographs of the lower cervical area and the neck of the scapula may help in the diagnosis and prognosis of the case.[19]

TREATMENT

Early treatment with steroids or other anti-inflammatory agents when a nerve is stretched or bluntly traumatized is important to reduce swelling and secondary anoxia and axonal damage quickly. Providing there is no complicating injury, the prognosis, other than the cosmetic appearance of the limb, is favorable. With lacerations or sectioning of the nerve at the neck of the scapula, surgical correction has been described for horses.[28] Attentive nursing care and physiotherapy can assist in total recovery from a partial injury.

Radial Paralysis

DEFINITIONS

Distal radial paralysis causes an inability to extend the carpus and digit. *Proximal radial paralysis* prevents an animal from extending its elbow, carpus, and fetlock in order to bear weight.

ANATOMY

The radial nerve arises from C7, C8, and T1 cord segments of the brachial intumescence. It innervates the extensor muscles of the carpus and digits and is a sensory nerve to the skin on the lateral side of the forelimb from the elbow to the carpus (see Figs. 13–2 and 13–3). The area of sensitivity distally moves to the dorsal aspect from the carpus to the digits. Lesions at the cervicothoracic junction involving the eighth cervical and first thoracic segment cause pronounced radial nerve deficits. Severe traction or concussive injuries of the scapulohumeral area often damage or even avulse some or all of the brachial plexus roots and give rise to proximal radial nerve injury (see Brachial Plexus Paralysis) (Fig. 13–5). The pressure caused by recumbency of large animals can also cause a radial nerve deficit. Very occasionally, ischemic infarction of the spinal cord at the level of the brachial intumescence (usually due to fibrocartilaginous embolism) can produce a pronounced radial nerve palsy in association with asymmetrical tetraparesis (author's observation).[32]

The *distal* radial nerve is vulnerable to injury in the musculospiral groove of the humerus, as a result of either fractures or deep soft tissue trauma (see Fig. 13–5). A lesion of the nerve proximal to the sulcus for the brachial muscle causes proximal radial paralysis.[33]

CLINICAL SIGNS AND DIAGNOSIS

The limb posture of proximal radial paralysis is characteristic (Fig. 13–6). The elbow is dropped, the carpus and fetlock in partial flexion, with the limb dragged, causing abrasion of the dorsum of the fetlock. In the absence of fractures and obvious muscle damage, difficulty in advancing the limb and inabil-

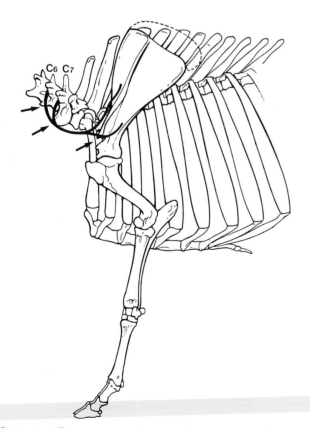

Figure 13–4. Root origins and course of the suprascapular nerve. Arrows indicate sites vulnerable to injury.

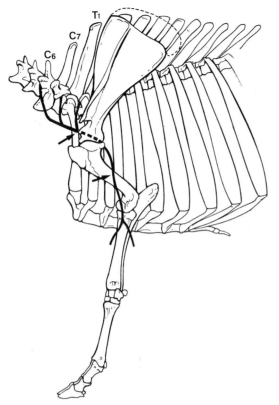

Figure 13–5. Root origins and course of the radial nerve. Arrows indicate sites vulnerable to injury. Note that injury at the level of the musculospiral groove of the humerus produces distal radial paralysis only.

ity to extend the elbow, carpus, and fetlock to bear weight confirm the radial nerve deficiency. On performing the flexor reflex, only a slight decrease in shoulder flexion may be observed. With proximal injuries, however, other nerves of the brachial plexus are often involved; thus, decreased elbow, carpus, and digital flexion may be present (see Brachial Plexus Injury). With total injury of the distal or proximal radial nerve, an area of analgesia may be detected over the dorsum of the metacarpus and phalanges of the bovine species (autogenous zone of the radial nerve) (see Fig. 13–3).[33] Distal radial paralysis (with intact innervation to the triceps group) leads to no elbow abnormality but paresis affecting the carpal and fetlock position. EMG and nerve conduction studies beginning 7 to 10 days after injury can be useful in evaluating the severity and extent of the nerve damage.

TREATMENT

With partial radial nerve damage, the prognosis is favorable and nursing care is most important. Many cases rapidly improve within days or a few weeks after injury. The dorsum of the fetlock and the contralateral limb must be protected from injury; bandaging may be necessary. In addition, anti-inflammatory treatment, confinement, secure footing, and adequate bedding are recommended. Passive manipulation, hydrotherapy, and massage can help to pre-

vent muscle contractures and stimulate blood flow to the flaccid musculature. If concurrent fractures or muscle damage has occurred, the prognosis becomes more guarded unless these complications are successfully resolved. Complete proximal radial paralysis with evidence of anesthesia in the autogenous zone augurs a grave prognosis unless a definite improvement occurs within the first 10 to 14 days after injury. Surgical exploration of the musculospiral groove may be attempted to free the distal branch of the radial nerve from callus or fibrous tissue entrapment in selected valuable stock.

Prevention of the iatrogenic partial radial paralysis caused by casting and recumbency on hard ground or an operating table involves

- Adequate padding below the dependent limb (e.g., foam rubber, inner tubes of tires, and so on)

- Maintenance of the lower limb in forward extension with a rope

- Avoidance of tightly fixing the upper limb to the operating table, an action that increases pressure not only on the thorax but also on the lower (dependent) limb. The upper limb is best maintained in moderate caudal extension

Brachial Plexus Paralysis

DEFINITION

Brachial plexus paralysis implies involvement of all the nerves of the brachial plexus and consequently paralysis of all the muscles of the forelimb. The radial nerve is the most important nerve for forelimb gait, and when it is intact, deficits associated with

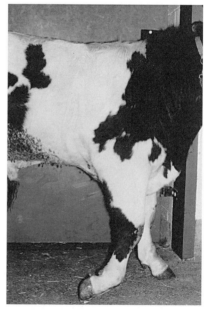

Figure 13–6. A young bull with the typical posture of radial paralysis. Note the dropped elbow, flexed carpus, and fetlock. (Photo courtesy of J. Ferguson.)

injury to other nerves of the brachial plexus are more subtle.

ANATOMY

The brachial plexus is formed primarily by the last three cervical segments and the first thoracic segment. C5 and T2 segments make minor contributions (see Figs. 13–1 and 13–5). Severe lesions such as a spinal abscess resulting in a pathological vertebral fracture or a localized meningomyelitis at the level of the cervicothoracic junction will involve the major roots and segments contributing to the brachial plexus. Axillary damage affects the nerves of the plexus as they intermingle between the scapula and the first rib. Severe foreleg trauma may actually avulse the entire plexus at the level of the roots. The nerves are also vulnerable when crushed between the forelimb and first rib during prolonged recumbency, especially during anesthesia or manual restraint with the animal in lateral recumbency.

CLINICAL SIGNS AND DIAGNOSIS

Total brachial plexus paralysis causes paralysis of the entire limb with no shoulder movement and no extensor or flexor ability. If the lesion is severe, the limb is totally anesthetic below the elbow and thus devoid of any voluntary or flexor reflex in response to noxious stimuli applied over all parts of the digits. If the more caudal nerves of the plexus are partially affected, weakness of the extensors of limbs results from radial nerve involvement and incomplete or absent flexion of the fetlock and carpus from median and ulnar nerve impairment. A more craniad lesion is more likely to produce absent or incomplete flexion of the elbow due to musculocutaneous nerve palsy. The radial nerve usually is also partially involved, but the median and ulnar nerves are relatively spared. If a Horner syndrome is apparent in the ipsilateral eye, the first thoracic or all of the first three thoracic ventral roots have been damaged or avulsed.

TREATMENT

The treatment and prognosis are the same as for proximal radial paralysis if the paralysis arises as a result of trauma. Anti-inflammatory agents may be given in early stages, and limb support is essential to minimize self-trauma. The prognosis for animals with abscesses and tumors expanding in the area is grave.

Median and Ulnar Paralysis

DEFINITION

Median and ulnar paralysis is defined as paralysis of the flexors of the carpus and digit.

ANATOMY

These nerves at the level of the brachial plexus are rarely affected alone unless a discrete tumor arises from one of them.[5] The ulnar nerve is vulnerable in the distal humeral region, where it passes subcutaneously over the large medial epicondyle.[33]

CLINICAL SIGNS AND DIAGNOSIS

The gait is slightly stiff, resulting in a goose-stepping stride. Hyperextension of the carpus, fetlock, and pastern may be apparent on weight-bearing. If motor damage is severe, flexion of the digit and carpus is detected on flexor reflex testing. Desensitization of the palmar and lateral aspect of the appendage from the elbow to the claw can occur with complete injuries[21] (see Fig. 13–3). The prognosis becomes guarded when the digits remain desensitized and septic conditions progress unobserved and untreated.

PELVIC LIMB

The components of the lumbosacral plexus that innervate the muscles of the pelvic limb arise from lumbar segments 4, 5, and 6 and sacral 1 and 2 (see Fig. 13–1). The most common clinical problem is injury of the *ischiadic* nerve or its *peroneal* branch, which causes an animal to stand or walk knuckled over at the fetlock. The femoral nerve, with its innervation to the quadriceps, which extends the stifle to allow weight-bearing, is rarely injured. The *downer cow syndrome* of neurological origin that was once attributed to obturator nerve paralysis is often a complicated injury involving lumbar root 6, which contributes to both the ischiadic and obturator nerves. Many affected animals also have primary muscle injury of the adductors and the muscles of ischiadic nerve innervation.

Femoral Paralysis

DEFINITION

Femoral paralysis is defined as paralysis of the quadriceps muscles, which extend the stifle to bear weight, and partial paralysis of the psoas major muscle, which flexes the hip.

ANATOMY

The femoral nerve arises from lumbar segments L4–L6, with L5 making the major contribution. A mid to caudal lumbar vertebral lesion can affect the femoral cord segments or the roots as they course through the intervertebral foramen (the mid-to-caudal cord segments lie slightly cranial to the corresponding vertebrae) (see Fig. 13–1). The nerve itself is not particularly vulnerable to injury along its course to the quadriceps. Cord lesions or direct trauma to the muscle are more likely causes of a reduced or absent patellar reflex. Femoral paralysis is also encountered as a unique stretch injury in large calves, more often beef breeds, with hip or stifle lock during parturition.[21] The saphenous branch of the femoral nerve is sensory to the medial aspect of the leg, a fact that is useful when evaluating pelvic limb paresis (see Fig. 13–3).

CLINICAL SIGNS AND DIAGNOSIS

Discrete femoral nerve palsy is mostly noted in newborn calves (e.g., Charolais, Simmental, other big-framed cattle) with a history of dystocia (Fig. 13–7).[21] Most cases result from dystocia in primiparous animals. Hyperextension of the fetal femur is postulated to result in severe stretching of the quadriceps femoris, resulting in both neural and vascular damage. The reduced quadriceps tone permits excessive patellar laxity. Some calves are observed at a few days of age to have a lateral patellar luxation; however, discrete quadriceps atrophy is usually evident. The patella may be easily replaced but may immediately reluxate. Femoral paresis may be unilateral or bilateral and produces a weight-bearing type of lameness that may not be defined until the patellar reflex is evaluated or until pronounced neurogenic atrophy develops in the quadriceps. The ambulatory problem and neurological assessment of the condition may also be complicated by general musculoskeletal trauma that occurred during dystocia and forceful delivery.

With unilateral femoral palsy, an animal has limited purposeful advancement of the limb, which collapses at the stifle on weight-bearing. The digit does not drag or knuckle over in uncomplicated cases, and the animal can flex the stifle and extremity. Decreased resistance is noted on passive manipulation, and the patellar reflex is diminished or absent. Sensation in the medial aspect of the limb is often still intact. Neurogenic atrophy appears within a week and progresses until the femur is easily palpable and the muscle replaced by fibrous tissue over

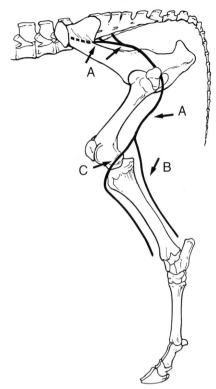

Figure 13–8. Course of the ischiadic nerve (A) and its division into the tibial (B) and peroneal (C) branches. Arrows indicate sites vulnerable to injury.

several months.[19, 21, 24] Animals with bilateral total paralysis will be recumbent.

The differential diagnosis includes femoral and pelvic fractures, coxofemoral dislocation, and muscle or tendon ruptures.

TREATMENT

The prognosis depends on the etiological diagnosis and degree of injury. With partial stretch injuries, the prognosis is fair to good if adequate nursing care can be given to a calf that has difficulty rising. Good-quality colostrum should be given as soon as possible after birth to a recumbent calf, which should be kept on clean, dry bedding and encouraged to stand. Analgesics and anti-inflammatory drugs have been advocated.[8] Vertebral lesions such as abscessation, fractures, or tumors tend to be untreatable.

Ischiadic Paralysis

DEFINITION

The ischiadic nerve provides innervation to the muscles that flex the stifle, extend the hock, and flex and extend the digits.

ANATOMY

The ischiadic nerve is vulnerable at the level of the pelvis and proximal femur, where fractures may encroach on the nerve as it courses over the greater ischiadic notch of the ileum and caudal to the femur

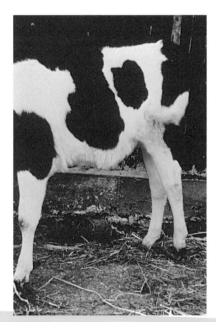

Figure 13–7. A heifer with severe quadriceps atrophy due to femoral nerve injury at parturition. (Photo courtesy of J. Ferguson.)

(Fig. 13–8). In thinly muscled, often young animals, injections deposited into the gluteals or caudal femur area may affect ischiadic nerve function. The nerve roots contributing to the ischiadic nerve may be affected within the vertebral canal, and lesions may involve the caudal lumbar and cranial sacral segments. Intrapelvic pressure damage during calving occurs when the sixth lumbar nerve is compressed against the prominent ridge on the sacrum before it joins the first two sacral roots to form the ischiadic nerve (Fig. 13–9). This can produce both an ischiadic and obturator nerve paresis, which is often characteristically found in a neurologically impaired postparturient cow with the downer cow syndrome.[12, 13, 19, 21, 33]

CLINICAL SIGNS AND DIAGNOSIS

Although complete ischiadic paralysis is rare, it may complicate coxofemoral trauma (e.g., fracture of femoral neck, acetabulum) and is noted as a component of calving paralysis (downer cow syndrome). Somewhat more common is an injection neuropathy in neonatal calves and poorly muscled growing stock.

Total unilateral ischiadic paralysis is recognized by a limb that tends to be dragged and advanced by flexion of the hip only; the stifle extends to bear weight but often on the dorsum of the fetlock. The posture of the hock is often perceptibly lower and overflexed compared with the normal limb (Fig. 13–10). The limb is analgesic except for the medial aspect (supplied by the saphenous branch of the femoral nerve). Thus, with total injuries, no flexion of the leg is produced on stimulation of the dorsal, lateral, and caudal surfaces of the metatarsus and the coronary bands. Stimulation of the upper medial metatarsus and thigh causes flexion of the hip only and a pain response (see Fig. 13–3). With chronic partial injuries, an animal sometimes develops a compensatory hypermetric movement of the distal extremity so that it jerks the limb up and flips the digit forward to land on the plantar aspect to bear weight. Acute partial injuries may cause an animal to knuckle over at the digit intermittently because of the weak exten-

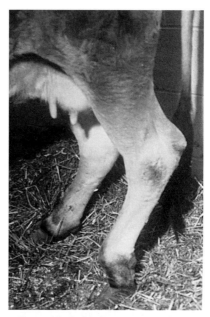

Figure 13–10. Cow with ischiadic nerve paralysis. Elongation of the gastrocnemius muscle with lowered hock position differentiates this from peroneal nerve palsy.

sors of the digits; the flexor reflex may be normal or diminished in hock flexion only. Sensation in this situation is usually normal, and the prognosis is favorable if the injury is due to trauma.

TREATMENT

Nursing care and palliative treatment for acute nerve trauma as described previously is indicated. If fractures are treated, the nerve function must be monitored to be sure that the nerve does not become entrapped during the healing process. The treatment and prognosis for chemical neuritis due to injection (injection neuropathy) injury depend on the nature of the substance. Aqueous forms of drugs may cause only temporary neuropraxis, but oil-based forms may cause irreversible damage. Unfortunately, a progres-

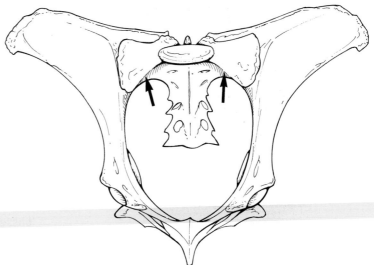

Figure 13–9. Cranial-ventral view of the pelvis of a cow. Arrows indicate the ridge on the wing of the sacrum where the L6 root may be compressed during parturition.

sive ischiadic deficiency may not be recognized before severe damage is done to the nerve. Otherwise, early treatment with anti-inflammatory agents or even surgical exploration of the injection site is indicated in special cases. Most animals with unilateral paresis or paralysis are ambulatory. Problems arise either when the contralateral limb becomes injured or more commonly severe abrasion and infection develop in the affected leg. Splints, casting, and bandaging of the distal extremity are indicated for partial ischiadic paresis, from which recovery is a good possibility.

Peroneal Paralysis

DEFINITION
Peroneal paralysis is defined as paralysis of the muscles flexing the hock and extending the digits.

ANATOMY
The peroneal nerve is the cranial division of the ischiadic nerve. It passes superficially over the lateral femoral condyle and the head of the fibula and thus is vulnerable to external trauma or pressure during recumbency.

CLINICAL SIGNS AND DIAGNOSIS
In cases with significant motor damage to the peroneal nerve alone, the animal stands with the digit knuckled over onto the dorsum of the pastern and fetlock joint; the hock joint appears overextended (Fig. 13–11). In mild peroneal nerve deficiency, the fetlock tends to knuckle over intermittently during ambulation. In more severe cases, the locomotor action is jerky, often with a goose-stepping compensatory motion as the dorsal surface of the digital area and hoof is dragged along the ground. Decreased sensation in the dorsum of the fetlock is often detected in severe cases (see Fig. 13–3).[14, 19, 21] Careful reflex examination reveals that the limb fails to flex

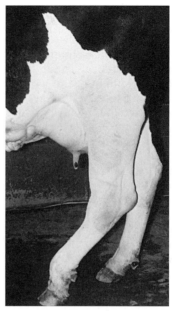

Figure 13–12. Holstein cow with tibial nerve paralysis. Note the overflexed and lowered hock position. The buckled fetlock continues to bear weight on the plantar surface.

at the hock, but the stifle and hip flexion are normal if the peroneal nerve alone is severely damaged.

Treatment and prognosis are the same as for ischiadic nerve injury. Protecting the limb from further injury and possible infection of the abraded surfaces is most important during convalescence, which could take many months.

Tibial Paralysis

DEFINITION
Tibial paralysis is defined as paralysis of the extensors of the hock and flexors of the digits.

ANATOMY
The tibial nerve is the caudal branch of the ischiadic as it divides into the tibial and peroneal branches caudad to the femur and at the level of the head of the gastrocnemius muscle (see Fig. 13–8). Its deeper location makes it less vulnerable to superficial injury compared with the peroneal nerve. Severe trauma to the gastrocnemius muscle is necessary to involve the tibial nerve discretely.

CLINICAL SIGNS AND DIAGNOSIS
In many natural cases of tibial paralysis, the hock joint is overflexed and the fetlock is partially flexed (Fig. 13–12).[19] It is postulated that partial flexion of the fetlock is due to loss of tonus in the extensors of the hock. Much tension is exerted on the largely tendinous superficial digital flexor, whose tendon passes over the tuber calcanei and ultimately inserts on the plantar aspects of the middle phalanges, causing a backward pull on the digits. Interestingly, this does not occur during therapeutic or experimental

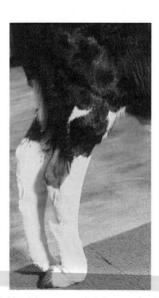

Figure 13–11. Calf with peroneal injury only. Note the normal position of the hock.

sectioning of the tibial nerve.[19] The gastrocnemius

area looks elongated and the hock hyperflexed, but the animal can walk with a jerky movement with weight-bearing on the plantar foot surface despite the buckled fetlock. With severe damage, sensation may be lost to the caudal surface of the limb below the hock (see Fig. 13–3). The appearance of the dropped hock syndrome must be differentiated from higher (ischiadic) nerve damage, gastrocnemius muscle rupture, and tibial tendon avulsion.

Treatment in the acute stages is the same as for other nerve injuries. Compared with peroneal nerve injury, the gait disturbance is mild, but the postural disturbance could be permanent. In weak and debilitated animals, struggling to rise in conditions with poor footing may predispose to muscle and nerve injury in this area. Care must be taken to avoid injecting drugs in the caudal-lateral stifle area.

Obturator Paralysis

As discussed earlier under Ischiadic Paralysis, paresis of the adductors innervated by the obturator nerve is an important problem with downer animals. The sixth lumbar nerve contributes to both the obturator and ischiadic nerve and is vulnerable to intrapelvic compression during calving (see Figs. 13–1 and 13–9). In addition to a base-wide stance when ambulatory, the animal may also show proprioceptive loss in the fetlock, which signifies the ischiadic nerve deficit. Severe adductor muscle injury may also occasionally stretch the nerve at the level of the muscle.[24]

Spastic Syndrome (Progressive Hind Limb Paralysis)

DEFINITION

Spastic syndrome is a neuromuscular disorder characterized by episodic involuntary muscle contractions or spasms involving the hind legs and often the epaxial thoracolumbar musculature. This gives rise to a postural disturbance and movement also described as crampiness, stretches, periodic spasticity, standings disease, and, misleadingly, progressive posterior paresis or hind limb paralysis.

INCIDENCE

Spastic syndrome occurs most frequently in Holstein and Guernsey cattle, with onset between 3 and 7 years of age. Other breeds (Danish Red, Hungarian Red) and both sexes are affected.[19, 35] Most reports arise from studies of bulls in artificial insemination units.[29]

ETIOLOGY

Spastic syndrome is regarded as a genetic disease, possibly due to an autosomal dominant gene with incomplete penetrance.[29] The pathology and pathophysiology of the disease remain obscure. In the limited number of histopathological studies published, all lesions have been attributed to secondary musculoskeletal and nerve injuries or the effects of aging.[35] No primary brain, spinal cord, nerve, or muscle lesions can explain the problem. Theories include functional disorder of the myotactic reflex or postural reflex mechanisms; one investigator has proposed muscle pain as the probable effector.[35]

CLINICAL SIGNS AND DIAGNOSIS

Muscle trembling and backward extension and abduction of both back legs tend to occur on rising. An affected animal cannot move forward, and severe lordosis of the back may be seen. The episodes vary in degree and duration. Various stimuli and movements may provoke an attack: rising from the recumbent position, excitement, sideways or backward movement, pressure on the sacrum, hitting of the back or jaws, manipulation of the teats, and so on.[19] The course may wax and wane, depending on the general health of the animal. Animals with sore feet or primary osteoarthritic conditions may develop progressively worse attacks, which in turn exacerbate arthritis and muscle atrophy of the pelvic limbs. Between attacks, the animal is normal neurologically but could be lame from the musculoskeletal changes.

No abnormality is evident when an affected animal is recumbent or when kept at pasture.

TREATMENT

Animals with spastic syndrome usually do not recover and tend to deteriorate progressively. In mild cases in productive animals, attentive health care may help to lessen the severity of the attacks. Treatment with mephenesin during severe attacks has alleviated the episodes of some cases for several weeks (30 to 40 mg/kg PO for 2 to 3 days).[21] Phenylbutazone cured 8 and improved 17 other cattle in another series of 34 cases.[19] Genetic screening, especially of bulls used for artificial insemination, is recommended.[21, 29]

Spastic Paresis (Elso Heel)

A. David Weaver *United Kingdom*

DEFINITION

Spastic paresis is a neuromuscular contracture disorder that causes a progressive unilateral or bilateral hyperextended posture and gait of the hock and stifle joints.

INCIDENCE

Spastic paresis occurs sporadically in both dairy (e.g., Holstein, Friesian, Brown Swiss, Ayrshire, and Danish Red) and beef breeds (Aberdeen Angus, Hereford, Murray Gray, Beef Shorthorn), rarely in crossbred cattle.[18, 19]

ETIOLOGY

Initial cases appeared to originate in descendants of a Dutch Holstein-Friesland bull called Elso II.

The inheritance of spastic paresis is currently considered to be by a recessive gene with incomplete penetrance, possibly involving multiple recessive genes. This hypothesis attempts to reconcile the conflicting observations and experimental results. The significance of this gene in breeding stock requires further study. Neither male nor female affected stock should be used for breeding.

In the United Kingdom, one bull that developed signs in adulthood had five daughters (of 50 heifers examined) with classical signs of spastic paresis (author's observation).

Most investigators believe its expression is multifactorial; animals with straight-legged conformation of the pelvic limbs are more commonly affected. The term *spastic paresis* is inappropriate in that no central or peripheral nerve lesions are consistently demonstrable. Most researchers of the disease agree it is a primary muscular disorder.[4]

Hypersensitivity of the myotactic reflex was involved in the pathogenesis when selective gamma-efferent nerve block relieved the condition in 20 affected calves.[15] In a subsequent study, sectioning the dorsal roots of L5 and L6 also alleviated the condition.[15] The neurophysiological explanation is that voluntary movement stimulates hyperactivity of the gamma-efferents to the caudal leg muscles, thus inducing impulses in the insertion activity afferents. These synapse on the alpha motor neurons, which cause the extrafusal fibers of the gastrocnemius muscle to contract and extend the tarsus. Because of the reciprocal mechanism through the peroneus tertius muscle, the stifle also extends. Some studies suggest that the caudal thigh muscles may also be involved. Additional theories include imbalances of neurotransmitter activity in cerebrospinal fluid and the role that magnesium and lithium may have in this disease.[1]

CLINICAL SIGNS

Signs can be noticed in calves aged 2 weeks to 6 months. Excessive tone and a spastic contracture of one or both hind legs primarily involving the gastrocnemius muscles lead to progressive overextension of the hock joint and to a lesser extent the stifle. The insidious first signs are of stiff movement and a straight hock. Mild overextension of the hock causes the distal part of the limb occasionally to be placed more caudally, and the limb is advanced in a swinging motion (pendulum fashion). Later the claws may not contact the ground, and the animal may stand on three legs, the more affected hind limb extended caudally. The less affected contralateral limb tends to be placed across the median line for balance, and bowing of the limb medially may be a secondary effect.

The tail head tends to be raised and may move spasmodically up and down. The forelimbs tend to be placed caudally to transfer more weight-bearing to the forequarters, resulting in an arched back. Manipulation of the hind limb is not resented. The gastrocnemius muscle group feels harder than normal as a result of the contracted state. Both hock and stifle may be flexed, but the limb immediately becomes extended again. The posture is unremarkable during recumbency. The spinal reflexes are intact, with an exaggerated patellar reflex. Limb sensation is unaffected.

Radiographic changes in the hock joint of affected calves reflect the effects of overextension. Features seen on lateral-medial projection include widening of the growth plate of the tuber calcanei, bowing forward of the dorsal and plantar aspects of the calcaneus, abnormal curvature of the distal tibial epiphysis with exostosis formation, and possibly osteoporosis.

In very early stages, the condition must be differentiated from infectious tarsitis and gonitis and upward patellar fixation. In later stages, the stance and gait are pathognomonic. True spastic paraparesis associated with a thoracolumbar lesion above the lumbosacral plexus results in bilateral motor weakness and general proprioceptive deficits.

TREATMENT

No medical treatment has been successful. Breeding animals should be culled because the current hypothesis states that spastic paresis may involve a recessive gene with incomplete penetrance, or possibly multiple recessive genes. Surgery can effectively alleviate the condition by appropriate effects on the overextension produced by the gastrocnemius muscle and tendon. Several techniques have been used. These are described next in chronological order.

Complete Tenotomy. Complete tenotomy of the gastrocnemius tendon inserting onto the proximo/caudal part of the calcaneus and partial tenotomy of the superficial flexor tendon results in a dropped hock; therefore, this technique has been discarded.

Complete Tibial Neurectomy. Five to eight branches of the tibial nerve innervate the gastrocnemius muscle. Under general anesthesia or sedation with epidural block, the tibial nerve or its branches are approached through a lateral incision between the two heads of the biceps muscle. The nerve lies close to the popliteal lymph node. The tibial nerve is distinguished from the other major branch of the ischiadic nerve, the peroneal, by electrostimulation (e.g., sterilized electrodes attached to an electric goad). Stimulation of the tibial nerve causes hock extension and fetlock flexion. The nerve is severed. Relief is immediately evident, and after operation, most animals are successfully reared to fatten. Complications in a minority have included gastrocnemius rupture and wound breakdown.

Partial Tenectomy.[34] Partial tenectomy of the two insertions of the gastrocnemius muscle onto the calcaneus, with section through the surrounding calcanean tendon sheath, has been proposed and adopted by French workers.[25, 26] Advantages over classical tenotomy (discussed earlier) include the absence of a dropped hock after surgery, a simpler and more superficial procedure than tibial neurectomy, and possibly better long-term results.

Surgery may be performed in a recumbent sedated calf or in a standing animal. Local infiltration analgesia is effective. The skin is clipped and prepared for sterile surgery over a 15-cm length proximal to the calcaneus. A 5-cm skin incision is made through skin over the lateral cranial border of the Achilles tendon. The superficial digital flexor tendon is identified as it twists around the superficial branch of the gastrocnemius tendon and is preserved intact. Blunt dissection reveals the two branches, superficial and deep, of the gastrocnemius to be relatively close together proximally and to separate distally. The deep branch is just cranial to the superficial flexor tendon. Each is enclosed with its own sheath. The calcaneal tendon sheath is incised longitudinally to expose the superficial branch of the gastrocnemius muscle. With the hock extended, the tendon is separated from surrounding tissue and transected first distally and then 2 cm more proximally. The 2-cm section is removed. The deep branch undergoes a similar tenectomy. The

calcaneal tendinous tissue is transected both laterally and medially around the tenectomy site. Care should be taken to identify and preserve the lateral saphenous vein. The subcutis is closed with a single continuous layer of number 1 chromic catgut, and the skin edges are apposed in a routine manner. The leg should be bandaged for 7 days to reduce postoperative wound swelling. If the other hind leg is also involved, similar surgery may be carried out 4 to 10 days later. Postoperative exercise should be encouraged. Clinical improvement is seen within 24 hours, and hind limb posture and gait should return to normal within 1 week.

Other signs of generalized spasticity, such as elevation of the tail head and forelimb (carpal, fetlock) flexion, rarely regress after any form of alleviative surgery, unless undertaken in very early stages.

Downer Cow Syndrome

A. David Weaver *United Kingdom*

DEFINITION

A *downer cow* is an animal that is, for unknown reasons, in sternal recumbency and is not showing obvious clinical signs of hypocalcemia or hypomagnesemia or any obvious limb or spinal injury. Most cases are related to parturition, occurring in the few days before or up to a week after calving.

ETIOLOGY

Typical traumatic causes of downer cow syndrome include sacroiliac luxation and subluxation (see p. 175), bilateral or unilateral coxofemoral luxation, and a pelvic fracture.

Metabolic causes include non-responsive hypocalcemia, hypomagnesemia, or hypokalemia, as well as fat cow syndrome. Neurological explanations include obturator, partial ischiadic, peroneal or tibial paralysis (bilateral) and lymphosarcomatic infiltration into the thoracic, lumbar, or sacral spinal canal and cord. The toxic infections category includes starvation, septic or gangrenous mastitis, septic metritis, or ruptured uterus with peritonitis, an acute abdominal disaster, or rarely bovine spongiform encephalopathy.

Pressure ischemia is likely to develop, as a secondary syndrome, within a few hours of recumbency on a hard surface. Continued struggling can result in secondary muscle or tendon injury such as gastrocnemius or adductor group trauma. The pressure damage is described as the *compartment syndrome*[11]; increased pressure develops in an osteofascial compartment after external pressure or the buildup of blood and edematous fluid within that space. Ischemia follows, and the crush syndrome with systemic effects becomes apparent.

INCIDENCE

The incidence of downer cows was 1.1% (within 30 days prepartum) in a 4-year study of 12 Holstein dairy herds in New York State.[10] Various surveys reveal a considerable range of values (3.8% to 28.2%)

for the incidence of downer cows after milk fever.[6] No less than 58% of cases developed within 1 day of calving, but a paradoxical lack of response to calcium borogluconate therapy for milk fever is not the sole cause.

An analysis[12] of causes of a primary recumbency revealed 46% to be due to dystocia and 38% to milk fever or other causes (16%). Not surprisingly, survey data show that half of all downers develop within 24 hours of parturition. Patients tend to be mature, high-producing cows, typically calving indoors in the winter. One survey revealed that nearly half (44%) of all downers died.[12]

CLINICAL SIGNS AND DIAGNOSIS

Because numerous etiological diagnoses are possible in a downer cow, the history of each case is of utmost importance—for example, duration of recumbency, details of parturition (duration, difficulty), whether she rose after calving only then to go down, treatment for milk fever, and the immediate and subsequent position of the cow when she went down, if observed.

Cows with severe lameness may become recumbent but can usually be stimulated to rise. Lameness associated with septicemia may be an exception and can cause a cow to remain down owing to the toxic infectious condition.

From a neurological point of view, rapid assessment of the animal is extremely important; heavy animals often quickly succumb to secondary muscle and nerve damage from the pressure of recumbency and struggling efforts when footing is poor. Once metabolic conditions have been identified and treated adequately, the animal should be elevated by slings or a hoist and evaluated for neurological signs. Observing for the degree of voluntary movement of each limb and finally actual voluntary support ability after placing the animal in a sling and slowly raising it is necessary for accurate evaluation. It can help in identifying monoparesis due to peripheral nerve damage, paraparesis of upper or LMN origin, or tetraparesis that could indicate cervical or cervicothoracic junction cord lesion. If the animal does not move while placed in a sling, it is important to apply adequate stimulus to produce struggling movements. An electric goad may be necessary.

In case of doubt about intact nerve function, sensation may be checked by needle prick and, if no reaction is noted, by pinching the skin with a hemostat, starting distally at the dorsal and volar aspects of the interdigital space and proceeding proximally. *Calving paralysis* involves damage to both the obturator and ischiadic nerve roots (L4–S2). It is now believed that obturator damage alone cannot account for calving paralysis in cows.

Very occasionally, the forelimbs may seem to be affected more than the hindquarters. This can occur with early lower cervical lesions or, even more rarely, bilateral brachial plexus injury, in which case pelvic limb function would be normal. The slinging maneuver may also precipitate a head tremor that could denote cerebellar incoordination or neuromuscular weakness of possible metabolic or toxic origin.

Alert downer cows that are afebrile, continue to eat and drink, and move their hind legs have the most favorable prognosis, and most will rise as long as they are nursed along on deep straw bedding.

At the opposite extreme, a cow barely able to maintain sternal recumbency, disinterested in food and drink, and with no spontaneous hind leg movements warrants a poor prognosis. Such a cow is probably starting to show signs of toxemia.

Examination reveals that some downers move around the floor (preferably deep straw) and can be termed "creepers." In such cows, the development of the compartment syndrome is delayed owing to the variable pressure exerted on the hindquarters musculature.

Dehydration develops slowly unless a water source is constantly available.

Mastitis. The udder should be palpated for signs of septic or gangrenous mastitis and milk taken for the California Mastitis Test (CMT).

Hemorrhage. The vaginal mucosa should be inspected for color. An occasional downer cow has severe internal hemorrhage of the middle uterine vessels after a complicated parturition.

Puerperal Problems
- Presence of a second fetus

- Pelvic damage (fracture, sacroiliac luxation, coxofemoral luxation)

- Early septic metritis

The bony promontories and hindquarters musculature should be palpated. The cow should be turned to permit palpation of the adductor muscle groups, which are at particular risk from any ataxia and slipping that may have preceded recumbency.

Laboratory examination of a downer cow is frequently carried out first after a repeat visit has revealed a failure to respond to further intravenous mineral (calcium, magnesium, phosphorus) treatment. The plasma mineral values in downer cows are inconsistent, some showing a persisting hypocalcemia, hypophosphatemia, and less commonly hypomagnesemia. The role and significance of hypokalemia are disputed. Release of potassium from damaged muscle cells does not necessarily result in hyperkalemia, because the usual coexistent hypocalcemia tends to lead to hyperkalemia.

Downer cows consistently show an elevated creatine kinase (CK) level, which is a specific marker of striated muscle damage. CK has a short half-life of about 4 hours; thus, CK determination is of more clinical value if the blood sample is taken shortly after acute muscle injury or later if the damaging process is continuous.[20] One study of CK in downer cows showed that the enzyme peaked at 24 hours after onset in cows that recovered to stand and at 48 hours in continuing downers.[7] Another study[11] casts doubt on its clinical usefulness, because serum CK level in cows that recovered and those that did not was not significantly different 12 and 24 hours after the experimental induction of recumbency (general anesthesia for 6, 9, or 12 hours).

Plasma aspartate aminotransferase (AST) level is also elevated in muscle-damaged cows, although the enzyme is also released in cardiac myopathies.

Clinical pathology after 48 hours of recumbency is likely to reveal proteinuria resulting from muscle breakdown and release of myoglobinuria, as well as ketonuria and bilirubinuria, from partial anorexia.

TREATMENT
The first requirement is to make an affected animal comfortable in a straw yard or, in appropriate climate and season, outside in a well-drained grass paddock. The cow should be turned from one side to the other at least four times daily. Attempts should be made at least once daily to raise the cow, not only better to assess any improvement but also to relieve stiffness, improve the circulation, and encourage the cow to move. Ample food and water must be provided.

Careful examination must be made for possible development of a toxic or gangrenous mastitis after a day or two. Systemic disease of this type, loss of appetite, pyrexia, and dullness are signs of an unfavorable prognosis.

Parenteral treatment includes repeated injections of solutions containing calcium, magnesium, and phosphorus, with added glucose and potassium. Additional potassium should only be given by stomach tube (e.g., 50 grams KCl daily). Tripelennamine HCl (12 mL solution IV) has been advocated as an effective stimulant and antihistamine that makes a downer cow appear brighter.[6] Use of analgesics such as phenylbutazone and flunixin meglumine should be restricted to cows showing signs of pain.

PROGNOSIS
A favorable prognosis is given on day 2 of recumbency to cows that have a good body condition score

(3.5+), are non-hypocalcemic, have lower CK and AST values than on day 1, show some hind limb movement, and are alert and eating well.

Creeper cows have a more favorable prognosis. Conversely, a cow that is raised by slings or clamp on day 1 after recumbency and that shows no movement in the hind limbs has an unfavorable prognosis.

Some cows take as long as 2 weeks to stand. Anecdotal accounts refer to cows' eventually recovering after 5 weeks of recumbency. All such cows will have had excellent nursing care and minimal development of decubital ulcers, as well as minimal weight loss.

CONTROL
Prevention is primarily directed at

- The prevention of milk fever
- Provision of non-slip, well-bedded surface for parturition
- Careful monitoring in the 48 hours before and after parturition
- Keeping the cow in the calving accommodation for 48 hours postpartum

NEUROMOTOR PSYCHOSIS

Definition

Neuromotor psychosis is a state during which an animal is physically able to rise but is not willing to do so because of fear of slipping, pain, or loss of motivation.

Etiology

Loss of motivation can occur if an animal is recumbent on a slippery surface and makes numerous futile attempts to rise. An animal is also deterred from attempting to rise if lunge space in front of it is insufficient. An animal that has been recumbent for several days probably has eaten very little and is weak. Reduced muscle function is also an expected sequel, particularly if the animal has not been turned regularly from one side to another (every 4 hours). Circulation to muscles may be compromised if an animal lies directly on cold ground for a prolonged period. The condition is mainly psychosomatic and usually a result of poor-quality nursing.

Management of Recumbency

Location. An animal suffering from neuromotor psychosis invariably is found in a hostile location. The quality of the environment must be improved, or the animal must be relocated to suitable accommodations.

Moving a Recumbent Cow. The least traumatic method of relocating a heavy cow is by means of a sled. Under farm conditions, a farm gate is likely to be the most useful device for this job. Some front-end loaders can be modified for this task. If the sled is to be a gate, it must be covered with a tarpaulin to prevent dependent parts of the animal (ears, tail, foot) from chafing on the ground. The cow is placed in lateral recumbency. The floor surface is well covered with straw to improve sliding, and the animal is moved onto the transportation device by pulling a rope attached to the underside forelimb.

Preparing the Location. The location must be unrestrictive to a cow lunging to rise. If the ground surface is concrete, at least 20 cm of wet or partially rotted manure must be used as a base. Whatever the base, manure or earth, insulation must be provided in the form of a 30-cm layer of dry straw. If dried peat, sawdust, chopped straw, or sand is available, it may be added to provide a grip. Protection from cold drafts or precipitation should be provided.

Nursing. The best results are obtained if the animal is turned from one side to the other at least every 4 hours. This procedure is difficult if the cow is heavy. A useful technique is to draw (with a sawing action) a rope under the animal's body. One end of the rope would appear beneath the shoulder on which the cow is lying, and the other end would appear just in front of the udder. The end nearest to the udder should be tied around the fetlock of the hind limb on which the animal is lying. Pulling on the other end of the rope pulls the underside limb beneath the body. At this point, the free end of the rope is moved across the shoulder and pulled from the other side. The animal rolls easily to lie on the other side.

Plenty of cold water should be accessible to the cow. Small amounts of choice hay should be supplied. Uneaten feed should be removed and replaced every 4 hours. A cow will not usually consume feed on which it has salivated.

Aids to Rising. Various hoisting and slinging devices are available to assist an animal to rise. A hoist that can be clamped across the tuber coxae is useful. It can be elevated by means of a pulley attached to a beam or tripod. Alternatively, some front-end loaders can be modified to perform the task. The preferred technique is to lift the animal until the hindquarters are just a little lower than the normal standing position of the animal. Assistants should then attempt to make the animal stand square on its forelimbs. With patience, the cow may make a few tentative efforts to stand on its own.

REFERENCES

1. Arnault GA: Bovine spastic paresis. An epidemiologic, clinical and therapeutic study in a Charolais practice in France. Efficacy of lithium therapy. World Association of Buiatrics. Proceedings of the 12th World Congress on Diseases of Cattle, Amsterdam, The Netherlands, 11:853–858, 1982.

2. Baker JC (ed): Bovine neurology. Vet Clin North Am Food Anim Pract 3:1–216, 1987.

3. Bargai U: Myelography in neonatal bovine calves. Veterinary Radiology Ultrasound 34:20–23, 1993.

4. Bradley R, Wijeratne WVS: A locomotor disorder clinically similar to spastic paresis in an adult Friesian bull. Vet Pathol 17:305–317, 1980.

5. Bundza A, Dukes TW, Stead RH: Peripheral nerve sheath neoplasms in Canadian slaughter cattle. Can Vet J 27:268–271, 1986.

6. Chamberlain AT: The management and prevention of the downer cow syndrome. Proc BCVA 20–30, 1987.

7. Chamberlain AT: Prognostic indicators in the downer cow. Proc BCVA 57–68, 1986.

8. Ciszewski DK, Ames NK: Diseases of peripheral nerves. Vet Clin North Am Food Anim Pract 3:193–212, 1987.

9. Cordy DR: Progressive ataxia of Charolais cattle—an oligodendroglial dysplasia. Vet Pathol 23:78–80, 1986.

10. Correa MT, Erb HN, Scarlett JM: Risk factors for downer cow syndrome. J Dairy Sci 76:3460–3463, 1993.

11. Cox VS: Nonsystemic causes of the downer cow syndrome. Metabolic diseases of ruminant livestock. Vet Clin North Am Food Anim Pract 4:413–433, 1988.

12. Cox VS, Marsh WE, Steuernagel GR, et al: Downer cow occurrence in Minnesota dairy herds. Prev Vet Med 4:249–255, 1982.

13. Cox VS, McGrath CJ, Jorgensen SE: The role of pressure damage in pathogenesis of the downer cow syndrome. Am J Vet Res 43:26–31, 1982.

14. De Lahunta A: Veterinary Neuroanatomy and Clinical Neurology, 2nd ed. Philadelphia, WB Saunders, 1983.

15. De Ley G, De Moor A: Bovine spastic paralysis: Results of selective gamma-efferent suppression with dilute procaine. Vet Sci Commun 3:289–298, 1979/1980.

16. Doige CE, Townsend HGG, Janzen ED, McGowan M: Congenital spinal stenosis in beef calves in Western Canada. Vet Pathol 27:16–25, 1990.

17. Dowling P, Tyler JW, Wolfe DF, et al: Thermographic and electromyographic evaluation of a lumbosacral spinal injury in a cow. Prog Vet Neurol 2:73–76, 1991.

18. Keith JR: Spastic paresis in beef and dairy cattle. Vet Med Small Anim Clin 76:1043–1047, 1981.

19. Greenough PR, MacCallum FJ, Weaver AD: Lameness in Cattle, 2nd ed. Philadelphia, JB Lippincott, 1981, pp 337–359, 360–365.

20. Lefebvre HP, Toutain P-L, Serthelon J-P, et al: Pharmacokinetic variables and bioavailability from muscle of creatine kinase in cattle. Am J Vet Res 55:487–493, 1994.

21. Mayhew IG: Large Animal Neurology. A Handbook for Veterinary Clinicians. Philadelphia, Lea & Febiger, 1989.

22. Oliver JE, Horlein BF, Mayhew IG: Veterinary Neurology. Philadelphia, WB Saunders, 1987.

23. Palmer AC: Introduction to Animal Neurology, 2nd ed. Oxford, UK, Blackwell Scientific Publications, 1984.

24. Paulsen DB, Noordsy JL, Leipold HW: Femoral nerve paralysis in cattle. Bovine Pract 2:14–26, 1981.

25. Pavaux C, Arnault G, Baussier M, Dumont M: Treatment of spastic paresis in cattle with Gotze's technique, triple tenectomy. Point Veterinaire 20:41–50, 1988.

26. Pavaux C, Saulet J, Ligneux IY: Anatomy of the bovine gastrocnemius muscle as applied to the surgical correction of spastic paresis. Vlaams Diergeneeskd Tijdschr 54:296–312, 1985.

27. Rebhun WC, de Lahunta A, Baum KH, et al: Compressive neoplasms affecting the bovine spinal cord. Comp Cont Ed Prac Vet 6:S396–S400, 1984.

28. Schneider RK, Bramlage LR: Suprascapular nerve injury in horses. Comp Cont Ed Prac Vet 12:1783–1789, 1990.

29. Sponenberg DP, Van Vleek LD, McEntee K: The genetics of the spastic syndrome in dairy bulls. Vet Med 80:92–94, 1985.

30. Steiss JE, Argue CK: Normal values for radial, peroneal and tibial motor nerve conduction velocities in adult sheep with comparison to adult dogs. Vet Res Commun 11:243–252, 1987.

31. Stuart LD, Leipold HW: Bovine progressive degenerative myeloencephalopathy ("weaver") of Brown Swiss cattle I, II. Bovine Pract 18:129–132, 133–146, 1983.

32. Taylor HW, Vandevelde M, Firth EC: Ischemic myelopathy caused by fibrocartilaginous emboli in a horse. Vet Pathol 14:479–481, 1977.

33. Vaughan LC: Peripheral nerve injuries: An experimental study in cattle. Vet Rec 76:1293–1304, 1964.

34. Weaver AD: Modified gastrocnemius tenectomy: A procedure to relieve spastic paresis in dairy calves. Vet Med 86:1234–1239, 1991.

35. Wells GAH, Hawkins SAC, O'Tool DT, et al: Spastic syndrome in a Holstein bull: A histologic study. Vet Pathol 24:345–353, 1987.

36. White ME, Whitlock RH, de Lahunta A: A cerebellar abiotrophy of calves. Cornell Vet 65:476–491, 1975.

Paul R. Greenough *Canada*

14

Applied Anatomy

In the past, many veterinarians graduated with insufficient knowledge of bovine digital anatomy to enable them to investigate and treat lameness problems logically. Advances in the understanding and treatment of bovine lameness have called for much more detailed knowledge of digital structure and function. The material presented here is primarily for general reading and review.

This chapter addresses only structures with special clinical significance. Sensory nerve supply to the distal limb is described in Chapter 4, motor innervation of the limbs in Chapter 13. For a more comprehensive review of the anatomy of the bovine axial skeleton, readers are directed to standard texts.[11, 12, 20]

ANATOMICAL NOMENCLATURE

More than 20 years ago, anatomists, having rationalized anatomical nomenclature, published it in successive editions of the *Nomina Anatomica Veterinaria* (NAV).[21] Nevertheless, many clinicians adhere to the older names. For example, confusion can arise if an anatomist uses the correct term *distal phalanx*, a surgical instructor *P3*, and an older practitioner *coffin bone*. The livestock industry naturally retains the traditional terminology such as leg, foot, stifle, pastern, hock, and so on. These terms are fine for general lay use if specific. They are used frequently and interchangeably throughout this chapter with NAV nomenclature. Some compromises are desirable for effective communication. Readers who encounter difficulty relating lay terms to scientific terminology should consult Table 14–1. For all structures without a commonly accepted traditional term, only NAV terminology is used.

The word *foot* is in well-established use in the livestock industry. Accordingly, Kainer[14] defines the equine foot as including the hoof (capsula ungulae) and all structures within it. Nickel and colleagues[20] apply the same definition to the word *claw*; this is the preferred term. Traditionally, the word *hoof* is applied to the comparable structure of a horse. In some clinical applications, the term *digit* or *digital region* is preferable.

The surfaces of the limb have been defined: That facing the midline of the animal is the medial surface, and that facing away from the midline is the lateral. *Cranial* and *caudal* apply to the limbs proximal to the carpus and tarsus. More distally, the cranial surface should be termed *dorsal*. The caudal surface of the distal limb is termed *palmar* (forelimb) and *plantar hindlimb*. The phrase *flexor surface* is proposed as more appropriate and less clumsy than the current term *palmar/plantar surface* in reference to both fore and hindlimb.

The claws are located on either side of the axis of the limb. The outer claw is the lateral, and the inner the medial. The claw surface facing the limb axis is the axial surface, and that facing away is the abaxial surface.

The dorsal surface merges with the axial surface at the dorsal flexure of the claw. The axial surface in turn meets the bulb at the axial groove. This groove is one of the thinnest areas of the entire claw capsule, is easily traumatized, and serves as a pocket for the activity of anaerobic organisms. The bulb joins the abaxial surface at the abaxial groove.

The sole and distal border of the wall of the claw together form the ground surface, which is divided into four segments: the apex, the subapical region, and the prebulbar and bulbar regions (Fig. 14–1). In practice, the words *heel* and *bulb* are used interchangeably. The heel is more accurately thought of as the external rounded surface of the flexor surface of the claw. The bulb is commonly considered to include the heel and its contents (digital cushion or pulvinus). For the purpose of identifying regions of the claw in which lesions occur, the structure has been divided into zones (see Fig. 1–2, p. 10).

THE ANATOMY OF THE DIGITS
(Fig. 14–2)

PHALANGES

Proximal and Middle Phalanges

The proximal and middle phalanges are similar in shape, but the proximal phalanx is about twice as long as the middle phalanx.

TABLE 14–1. ANATOMICAL NOMENCLATURE

Scientific Term	Common Lay Term	Alternative	French	Spanish	German
Thoracic limb	Forelimb	Front leg	Membre thoracique	Mano	Vorderbein Vordergliedmasse
Cubital joint	Elbow		Coude	Codo	Ellbogengelenk
Antebrachiocarpal joint	Knee		Carpe	Carpo rodilla	Vorderfußwurzelgelenk
Metacarpophalangeal joint	Fetlock		Boulet	Menudillo	Fesselgelenk
Proximal interphalangeal joint	Pastern		Paturon	Cuartilla	Krongelenk
Distal phalanx	Coffin bone	P3	Troisième phalange	Corona	Klauenbein
Distal interphalangeal joint	Coffin joint	Coronopedal joint		Aticulacion de la corona	Klauengelenk
Distal sesamoid	Navicular bone	Podotrochlear bone	Os naviculaire	Hueso navicular	Distales sesambein
Pelvic limb	Hindlimb	Back leg	Membre pelvien	Pie	Hinterbein
Coxal joint	Hip		Hanche	Cadera	Hüftgelenk
Tarsocrural joint	Hock		Jarret	Corvejon	Sprunggelenk
Tuber coxae	Hook			Tuberculo coxal	Hüftbeinhoecker
Great trochanter (femur)	Thurl		Grand trochanter	Trocantor mayor	Grosser Trochanter
Tuber ischiadicum	Pin		Tuberosité ischiatique	Tuberculo isquiatico	Sitzbeinhoecker
Calcanean tendon	Hamstring	Achilles tendon	Tendon d'Achilles	Tendon de aquiles	Achillessehne
Tuber calcanei	Point of hock		Point de jarret	Punta del corvejon	Fersenhoecker
Distal interdigital ligament	Cruciate ligament			Ligamento cruzado	Klauenkreuzbaender

The scientific term is the English translation of the Latin terminology used in the NAV. The common term is the term most frequently used in the English language. The alternatives cited should be avoided.

Distal Phalanx

The proximal surface is wholly occupied by the main articular surface, which is lightly keeled sagittally to accommodate a groove on the distal articular surface of the middle phalanx. The dorsal border is formed by a pronounced eminence, the extensor process. This structure protects the dorsal surface of the distal interphalangeal (coffin) joint and is an important landmark.

The distal sesamoid (navicular bone) extends the articular surface of the coffin joint. This bone is attached to the flexor surface of the distal phalanx by a very strong interosseus ligament. The navicular bone and the deep flexor tendon protect the coffin joint against penetration through the sole by a foreign body. The remainder of the flexor surface accommodates the insertion of the deep flexor tendon onto the flexor tubercle. The ground surface of the bone is slightly concave, giving added prominence to the flexor tubercle, which corresponds to the region of the sole in which pododermatitis circumscripta (sole ulcer) is usually located. The ground surface of the bone tends to become rougher as an animal ages.

Close to the flexor tubercle is a large axial foramen, through which the axial flexor artery passes to form the terminal arch. This arch anastomoses within the bone with smaller arteries entering through foramina on the abaxial surface.

LIGAMENTS
(Figs. 14–3 and 14–4)

The *distal interdigital ligament (cruciate)* inserts onto the axial aspects of the middle and distal phalanges as well as the distal sesamoid (navicular bone). Stretching of this ligament is allegedly associated with the occurrence of interdigital fibroma. Exostosis formation occasionally occurs at the sites of insertion. Some fibers of this ligament merge with the deep flexor tendon and the digital cushion. Others insert into the abaxial borders of the middle and distal phalanges and the distal sesamoid. The distal interdigital (cruciate) ligament and the distal interphalangeal collateral ligament provide substantial protection for the axial aspect of the distal interphalangeal joint. This protection is reinforced by the axial digital band and the dorsal elastic ligament. A proximal interdigital ligament binds the two proximal phalanges together. The locations of axial digital ligaments may be considered when deciding the level of a digit amputation.

The *abaxial collateral ligament of the distal interphalangeal joint* is a fan-shaped structure and is

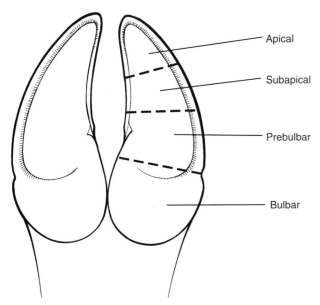

Figure 14–1. The regions of the sole.

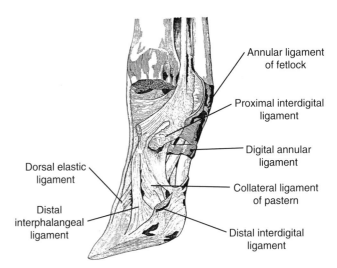

Figure 14–3. The ligaments of the axial surface of the digit. (From Ellenberger-Baum: Handbuch der Vergleichenden Anatomie der Haustiere. Berlin, Springer-Verlag, 1977.)

often the site of periarticular exostosis formation. Such an exostosis can exert pressure on the coronary dermis, thereby stimulating accelerated growth of the hoof wall (corkscrew claw, see Chapter 9).

The *flexor annular ligament of the fetlock* contains a fibrous plate for attachment of the accessory digits. The injection site for administering an axial regional nerve block is located distal to this plate.

SYNOVIAL STRUCTURES

Joints

Each digital joint capsule has a dorsal and flexor pouch. The pouches of the distal interphalangeal joint are of great clinical importance.

The *dorsal pouch* of the coffin joint is almost subcutaneous at a point axial and abaxial to the extensor process. The axial site is vulnerable to penetration as a complication of interdigital phlegmon (foot rot). The abaxial site is vulnerable to penetration from extension of a vertical fissure (sand crack).

The *flexor pouch* protrudes into the *flexor recess*, which is located proximal to the distal sesamoid and on the flexor surface of the middle phalanx. The pouch is close to the podotrochlear (navicular) bursa but separated from it and from the distal portion of the sheath of the deep flexor tendon by portions of the collateral ligament of the distal sesamoid. If one synovial structure becomes infected, the others are sufficiently close to be endangered.

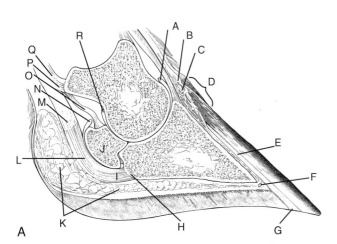

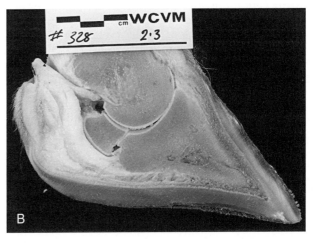

Figure 14–2. *A,* A sagittal section of the digit: A, Dorsal pouch of distal interphalangeal (coffin) joint; B, periople or perioplic dermis; C, coronary cushion; D, coronary band (perioplic epidermis); E, lamellae; F, marginal artery; G, zona alba; H, flexor process of distal phalanx; I, insertion of deep flexor tendon; J, distal sesamoid (navicular bone); K, digital cushion; L, deep flexor tendon; M, tendon sheath; N, podotrochlear bursa; O, suspensory ligament of distal sesamoid; P, retroarticular recess; Q, sheath of deep flexor tendon formed in part by superficial flexor tendon; R, flexor pouch of distal interphalangeal (coffin) joint. *B,* Photograph of a sagittal section of the digit.

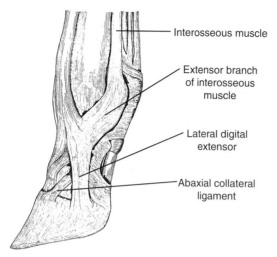

- Interosseous muscle
- Extensor branch of interosseous muscle
- Lateral digital extensor
- Abaxial collateral ligament

Figure 14–4. The ligaments of the abaxial surface of the digit. (From Ellenberger-Baum: Handbuch der Vergleichenden Anatomie der Haustiere. Berlin, Springer-Verlag, 1977.)

Tendon Sheaths

The *common digital extensor sheath* extends to the middle of the middle phalanx. Traumatic infection of this sheath occurs occasionally.

The *digital flexor tendon sheath* envelops both superficial and deep flexor tendons in the digital region. Inside the sheath, the superficial flexor tendon envelops the deep flexor tendon. The sheath and enclosed tendons are supported externally by the distal interphalangeal and distal and proximal annular ligaments.

The most distal portion of the digital flexor sheath is located proximal to the coronary band. It is therefore not compromised during resection of the distal sesamoid by an approach through the heel. The sheath is usually opened when the digit is amputated even at the lowest level. The medial and lateral sheaths communicate in a small percentage of cases. The sheath extends for a short distance proximal to the fetlock and is present in the groove between the flexor surface of the bone and tendon. If the tendon sheath becomes infected at the level of the coffin joint, palpable distention is commonly found proximal to the fetlock.

The *navicular (podotrochlear) bursa* (Fig. 14–5) is located between the distal sesamoid and the deep flexor tendon. The bursa has an extensive pouch, which extends into the retroarticular recess behind the middle phalanx, where it is close to the flexor pouch of the distal interphalangeal joint. The abaxial recess of the podotrochlear bursa is frequently infected from abscesses extending from the abaxial white line at the level of the sole-heel junction.

BLOOD SUPPLY TO THE DIGITAL REGION

Arteries

(Fig. 14–6)

The Forelimb. The digits of the forelimb receive their blood supply mainly from the median artery, which flows into the palmar digital common artery before dividing into the palmar proper axial digital arteries II and IV. The palmar common artery lies on the tendon groove dorsal to the flexor tendons, close to the medial metacarpal nerve. This vessel is substantial and superficial, particularly in the distal portion of the groove between tendon and bone, and extreme caution should be taken in placing needles.

The Hind Limb. The digits of the hind limb are supplied mainly by the dorsal metatarsal artery, which anastomoses with plantar common digital arteries III and IV before bifurcating to form the plantar proper axial digital arteries. Care should be taken in introducing a needle into the proximal interdigital space because the risk of entering the arterial complex at this point is quite significant.

Blood Supply to the Dermis

The proper axial digital artery enters the distal phalanx through a foramen on its axial face. Within the bone, the artery forms the terminal arch, which anastamoses with the proper abaxial digital artery entering on the abaxial surface.

The marginal artery has been referred to as the *circumflex artery* or the *artery of the rim of the sole.* It should not be confused with the terminal arch.

The marginal artery is a collection of small arched anastomoses connecting small vessels radiating from the terminal arch. It lies in the angle between the sole and the wall (see Fig. 14–2).

The dermis of the sole and much of the wall are supplied by this artery. Widened vascular channels and a tortuous course of the terminal arch were pres-

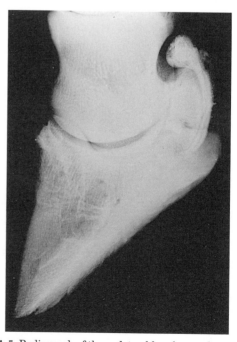

Figure 14–5. Radiograph of the podotrochlear bursa, demonstrating its size and location.

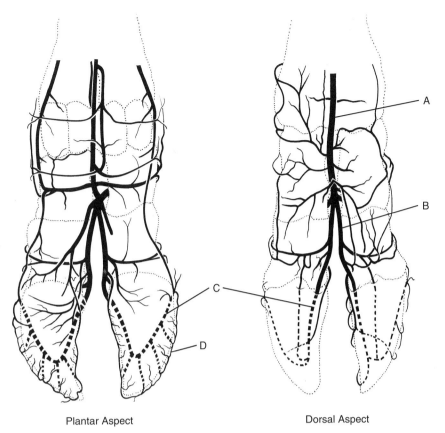

Figure 14–6. Blood supply to the digits. A, Dorsal metatarsal artery; B, (axial) proper digital artery; C, terminal arch; D, marginal artery. (From De Vos N, Morcos MB: De arteries van de achervoet bij hetrund. Vlaams Diergeneesk Tijdschr 29:241–246, 1960.)

Plantar Aspect   Dorsal Aspect

ent in the digits of the front limbs of barley-fed beef cattle.[16] Constrictions in the arteries radiating from the terminal arch were found[4, 8, 19] to be present in dairy cattle suffering from sole ulcers. Angiographic studies of hooves of horses affected with chronic[1] or acute laminitis[6, 13] showed irregularities in the lumen of the terminal arch. Boosman and colleagues[4] postulate that mural thrombosis may occur during episodes of subclinical laminitis and that organization of this mural thrombus could be a possible cause of intimal proliferation and arteriosclerosis.

lar depressions compatible with the presence, in life, of smooth muscle cells. These structures may be considered arteriovenous diverticula.

Function of an Arteriovenous Shunt

AVAs may function as mechanisms to accommodate changes in intraungular pressure during weight-bearing.[26] It is assumed that smooth muscles in the

Arteriovenous Anastomoses

MORPHOLOGY
An arteriovenous anastomosis (AVA) is a vascular connection between arteries and veins that allows the capillary bed to be bypassed. A smooth muscle constriction is present at the arterial end of the bridge. A marked difference in luminal diameter generally exists between the arterial and venous ends of AVAs, the latter being considerably wider. Some AVAs are referred to as *thoroughfare channels*, which, as the name implies, may shunt blood directly from arteriole to venule. When they are closed by smooth muscle activity, more blood is perfused through the dermis.[26, 27] Collections of AVAs are referred to as a *glomus*.

Some AVAs are extremely large, and scanning electron microscopic photographs (Fig. 14–7) reveal cellu-

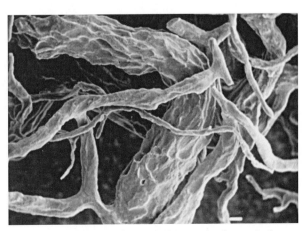

Figure 14–7. A scanning electron micrograph of an arteriovenous anastomosis. (From Vermunt JJ, Leach DH: A scanning electron-microscopic study of the vascular system of the bovine hindlimb claw. N Z Vet J 40:146–154, 1992.)

walls of the AVAs constrict and relax owing to a reflex mechanism associated with variations in pressure inside the claw.[23] Blood is thus shunted directly into veins to bypass the deepest arterioles (Fig. 14–8). Similarly, the arteriovenous diverticula open and close to assist in pressure equalization. Bicuspid valves in the small veins assist this mechanism.[26, 27]

It has been assumed that muscles in the arteriovenous shunts can be paralyzed by toxins in the blood. The subsequent increased intraungular pressure may damage the walls of the delicate small vessels, resulting in mural thrombosis.[4] This hypothesis may contribute to the understanding of the etiology of laminitis.

Because AVAs control the perfusion of blood within the corium, they are believed to have a temperature-regulating function, particularly in maintaining claw warmth during cold weather.

Veins

In each digit, the veins are situated more superficially than the arteries, the hind limb veins draining into the lateral saphenous vein and the forelimb into the palmar common digital vein, which drains into the cephalic vein. Although not constant in location, the palmar and plantar proper digital veins run subcutaneously dorsal to the dewclaws, and the dorsal common digital vein is located more or less on the axial side of the limb. The saphenous vein is subcutaneous as it crosses the hock. These superficial veins are ideal sites for intravenous regional nerve blocks or antimicrobial therapy (see Chapter 4). The superficial veins become distended during very acute laminitis.

THE INTERDIGITAL SPACE

Dorsally, the surface skin width, owing to its folds and loose attachment, is about 3 cm. The width is less between the heels, where the skin is more firmly attached. The surface is hairless and in the non–weight-bearing state has fine longitudinal folds. During weight-bearing, the dorsal aspect opens as the skin stretches, whereas the flexor section remains relatively closed and may even be compressed by the digital cushion. The interdigital space is considerably farther from the ground dorsally (5 cm) than between the heels (3 cm). The space is bounded by the axial claw wall and axial coronary band, by the heels in the flexor region, and by the hair-bearing skin of the dorsal surface of the digit. The thickness of interdigital skin varies with the particular region, breed, and age but averages about 4 mm. The stratum corneum is well developed in adults.

STRUCTURE OF THE CLAW

The term *claw* comprises the claw capsule (epidermis) and its contents. This includes the distal phalanx, the distal part of the middle phalanx, the distal sesamoid bone, the podotrochlear (navicular) bursa, the joint ligaments, and the terminal parts of the

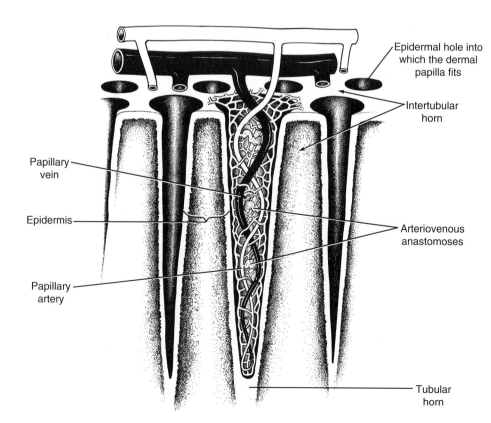

Figure 14–8. A diagrammatic representation of the arteriovenous shunt. (From Pollitt CC, Molyneaux GS: A scanning electron microscopical study of the dermal microcirculation of the equine foot. Equine Vet J 22:79–87, 1990.)

extensor and flexor tendons. The claw capsule also embraces the vascular dermis as well as the subcutis, which exists only in a modified form at specific locations to form the coronary and digital cushions.[25]

WALL OF THE CLAW

Epidermis

The epidermis of the wall, according to the NAV,[21] is divided into the perioplic, tubular, and lamellar parts. The current terminology for this region is inaccurate and misleading.

The *coronet*, the most proximal 1.5 cm of the claw, is produced by a specialized dermis located at the skin-claw junction. This groove is referred to by the NAV as the *limbus* or *periople*. The coronet is, therefore, a separate structure from the dermis of the wall, which lies beneath the coronet.[15] Also beneath the coronet is the coronary cushion. The coronet widens caudally to form the bulb of the heel. The similar character of the coronet and bulb is extremely obvious in a mature fetus.

The perioplic epidermis (epidermis of the coronet) consists of tubular and intertubular horn in which, compared with the wall, the cells are loosely packed. The structure is permeable to water and water-soluble materials. It is probably the softest part of the claw because the horn is easily worn away when an animal walks through grass, soil, and so on. The horn of the coronet is thickest where the wall horn (tubular part) is thinnest, and its primary function is to protect the underlying vulnerable tubular dermis. Coronary horn does *not* continue as the stratum externum of the wall. The cuticle (eponychium) in humans performs the same function and is analogous to the perioplic epidermis of the ox.[15]

The pathological changes in the coronary band can be observed before clinical lesions appear in the claw wall.

The *parietal epidermis* is the claw wall proper, which is divided into the stratum externum and stratum medium. The stratum internum is termed the *lamellar epidermis*.

The *stratum externum* is the outer layer of the wall consisting of non-tubular flat, keratinized cells. This layer decreases in thickness with age, can be mechanically abraded, and is characteristically diminished by chronic laminitic changes. The function of the stratum externum is probably to maintain a constant water content in the stratum medium. A low water content makes horn less prone to abrasive wear and lesions.[9, 10] The term *periople* has been applied to the stratum externum.

The *stratum medium* is predominantly a tubular structure. The tubules extend from the dermis distally and are larger in diameter and closer together toward the internal region of the wall. Evidence suggests that the hardness of the horn is related to the number of tubules per square millimeter. The average number of tubules in the tubular epidermis is 80 per mm².[10]

The claw wall grows from the coronary band at 0.5 cm (0.3 to 0.7 cm) per month at the abaxial groove in dairy cattle and 0.25 cm to 0.4 cm per month on the dorsal surface of the claws of beef cattle.[25] The rate of growth varies according to the temperature of the environment as well as the age and level of nutrition. As with the human nail, the claw wall moves distally to be worn away at the bearing surface.

Faint ridges (rugae) in the claw wall extend more or less parallel to the skin-claw junction (limbus). These ridges diverge slightly toward the heel, reflecting its more rapid rate of growth and wear. Changes in the quality of the ridges result from metabolic variables.

The *lamellar epidermis* is the fluted lining of the wall of the claw. The flutes increase very slightly in depth distally and merge with the sole horn to form the zona alba (white line). The lamellae are leaflike structures arranged perpendicularly to the inner surface of the wall. They increase the surface area of the inner surface of the wall to provide maximal anchorage for fibrous attachment to the distal phalanx.

HISTOLOGY

The innermost layers of the epidermis of the coronary band, sole, and wall show a gradual change from living to dead keratinized cells. The stratum basale adjacent to the dermis has a mitotic function. The next layer is the stratum spinosum, in the cytoplasm of which tonofibrils may be observed radiating from the desmosomes (intercellular adhesions).[7] By crisscrossing the cell, the tonofibrils form an internal cytoskeleton, which adds to the mechanical strength of the epidermal cell while retaining flexibility. In some texts, the tonofibrils are referred to as the *onychogenic substance*. The stratum granulosum and stratum lucidum are absent.[3]

A modified stratum basale is present in the lamellar dermis, where horn is produced very slowly. The lamellae apparently slide past the stationary cells of keratogenic layers. It is assumed that as in horses,[3] desmosomes joining the moving parts to the stationary parts break and re-form in a staggered ratchetlike manner so that load can still be supported. A junctional disruption between these elements causes failure of the bond between the claw and the distal phalanx, with serious pathological consequences.

Dermis

The dermis is divided into three parts corresponding to those of the epidermis. The coronary (perioplic), the parietal (tubular), and lamellar dermis are predominantly vascular. A reticular layer is present in the laminar dermis.[11]

The *coronary (perioplic) dermis* occupies a narrow recess at the limbus. It consists of highly vascularized papillae that are oriented toward the ground surface. The juxtaposed germinal cells produce the soft, non-tubular horn of the coronary band.

The *parietal dermis* is located beneath the coronet (perioplic dermis). Although referred to in the NAV as the *coronary dermis*, it contributes nothing to the coronet. The tubules arise from germinal cells that cover the distal and lateral portions of the papillae, which are elongated and oriented toward the bearing surface. The intertubular horn is elaborated from germinal cells around the bases of the papillae.

The *lamellar dermis* has few horn-producing cells but many dense reticular fibers. These fibers anchor the claw capsule to the distal phalanx. Although there is no evidence (no increase in thickness, no mitotic figures) that cells of the dermis contribute significantly to the lamellae, the reverse is true in abnormal conditions.[22] The stratum basale is capable of rapid proliferation when the wall is damaged (surgical wall stripping, trauma) or if the keratinized parts of the wall are separated from the keratogenic layers as in laminitis. These changes may well be similar in cattle.

THE SUBCUTIS

The subcutis is absent where the corium overlies the bones but exists in the bulb (torus) as a dense mass of fibroelastic tissue, the bulbar cushion. At the region of the coronary band, it is termed the *coronary cushion*.

The *coronary cushion (pulvinus limbi, coronae)* lies directly beneath the coronary band and is composed of a spongy network of veins and elastic tissues. It is hypothesized that during locomotion, the distal phalanx presses against the wall of the claw, thereby squeezing blood back into the systemic circulation. Exercise, therefore, is extremely important for a normal blood supply in this region.

The Digital Cushion

The soft and flexible horn of the rounded bulb originates from a flexor extension of the true periople and joins the wall at the axial and abaxial grooves. The bulb (torus ungulae) envelops the digital cushion (pulvinus digitalis), which fuses dorsally with the deep flexor tendon and axially with fibers from the distal interdigital ligament (cruciate ligament). This fibroelastic complex inhibits drainage of purulent material from the retroarticular recess, which is bounded by the deep flexor tendon, the distal sesamoid, and the middle phalanx.

The bulb has a significant shock absorptive function. When compressed during weight-bearing, it expands axially and abaxially, transferring the forces to the respective walls. Thus, vertical forces are directed horizontally, causing the walls to act as springs. Shock absorption is clearly compromised if the structure of the bulb is changed (heel erosion) or if the tensile strength of the wall is reduced (chronic laminitis).

SOLE OF THE CLAW

The bovine sole is leaf shaped and merges imperceptibly with the bulb. The periphery of the sole adheres to the wall by means of the zona alba (white line). The white line is composed of softer horn than is the sole and, in most breeds, tends to be whitish gray.

The tubules of the sole are fewer in number than in the wall (about 16/mm^2). The sole tubules run parallel to the dorsal wall of the claw—that is to say, diagonally, distally, and dorsally. If, in a sole composed of light-colored horn, the tubules become filled with blood during a laminitic episode, the structure has a striated (paintbrush) appearance. The normal sole has a water content of up to 32%.[2] Increased water content is probably responsible for physically softer horn in animals with laminitis.[17] A negative correlation has been reported between midsole hardness and lameness.[2, 18]

The distal border of the abaxial wall of the claw capsule together with 2 to 5 cm of the adjacent sole is the true ground (weight-bearing) surface of the claw. The ground surface at the abaxial bulb-wall junction of the hind claws receives the first impact of each step. It consequently wears more rapidly than other areas of the true bearing surface. The abaxial wall merges with the axial wall at the *dorsal flexure* of the toe.

The normal sole averages 7 mm in thickness. The sole is thicker at the junction with the bulb than it is at the apex.

PHYSICAL AND CHEMICAL COMPOSITION OF WALL, SOLE, AND HEEL HORN

Measurements on the central sole, the central bearing surface of the heel and the midwall horn revealed significant (P < 0.001) differences in hardness (Shore type D durometer) between all three areas (respectively, 43.7, 31.0, and 65.5 units). Moisture content (sole, heel, wall) averaged 32.5%, 38.1%, and 26.6%. Horn hardness was related to composition. Harder claw wall keratin contains more calcium, copper, zinc, and phosphorus, and less sodium, potassium, and iron. Zinc was lower in the horn of lame animals. No significant differences were found between lateral and medial claws of normal cows. The lateral claw of lame cows was significantly (P < 0.01) softer and had higher water, ash, and magnesium content than the medial claw.[2]

JOINT ENTRY SITES

A needle or other instrument may be inserted through the joint capsule for diagnostic or therapeutic procedures. Preliminary sedation (intravenous or intramuscular xylazine) may be advantageous.

ARTHROCENTESIS

Synovial fluid analysis may reveal characteristic changes (see Chapter 11, Table 11–1) that may assist diagnosis. Access to the joint permits intra-articular medication.

ARTHROSCOPY

It may be useful to enter a joint to see a lesion or to remove detritus from the synovial space (sse p. 238).

DIGITAL JOINTS
(Fig. 14–9)

Distal Interphalangeal Joint (Coffin Joint). The needle is inserted lateral to the common/long extensor tendon, which inserts into the extensor process of the distal phalanx. The entry point is just proximal to the coronary band.

Pastern Joint (Proximal Interphalangeal Joint). Insert the needle lateral to the extensor tendon.

Fetlock Joint (Metacarpo/Metatarsophalangeal Joint). The needle is directed downward close to the bone and between it and the interosseus (suspensory) ligament. Because this procedure may be painful, a nerve block at a higher level is recommended. The joint can also be entered from the dorsal surface in a manner similar to that for the distal joints. However, the flexor pouch is more capacious than the dorsal.

Digital Synovial Sheath (Sheath of the Deep Flexor Tendon). The needle is directed downward behind the interosseus ligament.

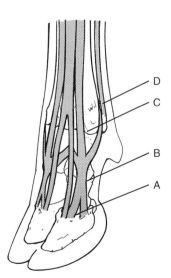

Figure 14–9. Access sites for the joints of the digital region. A, The distal interphalangeal joint (DIP joint); B, proximal interphalangeal joint (pastern); C, metacarpo/metatarsophalangeal joint (fetlock); D, sheath of deep flexor tendon.

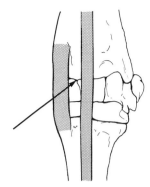

Figure 14–10. Carpal joint. The radiocarpal part of the joint does not communicate with the intercarpal compartment. (Some diffusion of the analgesic may reach the more distal compartments.) Penetration is easier if the joint is flexed, but the problem of forcing cattle to stand on three legs presents difficulties. The needle penetrates lateral to the tendon of the extensor carpi radialis and medial to the combined tendons of the common digital extensor and proper extensor of the digit.

CARPAL JOINT
(Fig. 14–10)

The antebrachiocarpal part of the joint capsule does not communicate with the intercarpal compartment, but some anesthetic may reach the more distal compartments by diffusion. Placing a needle in the synovial space is easier if the joint is flexed, although some cattle resist standing on three limbs. The site of entry is lateral to the tendon of the extensor carpi radialis and medial to the combined tendons of the two bellies of the common digital extensor muscle. The proximal border of the accessory carpal is a guide to the level of penetration.

ELBOW JOINT
(Fig. 14–11)

The needle should be inserted close behind the palpable lateral collateral ligament. Location can be facilitated by appreciating the lateral tuberosity of the

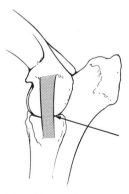

Figure 14–11. Elbow joint. The needle penetrates close behind the lateral collateral ligament, which can be palpated. Location can be facilitated by palpating the lateral tuberosity of the radius and entering just proximal to it.

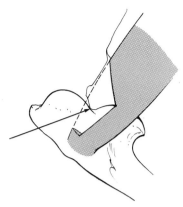

Figure 14–12. Shoulder joint. The needle penetrates just in front of the infraspinatus tendon, which can be palpated. Use of the major tubercle of the humerus and distal extremity of the scapular spine assists in the location.

radius and entering just proximal to it. An alternative site is cranial to the lateral collateral ligament.

SHOULDER JOINT
(Fig. 14–12)

The site is cranial to the palpable infraspinatus tendon. Landmarks are the major tubercle of the humerus and the distal extremity of the scapular spine.

HOCK JOINT (TARSAL JOINT)
(Fig. 14–13)

The site for entry is medial to the extensor tendons. The lateral malleolus is easy to palpate and is used to judge the level of penetration. This is the tibiotarsal part of the joint capsule, which communicates with the proximal but not with the distal intertarsal compartment. Some anesthetic may diffuse to the more distal compartment.

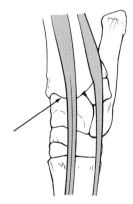

Figure 14–13. Tarsal joint (hock). The needle penetrates medial to the extensor tendons. This is the tibiotarsal part of the joint capsule, which communicates with the proximal intertarsal compartment but not with the distal intertarsal or tarsometatarsal compartment.

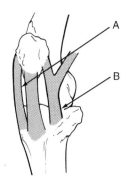

Figure 14–14. Stifle joint. It is advisable to use two sites, because sometimes the lateral femorotibial compartment does not communicate with the rest of the joint. The needle (B) penetrates close behind the lateral patellar ligament and is directed backward. The second needle (A) is inserted between the middle and medial patellar ligaments and is directed slightly down and toward the large medial lip of the trochlea.

STIFLE JOINT
(Fig. 14–14)

It is advisable to use two sites because the lateral femorotibial compartment may not communicate with the rest of the joint.

1 Site one is close behind the lateral patellar ligament (lateral femorotibial compartment). The needle should be directed caudally.

2 At site two, the needle is inserted between the medial and middle patellar ligaments and directed slightly down and toward the large medial lip of the trochlea (femoropatellar and medial femorotibial compartments).

HIP JOINT
(Fig. 14–15)

Palpate the prominent trochanter major and the insertion of the middle gluteus onto it. The needle penetrates in front of the trochanter major and just in front of the insertion of the middle gluteus and is directed caudally and medially.

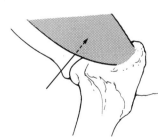

Figure 14–15. Hip joint. Palpate the prominent trochanter major and the insertion of the middle gluteus onto it. The needle penetrates in front of the trochanter major and close in front of the insertion of the middle gluteus muscle and is directed backward and inward.

The Physis

James G. Ferguson Canada

The basic structure of the growth plate and epiphysis is rather complex and requires considerable study if all aspects of its normal growth and pathological conditions are to be known. This area of bone has its own terminology to describe its anatomy and physiology as well as specific definitions and classification systems to describe disease conditions. In earlier literature from human and veterinary sources there has been confusion involving the terms physis, epiphysis, and epiphyseal growth plate. It is important to clarify these terms to prevent misunderstanding. The physis is the radiolucent area that separates the metaphysis from the epiphysis and is responsible for longitudinal bone growth by transforming cartilage into bone by the process of endochondral ossification. Since the physis contributes length to the metaphysis, it is incorrect to refer to it as the "epiphyseal growth plate." Histologically, the physis contains four zones of different cell types that provide an efficient method of bone growth by pushing the epiphysis farther from the metaphysis. The epiphysis is composed of the bony and cartilaginous structures between the physis and the joint (pressure epiphysis) or tendon (traction epiphysis) and has a complex method of growth to enlarge in circumference and surface area.

The relationship of the physis and epiphysis to the structures of the joint are specifically important in the consideration of septic conditions that may progress to adjacent structures and to axial abnormalities, which effect functioning of articular structures.

The many conditions affecting the physes of cattle have not been well described in the literature and most diagnoses are made by direct extrapolation of similar conditions that have been well documented in other species. A great deal of reliance is placed on conditions affecting the horse, dog, and man with regard to anatomy, physiology, and therapeutic approaches to such conditions as angular limb deformities, fractures of the growth plate, infections of the physes and epiphyses, and nutritional conditions affecting growth and conformation. While this may seem a somewhat superficial approach to diagnosis and therapy, it does provide a satisfactory basis for treatment in the majority of cases. As research and detailed evaluation of such conditions continue, the specifics of each condition will be identified along with pathogenesis and a rationale for treatment and prognosis.

The physis is made up of the resting, proliferative, transitional, and degenerative zones. The activity of the physis is under hormonal control and in the normal animal is fairly predictable relative to age and breed. In general its width is considered to be a function of the rate of bone production—the broader the physis, the more active the site. The resting zone is composed of progenitor chondrocytes that serve as a source of cells for the proliferating zone. These cells of the proliferating zone multiply in columns and form palisades. As proliferating cells continue to grow, their size and shape change and give rise to the third zone termed the transitional or hypertrophic layer. At the end of the process of maturation and degeneration of the hypertrophic cells, they become calcified (zone of calcification) and merge with the metaphysis to complete the process of endochondral ossification and thus provide bone growth in a longitudinal direction (Fig. 14–16).

As the animal matures and hormonal changes progress, the physis ceases to produce new bone and becomes narrower. With time the radiolucent area disappears leaving only a faint line or physeal scar on radiographs. When the physis is no longer distinctly visible, it is considered to be "closed" or "fused" and the potential for growth terminated. In reality, cessation of bone growth probably does not exactly coincide with radiographic "fusion." It is likely that considerable time elapses between the point at which significant axial growth ceases and ablation of the physis by osseous substance becomes evident.

Table 14–2 is a list of generally accepted physeal closure times of commonly affected bones by location and age.

The vascular supply to the region of the physis

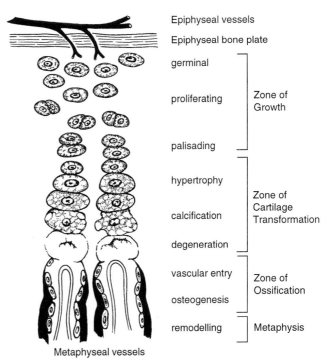

Figure 14–16. Schematic of the physis illustrating the relationship of the zones of chondrocyte differentiation, perichondrium, and vascular regions of the distal metaphysis.

TABLE 14–2. FORELIMB, HINDLIMB, AND AXIAL SKELETAL CLOSURE TIMES

Bone	Physis	Closure Time
Forelimb		
Middle phalanx	Proximal	15–18 months
Proximal phalanx	Proximal	18–24 months
Metacarpus	Distal	2–2.5 years
	Fusion of MC3 with MC4	6 months
Radius	Distal	3.5–4 years
	Proximal	12–15 months
Ulna	Distal	3.5–4 years
	Proximal	3.5–4 years
Humerus	Distal	15–20 months
	Proximal	3.5–4 years
Scapula	Supraglenoid tubercle	7–10 months
Hindlimb		
Middle phalanx	Proximal	15–18 months
Proximal phalanx	Proximal	18–24 months
Metatarsus	Distal	2–2.5 years
	Fusion of MT3 with MT4	6 months
Calcaneus	Tuber calcaneus	30–36 months
Tibia	Distal	2–2.5 years
	Proximal	3.5–4 years
Patella	Ossification time	3.5 years
Femur	Distal	3.5–4 years
	Proximal	3.5 years
Axial Skeletal		
Pelvis	Ilium, ischium, pubis	7–10 months
	Tuber ischii	5 years
	Tuber coxae and sacrale	5 years
	Pelvic symphysis	5 years

Modified from Greenough PR, MacCallum F, Weaver AD: Lameness in Cattle. Bristol, England, Wright Scientechnica, 1981.

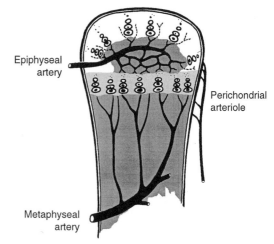

Figure 14–17. Diagrammatic representation of the vascular supply to the distal metaphysis, physis, and epiphysis in the immature animal.

The typical response of the physis to abnormal stimuli or nutritional factors is termed "epiphysitis" despite the fact that the physis rather than the epiphysis is the structure responsible for the majority of the changes and, strictly speaking, the process plays an important role relative to both infectious processes and to healing potential. Before the growth plate closes, there is a separate blood supply to the metaphyseal and epiphyseal areas. While there may be some blood vessels that cross the physis, they are considered to be very few in number and to play a minor role in supply of nutrients to the area. The metaphyseal side is supplied from within the bone by branches of the metaphyseal artery that enters the bone via the nutrient foramen. Externally, the periosteal vessels supply nutrition to up to one third of the outer cortex of growing bone (Fig. 14–17). The perichondral ring that surrounds the bone at the level of the physis is supplied by perichondral vessels that usually originate from the main metaphyseal arteries. Epiphyseal arteries supply nutrition to the epiphysis and, by diffusion, to the physis. As a result, interruption of the epiphyseal blood supply results in interference with chondrocyte proliferation of normal growth.[5] The origin and vulnerability of all of these vessels play an important role in the amount of damage that results from disruption of the vascular supply to both the physis and epiphysis of growing animals.

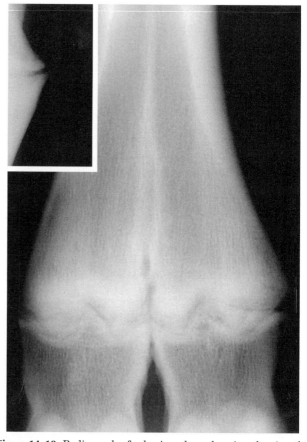

Figure 14–18. Radiograph of a bovine physeal region showing the typical signs of "epiphysitis." Widening of the growth plate and sclerosis of the distal metaphysis are shown in the larger radiograph; "lipping" at the periphery of the growth plate is shown in the inset.

is not one of inflammation. Many physes are affected but the most clinically apparent sites are the fetlocks of all four limbs. Affected animals have an upright conformation and enlargement of the fetlock, and varying degrees of lameness. Early on in the disease, there is widening and irregularity of the physis. With time, there is widening of metaphyseal and epiphyseal bone by periosteal proliferation, which appears as "lipping" of opposing osseous tissues at the periphery of the physis. Sclerosis, narrowing of the growth plate, and regions of bony bridging may also be evident (Fig. 14–18).

Fractures involving the physis in humans were described in a classic paper by Salter and Harris in 1963, which resulted in a classification system that combines location and configuration with prognosis (Table 14–3).[24] This system is used universally to describe fractures involving the physes of all species. Basically, fractures occur by separation of the epiphysis from the physis, by crossing the physis, by compression of the physis, or by a combination of these conditions. While interference with physeal growth can produce serious conformational problems, separation as a result of transverse forces usually results in disruption at the interface of calcified and uncalcified cells. This fortunately does not affect the resting and proliferating cells that remain attached to the epiphysis. With an intact vascular supply, these cells will continue to function if axial alignment is restored and maintained, the limb will continue to grow normally and reach its full potential.

Methods of correcting physeal abnormalities of an-

TABLE 14–3. CHARACTERISTICS, APPEARANCE, AND PROGNOSTIC FEATURES OF THE MOST COMMON FRACTURES AFFECTING PHYSES AS CLASSIFIED BY THE SALTER-HARRIS SYSTEM

Salter-Harris Type	Description	Appearance	Prognosis
1	Simple separation caused by transverse forces, minimal displacement		Good
2	Most common type involves the physis and metaphysis characterized by the Thursten-Holland sign		Good
3	Fracture involves the physis and epiphysis resulting in an articular component		Reasonable prognosis if open reduction results in smooth and stable cartilaginous surface
4	Fracture line runs from the articular surface, through the physis, and into the metaphysis		Prognosis is guarded even with effective open reduction because of the residual effects of the initiating trauma
5	Compressive forces acting on the physis act to damage the proliferating and progenitor cells resulting in premature closure of the physis		Poor prognosis if significant growth was expected to occur from the affected physis. The closure is not seen until too late

gular limb deformities in cattle follow the same principles as advocated for other species and are selected on the basis of degree of angulation, age, remaining growth potential of the involved physis, and experience of the veterinarian. Methods used to correct minor deviations may involve only manual alignment and rigid splinting or casting of the limb. These forms of external support have given variable results and are not universally utilized. Surgical growth stimulation by means of periosteal stripping on the concave aspect of the deformity has been used successfully provided that enough growth potential remains to permit the animal to correct the deviation by physeal growth. Immediately following transection of the periosteum there is retraction of this tissue, which is considered to have restricted normal bone growth by acting as a "spring" on the concave surface of the affected bone. In species that have an intact ulna, which is the case in cattle, this structure may also act as a "bowstring" on the concave surface of the deviated bone. In such instances it may be advantageous to resect a section of the ulna to remove any forces that act in this manner. Unless all of the ulnar periosteum of the resected segment is removed, the defect will quickly be filled with osseous tissue that may restore the bowstring effect.

Correction of angular deformities may also be achieved by growth retardation of affected bones by means of transphyseal bridging on the convex surface. The most appropriate method is to place 4.5 mm cortical screws on either side of the physis and bridge the physis with two figure of eight wires under tension. This technique will inhibit growth on one side of the physis and allow the other side continual growth, which will result in straightening of the limb. Owner cooperation is required to determine when the limb has regained its normal conformation, at which time the implants must be removed to prevent overcorrection of the physis. Details of surgical considerations and techniques for angular limb deformities are covered in Chapter 16.

REFERENCES

1. Ackerman N, Garner HE, Coffman JR, Clement JW: Angiographic appearance of the normal equine foot and alterations in chronic laminitis. J Am Vet Med Assoc 166:58–62, 1975.
2. Baggot DG, Bunch KJ, Grill GR: Variations in some inorganic components and physical properties of claw keratin associated with claw disease in the British Friesian cow. Br Vet J 144:534–542, 1988.
3. Banks WJ: Applied Veterinary Histology. Baltimore, Williams & Wilkins, 1981.
4. Boosman R, Németh F, Gruys E, Klarenbeek A: Arteriographical and pathological changes in chronic laminitis in dairy cattle. Vet Q 11:144–155, 1989.
5. Breur G: Injury and repair of the growth plate: Application of research models to clinical disease. Proceedings of the Fifth ACVS Veterinary Symposium, Chicago, 1995, pp 223–224.
6. Coffman JR, Johnson JH, Guffy MM, Finochio EJ: Hoof circulation in equine laminitis. J Am Vet Med Assoc 156:76–83, 1970.
7. Dellman H-D, Brown EM: Textbook of Veterinary Histology. Philadelphia., Lea & Febiger, 1976.
8. De Vos N, Morcos MB: De arteries van de achervoet bij hetrund. Vlaams Diergeneesk Tijdschr 29:241–246, 1960.
9. Dietz O, Naumann J, Prietz G: Inorganic composition and physical properties of bovine digital horn. Proceedings of the 5th International Symposium on the Disorders of the Ruminant Digit. Dublin, Ireland, 1986, pp 24–31.
10. Dietz O, Prietz G: Klauenhornqualität-Klauenhornstatus. Mh Vet Med 36:419–422, 1981.
11. Dyce KM, Sack WO, Wensing CJG: Textbook of Veterinary Anatomy. Philadelphia, WB Saunders, 1987.
12. Ellenberger-Baum. Handbuch der vergleichenden Anatomie der Haustiere. Berlin, Springer-Verlag, 1977.
13. Hood DM, Amoss MS, Hightower D, et al: Equine laminitis I: Radioisotopic analysis of the hemodynamics of the foot during acute disease. J Equine Med Surg 2:439–445, 1978.
14. Kainer RA: Clinical anatomy of the equine foot. Vet Clin North Am Equine Pract 5(1):1–27, 1989.
15. Kempson S: Personal communication, University of Edinburgh, 1995.
16. Maclean CW: A post-mortem x-ray study of laminitis in barley beef animals. Vet Rec 86:457–462, 1970.
17. Maclean CW: The long-term effects of laminitis in dairy cows. Vet Rec 89:34–37, 1971.
18. Manson FJ, Leaver JD: The influence of dietary protein intake and of hoof trimming on lameness in dairy cattle. Anim Prod 47:191–199, 1988.
19. Morcos MB: Nature and etiology of the ulceration of the claw in the bovine. Mededelingen Veerartsenijschool, Rijksuniversiteit Gent 4(3):1–30, 1960.
20. Nickel R, Schummer A, Seiferle E: The Anatomy of the Domestic Animals, vol 3: The Circulatory System, the Skin and the Cutaneous Organs of Domestic Mammals. New York, Springer-Verlag, 1981, pp 524–536.
21. Nomina Anatomica Veterinaria and Histologica, 4th ed. Ithaca, NY, International Committee on Veterinary Gross Anatomical Nomenclature, 1994.
22. Pollitt CC: Clinical anatomy and physiology of the normal equine foot. Equine Vet Educ 4:219–224, 1992.
23. Pollitt CC, Molyneux GS: A scanning electron microscopical study of the dermal microcirculation of the equine foot. Equine Vet J 22:79–87, 1990.
24. Salter RB, Harris RW: Injuries involving the epiphyseal plate. J Bone Joint Surg Am 45A:3A, No. 3, 1963, 587–621.
25. Vermunt JJ: Lesions and structural characteristics of dairy heifers in two management systems. M.V.Sc. Thesis, University of Saskatchewan, Saskatoon, Saskatchewan, Canada, 1990.
26. Vermunt JJ, Leach DH: A macroscopic study of the vascular system of the bovine hindlimb claw. N Z Vet J 40:139–145, 1992.
27. Vermunt JJ, Leach DH: A scanning electron-microscopic study of the vascular system of the bovine hindlimb claw. N Z Vet J 40:146–154, 1992.

Surgical Procedures

James G. Ferguson   *Canada*

15

Principles of Bovine Orthopedics

SPECIFIC CONSIDERATIONS

AGE

Many fractures occur in calves, particularly in the first few days of life. Lameness associated with fractures in young calves may dramatically affect gait and muscle development. Changes in conformation and adhesions of adjacent structures may occur during the healing phase, and permanent deformity may result. Flexor tendon laxity, quadriceps tie-down, and other related conditions frequently result from excess stresses placed on contralateral and ipsilateral limbs. Trauma associated with the fracture, its surgical repair, or the postoperative activity of the animal also causes impaired function. Bowing of the contralateral limb, knuckling of the carpus, muscle atrophy over the affected limb, and decreased range of motion of the femorotibial joint are common sequelae of femoral fractures that have been treated using internal fixation techniques.

Young animals have an amazing ability to heal, particularly in terms of callus production. This property may be used to advantage when external fixation devices are being considered as the treatment modality.[14] Depending on the type of fracture, some calves may have their casts removed after 3 weeks and be allowed unrestricted activity without risk of refracture. More mature animals usually require a more protracted healing period before external devices may be safely removed.

The neonatal periosteum appears to have extraordinary ability to respond to trauma and limited motion at a fracture site, provided that vascularity is intact. The bovine periosteum is a relatively substantial structure. In calves, it is capable of producing a fibrous response within a few days. This tissue rapidly grows and becomes calcified to form an effective stabilizing structure. This response may be relied on to produce a successful end result in the majority of cases of metacarpal and metatarsal fractures treated with plaster casts and tibial fractures treated using Thomas-Schroeder splints. The characteristics of periosteal attachment can vary between bones, and in the femur in particular, the periosteum has a propensity to become detached from the cortex as a result of overriding and posttrauma muscular movement before reduction is attempted.

Metacarpal and metatarsal fractures in calves that have been delivered with the assistance of chains and a calf-puller may incur marked vascular damage at the site of chain application. The effects range from a delayed healing response to loss of the limb due to complete destruction of the distal blood supply. The severity of the damage depends on the application technique and the amount of force applied.

SELECTION OF IMPLANTS

The selected implant must match the holding potential of bone because of the extreme differences in cortical thickness and bone consistency between various bones of the neonate and adult. For example, the cortical thickness of the distal neonatal femur has the dimension of approximately one screw interthread distance (Fig. 15–1) at a common fracture site. Because the bone has not experienced significant stress and strains *in utero,* it has poor inherent strength.

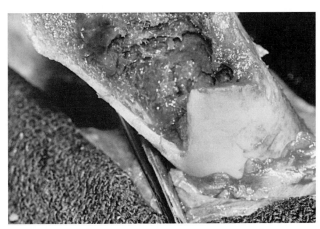

Figure 15–1. Intraoperative view of a distal femoral fracture in a newborn calf, illustrating the thin cortex that is without periosteum at the fracture site.

ECONOMICS

The cost of internal versus external fixation must be carefully evaluated. Repeated application of casts with associated transportation costs, the expense of casting materials, the time associated with cast removal, and anesthetic and recovery costs frequently approach the cost of plate and screw fixation.

PROGNOSIS

Each fracture is characterized by a probable prognosis and time frame that depend on the selected treatment. These characteristics vary with the age, size, and temperament of the subject. Knowledge of and experience with these variables allow discussion with the owner about the most appropriate method.

ATTITUDE OF THE OWNER

Present-day livestock owners are aware of the potential pain and suffering associated with leaving certain conditions untreated. Today's owners have an increased willingness and sense of responsibility to seek advice and treatment for animals suffering from traumatic and degenerative conditions.

IMMUNOLOGICAL MATURITY

Neonates presented for fracture treatment may have been affected since birth and may have been unable to stand and nurse properly. Many will have failed to receive adequate amounts of colostrum and have suffered considerable stress before treatment. These immunologically immature animals are unable to withstand the challenges of infectious agents as effectively as older, immunologically protected individuals. This factor worsens the prognosis and increases time spent on nursing management. The loss of up to 25% of the circulating blood volume into a hematoma, occurring in some femoral shaft fractures, affects the individual's ability to fend off secondary disease.

SIZE OF THE PATIENT

Surgical procedures involving the upper limbs may be limited owing to the size of the animal. Surgical approaches may be limited by the physical mass of tissue. Mechanical devices that facilitate fatiguing and levering may be appropriate (Fig. 15–2). Extra personnel may sometimes be needed in the surgical team.

RADIOGRAPHIC EXAMINATION

Positioning an animal for radiographic studies of the upper limb requires special attention. Unique radio-

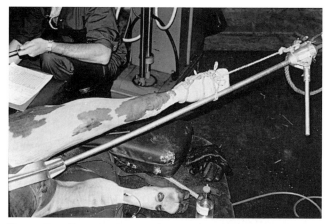

Figure 15–2. Preoperative positioning of a young bull with a humeral fracture. Note the positioning of an abdominal sling, block and tackle, and calf-puller used to facilitate the reduction of a fracture.

graphic views must be considered in addition to the requirement for prolonged exposure times, particularly for regions of the hip, sacrum, shoulder, and spine of larger animals. In many such instances, general anesthesia or deep sedation is needed to provide adequate control of the animal and immobilization during the process. Thus, food and water must initially be withheld for an appropriate interval. Medial-to-lateral views of the scapulohumeral and coxofemoral joints require exposure times frequently exceeding 1 second. Total control of the animal and removal of people from the vicinity of the x-ray source are thus required. Such animals may need to be held in unusual positions with their limbs extended using weights, wedges, ropes, or a combination of these devices (Fig. 15–3).

SELECTION OF TECHNIQUE FOR FRACTURE STABILIZATION

EXTERNAL FIXATION

Plaster of Paris casting material is both economical and adequate for younger animals provided that

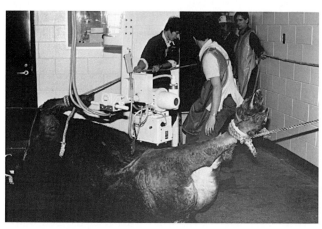

Figure 15–3. A sedated animal is positioned on its back and stabilized by means of ropes to allow for long radiographic exposure times to minimize radiation risk to staff.

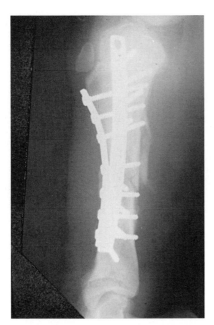

Figure 15–4. Radiograph of an open, comminuted tibial fracture in a mature dairy cow. The fracture has been stabilized with two orthopedic plates. Despite this open fracture with prolonged exposure of the implants, the animal recovered successfully.

housing and maintenance are consistent with good cast care. Even older, heavier cattle may have plaster included in the external fixation device if other materials are incorporated into the cast to overcome the shortcomings of excess weight and limited final strength inherent in plaster. The use of an aluminum walking bar or combinations of plaster and fiberglass are two methods of overcoming such limitations.

Fiberglass cast material alone provides excellent strength with minimum weight. It has had the disadvantage of increased cost and less than optimum conforming and molding characteristics. Innovative products have largely overcome these last two problems.

Supplementary fixation devices such as the Thomas-Schroeder splint, leg braces, modified Robert Jones bandages, and spica and polyvinyl chloride (PVC) splints are examples of devices that have been modified for cattle.

INTERNAL FIXATION

The technology used in other species has been modified for cattle. The incorporation of multiple pins within the medullary cavity (stack pinning), the use of two or more plates for long bone fractures (Fig. 15–4), the use of the larger-diameter screws, and modification of the number of wires and points of fixation in tension band wiring are examples of techniques developed to meet demands by some methods modifying the use of existing materials.

PRINCIPLES OF EMERGENCY FRACTURE MANAGEMENT

The circumstances surrounding the initiation of a fracture may involve excitement of the animal and the potential for severe self-inflicted damage. An animal's attempts to ambulate compound the damage to the affected area and must be minimized by applying some form of external support. Without such support, the loading and transport of an animal worsens the surgical prognosis and increases the risk of complications. A support device applied before transport or treatment is a sound investment in time and effort. An external supportive device is also advocated on humane grounds, because minimal pressure over the site of the wound and control of a flailing limb reduce suffering. Open wounds associated with fractures are also kept cleaner than if exposed to the contaminated environment of many stables, trailers, and holding facilities. Every attempt should be made to provide stabilization and support of all fractures below the humerus and femur.

Fractures and dislocations distal to the mid-metatarsal or metacarpal bones respond well to casting using plaster or fiberglass. A less effective but nevertheless helpful alternative is the modified Robert Jones bandage. PVC pipes cut in half longitudinally and applied to the dorsal or plantar surface of these bones provide excellent temporary support (Fig. 15–5). Fractures of the radius and ulna or tibia are well protected by either a modified plaster spica or Thomas-Schroeder splint. Adequate padding must be applied over pressure sites between the limb and the splint surface.

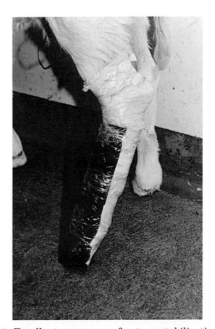

Figure 15–5. Excellent emergency fracture stabilization in a calf with a distal metatarsal fracture using polyvinyl chloride tubing, sheets for padding, and clear packing tape. This support was applied by the owner before transport to the clinic.

COMMON ERRORS IN HANDLING FRACTURES

- Inadequate advice given to owners about restraint until veterinary assistance arrives, as well as failure to emphasize its importance
- Failure to understand the importance of emergency immobilization
- Lack of materials to construct external support devices at the site where the injury occurred
- Failure to select and apply an appropriate form of support to the fractured limb
- Failure to begin antibiotic treatment in the early posttrauma period, especially indicated in open fractures
- Administration of drugs for restraint or control of infection when economics and the nature of the fracture dictate or strongly suggest the need for emergency slaughter
- Failure to radiograph proximal limb problems before transport or referral
- Failure to advise owners about the cost of treatment, the immediate postoperative care required, and the long-term prognosis

PRINCIPLES AND USE OF ARTHROSCOPY

DEFINITION

Arthroscopy is a system by which instruments (Fig. 15–6) may be inserted into a joint for diagnostic purposes or to undertake certain surgical procedures.

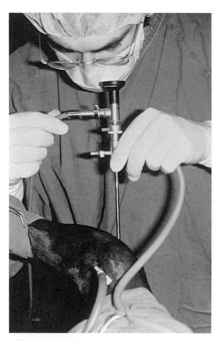

Figure 15–6. Direct visualization of the joint space and articular surfaces by the arthroscopic method. Note the sterile technique necessary for safe entry into an articulation.

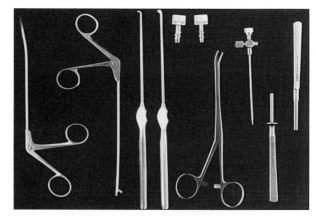

Figure 15–7. A selection of arthroscopic instruments used to enter the joint space and perform surgical procedures.

TECHNIQUE

To visualize intra-articular structures, the joint capsule must be distended. This is usually done by continuous infusion of a sterile physiological fluid such as Ringer's solution into the joint under controlled pressure.

Both diagnostic and therapeutic procedures may be performed using small cannulas (usually two), which are inserted through separate stab incisions into the joint space. The joint can thus be flushed to maintain a clear field by removing blood, undesirable debris, and products of infection and inflammation. This is a very beneficial procedure, particularly in septic arthritides.

Arthroscopic telescopes are available in various diameters and viewing angles and should be selected to provide the optimal visibility and ease of insertion for the particular joint. Many instruments are available for performing specific surgical procedures (Fig. 15–7).

The joints most commonly entered in cattle are the femoropatellar, femorotibial, and tibiotarsal and less commonly the radiohumeral, scapulohumeral, radiocarpal, and metacarpophalangeal. Readers are referred to the work of Hurtig[6] for more detail on approaches, equipment, and arthroscopic anatomy.

INDICATIONS

The use of an arthroscope in treatment of septic arthritis allows visualization of affected tissues and active, aggressive flushing of cavities in a much more selective and thorough manner. Large volumes of fluid applied under direct visualization provide better therapy than simple active distention and passive release of fluids from a joint space such as occurs using medium-bore needles.

Bone and cartilage fragments, as well as synovial tissues, are readily removed by arthroscopic techniques.

ORTHOPEDIC BIOMECHANICS

DEFINITIONS

Biomechanics is the study of the forces and accelerations acting on the bones and soft structures of the abaxial skeleton.

Stress is a force per unit area acting on material in a specific plane.

Strain is the resulting deformation or change in the dimension of the material. A characteristic interaction of stress and strain of a particular material is typically represented as a stress-strain curve (Fig. 15–8). Strain may be produced by stresses of tension, compression, or sheer.

Compression is a force such as weight-bearing that tends to reduce the dimension of the plane in which it operates.

Tension is a force that tends to increase the dimension of the plane in which it operates. The tensile strength of a material is defined as its ability to resist breaking when subjected to tension.

Shear stresses are generated when opposing forces operate in different regions of the same plane. Bending of a structure creates deformation and therefore a concave surface, which experiences compressive stress, and a convex surface, which experiences tensile stress. Shear forces exist in that structure. Bending is a dynamic, ever-changing condition in the living body.

BASIC PRINCIPLES

Bone throughout the body is constructed with economy of material, and the shape of each bone and its internal structure are devoted to this objective. The presence of a medullary cavity in tubular bones reduces bone weight without loss of resistance to either compressive or tensile forces and results in increased resistance to shear stresses.

These forces of tension and compression are frequently represented in a simplistic manner with only two dimensions being described, but in fact the relationship is rather complex, even in a standing animal. Depending on bone shape and loading characteristics, different aspects of weight-bearing bones have regions of compression and tension forces. These regions are frequently termed the *tension* and *compression* sides of that bone and are critical to the placement of implants for effective immobilization.

Because metal implants have their greatest strength in tension, they must be placed on the tension side of the affected bone to result in fixation. Inappropriately placed implants quickly fail when subjected to the large forces generated in even small calves.

Tension band technology is an engineering concept used in orthopedics to convert tensile forces into compressive forces at the fracture site by using strategically placed implants and the normal forces generated in the body.

Compression plating techniques produce compression at the fracture site by applying the tension band principle and plates placed under tension. Compression of the fracture fragments only provides for stabilization of the components, which allows for healing, minimizes callus formation, and permits early controlled ambulation.

Anisotropy refers to the property of bone that relates orientation of bone microstructure to direction of greatest strength. Cortical bone thus is stronger in its longitudinal direction than its transverse direction because its osteons are oriented longitudinally.

The trabeculae of spongy bone are more numerous and prominent in areas of normal stress, where they align themselves in the direction of physiological strain.[13] Configuration of fracture fragments is a result of bone shape and characteristics of forces acting on the skeletal components. The presence of open physeal growth plates and the spiral configuration of such bones as the humerus have obvious effects on fracture appearance, but when a bone approaches the shape of a tubular structure, general statements may be made about how force characteristics are manifested in the shape of bone fragments.

FRACTURE MECHANICS

- Under eccentric compression (simultaneous compression and tension), shear forces are set up at 45° to the direction of compression and are capable of causing a fracture in this configuration (Fig. 15–9).

- Bone under tension tends to break in a direction perpendicular to that of the tensile force.

- Pure compressive forces tend to cause fractures at 45° to the long axis of bone.

- Shear stresses due to compression and torsion produce spiral configuration fractures with the point of initiation of the fracture parallel to the long axis of the bone.

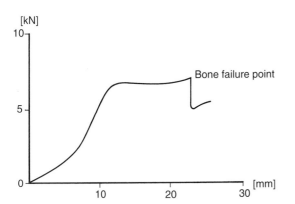

Figure 15–8. A stress-strain curve demonstrating the forces involved in testing a newborn calf femur in compression in an Instron testing machine. The curve illustrates a relatively linear portion followed by a flat segment, suggesting occurrence of microfractures followed by a distinct failure point.

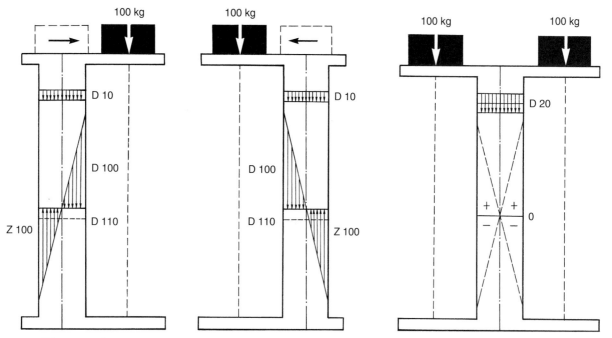

Figure 15–9. Schematics demonstrating the effect of eccentric loading of a column, which produces shear forces within the structure. When the forces are not eccentrically loaded, the shear forces are neutralized and simple compression is created. D, axial compression; Z, tensile stress. (Redrawn from Pauwels F: Biomechanics of the Locomotor Apparatus. New York, Springer-Verlag, 1980.)

• When bending and compressive forces are combined, the fracture configuration tends to be transverse, with a butterfly component at the compression side of the affected bone (Fig. 15–10).

• Torus fractures are found at the interface of meta-

physeal and diaphyseal bone at the point where cortical bone changes from dense lamellar bone to woven, more cancellous bone. It is believed that this junction of two bone types provides a biomechanical transitional region that is less capable of absorbing stresses such as are created by axial loading. These fractures typically have a plastic deformation or buckling on one side of the cortex and a fracture with minor displacement on the opposite cortex (Fig. 15–11). They are the usual fracture type created in the distal femur by experimental application of compressive forces on the neonatal femur.[3]

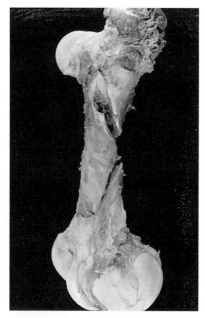

Figure 15–10. A fractured femur from a 450-kg bull demonstrating a large midshaft butterfly fragment suggestive of simultaneous compressive and torsional forces being applied to the limb. This is not the typical (torus) configuration of femoral shaft fractures seen in newborn animals.

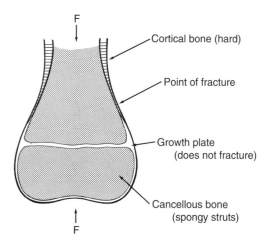

Figure 15–11. Schematic illustration of the forces applied, area of stress concentration, and fracture site of the typical torus fracture seen in newborn calves that have had assisted delivery.

CALLUS STABILIZATION

The biomechanical effect of callus on stabilization of fractures is primarily a function of the periosteum, which forms from the cambium layer of the cortex. The mass and shape of the external callus is formed in response to movement at the fracture site. The greater the motion, the greater is the diameter of the callus. Callus is initially formed from vascular components that are invaded by fibroblasts and result in bridging of the gap by fibrous tissue. The fibroblasts provide early resistance to motion. As movement is further reduced, cartilaginous tissues replace the fibrous tissue. With time and further stability, the callus becomes mineralized, and bone remodeling eventually occurs. The end result is a healed fracture site with bone strength and orientation approaching that of the original bone. The progression of the healing process sequentially places at the callus site those tissues that are best able to function with the degree of mobility present at the time. The distribution of callus material in a circumferential location best uses principles of mechanics by locating the relatively weak early tissues at a greater distance from the axis of the bone, thus increasing the mechanical advantage of the callus. The greater the motion at the site, the greater is the distance from the axis and, therefore, the larger the external callus. Fractures with little or no movement at the fracture site develop minimal callus.

NEONATAL BONE

Biomechanics of developing bone is important in bovine orthopedics because a relatively high proportion of problems occur in neonates. In general, bone from young animals is considered to have less strength in tension and degree of elasticity.[2] Maturing bone becomes more stiff in response to physical stresses, particularly in the diaphysis and metaphysis. With time, the orientation of collagen fibers along lines of normal forces further strengthens developing bone. In general, the more porous nature of the immature metaphysis renders the bone more susceptible to failure in compression than in an adult. However, developing bone is thought to have a greater ability to absorb energy before failure and to absorb more energy after the fracture has been initiated. It may also respond to loading more rapidly than adult bone and therefore may remodel faster.[1] Bone that does not have optimal ratios of mineral and collagen components has a reduced strength and is thus less able to resist forces acting on it.[13] Neonatal bone has not had sufficient time, stimulation, or degree of mineralization to be of optimal quality. Young animals generally have a relatively high proportion of cancellous to cortical bone. Consequently, inherent strength and implant holding power of bone in neonates are compromised. It is essential that these factors be considered in the treatment and prognostic decisions involving young calves.

ILIOTIBIAL TRACT

DEFINITION

The iliotibial tract (ITT) functions as a tension band to protect the femur from the shearing forces that occur during the limb stance phase or during contraction of the quadriceps.

The structural and functional components of the ITT in cattle are

- Gluteobiceps
- Deep and superficial fascia of biceps femoris
- Tensor fascia lata
- Fascia lata
- Lateral femoropatellar ligament
- Tendon of the biceps femoris
- Lateral ligament of the patella
- Middle patellar ligament
- Extension of the retinaculum of the stifle joint

FUNCTION OF THE ILIOTIBIAL TRACT

The bovine femur, when loaded in compression during normal weight-bearing, is under considerable shearing stress. Pauwels[9] states that the action of the ITT is to reduce stress on the femur by neutralizing shearing forces resulting from loading of the femur by its contact with the acetabulum. Maximum strength is provided with minimum bony material by counterbending the femur through the active contraction of the muscular components of the tract.

In addition, as the quadriceps femoris muscle contracts and expands, the tract is displaced laterally and thus exerts an additional tensile force along the system.

In its middle portion, the ITT is anchored to the femur by the intermuscular septum and is anchored distally to the lateral condyle of the tibia. Just before it attaches to the tibia, it blends with the aponeurotic extension of the vastus lateralis and the lateral fibers of the retinaculum of the knee.

A study of the diversity of function of the human tensor fascia lata[8] provides a detailed account of the role of the ITT, pointing out the different roles of the tensor fascia lata muscle depending on the gait phase and location of the fibers being examined. Further, several references discuss the part that the muscles and the ITT may play to control anterolateral instability of the knee.[9]

In contrast to human technology, the use of fascia in stifle joint reconstruction by veterinary surgeons has not been considered in its relationship to the ITT. Many human surgical references describe stabilization of the knee by use of part of the iliotibial band and the interrelationships of the tendinous structures in the lateral aspects of the knee.[10]

It appears that the component lateral to the stifle

acts as a stabilizing structure preventing medial displacement of the patella and ensuring proper seating of the patella within the intertrochlear groove during contraction of the quadriceps. This structure also maintains the insertion of the ITT on the lateral aspect of the tibia, especially during flexion or medial rotation of the limb (i.e., outward rotation of the hock).

Design and placement of implants and prostheses, as well as selection of surgical approaches to the femur and structures surrounding the stifle joint, are best served by an appreciation of structures acting to protect and stabilize the upper hind limb. The ITT may be an important consideration in gait analysis, lameness diagnosis, conformation, and selection of surgical procedures.

MECHANISMS OF BONE GROWTH

Increase in bone length primarily results from the process of endochondral ossification taking place at the growth plate (metaphyseal growth complex,[7] separating the epiphysis and metaphysis). This structure (see p. 229) is important when considering the etiology, treatment, and prognosis of fractures involving the growth plate, frequently termed Salter-Harris fractures. The growth plate must transfer all forces from the shaft of the bone to the epiphysis and is a structurally weak link in the immature skeleton. The epiphysis is connected to the metaphysis by a network of collagen fibers that span the growth plate[12] and provide circumferential support.

Longitudinal bone growth at the metaphyseal growth plate occurs by widening of the plate by the process of endochondral ossification. The cells responsible are chondrocytes that originate from the metaphyseal side of the plate (resting zone), multiply (proliferating zone), hypertrophy, calcify (transitional zone), and mature. The amount of growth is directly related to the number of cell divisions and the degree of chondrocytic hypertrophy. The mature chondrocytes degenerate and calcify before being invaded by metaphyseal blood vessels, which carry in primitive osteogenic cells and eventually convert the tissue into bone. Invasion of the vessels is facilitated by the columnar arrangement of the chondrocytes originating in the proliferating zone.

Growth in bone circumference is accomplished by periosteal activity, which deposits new bone on the outer surface of the bone at the same time bone is being resorbed on the inner surface.

Immature bone has an internal structure that reflects an unorganized arrangement of collagen fibers and osteocytes and is termed *woven bone*. The majority of immature bone is formed *in utero* or in the neonatal period and is the type of bone involved in fractures and healing in most very young animals. Woven bone is a temporary type of bone that is typically laid down in response to some stimulus and replaced at a later date by lamellar bone. Immature bone is less dense and less well mineralized than mature bone. However, it may be more effective in absorbing compression forces before and during the development of a fracture.

Mature bone is purposefully constructed and has a specific internal structure and orientation. This lamellar bone can be either cancellous or cortical and is characterized by collagen sheets and osteocytes arranged in the three-dimensional form (haversian system). Mature bone is more dense, more structurally organized, and hence inherently more capable of functioning effectively with internal fixation devices.

Bone remodeling occurs on a constant basis in response to changes in biomechanical, nutritional, and endocrine status. It occurs by the addition and removal of bone in existing structures by osteoblasts and osteoclasts. Bone responds to stress or demands placed on it in a manner that modifies its structure and form (Wolff's law, 1896, paraphrased).[15]

As an animal grows, the bone diameter, its cortical thickness, and the diameter of the medullary cavity depend on osteoblastic and osteoclastic activity. Appropriate ratios are maintained to ensure maximum strength with minimum weight. Allowance is thus made for adequate medullary volume to ensure hematopoietic function.

The remodeling of woven bone from callus or its early formation occurs within the tissue itself by use of a cutting cone mechanism (Fig. 15–12), which functions to remove existing bone tissue and replace it with mature, lamellar bone in the haversian format. This mechanism removes bone using osteoclasts and replaces it with mature bone at the rate of 50 to 100 μm/day.

PERIOSTITIS

DEFINITION

Periostitis is an inflammatory reaction of the tissue immediately overlying bone.

PATHOGENESIS

Complications of an infectious nature may be either osteitis or osteomyelitis. Periostitis may also be caused by trauma, neoplasia, or metabolic conditions. The bovine periosteum is a very responsive tissue and is capable of producing large amounts of fibrous, cartilaginous, and bony tissues when stimulated by any number of factors. This response is particularly evident in calves, provided that the vascular supply is not compromised.

OSTEOMYELITIS

DEFINITION

Osteitis is an inflammation of the cortical area of bone only. *Osteomyelitis* is involvement of both the cortex and medullary cavity.

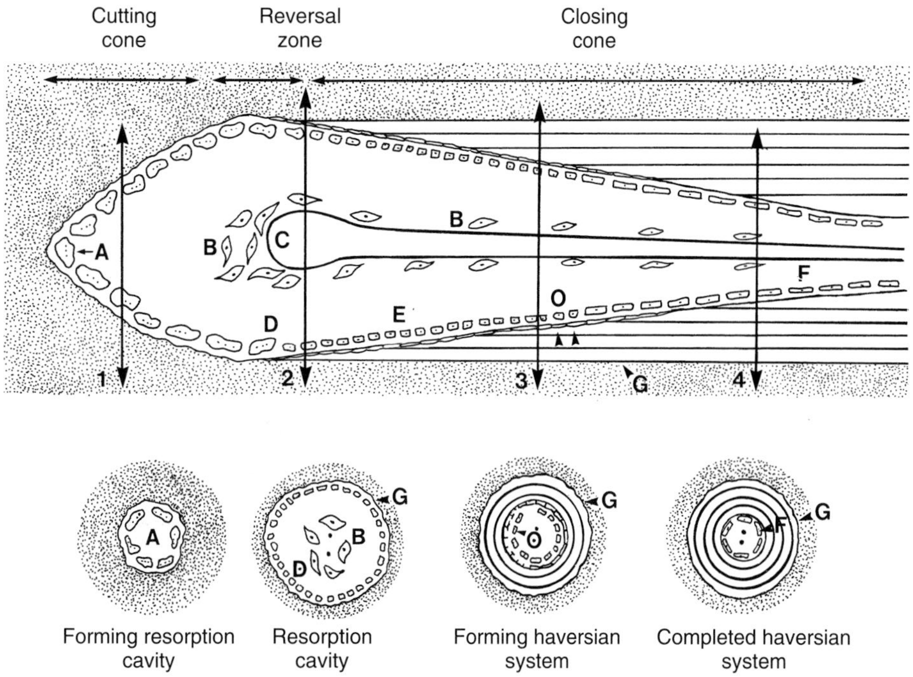

Cutting cone   Reversal zone   Closing cone

Figure 15–12. Diagrammatic representation of bone remodeling by the cutting cone and its associated activities. 1, 2, 3, and 4, the planes of transection used to produce the four cross sections; A, advancing osteoclasts; B, undifferentiated mesenchymal cells; C, capillary; D, cells in transition at the maximum core width; E and O, osteoclasts filling in the culling cone; F, flattened haversian lining cells; G, the cement line separating new bone from old bone. (Redrawn from Parfitt AM: The action of the parathyroid on bone: relation to bone remodelling and turnover, calcium homeostasis and metabolic bone disease. Metabolism 25(7):809–844, 1976.)

Forming resorption cavity   Resorption cavity   Forming haversian system   Completed haversian system

ETIOLOGY

Organisms may be carried to the site via the bloodstream during a bacteremic episode from a focus originating elsewhere in the body. In young animals, the common source is the umbilicus. Localization of hematogenous spread of organisms tends to be in the small, end vessels of the metaphyses and epiphyses of the long bones, where blood flow slows (sludging) and colonization of the vessel walls by bacteria is facilitated.

Local spread of infection from adjacent tissues and inoculation of organisms by trauma and foreign bodies represent other routes of spread of osteomyelitis.

The inflammatory process parallels that in soft tissue, with thrombosis, edema, fibrin production, invasion of the area by white blood cells, and necrosis of the marrow tissue and cortex, which results when pressure within an unyielding structure forces infected and necrotic tissues through the cortical channels. When the infection migrates radially toward the periosteum, it applies pressure at the interface, resulting in periosteal elevation from the cortex and considerable interference with local cortical blood supply, which has a particularly pronounced effect in younger animals. Bone is limited in its ability to resorb necrotic foci, particularly when that tissue is mineralized. Trabecular bone is more readily removed than devitalized, mature cortical bone.

The metaphyseal growth plate in immature animals tends to limit the progression of the infection into the epiphyses, whereas no such barrier is present in adult animals with closed growth plates. Infection originating from the epiphysis tends to advance into the joint space, leading to septic arthritis.

Hematogenous osteomyelitis in cattle has been classified[5] as being primarily of two types, either physeal or epiphyseal. In the former, the origin of the infection is said to be in the growth plate, usually in the distal metacarpus, metatarsus, radius, or tibia. Epiphyseal osteomyelitis is initiated in the subchondral bone and immature epiphyseal joint cartilage, usually by *Salmonella* organisms, and has a relatively poorer prognosis than the physeal type (Table 15–1).

CLINICAL SIGNS

Early stages of infection present a variable spectrum of clinical signs. Lameness may not be overtly demonstrated in all cases but may develop progressively over days. Likewise, fever and a leukogram may not always suggest a bone infection in the early stages of the disease. Pain on palpation may prove helpful in diagnosis. As the condition advances, the clinical signs listed earlier become more obvious and radiographic examination may reveal typical changes associated with osteomyelitis, as described in Chapter 3.

DIFFERENTIAL DIAGNOSIS

Table 15–1 summarizes the differences and similarities between the two types of osteomyelitis in cattle.[5]

TREATMENT

Osteomyelitis is a difficult condition to overcome and may prove to be virtually impossible to treat economically in cattle. With regard to the basic problem, infected and necrotic material is contained within

TABLE 15–1. PHYSEAL VERSUS EPIPHYSEAL OSTEOMYELITIS IN CATTLE

	Physeal	Epiphyseal
Location	Metaphyseal bone near the physis	Below the articular cartilage
Organism	*Actinomyces* spp., *Salmonella* and other species	*Salmonella* spp.
Affected bones	Distal metatarsal, metacarpal, radius, ulna	Distal femoral epiphysis, patella, distal radius
Age affected	*Salmonella* <12 months: *Actinomyces* >6 months	*Salmonella* <12 weeks
Prognosis	Satisfactory	Grave
Surgery	Drain abscesses, sequestrectomy	Delay surgery, then perform sequestrectomy
Radiographic signs	Lucency on metaphyseal side, localized to the physeal region; pathological fractures possible; sclerotic zones possible	Cyst or lucency at subchondral cartilaginous interface, sclerotic zones possible

tissue that is poorly vascularized and readily harbors infectious organisms. It is therefore very difficult for normal defense mechanisms to overcome this type of infection. Because of the very serious implications inherent in the condition, any diagnosis of cortical and medullary infection should be viewed with considerable concern.

Medical antibiotic therapy may control the infectious organisms, but surgical removal of the affected bone and surrounding tissues and provision of drainage are usually required for successful long-term results. Although medical therapy alone may be sufficient in cases of acute osteomyelitis, in the vast majority of cattle, the condition is well advanced by the time they are seen by a veterinarian.

Medical Treatment. Medical treatment involves attempts to isolate and identify the offending organism by means of blood cultures, examination of cultures taken from draining tracts, or biopsy samples. Because many animals have already received previous treatment by the owner, these investigations may not provide accurate results. These results may be compared with later samples in cases in which therapy appears to produce a disappointing response.

The most likely organism or class of organisms may be implicated on the basis of the location of the process or the suspected cause. The animal should receive antibiotics as soon as possible; selection of a "best-guess" drug is often necessary.

Surgical Treatment. Surgical treatment of all but very acute cases of osteomyelitis should be considered in addition to antibiotic therapy. The decision to operate should be based on either a failure of response to antibiotic therapy or a primary specific indication for surgery. The objectives of surgical intervention are to remove all dead and devitalized bone and associated material, remove the source of infection to the immediate area, remove tissues of questionable vascularity, and provide the opportunity for drainage and lavage. Removal of fibrous tissue near the site of osteomyelitis facilitates replacement with well-vascularized tissue better capable of combating infection. Drainage is provided by the placement of devices that allow for irrigation and suction of material from the defect.[12] Another technique that

may be used to provide drainage from the site is delayed closure of the tissue over the infection site.

Amputation of a digit results in removal of infected bone and soft tissue, allows for incorporation of well-vascularized granulation tissue into the site, and provides for effective drainage of the area. Although long-term results may not be optimal, amputation provides for simple, economical treatment of osteomyelitis (and frequently septic arthritis) of the distal digit.

The more conservative approach to surgical treatment of osteomyelitis involves the removal of infected tissues without amputation of the part. In this technique, the site of infection is approached directly over the involved tissues, and any fistulous tract is resected. A wide exposure is made, and fibrous tissue is removed when it overlies the site. The area is lavaged thoroughly before placement of drains. The defect may be lavaged on an intermittent or continuous basis with physiological solutions to facilitate healing. Dressings and external support should be used as required to maintain a clean field and prevent pathological fractures from occurring.

MECHANISMS OF BONE HEALING IN FRACTURE REPAIR

PRIMARY BONE HEALING

Definition

Primary bone healing is the process of bone repair associated with internal fixation in which direct or primary healing proceeds without callus formation.

Pathophysiology

Compression of the fragments is not an essential prerequisite for primary bone healing but does ensure that rigid fixation and bone-to-bone contact are maintained.

No radiographic evidence of periosteal callus formation occurs in classical primary bone healing, although damage to the periosteum and surrounding tissues usually occurs in clinical situations. Fibrous and calcified tissue, which is unrelated to purposeful callus formation, can be produced. The mechanism of primary bone healing is a function of cells growing from viable bone on one side of the fracture site, directly across the necrotic bone regions, through the fracture itself, and back into healthy bone on the other side of the defect. Callus formation is not required. New bone is formed at about the same rate as the dead bone at the fracture ends is resorbed. The net effect is that no fracture gap is visible radiographically. The union has less initial strength than if a callus were formed, but the original mechanical properties are eventually attained. In contrast, a callus, once mineralized, attains greater strength earlier. A major advantage of primary bone healing lies in its facilitation of an early return to normal locomotion. In addition, deleterious effects of prolonged external fixation tend to be less, because articular range of motion is not affected and muscle tie-down and muscle atrophy do not occur. A slight risk is that excessive callus formation may interfere with proper nerve function in some locations where healing is accompanied by excessive callus production.

SECONDARY BONE HEALING

Definition

Secondary bone healing is bone repair involving the formation of a callus that is responsible for stabilization of the fracture ends.

Pathophysiology

Displacement of bone ends and variable distraction of periosteal and muscle attachments leading to local hemorrhage occur immediately after a fracture. The bones later are frequently moved to abnormal configurations as a result of muscular forces that act in characteristic patterns, usually typified by flexor muscles overpowering extensors. This configuration is well illustrated in distal femoral fractures, which almost always have significant overriding, with the coxofemoral joint and femorotibial joints flexed regardless of the nature of forces causing the fracture.

Within a few days, a granulation tissue mass forms in the area that will become the callus. It contains fibroblasts, fibrocytes, and early vascular elements. This granulation tissue is replaced by a connective tissue mass, which later changes to fibrocartilage. The source of the fibroblasts and chondroblasts is the periosteal, endosteal, and medullary osteogenic cells, which respond to the fracture by rapid multiplication and differentiation.

As the callus becomes more rigid, conditions become more appropriate for invasion of larger blood vessels, which aid more effective bone formation. During the transformation to connective tissue and cartilage, the callus becomes mineralized and develops into a relatively strong cancellous structure. The callus and bone in the immediate area are then remodeled, and lamellar bone is laid down in this process.

This constantly changing callus also has a role in removing avascular bone tissue resulting from loss of bone integrity. After stabilization, haversian remodeling occurs, restoring the bone to its initial strength. The bone is thus returned, more or less, to its initial shape as a result of modification of the callus.

BONE SEQUESTRA

Definitions

A *sequestrum* is a piece of necrotic bone that is separated from the surrounding healthy bone. An *involucrum* is an area of new bone formation surrounding necrotic bone. It is laid down in response to the inflammatory process associated with the devitalized tissue.

Pathophysiology

The new bone is laid down as membranous bone and is initially associated with a fibrous tissue response. On palpation, the tissue is very hard and cannot be distinguished from bony reactive tissue.

A *cloaca* is an opening or drainage tract (sinus) that connects the area of purulent fluid surrounding the sequestered bone to the outside and functions to allow drainage. This tract may be followed from the skin to find the sequestrum, which may be difficult to localize clinically. The tract may also be identified and characterized using contrast medium as a fistulogram.

In the early stages, radiographs show no evidence of the formation of a bony envelope nor the presence of a radiolucent lake surrounding the isolated fragment. Within about 2 weeks, the inflammatory process results in the development of purulent debris surrounding the dead bone, and a fistulous tract often forms, allowing drainage to the outside.

The author believes that the etiology of a bone sequestrum in young animals is related to the competence of the immune system and the relatively high incidence of infectious disease in the young. The bone is probably infected via an embolic process and dies as a result of the infection. The dead bone then initiates the inflammatory process, which produces thrombosis of the region, causing the local bone to die and a sequestrum to result. The dead bone is then separated from the living bone by purulent material.

Clinical Signs

Adult cattle frequently have sequestra located in distal extremities (Fig. 15–13). These sequestra result from a traumatic incident[4] that causes necrosis of

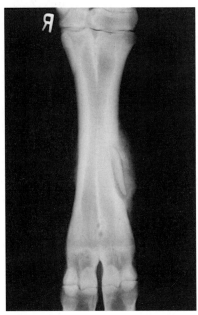

Figure 15–13. Radiograph of a sequestrum and reactive involucrum in a dairy cow. The cow had evidence of pre-existing trauma to this area. The necrotic bone was successfully removed surgically.

bone, presumably because of interference with vascularity or infection. These lesions are classically found in the greater metacarpal and greater metatarsal bones.[4] They are characterized by pain and swelling of the region, evidence of trauma, and, in chronic cases, a fistulous tract. The presence of a sequestrum is confirmed by plain radiographs and sinography when indicated.

Young cattle frequently have sequestra in the long bones of the upper limb such as the radius, humerus, or femur. These bones are relatively protected from direct insult, and in most cases, trauma does not appear to be a prominent factor in the history or development of the condition.

A specific type of hematogenous infection of metaphyseal bone is a Brodie's abscess, which is an infected area segregated by fibrous inflammatory tissue and woven bone. In a long bone (e.g., metacarpus), surgical curettage and drainage is usually successful.

Treatment

Affected animals should be anesthetized using local intravenous methods or general anesthesia if the lesion is located in the proximal forelimb. If the proximal hind limb is involved, epidural anesthesia may be used. A tourniquet should be applied when the lesion is distal to the hock or elbow to control hemorrhage, which may obscure the operative field.

Physical landmarks are carefully identified to determine the extent of the surgical excision required. When a fistulous tract is present, the tract should be resected, including some tissue overlying the involucrum. Care should be taken to conserve enough tissue to allow the incision to be covered. Radiographic examination may include the placement and documentation of radiopaque markers for surgical refer-

ence. The location of the sequestrum is frequently obscured by a fibrous or periosteal bone response over the site and the variable course of the draining tract.

Simple, early or small sequestra may be removed by sedating the animal, providing local intravenous anesthesia to the limb, and resecting the offending necrotic bone. An elliptical skin incision is made over the sequestrum, and sharp dissection is used to remove all soft tissue over the site. Bone gouges, chisels, and curettes are used to remove the new bone over the sequestrum. Healthy cortex can be differentiated from the sequestrum, which is typically yellow (Fig. 15–14). Purulent or granulation-type tissue separates the sequestrum from the surrounding healthy cortex and overlying new bone. The dead bone is removed, and its necrotic tissue bed curetted down to healthy, bleeding bone before closure. Placement of a drain is frequently advantageous. The defect is closed and bandaged in a routine manner.

Prognosis

The prognosis for successful treatment of a bone sequestrum is good to excellent, depending on the size of the necrotic portion, the duration of its existence, and the degree to which other nearby structures such as joints have been compromised. When a sequestrum involves the full cortical thickness and has significant longitudinal or circumferential dimensions, its removal may jeopardize the ability of the long bone to resist normal forces. A pathological fracture may result. In most cases, the developing involucrum has a callus-like effect, which contributes to bone strength, enabling it to resist normal forces in the postoperative period.

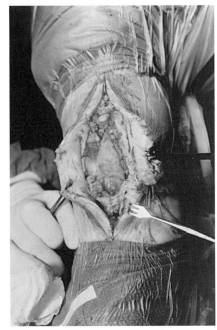

Figure 15–14. Intraoperative view of a bony sequestrum and involucrum, which was removed. The limb subsequently healed uneventfully.

Whenever a significant amount of bone is removed, some form of external support should be provided in the recovery period and the first few weeks of ambulation. Selected cases may require support using internal fixation devices.

REFERENCES

1. Chamay A, Tschantz P: Mechanical influences in bone remodeling. J Biomech 5:173–180, 1972.
2. Curry JD: Mechanical properties of bone tissues with greatly differing functions. J Biomech 12:313–319, 1979.
3. Ferguson J: Clinical investigation on the newborn calf femur: bone strength, density, and fracture biomechanics (DMV thesis). Vienna, Veterinary University of Vienna, 1987.
4. Firth EC: Bone sequestration in horses and cattle. Aust Vet J 64:65–69, 1987.
5. Firth EC, Kersjes AW, Dik KJ, Hagens FM: Hematogenous osteomyelitis in cattle. Vet Rec 119:148–152, 1987.
6. Hurtig M: Recent developments in the use of arthroscopy in cattle. Vet Clin North Am Food Anim Pract 1:175–193, 1985.
7. Mase C: The anatomy and response to surgical manipulation of the distal radial growth plate in foals (MSc Thesis). Saskatoon, SK, University of Saskatchewan, 1986.
8. Pare EB, Stern JT, Schwartz JM: Functional differentiation within the tensor fascia latae. J Bone Joint Surg Am 63:1457–1471, 1981.
9. Pauwels F: Biomechanics of the Locomotor Apparatus. New York, Springer-Verlag, 1980.
10. Scott WN, Ferriter P, Marino M: Intra-articular transfer of the iliotibial tract. J Bone Joint Surg Am 67:532–538, 1985.
11. Smith JA, Williams RJ, Knight AP: Drug therapy for arthritis in food-producing animals. Comp Cont Ed Pract Vet Food Anim 11:87–94, 1989.
12. Speer DP: Collagenous architecture of the growth plate and perichondral ossification groove. J Bone Joint Surg Am 64:399–407, 1982.
13. Sumner-Smith G: Bone in Clinical Orthopedics: A Study in Comparative Osteology. Philadelphia, WB Saunders, 1982.
14. Tulleners EP: Management of bovine orthopedic problems. Part I. Fractures. Comp Cont Ed Pract Vet Food Anim 8:69–80, 1986.
15. Wolff J: Das Gesetz der Transformation der Knochen. Berlin, Verlag August Hirschwald, 1892.

16

Surgery of the Distal Limb

The distal limb is that region below the metacarpus and metatarsus. Each limb has two metacarpophalangeal (and metatarsophalangeal) joint capsules, which communicate through a small window in the joint capsule in the normal, healthy state. In diseased states, this communication is not usually open.

Distal to the metacarpophalangeal and metatarsophalangeal joints, the digits are arranged in tandem, thus allowing for unique approaches to surgical treatment of these structures. One digit can be rested while the other provides full support and function. Devices such as wooden blocks affixed to the weight-bearing surface of the sound digit can relieve pressure, reduce motion of the diseased digit, and facilitate the repair processes. As a result, amputations, arthrodeses, fracture repair, tendon resection, and pseudoarthrodeses are possible and readily achieved in cattle.

OSTEITIS/OSTEOMYELITIS OF THE DISTAL PHALANX

DEFINITION

The terms *osteitis* and *osteomyelitis* are frequently used interchangeably; however, infection and inflammation of the distal phalanx is an osteitis because the process does not involve either a medullary cavity or a physis.

ETIOLOGY AND PATHOGENESIS

Although infection of the distal phalanx may result from hematological sources, the most common cause is bacterial invasion through the sole or sole-horn junction. This may result from penetration by sharp objects or direct spread of infection from solar abscesses and white line disease. With severe laminitis and rotation of the distal phalanx, the apex may penetrate or may be exposed through the sole and thus develop an infectious process (see p. 108, Fig. 8–18, and Chapter 18). The phalanx may also be unprotected when moist and soft claws are suddenly exposed to extremely abrasive surfaces, resulting in excessive wear and exposure.[13]

CLINICAL SIGNS

Lameness is frequently severe, resulting from pain produced by increased pressure and inflammation. Some animals show only minor gait and weight-bearing abnormalities. Swelling is minimal because the problem is within the hoof. When the sole is open, a hemorrhagic and necrotic distal phalanx may be suspected but may be confidently identified only when the necrotic debris is removed by curettage.

The diagnosis frequently is obvious when the sole is trimmed and the distal phalanx is probed and examined visually. Bony fragments may be unattached to the parent bone, or curettage may disclose obvious areas of necrosis, which are easily removed from the healthy bone. The full extent of the infectious process is best defined by a radiographic study with dorsoplantar/palmar and interdigital views. The apex of the distal phalanx is most commonly affected.

TREATMENT

Treatment and postoperative care depend on the degree to which the third phalanx is affected. In those instances in which the bone can be debrided and all necrotic tissue removed, the area should be packed with an antiseptic or antibiotic compound and a bandage applied. The dressing should be changed weekly. Repeat radiographs aid assessment of the progress of the osteitis. Systemic antibiotics are administered for 7 to 10 days. The antibacterial dressing is applied until a granulation tissue layer has completely covered the previously exposed bone. The defect is eventually repaired with fibrous tissue, and the sole is completely regenerated to provide protection to the bone and to permit complete clinical resolution. The prognosis in such cases is favorable, and the animal can become sound within a few weeks.

When the septic process is far advanced, amputation may be performed at the level of the distal interphalangeal (DIP) joint or through the middle or proximal phalanx.

An alternative to amputation is to resect all or part of the diseased distal phalanx through a distal approach, pack the defect, and allow granulation tissue to fill the cavity. The hoof wall is preserved with this alternative procedure.

FRACTURES OF THE DISTAL PHALANX

INCIDENCE

Fractures of the distal phalanx are not uncommon in cattle. Only one digit is usually involved, although multiple fractures have been reported. Fractures of both distal phalangeal bones of the same limb are rare. In free-ranging animals, when a fracture occurs in a forelimb, the medial claw is most frequently affected. Petzoldt[17] has reported a very high proportion of hind limb involvement in housed animals, with the lateral claw being most commonly affected. This is probably because of the increased proportion of weight born by that digit. Fractures are usually intra-articular and extend to the solar surface. Minimal displacement occurs initially, but distraction of fracture fragments increases with time, presumably as a result of tensile forces exerted by the deep digital flexor tendon and bone resorption at the fracture site (Fig. 16–1).

ETIOLOGY

Fracture of the distal phalanx has been associated with trauma, osteomyelitis, fluorosis, heavy body type, and low copper levels. When severe osteitis of the distal phalanx is present, avulsion of a fragment may be associated with the site of insertion of the deep digital flexor tendon. Problems related to slippery flooring or hard walking surfaces may predispose to the condition. The cause is unknown in most cases.

CLINICAL SIGNS

Animals are evidently in acute pain and are reluctant to bear weight on the affected digit. Those with bilateral fractures on contralateral limbs frequently assume a cross-legged stance in response to pain originating from both medial claws of the forelimb. Animals with severe pain may also prefer to kneel and crawl to reduce weight-bearing. Regardless of treatment, stance and gait improve gradually. The problem may be identified by compression of the claw with hoof testers and percussion. Little swelling is found because of restriction of the hoof wall, but heat may be felt. Lateral radiographs placing a non-screen film in the interdigital space can confirm the diagnosis.

TREATMENT

Therapy is aimed at relieving pain and minimizing the distractive forces of the flexor tendons by resting the affected digit by means of a wooden block affixed to the sound digit. The fractured phalanx then heals without additional fixation. Radiographic changes occur slowly and may fail to demonstrate bony union for several months.

If the rare double fracture occurs on the same limb, the distal limb is completely enclosed in a short

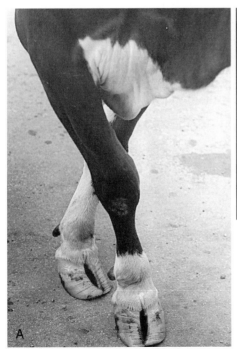
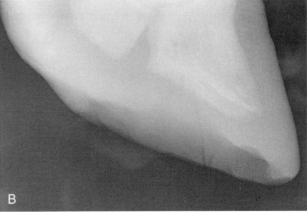

Figure 16–1. *A,* Cross-legged stance resulting from pain in the medial digits of both forelimbs, which can be due to bilateral fracture of the distal phalanx, although in this case the etiology involved deep intradigital sepsis. *B,* Radiograph of a distal phalangeal fracture showing widening of the fracture line as a result of bone resorption at the fracture site and distraction due to forces exerted by the deep flexor tendon.

fiberglass cast to the level of the proximal metacarpal bone. The use of a metal walking bar and fixing the distal limb in partial flexion facilitate ambulation and minimize distractive forces acting across the fracture site. Clinical healing occurs in 4 to 8 weeks, and weight-bearing and gait gradually improve. The animal should be confined to a small box stall for 1 to 2 months for best results.

Very rarely, articular fractures require treatment by arthrodesis of the DIP joint. Amputation should be reserved only for cases such as pathological fractures that occur as a result of, or in association with, infection of the distal phalanx. Amputation of the tip of the distal phalanx has been successful in treatment of limited osteitis.[14] The animal can then bear weight on the limb within a few days and becomes sound within a few weeks, thus facilitating finishing the animal for slaughter.

SEPTIC ARTHRITIS OF THE DISTAL INTERPHALANGEAL JOINT AND ADNEXA

INCIDENCE

Infection of the DIP joint is relatively common in cattle.

ETIOLOGY AND PATHOGENESIS

The proximity of structures and the ease of penetration along tissue planes make areas susceptible to bacterial localization (joints, synovial structures, and soft tissue) easy targets for infectious organisms. The anatomical relationship of the DIP joint, the navicular bursa, the distal sesamoid, and the tendons and their sheaths are illustrated in Figure 16–2.

Infection may enter the DIP joint by three main routes, discussed next.

Route One: Interdigital Route. Necrosis, infection, or trauma occurring on the dorsal axial skin of the interdigital space is perhaps the most frequent cause of septic arthritis of the DIP joint. The dorsal pouch of the joint capsule is located subcutaneously at this point and is extremely vulnerable to penetra-

tion. Cutaneous lesions at this site should be treated with considerable caution. Routine cleansing, a topical dressing, and protection are appropriate.

Route Two: Dorsoabaxial Route. At the dorsoabaxial coronary band, the dorsal pouch of the DIP joint is superficial and vulnerable to damage. Trauma or more frequently small vertical fissures and associated secondary infection are commonly implicated.

Route Three: Plantar/Palmar Route. Direct penetration of the joint from a distal direction is very unlikely because of the anatomical arrangement of the joint and associated structures. Infection entering the joint from the sole tends to pass along the plane between the distal phalanx and the wall.

The most common distal route is via the abaxial white line. Infection may pass from the white line via the lamellar spaces and establish a sinus at the coronary band. En route, the tract of infection passes either the joint or the navicular bursa. The joint is protected to some extent by its collateral ligament. The bursa has some protection from the abaxial insertions of the DIP ligament. These fibrous structures appear to delay further inward spread of infection for as long as about 38 hours. A coronary sinus, therefore, can develop without involvement of either the joint or bursa. Late presentation of the case, failure to diagnose the disease process, or inadequate treatment invariably leads to joint involvement.

Once the joint is infected, progressive tissue destruction occurs for a prolonged period. If the infection is untreated, marked periarticular exostosis formation occurs, with massive distortion of the pastern (clubfoot). Avulsion of the insertion of the deep flexor tendon is a common sequela.

CLINICAL SIGNS

The first sign is progressively increasing lameness. The region proximal to the dorsal coronary band becomes swollen and often erythematous. The enlargement usually continues to expand regardless of antibiotic treatment. The heel and the region of the flexor tendon sheath proximal to the fetlock may eventually become swollen. A fistulous tract frequently appears just above the coronary band (Fig. 16–3).

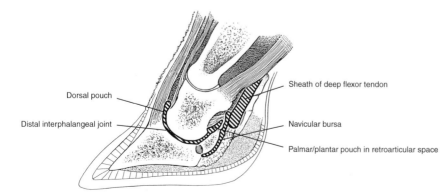

Dorsal pouch

Distal interphalangeal joint

Sheath of deep flexor tendon

Navicular bursa

Palmar/plantar pouch in retroarticular space

Figure 16–2. Schematic drawing of the structures of the distal digit, which are frequently involved in the process of septic arthritis as a result of their close spatial relationship.

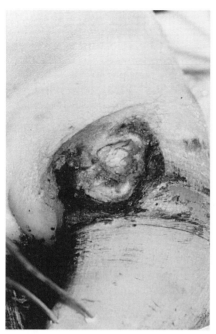

Figure 16–3. A digit with septic arthritis of the distal interphalangeal joint with a large fistulous tract at the level of the coronary band.

Radiographic examination in the early stages may reveal either no obvious abnormalities or only slight widening of the joint space. Later, further widening of the space indicates destruction of the articular cartilage and subchondral bone of the joint (Fig. 16–4). Concurrent with the bone and cartilage destruction is the production of new bone at the joint margin in what appears to be an attempt to stabilize the articulation or control the infection. As the disease process advances, the animal prefers recumbency

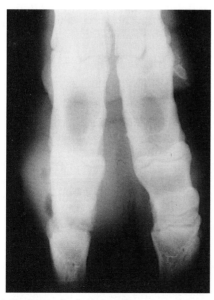

Figure 16–4. Radiograph of advanced septic arthritis of the distal interphalangeal joint showing soft tissue swelling, destruction of the joint cartilage, and gas production.

and loses its appetite, resulting in reduced milk or meat production.

The dorsal pouch of the joint capsule of the DIP joint extends proximal to the extensor process of the distal phalanx and is accessible at the level of the coronary band. A joint tap may be performed using an 18-gauge needle inserted 1 cm from the abaxial aspect of the extensor tendon and at 90° to skin surface. The animal should be restrained in a chute or tilt table and the area surgically prepared before entering the joint. Aspiration of the joint produces several milliliters of fluid, which may be evaluated using standard laboratory methods. After aspiration, the joint may be blocked with a local anesthetic, and because the space is relatively large, a volume of 10 mL or more is recommended. This technique is useful in cases in which the clinical examination has not provided a clear definition of the location of the site of lameness and further information is required.

TREATMENT

Antibiotic Therapy

The recommended treatment for early and suspected joint sepsis is systemic administration of one or more broad-spectrum antibiotics. In countries where antimicrobials are readily available to farmers without prescription, few animals have not received this form of treatment before veterinary care is requested.

For those cases in which a veterinarian attends the animal before any therapy has been initiated, the same approach is frequently taken, often without performing a detailed diagnostic procedure. Antibiotics should be administered at high doses for a maximum of 5 days. If resolution is not noticeable, the pathology present should be re-evaluated.

Trent and Plumb[21] recommend use of the intravenous route for the first few days of therapy. Intramuscular injections are begun as soon as culture and sensitivity results are available. The use of high levels of procain penicillin (44 to 66 mg/kg twice daily) is an appropriate initial treatment regimen when gram-positive organisms are suspected. Alternatively, gentamicin is recommended when gram-negative organisms are involved or when the identity of the organism on Gram stain cannot be determined. It is also suitable to combine penicillin and gentamicin if the tentative diagnosis and economics suggest that a broad spectrum of coverage is necessary. Other antibiotic choices that have been shown to be efficacious for septic arthritis are trimethoprim-sulfa or oxytetracycline given in the appropriate concentrations. Administration of intra-articular antibiotics has been both advocated and criticized in the veterinary literature within the past decade (see p. 68). Arguments against their use have focused on the potential damaging effects of the solution on synovium and cartilage when injected directly into the joint space because of the pH of the carrier solutions and the proposed direct effects on cartilage surfaces.

In general, in recent years, instillation of antibiotics into joints has been more favorably viewed, as has the use of mild disinfectant solutions as lavage media.

Administration of local intravenous antibiotics, in conjunction with a tourniquet, to treat limb infections has been advocated for cattle since 1965.[2] The advantages of this modality are related to the delivery of high concentrations of antibiotic to the region primarily affected, the ability to use low doses of drug relative to the overall mass of the animal, the probable reduction in drug residue levels, and the economic advantage of using small doses of expensive antibiotics. Pharmacokinetic studies[6] have demonstrated that when 250 mg of cefazolin is given to normal cows (1/40 of the systemic dose), therapeutic concentrations are obtained in the synovial fluid. Intravenous antibiosis (10 × 10^6 IU benzylpenicillin dissolved in 10 to 15 mL 2% lidocaine HCl) has caused serious postsurgical complications (extensive thrombosis necessitating slaughter) in 2 of 15 cows. Direct toxicity of the antibiotic solution was probably responsible.[20]

The principles and use of anti-inflammatory drugs are addressed in Chapter 5.

Criteria for Selecting Surgical Modalities

- How valuable is the animal?
- How long does the owner expect to keep the animal in the herd?
- Will the animal be retained for milk or meat or as a breeding animal or ovum donor?
- Will the animal be required to walk significant distances at pasture?
- Will the animal be maintained on solid ground, slippery surfaces, or slatted floors?
- What is a reasonable amount of time and money for the owner to spend?
- What postoperative care can the owner give?
- What other tissues or regions are involved (i.e., infected tendons, tendon sheaths, cellulitis, polyarthritis)?

Options

- Emergency slaughter.
- Allow natural resolution. This option, if likely to subject a patient to prolonged pain, should not be recommended by a veterinarian.
- Amputation of the affected part provides a short-term but economical technique for removing damaged or infected digital structures. A rapid reduction in pain, removal of infected tissues, and provision of surgical drainage are achieved by a relatively simple surgical procedure.

- Arthrodesis or resection techniques are advocated for very valuable animals. Long-term success is better achieved by selecting a surgical procedure that removes the infected tissues and supports the body's natural attempts to fuse the joint and provide pain-free, functional movement.

Surgical Indications

- Retroarticular abscess
- Necrosis of the deep flexor tendon and tenosynovitis
- Severe hoof wall defects and avulsion of the hoof wall
- Fractures or osteitis of the middle and distal phalanges
- Septic arthritis of the proximal or distal interphalangeal joints

Digital Amputation

CRITERIA TO BE CONSIDERED
Removal of hind claws of bulls intended for breeding is not recommended because extreme forces are transferred to the hind limbs during mounting. Alternatives to amputation of the digit should be carefully evaluated if a bull has valuable breeding potential.

Major weight-bearing occurs on the medial claw of the forelimb and the lateral claw of the hind limb and corresponds to the relative distribution of digital lesions. Whenever these structures are considered for amputation, their significance in weight-bearing and thus their effect on prognosis must be considered.

Several investigators have reported on longevity in cows after digital amputation. Although individual animals may function effectively for several years in certain environments, those with an amputated claw commonly leave the herd within 18 to 24 months after surgery.[4]

SURGICAL TECHNIQUE
The site of amputation may be at the DIP joint, through the middle phalanx (at the coronary band), at the level of the proximal interphalangeal joint, or through the proximal phalanx.[16, 22]

Kofler[12] compared amputation through the middle phalanx, using obstetrical wire, to exarticulation of the proximal interphalangeal joint and found both methods to be equally effective.

I prefer amputation at the level of the lower one third of the middle phalanx distal to the level of the nutrient artery. The procedure may be performed on quiet cattle with the animal standing, after the use of nerve blocks.

Alternatively, a patient may be cast on thick bedding after deep sedation. Ideally, a mechanical or hydraulic table places the animal in lateral recum-

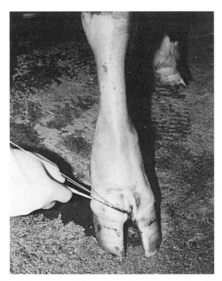

Figure 16–5. Claw amputation in a standing animal showing the skin incision and the initial placement of the obstetrical wire used to transect the bone. After the wire is seated, it is directed to cut through the distal region of the middle phalanx in the same plane as the skin incision.

bency while regional intravenous anesthesia distal to a tourniquet provides humane and effective control of the animal. After routine surgical preparation of the digit, a skin incision is made with a scalpel from the dorsal interdigital space to the plantar/volar aspect of the claw approximately 0.5 cm above the coronary band. This incision delineates the level of transection of the middle phalanx and facilitates operation of the obstetrical wire saw, which effectively cuts the digit at an oblique angle (Fig. 16–5). Skin flaps (recommended by other workers) are not created, nor are sutures applied to the wound. The tourniquet functions to control overt hemorrhage and should remain in place until a tight bandage has been applied. A topical dressing is applied to the open wound, and the digit is firmly bandaged to control bleeding and facilitate healing of the exposed stump.

Dressings may be changed every few days for a matter of weeks or may be applied and left alone until they are spontaneously lost. In uncomplicated cases, the stump is covered with granulation tissue within about 2 weeks and is completely healed in 5 or 6 weeks. Expected postoperative course of healing is related to the rate of granulation tissue production over the exposed bone, the rate of re-epithelialization, and the extent of concurrent disease of the surrounding tissues including the tendons and tendon sheath. Uncomplicated cases have a significant improvement in gait and reduction in pain within a few hours of surgery. If relief is not obvious within the first week, careful re-evaluation should take place. A patient should be using the limb normally by 3 weeks.

COMPLICATIONS

Although complications are rare, an animal may lose body condition or show signs that infection has not

been contained. During surgery, routine sampling of the diseased structures with a swab and testing for antimicrobial sensitivity are useful. The owner should remain alert for an ulcer that may develop on the remaining claw of the same limb. A limited number of cases of necrosis of the proximal portion of the middle phalanx are thought to be related to accidental resection of the nutrient artery supplying the bone, leaving the remaining bone without an adequate blood supply. This possible complication points out the need for amputation through the middle phalanx to involve only the distal portion of the bone.

Arthrodesis

DEFINITION
Arthrodesis is the surgical fusion of a joint. The procedure promotes the proliferation of osteocytes to bridge the defect.

APPLICATION
Antibiotic therapy for infection of the DIP joint and surrounding soft tissue is frequently unsuccessful. Digital amputation may be inappropriate for valuable animals. In these cases, the most favorable prognosis is obtained through surgical intervention aimed at controlling infection, removing necrotic tissues (cartilage, subchondral bone, synovial, and periarticular tissues, Fig. 16–6), and the promotion of fusion of the bones involved.[8] This procedure has also been referred to as *joint resection.*[15] The arthrodesis thus produced creates a pain-free union that is capable of functioning effectively for prolonged periods.

TECHNIQUE
Palmar/Plantar Approach. The animal is best maintained on a tilt table in lateral recumbency, with the affected limb uppermost. The limb is prepared for surgery by clipping it from above the fetlock distally and thoroughly cleaning the digits, claws, and interdigital region. Two holes are drilled into the tip

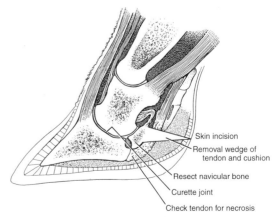

Skin incision
Removal wedge of tendon and cushion
Resect navicular bone
Curette joint
Check tendon for necrosis

Figure 16–6. Schematic representation of a flexotransverse approach to the distal interphalangeal joint, which provides access to the region and facilitates removal of infected intra-articular and periarticular tissues.

of the affected claw to allow placement of wire, which is used to hyperextend the digit during surgery and later to fix the claw in flexion.

After local intravenous anesthesia distal to a tourniquet, a transverse incision is made from the axial to the abaxial borders for approximately 180° (Fig. 16–7). A wedge of tissue is removed from the digital cushion, including some of the deep digital flexor tendon (distal to the level of the tendon sheath), the podotrochlear bursa, and the distal sesamoid bone (Fig. 16–8). Once the DIP joint is entered, a hand curette is used to remove all the accessible articular cartilage. If extensive tissue necrosis is present, the curette is then used to remove all the devitalized material down to the subchondral bone. The fistulous tract is debrided to remove all infectious material. Swabs should be taken from the infected areas for antimicrobial sensitivity testing. The skin incision is closed with non-absorbable interrupted sutures.

A drain is recommended if all necrotic or devitalized tissues cannot be removed with certainty. The resected joint should be continuously flushed with physiological electrolyte solution supplied to the drainage/irrigation tube from a 10-liter tank suspended over the animal.

Once the deep flexor tendon has been resected, the digit should be protected from weight-bearing and fixed in flexion to permit the heel bulb incision to heal and the tendon to be bridged by connective tissue. This step involves fixing a wooden block to the unaffected claw and wiring the affected digit to the block in flexion. This fixation may be supplemented by incorporating both digits in a polymethyl methacrylate shoe (Fig. 16–9).

The animal should be confined to a box stall for

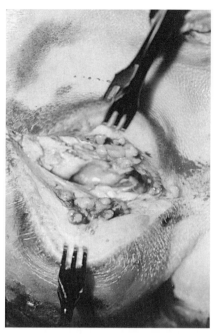

Figure 16–8. View of the flexor aspect of the digit showing how removal of a wedge of tissue has opened up this area of the distal interphalangeal joint and provided good access for curettage of the intra-articular structures.

the first 1 or 2 weeks postoperatively and after 1 month allowed more exercise. In uncomplicated cases, the animal should be relatively pain free after 1 month and sound after 3 months. It is important that an owner be advised, before surgery, of the relatively protracted recovery period. Figure 16–10 illustrates the ability of the bovine digit to produce an abundance of new bone and to heal by arthrodesis within a few months. Extensive production of new bone is expected after an initial lag period.

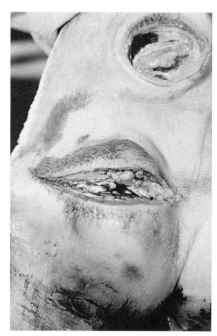

Figure 16–7. View of the flexor aspect of the digit showing the extent of the transverse skin incision that provides access to the joint.

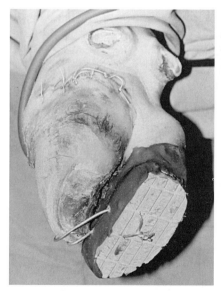

Figure 16–9. View of the digit showing the closed suture line, wooden block, and flexed digit with wire incorporated into the wooden block. Technovit is then applied to both digits, incorporating the wooden block.

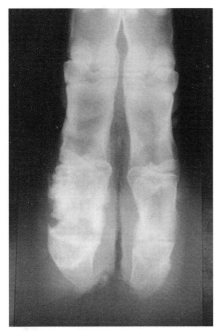

Figure 16–10. Radiograph 2 months after surgery for arthrodesis of the distal interphalangeal joint. The animal is sound at the walk and demonstrates effective bony bridging of the arthrodesis site.

A modification of this technique[15] advocates a different skin incision and not suturing the wound or using a drain for irrigation postoperatively. The results proved to be excellent in almost 80% of animals having surgery. Their complications included development of an ulcer beneath the block (8%) and wound infection (8%). Kersjes and colleagues[10] describe an approach to surgical joint fusion via a distal and dorsolateral approach and recommend preservation of the distal sesamoid bone.

Abaxial/Axial Approach. An approach to the joint through the abaxial wall is indicated if the retroarticular structures are not involved in the pathology. The site of original infection is then generally through the dorsal commissure of the interdigital space.

Clinical Signs. The presence of a granulating lesion on the edge of the dorsal commissure of the interdigital space should be considered as a possible entry site for joint infection. Edema and erythema arcund the dorsal surface of the digit adjacent to the coronary band are seen in such cases.

Technique. The patient is prepared for surgery, and the digit anesthetized. Using a 1.5-cm surgical drill, a channel is made through the joint from a point in the center of the abaxial wall 4 cm distal to the skin-horn junction. The drill is directed slightly proximad and dorsad so that the tip emerges at the fistula. The tissues in the center of the channel should be swabbed and evaluated for antibiotic sensitivity. A curette is then introduced into the channel, and both

the joint cartilage and a distal portion of the middle phalanx are removed.

A fenestrated tube drain is inserted through the channel (Fig. 16–11). The end of the tube emerging from the abaxial wall is folded over and secured. The digits are then bandaged and covered with adhesive tape.

The tube is then attached to a physiological saline reservoir and continuously irrigated for 2 to 4 days. The fluid escapes distally through a small hole cut in the bandage.

The bandage and tube should be removed not later than 4 days after surgery. The digits are then immobilized in a fiberglass cast to which a wear plate of methyl methacrylate is applied distally. A 4-cm-diameter opening may be left in the cast over the causative lesion to permit inspection and the injection of antibiotics into the channel if necessary. This window should be kept closed by a waterproof bandage between inspections.

Abaxial/Interbulbar Approach. This approach is indicated if a retroarticular abscess presents as a complication of ascending tracts from an abaxial white line lesion at the sole-heel junction. This complication may precede joint infection or may be associated with tenosynovitis of the deep flexor tendon sheath.

Clinical Signs. One heel typically is swollen and inflamed. This condition is frequently misdiagnosed as interdigital phlegmon. After prolonged antibiotic therapy, the case may be presented as non-resolving foot rot. Radiography may reveal a gas pocket in the heel region. Exploration of the white line reveals a tract that should be followed by removing adjacent wall. A fistula is usually revealed to be entering the heel.

Technique. The digit should be prepared for aseptic surgery. The retroarticular abscess should be entered by enlarging the opening of the sinus with a scalpel. The opening should be large enough to admit a finger. Palpation may reveal necrotic bone or other de-

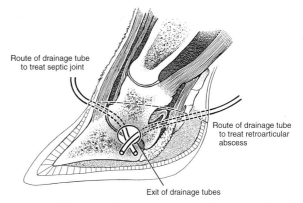

Figure 16–11. Schematic illustration of tube placement after drilling into the distal interphalangeal joint for the treatment of septic arthritis or a retroarticular abscess.

bris, in which case a modified plantar/palmar approach should be instituted.

If the abscess is uncomplicated, a probe should be directed through the cavity of the abscess and pressed into the axial wall of the bulb. An incision is cut down onto the probe, and a drainage/irrigation tube passed through the area. Continuous irrigation should be instituted as for the plantar/palmar approach. The tendon frequently is necrotic and avulsed. In such cases, the toe of one claw is hyperextended (turned-up toe). For this reason, blocking the sound claw and fixing the affected digit to it with wire and methyl methacrylate are appropriate. These cases invariably resolve rapidly and completely.

FRACTURES OF THE PROXIMAL AND MIDDLE PHALANX

INCIDENCE

Fractures of the proximal and middle phalanx are not common in cattle and are generally associated with slippery footing.

PATHOGENESIS

Because of the presence of ligamentous structures, thick and durable skin, and the fact that most injuries do not occur at speed, the fractures are usually closed.

CLINICAL SIGNS

Immediately after the traumatic incident, the animal appears to be very lame and may be totally non–weight-bearing. Pain is elicited on palpation, and visual and palpable abnormalities are identified. Radiography is required to characterize the fracture fully and to assess the appropriate treatment and prognosis.

TREATMENT

Although some phalangeal fractures may heal without treatment, reduction and stabilization of the affected region are strongly advised. Treatment is best accomplished by means of a plaster or fiberglass cast with a metal walking bar after physical and chemical restraint. It may be necessary to provide local anesthesia by means of intravenous injection distal to a tourniquet. The cast should completely incorporate the distal limb and extend to the proximal part of the metacarpal or metatarsal bone. The cast should be changed at 3- to 4-week intervals until healing takes place.

An alternative therapy is to elevate the sound digit with a wooden block affixed to the sole of the hoof. This removes many of the destabilizing forces that can act on the fracture site and allows the animal to produce exuberant callus, which can eventually result in a bony union of the fragments. It should be remembered, however, that the ligamentous association between the two digits continues to allow some movement at the level of the fractured bone. A low walking cast may supplement the wooden block to improve stability.

The prognosis is good for closed fractures that do not involve articular surfaces. Fractures that involve joints or are open have a poorer prognosis.

SEPTIC ARTHRITIS OF THE FETLOCK

INCIDENCE

Septic arthritis of the fetlock joint is more common in calves than in mature animals.

CLINICAL SIGNS

Most animals are presented within the first few months of life, and all breeds appear to be susceptible. Young animals usually have severe lameness and swelling of the affected fetlock. The skin over the swelling is warm and very sensitive to pressure. Older animals may not show the severe soft tissue swelling noted in younger animals, but the lameness is just as marked.

Radiographic examination confirms the obvious soft tissue swelling. In early cases, the joint space may not be grossly enlarged, but in more advanced cases the distance becomes increased and bony involvement may be apparent. Gas and fluid lines may be observed (Fig. 16–12).

TREATMENT

In the past, calves with septic arthritis of the fetlock were treated medically using antibiotics when the condition was diagnosed early in its course. Joint lavage was occasionally performed, particularly when the condition was more advanced. The success rate in such procedures is poor or moderate, and surgical intervention to remove infected and devitalized tissues should be considered when a few days of medical treatment alone proves to be inadequate.

ARTHROTOMY

Affected animals are administered appropriate systemic antibiotics before surgery. Anesthesia is accomplished by either general anesthetic or marked sedation with xylazine in combination with a local intravenous anesthetic of lidocaine applied distal to a tourniquet.

The metacarpophalangeal area of the affected limb is clipped and prepared for aseptic surgery in a rou-

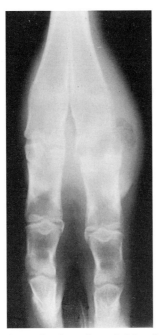

Figure 16–12. Radiograph of septic arthritis of the fetlock in a young calf. Note the presence of extensive soft tissue swelling, gas production, and destruction of cartilage and subchondral bone. The paired half of the fetlock remains free from the septic process.

tine manner. A lateral metacarpophalangeal arthrotomy is performed by making a 5-cm incision through the skin, subcutaneous tissue, and the joint capsule, at right angles to the axis of the limb. The joint space is opened up, and an initial irrigation carried out. The articular cartilage and all affected subchondral bone on the distal third and fourth metacarpal and proximal first phalangeal condyles are removed with number 4 curette (approximately 3 cm wide), and the joint is then lavaged with normal saline to remove all cartilage and bone fragments.

The joint capsule and the subcutaneous tissue are sutured in one layer using size 0 polyglycolic acid suture material in a simple continuous pattern followed by skin closure with size 1 nylon suture material in a cruciate pattern. After the arthrotomy incision is closed, a non-adhesive pad is placed over the suture line and a light bandage is applied, extending from the carpus down to the hoof.

Swelling around the fetlock is usually reduced within 24 to 48 hours. The affected limb is then cast from the level of the proximal metacarpus or metatarsus to the hoof. Standard cast management protocol is followed for the next 21 days, after which the cast is removed and a light bandage applied.

The curettage results in a clinically movable joint or a pseudoarthrosis. According to the classification established by Jubb and colleagues,[9] the simplest form of pseudoarthrosis occurs when a fibrous union between the two bones exists as a result of any cause. An extension of this case is the stage at which either fibrous or hyaline cartilage develops within the uniting fibrous tissue. In the highest stage of refinement of a pseudoarthrosis, clefts form in the cartilaginous

interface and a synovial-like tissue forms and lines the new joint, including capsular connective tissue on one surface and hyaline cartilage on the apposed surface. This final form of pseudoarthrosis may be termed a *neoarthrosis*. The foregoing sequence of events, if surgically induced, does not have the pathological connotations frequently associated with a pseudoarthrosis.

This "field quality" surgical procedure is clinically effective (Fig. 16–13) and economical and results in an animal's return to normal productivity.

ANGULAR DEFORMITY OF RADIOCARPAL AND TIBIOTARSAL JOINTS

DEFINITION

An angular deformity of the radiocarpal and tibiotarsal joints is defined as lateral deviation of the limb from the level of the carpus or hock distally.

INCIDENCE

Young growing animals from 1 to 7 months old are primarily affected. The condition is usually bilateral, but the relationship between angular deformity of the forelimbs and hind limbs is not known.

PATHOGENESIS

Trauma has been circumstantially implicated by some investigators.[1] Unlike other species in which

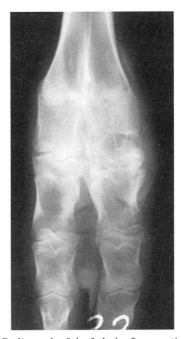

Figure 16–13. Radiograph of the fetlock after creation of a pseudo-arthrosis as a treatment for septic arthritis. Note the production of new bone around the joint. Although the joint appears to be fused, it is readily flexed, conformation is good, and the gait is normal.

angular deformities are recognizable in the early stages of the condition, cattle are considered to have a "normal" degree of medial deviation at the level of the carpus and hock, as well as normal external rotation of the lower limb, which would be considered to be abnormal in other species.[7] As a result, the condition tends to be missed in its mild forms or in early stages of development. Little if any work has been done to define factors resulting in angular deviation or to investigate the optimal time for corrective intervention.

CLINICAL SIGNS

The tentative diagnosis of angular limb deformity is made by clinically examining the limb for excessive lateral deviation from the level of the carpus. When viewed from the front, an affected animal appears to be knock-kneed. The area should be radiographed from the dorsopalmar view as described in Chapter 3. The degree of deviation is calculated from radiographs using the angle of intersection of the two lines representing the long axis of the greater metacarpal bone and the long axis of the radius. The level at which these lines intersect represents the source of the deviation and provides an objective measurement of the degree of angulation. The same radiographic view is used to evaluate the degree of correction of the deformity during or after treatment. Radiographs of the affected joints may reveal wedge-shaped distal radial epiphyses, with the narrow aspect of the wedge located laterally. A flared appearance is frequently seen in the distal radial physes and may also occur in other bones. The deviation distal to the carpus is usually lateral, hence, the term *carpal valgus* is applied to the condition. Cattle have a complete ulna.

TREATMENT

Treatment of the deviation is undertaken by any one or a combination of protocols and depends in part on the degree of potential growth remaining in the distal radial physis, because all methods except wedge osteotomy rely on altering growth rates of the medial and lateral physeal regions to produce a normal shape of the distal radial epiphysis and to correct the deviation.

Very young animals may return to a normal conformation after corrective trimming of the hoof. To correct a lateral deviation, the outer claw is trimmed shorter than the medial claw. Straightening and derotation of the limb result. Because very young animals may not have adequate hoof wall for effective trimming, the same effect may be produced by putting methyl methacrylate onto the weight-bearing surface of the medial claw.

Tube casts, which extend from the pastern to the proximal radius, have been used as a means of straightening the limb, with variable results.

Technique for Periosteal Stripping

The technique of periosteal stripping is borrowed from equine practice and is effective in early cases of angular limb deformation. For valgus deviations, a curved incision, with the base of the flap directed dorsally, is made on the concave (lateral) side of the limb over the radiocarpal joint. The soft tissues are dissected to expose the periosteum, which is incised vertically for 5 cm proximal to the level of the distal radial physis. The periosteum is then transected at right angles to the first incision for approximately 150°, and the flaps thus created are elevated to maximize periosteal mobility. The periosteum is usually seen to retract within minutes of transection. The axial tension on the periosteum is thus released, and the wound is closed by a simple continuous pattern involving subcutaneous tissues. The skin is closed in a separate layer. The wound is bandaged for 1 week. No further treatment is required because the limb cannot correct past the normal degree of angulation.

Technique for Transphyseal Bridging

Transphyseal bridging is performed in more severe cases or in animals thought to be past the rapid growth phase of the radius and ulna.[1] This technique is recommended for animals older than 5 months. The objective is to slow growth on the medial aspect of the limb by restricting growth of the distal radial physis.

A curved incision is made on the medial aspect of the limb at the level of the distal radius, the base of the skin flap facing dorsally. The soft tissues are reflected, and the distal radial physis located by inserting an 18-gauge needle into the growth plate and confirming its position radiographically. Using the needle as a landmark, a 4.5-mm cortical screw is placed in the epiphysis and diaphysis and a single or double figure-of-eight wire is placed and tightened. The screws are then set to tighten the wire further and minimize protrusion. The subcutaneous tissues and skin are closed separately, and a light bandage is applied for 1 week. The implants must be removed when the limb achieves normal conformation to prevent the development of a varus (bowlegged) deformity. Periosteal stripping is frequently performed at the same time to increase the possibility of full correction in animals with severe deviations or in animals nearing the end of their radial growth phase.

Technique of Wedge Osteotomy

Wedge osteotomy of the radius may be performed in advanced cases of deformity or in cases with deviation due to trauma and malunion.[5] The site and orientation of the wedge should be determined by careful clinical and radiographic examination. The limb must be stabilized by internal fixation by plate and screws for an extended postoperative period.

FRACTURES OF THE METACARPAL AND METATARSAL BONES

INCIDENCE

Fractures of the greater metacarpal and metatarsal bones may account for 50% or more of all fractures encountered. The forelimb is more commonly involved. In beef areas, the majority of cases involve newborn calves. This incidence reflects the management practices associated with dystocia.

ETIOLOGY AND PATHOGENESIS

Fetal extraction with excessive forelimb traction causes a significant number of fractures. The majority of metacarpal breaks occur in the distal diaphysis just above the growth plate. The most serious complicating factor in neonates is the soft tissue damage and resultant interference with vascular supply distal to the fracture site caused by the use of calving chains. When circulation to the distal limb is seriously compromised, the prognosis becomes poor or grave, although many limbs have healed successfully by the process of delayed union (Fig. 16–14).

CLINICAL SIGNS

Diagnosing these fractures is very simple because of the obvious lameness and angular deformity at the

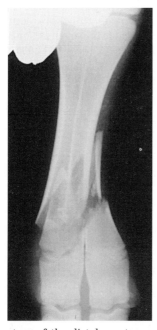

Figure 16–14. Fracture of the distal greater metacarpal bone at the level of chain application during forced extraction for dystocia. Although such views cannot be used to evaluate vascular supply to the distal limb, moderate to severe trauma to the major vessels should be expected and delayed healing anticipated. With complete vascular disruption, the distal limb undergoes ischemic necrosis.

fracture site. Swelling, edema, and pain occur in the region. If considerable time has elapsed before fixation can be applied, it may be necessary to apply a tension/support bandage to provide temporary support and reduce the swelling before placing the final external fixation apparatus. It is important to establish whether or not the animal received adequate passive immunity, because most calves with fractures are unable to suck unassisted, and the incidence of infectious disease compromises the overall success rate.

TREATMENT

In the vast majority of cases in newborn calves, external fixation by cast provides the necessary stabilization for healing. Only rarely is internal fixation required. Newborn calves fare very well with plaster casts, provided that the postoperative environment is kept dry and clean.

Older animals also fare well in plaster casts if walking bars are incorporated into the fixation to add strength, reduce wear and cast weight, and facilitate ambulation. Fiberglass casts reach maximum strength almost immediately, are much more resistant to breaking when used on larger animals, and are not affected by moist conditions. They are not resistant to abrasion, however, and may require methyl methacrylate, wood, rubber, or a metal walking bar to prevent destruction of the bottom of the cast when the animal walks on concrete or other abrasive surfaces. The significant difference in the cost of plaster and fiberglass casting materials is an economic consideration in the selection of cast materials.

Casts must generally be replaced every 3 weeks in young calves but may remain in place for 4 to 6 weeks in slower growing, more mature animals. Uncomplicated fractures usually have two or three casts applied. In the case of vascular compromise, the healing process should be rigorously monitored radiographically and casts applied accordingly.

If internal fixation is required, the use of 6.5-mm cancellous screws in both the metaphyseal and diaphyseal regions of the bone is advocated.[11]

Fractures that occur shortly after birth as a result of trauma by the dam or other factors usually have a favorable prognosis unless the site is open and subsequently becomes infected. Many of these cases involve the distal physis and may be classified as Salter-Harris type I or II fractures. Calves have a great ability to produce periosteal new bone and very quickly produce a substantial callus. Healthy, well-vascularized bones heal to functional union as early as 3 weeks after the original incident and usually do not result in abnormal conformation of the limb in types I and II fractures. Older, heavier animals have a somewhat less favorable prognosis.[18]

Older animals frequently have midshaft metacarpal and metatarsal fractures. The cause is invariably trauma. These bones are often comminuted and may be obviously open or at least have an adjacent skin defect. Comminution alone does not create any major problems, apart from a tendency for more prolonged healing. These cases may require internal fixation devices to assist the healing process, particularly because the incidence of comminution appears to be higher in this age group. Because of the size of the animal and the extreme forces generated, single or double plating is recommended using 4.5- or 5.5-mm screws.[3, 19] In addition, external support devices may be applied for the recovery period or longer when the integrity of the internal fixation system is questionable. The clinical result using double plates in mature cattle is usually excellent, and double plates are highly recommended whenever financial circumstances permit.

FLEXURAL DEFORMITIES OF THE DISTAL LIMB

PATHOGENESIS AND ETIOLOGY

Not all calves with contracted tendons are candidates for corrective intervention (Fig. 16–15). When the etiology involves arthrogryposis or lupine ingestion by the dam, surgical procedures are not recommended. Many calves, that are born normally have some carpal flexion associated with taut flexor tendons that prevent the extension of the limb by the animal or stockperson. Such cases usually appear sporadically and without apparent cause. The abnormality is usually considered to be an expression of a form of complex, recessive inheritance or is associated with a physical or nutritional cause *in utero*.

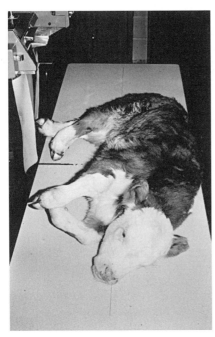

Figure 16–15. Flexural deformities in a calf with multiple joints affected. Such animals are not candidates for surgical correction.

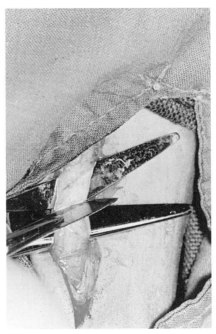

Figure 16–16. Contracted tendons in a calf. The superficial flexor tendon has been isolated and is being transected. Care must be taken to preserve vascular supply to the limb, because major vessels are closely associated with the tendons.

CLINICAL SIGNS

Flexion of the distal limb can have a wide range of manifestations and degrees of involvement. The spectrum of flexural deformities of the limb is wide and ranges from slight flexion of the limb at the level of the fetlock or carpus to severe contraction of the limbs, involvement of more than one joint of each limb, and an element of outward rotation.

Owners may report that the animal was normal at birth but developed the flexural deformity within hours or a few days. This deformity frequently occurs in association with an incidental condition that results in an inability to stand normally in the neonatal period. The forelimbs are more commonly affected.

TREATMENT

The method of treatment and prognosis depends largely on the severity of the flexural deformity and the amount of rotation of the limb. The more extensive the deformities, the more invasive is the corrective procedure and the poorer the prognosis. Mildly affected calves may recover spontaneously provided they are robust, have good footing, and are able to spend extended periods in the standing position, resulting in stretching of the flexor tendons.

The treatment for animals unable to bear weight on the toe of the digit and thus apply tension on the tendons is directed to splinting the limb from the level of the proximal radius to the fetlock distally.

Ideally, the distal limb should be left unsupported and is allowed to extend under the pressure of weight-bearing. If the fetlock joint is also contracted, the full limb may be included in the splint. Application of such a splint for 24 hours usually results in stretching of the tendons to the point where the claws can be left out of the bandage to serve a more physiological role. Splints should be changed on a daily to twice-daily basis and applied with enough tension to produce a non-contracted limb within 2 to 3 days. A simple and effective splint can be made from appropriately sized polyvinyl chloride (PVC) tubing cut in half and padded to prevent chafing of the limb. When both forelimbs are involved, the calf may initially require assistance to stand.

When rotation is present, a functional splint is difficult to maintain. In such cases, an alternative is to fatigue and then manually extend the limb and incorporate it in a plaster cast. In such instances, care should be taken to ensure that no pressure points occur at the skin-cast interface.

In more severely affected animals, surgical transection of the flexor tendons may be required to allow for extension of the limb. These animals warrant a more guarded prognosis and require a splint or cast applied to support and control the limb after surgery. The animal is first sedated with xylazine, 0.1 to 0.2 mg/kg of body weight IM, and the limb is clipped and surgically prepared and draped for surgery. After local instillation of local anesthetic, the limb is extended to allow palpation of the flexor tendons. The tendons are bluntly isolated via a medial or lateral incision, with care taken not to include the vascular supply to the digit, which is in close association with the tendons. With the tendons thus visualized (Fig. 16–16), the superficial flexor tendon is first transected, and the limb evaluated for improvement. The deep flexor tendon may also be transected if necessary. Deeper structure such as the suspensory apparatus or the carpal joint capsule may occasionally interfere with full extension and must therefore be cut to provide full range of motion of the limb. Padded PVC tubing may be applied over a bandage and changed daily.

Even this extensive surgery sometimes does not permit full extension of the forelimb, and although skeletal abnormality of the carpal bones may be suspected, radiography has consistently failed to demonstrate any such congenital changes.

REFERENCES

1. Adams SB, Amstutz HE: Surgical correction of angular limb deformity of the forelimbs of a seven month old calf. Vet Surg 12:58–61, 1983.
2. Antalovsky A: Technik der intravenösen lokalen Schmerzausschaltung im distalen Gliedmassenbereich beim Rind. Vet Med (Prague) 7:413–420, 1965.
3. Auer JA, Steiner A, Iselin U, Lischer C: Internal fixation of long bone fractures in farm animals. VCOT 6:36–41, 1993.
4. Baxter GM, Lakritz J, Wallace CE, et al: Alternatives to digit amputation in cattle. Comp Cont Ed Pract Vet Food Anim Pract 13:1022–1035, 1991.
5. Edinger H, Kofler J, Ebner J: Angular limb deformity in a calf treated with periosteotomy and wedge osteotomy. Vet Rec 2:245–246, 1995.
6. Gagnon H, Ferguson JG, Papich M, Bailey JV: Single-dose pharmacokinetics of cefazolin in bovine synovial fluid after intravenous regional injection. J Vet Pharmacol Ther 17:31–37, 1994.
7. Getty R: In Sisson S, Grossman JD (eds): The Anatomy of the Domestic Animals, vol 1, 5th ed. Philadelphia, WB Saunders, 1975, p 751.
8. Greenough PR, Ferguson J: Alternatives to amputation. Vet Clin North Am Food Anim Pract 1:195–204, 1985.
9. Jubb KVF, Kennedy PC, Palmer N: San Diego, Pathology of Domestic Animals, Academic Press, 1993, p95.
10. Kersjes AW, Nemeth F, Rutgers LJE: Atlas of Large Animal Surgery. Baltimore, Williams & Wilkins, 1985.
11. Kirpensteijn J, St.-Jean G, Roush JK, et al: Holding power of orthopaedic screws in metacarpal and metatarsal bones in young calves. VCOT 5:100–103, 1992.
12. Kofler J: Zur Therapie der Arthritis Infectiosa Articulationis Interphalangeae Distalis beim Rind: Vergleich der Operations-methoden "Amputation im Kronbein" und "Exartickulation im Krongelenk" (inaugural dissertation). Vienna, Veterinary Medical University of Vienna, 1988.
13. Miskimins D: Bovine toe abscesses. Proceedings of the 8th International Symposium on Disorders of the Ruminant Digit. Banff, Canada, 1994.
14. Müller K: Resection of the tip of the bovine claw. Tierarztl Prax 12:1112–1113, 1991.
15. Nuss K, Weaver MP: Resection of the distal interphalangeal joint in cattle: An alternative to amputation. Vet Rec 128:540–543, 1992.
16. Osman MAR: A study of some sequelae of amputation of the digit using three operative techniques. Vet Rec 87:610–615, 1970.
17. Petzoldt FJ: Fractures of the distal phalanx in the bovine (inagural dissertation, Faculty of Veterinary Medicine). Munich, Germany, Ludwig-Maximilians-Universität, 1985.
18. Steiner A, Iselin U, Auer JA, Lischer CJ: Physeal fractures of the metacarpus and metatarsus in cattle. VCOT 6:131–137, 1993.
19. Steiner A, Iselin U, Auer JA, Lischer CJ: Shaft fractures of the metacarpus and metatarsus in cattle. VCOT 6:138–145, 1993.
20. Steiner A, Ossent P, Mathis GA: Intravenous regional anesthesia and antibiotic therapy applied to the limbs of cattle: Indications, techniques, and complications. Schweiz Arch Tierheilkd 132:227–237, 1990.
21. Trent AM, Plumb D: Treatment of infectious arthritis and osteomyelitis. Vet Clin North Am 7:747–778, 1991.
22. Weaver AD: Performing amputation of the bovine digit. Vet Med 86:1230–1233, 1991.

James G. Ferguson *Canada*

17

Surgical Conditions of the Proximal Limb

SURGICAL TREATMENT OF SEPTIC ARTHRITIS OF THE CARPUS

The definition, etiology, clinical signs, and diagnosis of septic arthritis of the carpus are discussed in Chapter 11.

The majority of infected carpi are treated conservatively in the early disease stages by systemic antibiotic administration or, less frequently, by joint lavage using large-bore needles with or without joint distention. Joint irrigation is directed at removal of organisms, debris, and products of inflammation that contribute to joint destruction. The more effective technique of joint lavage with or without synovial resection by means of arthroscopic intervention is not commonly used owing to its cost, lack of necessary equipment, or unfamiliarity with the technique. As a result, many animals are presented for treatment in advanced stages of septic arthritis with extensive hard and soft tissue involvement.

Conservative therapies often fail because of inherent problems related to the complex structure of the carpal joint and because of the difficulties in flushing organisms from the synovial tissues and other soft tissues associated with the infected joint.[27]

In a 5-year study[28] of surgical and conservative treatment of septic arthritides in several joints, surgical intervention almost doubled the chances of recovery of animals with severely infected joints. Surgical treatment is directed at removal of infected and devitalized structures and stabilization of the joint to facilitate the repair process.

The surgical procedure depends on the extent and invasiveness of the septic process, and both have a direct bearing on the success rate. Selection of the appropriate technique requires careful clinical and radiographic examination to determine the extent of invasiveness required to produce joint arthrodesis. The carpal joint is approached from the cranial aspect by means of a transverse incision that transects all structures including skin, extensor tendons, and periarticular soft tissue to expose the interior of the joint. Flexion of the carpus provides increased visibility and access to the articular structures and synovial recesses of the site. The incision may be modified

to provide entry to the area of primary involvement of the joint. When the disease process is limited to synovial tissues and articular cartilage, synovectomy and resection of articular cartilage controls infection and promotes arthrodesis. When carpal bones are infected, a single row or both rows of bones are removed to maintain correct limb alignment (Fig. 17–1). After lavage and skin closure, the limb is cast from the elbow distally, including the complete digit.

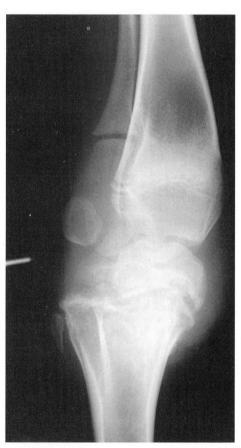

Figure 17–1. Lateral radiograph of the carpus of a heifer calf treated for septic arthritis by removal of the distal row of carpal bones 7 weeks previously. Note that fusion is almost complete and swelling is minimal. This animal was fertile and able to perform normally in pasture conditions.

A cast should provide support for at least 3 weeks. When both rows of carpal bones are removed, it is advisable to compress the remaining osseous tissues with transfixation pins and to include the device and the limb in a cast. The cast should be changed regularly until 5 months postoperatively. Analgesics should always be given to provide pain relief and to facilitate healing. The process of arthrodesis may be monitored on the basis of clinical and radiographic findings.

Appropriate techniques lead to a good success rate, even for chronic cases of septic carpal arthritis, particularly in animals requiring only moderate surgical intervention.

FRACTURES OF THE RADIUS AND ULNA

DEFINITION

Most fractures of the mid-forelimb of cattle involve both the radius and ulna. It is less common for either the radius or ulna to be affected alone. Concomitant fracture of both bones is attributed to the fact that the ulna is complete in cattle and that the radius and ulna are in close contact throughout their length through a strong interosseous ligament along the shaft and firm attachments distally. Although these fractures are encountered at any age, younger animals are most commonly affected.

ETIOLOGY

Trauma is always a factor. Owners frequently implicate other animals, although most animals are not observed at the time of injury. Very young animals may be stepped on, older animals may be caught in mechanical devices or rigid fencing, or other forces of unknown origin may be the cause.

CLINICAL SIGNS

Animals with radial and ulnar fractures exhibit a severe, non–weight-bearing lameness with obvious swelling over the affected site. The limb may appear deviated and is usually very painful on palpation. Crepitus is commonly evident when the limb is manipulated. Although skin abrasions may occur in such cases, the majority of animals do not have open fractures of these bones. Most fractures are in the mid to distal radial diaphysis.

DIAGNOSIS

The diagnosis is readily made on the basis of overt clinical signs. Radiographic evaluation is useful in further characterizing the fracture in terms of its location, degree of comminution, appropriate types of treatment, and prognostic criteria.

TREATMENT AND POSTOPERATIVE CARE

The radius is considered to be the main weight-bearing component and as such is more important in internal fixation procedures. The ulna is stabilized only when it is the only element of the pair that is affected (e.g., proximal ulnar fractures). A wide variety of methods have been used to stabilize radial and ulnar fractures. External fixation devices such as Thomas-Schroeder splints,[1] modified Robert Jones bandages with supplemental rigid splintage, walking casts with transfixation pins,[17] and other external fixators have been reported to be effective in selected cases. The type of transfixation pinning and cast length depend on the location of the fracture relative to the radiohumeral and radiocarpal joints. Casts or splints that bridge the elbow, carpal, or fetlock joints result in some temporary stiffness and reduction in joint mobility for a few weeks after removal of the external fixation device. Short casts combined with transfixation pins may provide adequate fixation without interfering with carpal function during the healing period.[20] Whenever transfixation pins or plates are applied, anesthesia and close attention to sterile technique are required. The Thomas-Schroeder splint may be the method of choice, particularly in younger animals, despite the difficulties in its construction, application, and maintenance, because it can be applied and adjusted without the need for general anesthesia.

Internal fixation of the radial fracture remains the most effective method for complete alignment and fixation of the radius when economics permit. General anesthesia is required, along with a full complement of broad orthopedic plates and 4.5- or 5.5-mm cortical screws. Cancellous screws may be used in the most distal holes of the plate. The ulna may interfere somewhat with reduction of the radius but need not be included in the fixation system because its periosteal response usually results in a synostosis at the fracture site. In growing animals with very distal shaft fractures in which a limited amount of diaphysis is available for plate application and screw placement, it is possible to extend the plate across the radial physis and apply one or more screws into the epiphysis to stabilize the fracture adequately (Fig. 17–2). Although this contravenes basic orthopedic principles, adverse effects have not been observed in several cases provided that the screws in the epiphysis are removed within 3 to 4 weeks. This technique provides for more rigid fixation in the critical immediate postoperative period. The screws may be removed under sedation and local anesthesia. Larger animals may require application of more than one plate or supplemental use of external support.

Postoperative care for patients with external or internal fixation devices involves proper bedding, non-slippery flooring, and restricted exercise.

PROGNOSIS

The prognosis for young animals with internal fixation is very favorable. Older or fractious animals

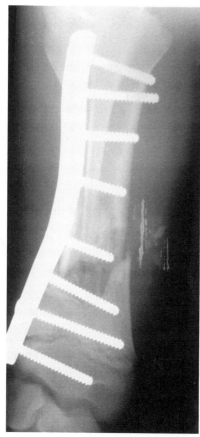

Figure 17–2. Reduction and fixation of a comminuted radial and ulnar fracture in a calf. Owing to the distal location of the fracture, the most distal screw was placed in the epiphysis (bridging the distal radial physis) to obtain stability of the fixation system. The distal screw was removed 6 weeks after reduction, and angular deformity or shortening of the limb did not result.

may exceed the capabilities of the implants unless additional support is provided. Effective use of the Thomas-Schroeder splint requires careful construction and knowledgeable application techniques to fully meet the potential of this modality.

HUMERAL FRACTURES

Fractures of the humerus account for about 5% of all fractures in cattle. The majority of cases involve either young calves or young bulls at pasture. Females from the breeding herd are less commonly affected. Although the cause of the fracture in individual animals is frequently unknown, in young calves it is thought to be related to trauma inflicted by other adult animals, including the dam, or contact with moving machinery. Young bulls may fracture the humerus as a result of inexperienced breeding activity, primarily during mounting or dismounting. A history of the affected animal's fighting with herd mates or intruding bulls is occasionally reported. The typical case is a spiral midshaft fracture relating to the spiral anatomy of the bone. Because of the relatively large muscle mass, the fragment ends are overriding,

and early surgery is needed for successful reduction. This is particularly true in larger animals. The radial nerve is usually involved either because of the initial trauma or as a result of secondary trauma due to overriding bone ends or swelling, edema, and inflammation in the immediate area of the fracture. Because the radial nerve innervates all extensors of the elbow, carpus, and digit, the limb cannot support weight unless the fetlock is extended manually or by a support device.[6]

CLINICAL SIGNS

Affected animals demonstrate severe lameness, localized swelling, and pain on manipulation. Some animals bear a limited amount of weight if the fetlock is manually extended. Examination usually reveals some degree of crepitation. An obvious lateral movement at the level of the mid-humeral region is evident when the distal limb is abducted by the examiner. The exact location of the fracture may be difficult to determine by palpation in larger animals. The neurological deficit is largely responsible for the clinical profile. The carpus and digits are in a flexed position, and the elbow is carried lower (dropped) as a result of loss of triceps muscle function. The animal may have difficulty in advancing the limb. Analgesia to the cranial and lateral aspects of the antebrachium and to the dorsal digit is usually noted.

Diagnosis is based on the clinical signs related to the neurological deficit as well as findings on manipulation and palpation. Lateral radiographs of the upper limb confirm the diagnosis. In heavy animals, radiographs are taken with the animal sedated and restrained in lateral recumbency with the affected limb down and drawn forward. The radiographic film is placed under the fracture site, and the beam is directed from medial to lateral. Anterior-to-posterior radiographs are not readily obtainable except in smaller animals. The typical fracture configuration has the proximal segment overriding the distal component cranially. In severe cases, the flexor surface of the elbow joint may become compromised by the displaced proximal bone end.

TREATMENT

Treatment options are related to the animal's value, size, and temperament, the duration of the fracture, and the long-term expectations of the owner.

Most animals heavier than 250 kg are difficult to treat successfully because of the larger muscle mass overlying the lateral aspect of the upper limb. The fracture ends prove difficult to reduce if the fracture is several days old. Such fractures heal well if the animal is confined to a small box stall for several weeks while a substantial callus forms. It is important to prevent trauma to and contraction of the flexed fetlock by means of a firm support wrap. Restriction to a small area prevents breakdown of the contralateral limb during the healing period. Severe overriding may reduce the range of motion of the elbow, giving a poorer prognosis. Animals left to heal without internal or external fixation begin to bear weight within 2 weeks and progressively become functionally mobile within 2 or 3 months. Radiographic evaluation shows exuberant, extensive callus formation and a degree of axial or rotational deviation. However, as a salvage procedure, this conservative form of treatment is a viable alternative to immediate euthanasia or slaughter due to inability to reduce the fracture (Fig. 17–3). The neurological deficit usually disappears within a few weeks.

Surgical intervention may be indicated in valuable animals or in older, larger individuals that the owners are not interested in salvaging for slaughter. When young animals are presented for repair shortly after the fracture has occurred, the prognosis is usually very good.[21] A lateral approach to the humerus may be used to reduce and fix the fracture site. Recommended implants are 4.5- or 5.5-mm lag screws or cerclage wires or a combination. Because most calves protect the traumatized limb and healing takes place quickly, such internal fixation is both effective and economical. Healing occurs within 6 weeks, and the implants are not usually removed.

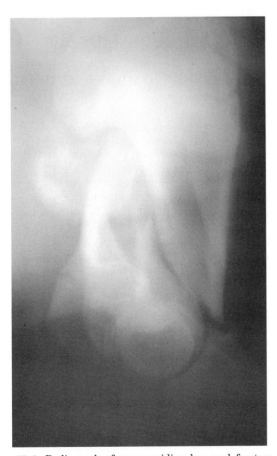

Figure 17–3. Radiograph of an overriding humeral fracture in a 400-kg bull calf approximately 2 weeks after onset. Despite general anesthesia and aggressive mechanical intervention, it was impossible to reduce this fracture. Note the position of the proximal fragment relative to the elbow joint and the periosteal reaction on the caudal aspect of the fracture line.

A lateral humeral approach does not provide adequate exposure for reduction and application of internal fixation devices in mature, well-muscled animals. A cranial approach has been reported by Rakestraw and coworkers.[18] The reported advantages of this approach include adequate access to the most common fracture sites, the ability to apply a long plate over most of the length of the humerus, and the potential for placement of more than one plate in larger animals. Although extensive dissection is needed to expose the humerus, this approach for compression plating should be considered in larger animals. Calves with limited muscle mass do not require a cranial approach for the application of cerclage wires or lag screws to the humeral midshaft area.

CONDITIONS OF THE SCAPULAR REGION

Conditions of the bovine shoulder and scapular region are uncommon and have not been well documented in the literature. Veterinarians must therefore rely on diagnostic and treatment options used in other species. Owners frequently present animals for treatment of a "shoulder problem," but the cause is more likely to be a digital lesion. Fractures of the scapula, dislocations of the scapulohumeral joint, and injury to the soft tissues of the region are responsible for most shoulder problems.

Rare fractures may involve the glenoid, neck, or body of the scapula. They tend to be due to direct trauma to the shoulder region by strong forces (motor vehicle accidents, cyclones, and contact with other, larger animals). Signs of scapular fracture include severe lameness, localized swelling, and crepitus. Diagnosis is based on clinical signs and radiographic evaluation. Roentgenological examination is difficult in larger animals. The best results are obtained with posterior-to-anterior oblique views. Only in smaller animals can diagnostic radiographs be produced from lateral projections.

Fractures of the body of the scapula are difficult to treat with external or internal fixation and heal spontaneously without support after enforced stall rest. Internal fixation with various plating techniques might be attempted in exceptional instances in cattle, but most fractures of the body of the scapula can be conservatively treated with acceptable results.

Fractures of the scapular neck should be handled conservatively. Implants are difficult to place, the fragments are resistant to reduction, and implant strength is inadequate to counteract the large biomechanical forces. Articular fractures have a dismal prognosis, and salvage by slaughter is recommended.

Luxation of the scapulohumeral joint is rare in cattle. Manipulative reduction has been successful in some cases. It is suggested that an open surgical approach be used to reduce and stabilize the joint following small animal techniques.

CONDITIONS AFFECTING THE HOCK

The hock joint is composed of the tarsometatarsal, distal intertarsal, proximal intertarsal, tarsocrural, and tibiotarsal joints. Fractures and dislocations of the hock joint are relatively common despite the paucity of relevant veterinary publications.

Luxations of various components of the tarsus may occur as a single condition or may be associated with a fracture of one or more tarsal bones.

Fractures and fracture-dislocations may involve any of the bones of the hock, but fracture-dislocation of the tibiotarsal bones has the most guarded prognosis. Fracture of the fibulotarsal bone is occasionally encountered in cattle.

Affected animals have a severe, non–weight-bearing lameness. Minimal swelling is noted initially, but within a few hours the region becomes distended and warm. Obvious instability and angular displacement are observed on manipulation or on attempting to walk. Crepitus is evident in the region of the fracture. Welker and coworkers[30] reported on two animals with tarsal fractures that caused the affected limbs to be locked in flexion by lodging of the fracture fragments within the joint. The fractures or luxations are caused by strong traumatic forces, although the inciting incident is rarely observed unless it is associated with farm vehicle misadventure.

Diagnosis of hock fractures is made by clinical signs and confirmed by radiography (Fig. 17–4). The prognosis can vary considerably. Valuable information may be provided by careful examination of a complete set of radiographs that characterize the fracture from several views.

Treatment of tarsal fractures has been described for certain situations. Fracture of the fibulotarsal bone may be repaired with wires using the tension band principle.[6] Immobilization by means of full leg casts or Thomas-Schroeder splints has been suggested by Tulleners,[26] who cautioned about the possible development of stiffness, pain, degenerative arthritis, and periarticular fibrosis. A tarsal bone fracture occasionally may, by virtue of its configuration, lend itself to repair by interfragmentary compression, although this has not yet been described in cattle.

TIBIAL FRACTURES

Fractures of the tibia in cattle are relatively common; one unpublished survey reported a 12% incidence of all fractures encountered.[6] All ages may be affected, from newborn calves to mature breeding animals. One unusual case is of a healed intrauterine tibial fracture.[4] Considerable forces are always required to disrupt the integrity of the bone. Young animals may be stepped on by the dam or other larger herd animals. Mature cattle have been seen to fracture the tibia during attempts to escape confinement when they try to accelerate and step on a slippery surface. Adult bulls are reported to have broken the tibia

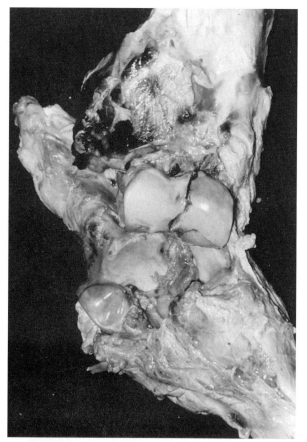

Figure 17–4. Fracture of the talus of a mature cow. The minimally displaced fragments are contained within reactive periarticular fibrous tissue.

during fighting. Contact with farm power implements and highway vehicles is also a potential cause. Because of the magnitude of the initiating forces, the size and temperament of the animal, and the transportation problems involved, the bone is frequently comminuted (Fig. 17–5). The fracture site may be open unless support devices such as a Thomas-Schroeder splint are applied soon after the fracture has occurred and before transportation. One advantage that cattle have over some other species is that their relatively thick skin serves as a protective barrier and usually prevents the fracture from becoming open.

Clinical signs of tibial fractures are relatively obvious: swelling, pain, non–weight-bearing, and usually excess mobility distal to the fracture site. The fracture location is best determined by palpation medially. Crepitus can be felt and auscultated with manipulation in most animals. The diagnosis, suggested treatment, and prognosis are based on radiographic evaluation and clinical signs, particularly when the break involves the proximal or distal ends of the tibia (Fig. 17–6). Luxations and fractures may be difficult to differentiate on clinical examination alone. The distinction is even more critical when the fracture incorporates the articular surface. The posterior aspect of the tibial plateau may occasionally sustain casts of plaster or fiberglass may also produce favorable results and allow for a degree of flexibility in pin placement, which may be an advantage over the less versatile external fixator systems[21] and compression plating modalities. The majority of tibial fractures treated by plating or transfixation pinning heal satisfactorily provided that good sterile orthopedic techniques are used.

Because of the great healing potential of bovine bone, even suboptimal treatment regimens can result in satisfactory healing of tibial fractures. Judicious use of a Thomas-Schroeder type of splint, primarily an emergency management tool, can provide enough support for healing of tibial fractures, particularly in animals weighing less than 150 kg. Success has been recorded in animals heavier than 350 kg,[9] but caution is advised when using splints in animals approaching this weight. The advantages of this type of treatment are that sterile surgical facilities are not required, plans and materials for splint construction are readily available, and adjustments to the splint may be made in the postoperative period. Disadvantages include the lack of rigid support for the fracture, pressure sores associated with weight-bearing surfaces of the splint, and ambulation difficulties. A Thomas-Schroeder type of splint and casts are recognized as useful forms of supplemental support to internal fixation during the immediate postopera-

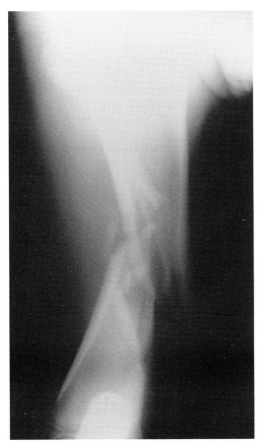

Figure 17–5. Radiograph of a severely comminuted tibial fracture in a mature bull. Because of the bull's size and difficult temperament, a decision was made to send the animal to slaughter rather than to repair the fracture.

fractures from abnormal femoral forces acting in the stifle joint in animals with rupture of the cranial cruciate ligament (Fig. 17–7).

Treatment of tibial fractures begins with immobilization of the limb before transporting the animal to a veterinary facility. This is best accomplished by means of an external splint that fully controls the limb from above the stifle to the digit. In the author's opinion, the best device is a Thomas-Schroeder splint, which, despite its difficult construction, is a sound investment. Once the limb has been splinted and radiographed, the most appropriate method of repair may be considered in a non-emergency framework.

The best repair technique for tibial fracture is internal fixation using plates and screws.[29] Compression plating using appropriate biomechanical principles produces the most stable fixation with the earliest return to function. When economics and facilities allow, these techniques are the methods of choice. Younger, lighter animals may require only one plate, whereas older, heavier cattle may need two or even three plates to provide the necessary support (Fig. 17–8). Plating is highly recommended when the fracture is open and osteomyelitis is a likely complication of bone healing. Transfixation pinning in conjunction with external fixators[10] or

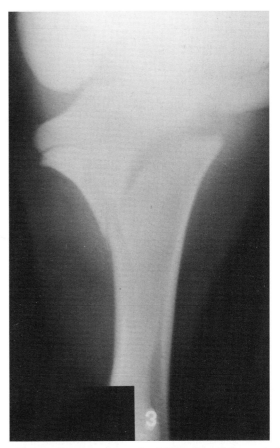

Figure 17–6. Radiograph of a proximal tibia of a calf demonstrating a Salter-Harris type II fracture configuration. This fracture was successfully repaired by means of a Thomas-Schroeder splint.

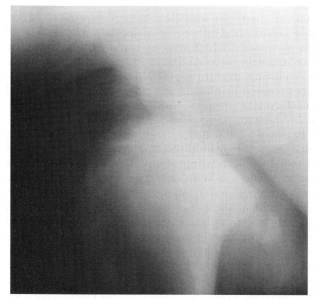

Figure 17–7. Radiograph of the stifle of a bull with anterior (cranial) cruciate ligament rupture. Fracture fragments from the posterior aspect of the tibial plateau are caused by weight-bearing of the femur on the cranially displaced tibia.

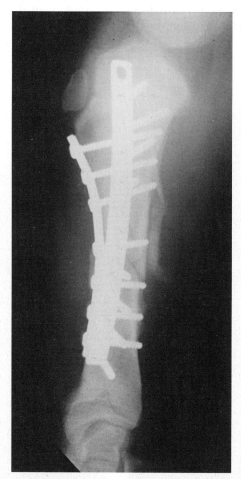

Figure 17–8. Radiograph of an open comminuted tibial fracture in a mature cow. Several plates were used to stabilize the fracture, and successful healing resulted despite a protracted convalescence.

tive period. With the possible exception of very distal tibial fractures, casts are not appropriate as a sole means of stabilization of this bone.

Not all tibial fractures are amenable to repair when economics, the animal's size or temperament, humane aspects, and fracture type are considered. When adult animals with good salvage value, severely comminuted fractures, and temperaments that interfere with postoperative treatment and preservation of fixation devices are presented for treatment, it is wise to consider slaughter.

STIFLE JOINT

The stifle joint is a complex structure from the anatomical and biomechanical points of view, and a thorough knowledge of its physical makeup is essential for effective understanding of both problems and potential solutions associated with treatment of disease conditions. Understanding the functional implications of radiographic examination, surgical procedures, and arthroscopic manipulations requires a working knowledge of the region. The stifle still provides a challenge to those who have not made a point of frequent dissection and review of the joint. Some inaccuracies in the veterinary literature regarding the meniscal and ligamentous anatomy further confuse readers.

From a gross clinical perspective, the stifle does not seem to reveal much information on palpation. However, the investigator should take every opportunity to examine this region in healthy animals of different ages, weights, and breeds. Fine-boned young dairy cows have an obvious tibial crest; middle, medial, and lateral patellar ligaments; non-distended medial and lateral synovial compartments; and patellar outline on palpation. These features are frequently more difficult to delineate in older dairy cattle and in mature beef animals. Mature bulls, because of their greater size and muscle/tendon mass, are the most difficult to palpate accurately. Acute trauma or inflammation of the joint is demonstrated by an inability to identify the patellar ligaments readily or by diffuse swelling of the synovial cavities between these ligaments. Later production of periarticular fibrous and connective tissue may totally prevent palpation of any normal anatomical structures.

Radiographic studies provide considerable information about even large individuals if restraint permits proper placement of the cassette and adequate exposure times. The cassettes can frequently be placed high enough inside the thigh to allow for complete visualization of the distal femur, patella, and proximal tibia in both the lateromedial and posteroanterior views of a standing animal. Consistently good results can be obtained from mediolateral and anteromedial exposures of a recumbent animal.

Anatomical features to note are that contrary to previous information, the medial meniscus is only loosely attached to the medial collateral ligament, which is not evidently associated with medial meniscal damage,[16] and the cranial cruciate ligament is composed of two distinct bands. The medial meniscus is probably more mobile than previously believed. This may explain the relatively high incidence of trauma and destruction of this structure. The two-component nature of the cranial cruciate ligament must be taken into account when an arthroscopic diagnosis of its rupture or insufficiency is made, because failure of one component may not result in complete joint instability. The cranial cruciate ligament originates on the anterior aspect of the tibial plateau and attaches on the posterior aspect of the femoral intercondylar fossa. It is located laterally to the caudal cruciate ligament. The compartmentalization and location of the fat pad are important considerations for arthroscopy and arthrocentesis.

UPWARD FIXATION OF THE PATELLA

The condition of upward fixation of the patella is commonly observed in draft animals in India and Egypt but has few references in the North American literature.[3] The incidence is low in both sexes of *Bos taurus* and *Bos indicus* breeds, with one report implicating an increased incidence associated with Brahmin breeding. In Canada, the condition is occasionally encountered in beef and dairy cows in sound physical condition. It may be possible that the condition is precipitated in individual animals with changing body condition, late gestation, changes in muscle tone and development, or different management practices. The etiology is not the same as that in horses, because the bovine femur lacks the prominent notch on the medial trochlear ridge and the patella does not have the same protuberance as the equine. Instead, the limb is intermittently locked in extension by the middle patellar ligament acting in concert with the medial patellar ligament, thus causing the patella to become fixed over the medial femoral trochlear ridge.[3]

CLINICAL SIGNS

Lameness is sudden in onset and intermittent. It frequently affects both limbs, although at the time of examination, one is usually more severely involved. The gait may remain normal for varying intervals of time, and lameness may disappear on presentation to a clinic after several hours' transport. Signs are occasionally much less severe than initially reported. Some animals delivered to a clinic with a different environment in terms of flooring or distracting factors may improve significantly within a few hours.

Affected animals have a typical gait characterized by intermittent extension of the limb to the rear or laterally. The dorsal aspect of the hoof is seen to remain in contact with the ground surface. In animals housed where the flooring has been abrasive (i.e., concrete), the hoof is worn away at the toe. The

fixation usually resolves spontaneously ("unlocks") but soon recurs. The condition may result from sudden movements initiated by the handler or from sharp turns. As the condition first develops, the animal may appear stiff. The limb may eventually be held in permanent extension. Palpation of the stifle does not reveal any obvious abnormalities. No pathognomonic radiographic features have been identified.

The signs are typical. Diagnosis is based on the usual posture of the limb during the period of fixation and the presence otherwise of a normal gait.

TREATMENT

Surgical correction of this condition by medial patellar desmotomy provides immediate and long-lasting relief without any significant long-term complications. It may be performed in a standing or laterally recumbent animal, depending on its temperament, udder size, and the agility of the operator. The medial area over the stifle is clipped and surgically prepared before instillation of 5 to 10 mL of 2% lidocaine into the skin and subcutis. Tail elevation or nose tongs may facilitate the anesthetic and surgical procedures. A 3- to 4-cm vertical skin incision is made over the medial patellar ligament, and blunt dissection is continued toward its point of insertion to the proximal tibia. A stout, sharp, curved bistoury is then introduced medially to the medial patellar ligament, rotated, and applied to section the ligament by short reciprocating strokes (Fig. 17–9). Moderate but insignificant bleeding may be expected in some cases. After complete transection, the total structure becomes non-palpable. If part of the ligament is felt in its normal position, the bistoury should be reintro-

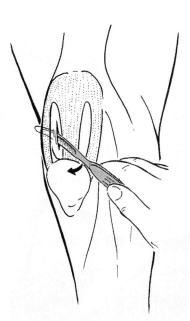

Figure 17–9. The surgical treatment for upward fixation of the patella in cattle. The bistoury is placed through a small skin incision and used to transect the medial patellar ligament, thus allowing the patella to move freely in its normal manner.

duced and the transection completed. The skin is then closed with simple interrupted or cruciate sutures. The animal should resume a normal gait immediately after surgery. Bilateral cases should have both stifles corrected at one session.

Surgical transection of the vastus medialis tendon may also be performed, but this procedure is recommended only for those cases in which a properly performed medial patellar desmotomy fails to result in immediate correction.

Systemic prophylactic antibiotics are usually administered owing to possible contamination during surgery (especially in a standing animal) and the proximity to the stifle joint. Postoperative exercise is considered by some clinicians to be very important in preventing recurrence, but this remains controversial. The prognosis is excellent, recurrence of the condition is not considered to be a problem, and complications are rare.

LUXATING PATELLA AND FEMORAL NERVE DEGENERATION

Degeneration of the femoral nerve occurs most commonly in neonatal calves after assisted traction and is thought to be due to excess tension on the nerve resulting in paralysis of its innervated muscles.[25] Most affected calves have been delivered by severe traction, usually with a calf-puller. Sporadic verbal reports have described development of the condition in calves born without assistance. The quadriceps muscle group receives its major innervation from the femoral nerve. Injury to the nerve results in loss of

quadriceps tone, which allows the patella to move out of the intercondylar groove of the distal femur and to be easily displaced laterally, hence the association of femoral nerve degeneration with patellar luxation. Not uncommonly, both limbs are affected; however, the right is often more seriously involved.

The major clinical sign is an inability to bear full weight on one or both hind limbs. Although the forelimbs are fully capable of normal function, the hindquarters cannot be supported by a complete extension of the stifle. Although the calf appears to crouch when encouraged to stand (Fig. 17–10), it usually prefers to remain recumbent. Severely affected animals are completely unable to support the hindquarters. In the first few days of life, the quadriceps muscles may appear more flaccid than normal. Neurogenic atrophy is evident about 1 week after birth. The degree of muscle atrophy progresses and becomes very obvious on palpation and visual observation.

No radiographic signs are seen initially. Fractures of other limbs such as the opposite hip, vertebrae, and ribs may be detectable, because it is common to find them related to the trauma of forced extraction. Various degrees of analgesia may be noted on the medial aspect of the thigh and leg. These areas correspond to the area innervated by the saphenous branch of the femoral nerve. In general, the history and typical clinical signs make diagnosis easy.

In the past, surgical treatment has been patellar stabilization procedures such as joint capsule and retinacular imbrication, along with stall rest and careful nursing. This symptomatic surgical treatment may result in only temporary relief of the clini-

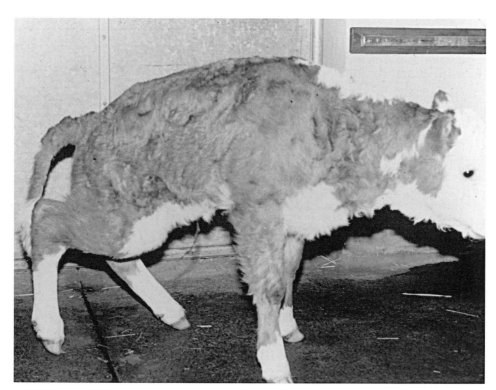

Figure 17–10. A calf with femoral nerve degeneration and resulting luxation of the patella. Note the typical posture with inability to support the hindquarters adequately. Both hind limbs are affected.

cal signs without producing a permanent solution. It does not correct the primary problem of the neurological deficit to the quadriceps muscle group.

Stall rest and attentive nursing care are recommended for milder cases. A minority progressively bear more weight and may be salvaged for slaughter at a relatively early age. This conservative protocol allows for such occasional animals to be given a reprieve that allows the owners to decide on the final fate of each. Severely affected animals should be destroyed early in the course of the problem on humane grounds.

It is not known if a genetic basis exists in the incidence of this condition. The problem is probably more frequent in beef breeds such as the Simmental, Charolais, and Maine Anjou. The importance of this condition with respect to culling is uncertain.

FEMORAL SHAFT FRACTURES

Fractures of the femur are a common orthopedic problem in bovine practice, and the femur is the first or second most commonly fractured long bone.[5] The most usual location is the femoral shaft, particularly the (distal) supracondylar region.[8] The high incidence is directly associated with forced extraction of relatively large calves with excessive forces using a calf-puller or block and tackle. Fractured femurs in older calves are usually related to restraint procedures involving a chute or head gate. Mature animals in range management conditions or confinement situations rarely fracture the femur.

Femoral fractures diagnosed after assisted traction may have two different causes. When calves in posterior presentation are pulled and become lodged by the hips within the maternal pelvis, the calving jack is frequently forced down and may cause the femur to make contact with the cow's pelvis, with transverse forces acting on the distal femur resulting in a fracture. Calves in anterior presentation can become stifle locked when the stifle enters the maternal pelvis before the hips,[15] resulting in axial compression along the femur as mechanical traction is being applied. There are no descriptions of fetal calf posturing during normal parturition. However, Husa and colleagues[13] analyzed the situation in sheep and described positioning of the fetal stifle relative to the maternal pelvis that would support the potential for stifle lock during parturition. Many factors may act to increase the magnitude of the compressive forces along the femoral axis. The second category of fracture closely resembles the torus fracture occurring in the distal femur of young children.[7, 14]

The clinical signs are always associated with a history of forced extraction of variable magnitude. An affected neonatal calf is reluctant or unable to stand and suck, partly because of the trauma and stress of a difficult delivery as well as the fracture itself. Crepitus is often absent owing to severe overriding of the two fracture fragments. The flexors of the hip and stifle cause the fragment ends to be

displaced, and the large muscles of the thigh produce an obvious shortening of the upper limb (Fig. 17–11). The distal end of the proximal fragment is usually palpable percutaneously just above the patella. An obvious femoral discontinuity is readily discernible on palpation along the medial aspect of the shaft. A large visible hematoma develops around the distal femur as a result of lacerated large muscle groups. Lateral deviation is seen during the calf's attempt to stand.

The clinical diagnosis is readily confirmed by radiographic examination. In order to visualize the full femoral length as well as the hip and the stifle, the animal should be placed with the affected limb down and the beam directed from medial to lateral. It is important to evaluate the opposite limb at the same time because luxation or fracture may also be present in the opposite leg.

Regardless of the cause, the surgeon should consider the factors that affect the prognosis and dictate the most suitable method of repair. The existence of concurrent disease in a young animal, such as diarrhea or pneumonia, reduces the chances of successful treatment by approximately 50%. The presence of

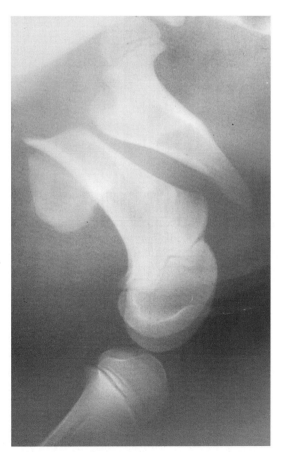

Figure 17–11. Radiograph of a femoral fracture in a calf showing the typical effect of dominant flexor muscles of the hip and stifle. Overriding of the fracture ends with shortening of the limb, seen here, frequently results in periosteal stripping. Note the normal appearance of the scrotum, which may be confused with callus formation in postoperative animals that have been treated with internal fixation.

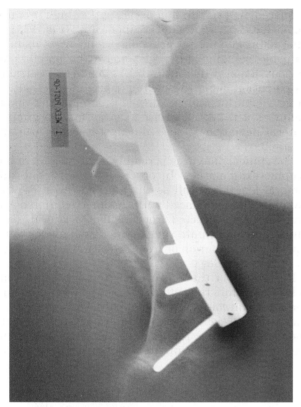

Figure 17–12. Radiograph of a femoral fracture in a calf. The fracture has been reduced and stabilized with a plate and screws. Exuberant callus formation is seen around the posterior aspect of the fracture site. Complications demonstrated in this figure are seen as lucencies around the distal screws, loosening of distal screws, and the presence of an untreated proximal femoral epiphyseal fracture.

any other orthopedic trauma such as other fractures also reduces the success rate by about 50%. A common complicating factor is the failure of passive transfer. It is, therefore, imperative to collect an accurate history on the colostrum intake and to administer blood or serum if it appears that serum protein levels are less than 50 mg/liter. Serum electrophoresis results indicative of inadequate immunoglobulin uptake can also be used when laboratory facilities are available. Long-term success rates have ranged from less than 50% to greater than 80%.

External fixation is inadequate because of the impossibility of achieving either reduction or stabilization of the fracture ends, in treatment of femoral fractures in calves. Treatment without any form of support is also inappropriate. Three types of internal fixation have been used in calves, with various degrees of success. Little has been published about the efficacy of half-pin splintage on calf femurs, but it is not currently considered the treatment of choice. Intramedullary pins or plates and screws (Fig. 17–12) have been the most accepted means of stabilizing femoral shaft fractures.[2, 22] The use of multiple pins or double plating is advocated whenever possible. Plate luting with polymethyl methacrylate or the use of the interlocking nail technique[24] for intramedul-

lary fixation may further improve the future success rate of femoral fracture repair.

The major impediments to healing are the severe degree of periosteal stripping from the femoral shaft, thin cortices, relatively soft bone, and wide intramedullary cavity, which dictate a prolonged healing time and a limited ability to maintain implants in their correct functional position.

To increase the likelihood of a favorable outcome, practitioners are encouraged to

1 Evaluate the immune status of the calf.

2 Treat any concurrent disease.

3 Diagnose concurrent trauma.

4 Initiate surgery as soon as possible using internal fixation with one or two plates or multiple pins.

5 Recognize the likelihood of delayed healing with excessive periosteal stripping.

6 Recognize the limitations of the thin distal femoral cortex to hold screw threads for prolonged periods.

7 Provide intensive postoperative nursing support, nutritional care, and monitoring of the healing process.

SLIPPED CAPITAL FEMORAL EPIPHYSIS

The condition of slipped capital femoral epiphysis has several causes in cattle and inflicts a severe lameness that occasionally involves both hind limbs. The most common situation involves a fracture of the proximal femoral growth plate; as a result, the femoral head remains within the acetabulum, and variable separation of the neck and the distal component occurs. Many such fractures follow forced extraction of relatively large calves that have been judged to be hip locked. It is assumed that forces initiated by a mechanical device such as a calf jack create shearing forces across the physis (Fig. 17–13).

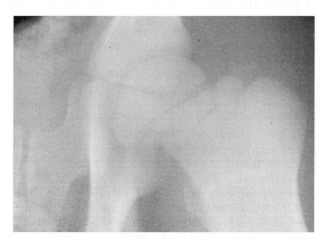

Figure 17–13. Radiograph of a slipped capital femoral epiphysis related to forced extraction of this newborn calf. Note the presence of open physes in the pelvis, a normal finding in an animal of this age.

The condition is more usual in the large or exotic breeds (Maine Anjou, Charolais, and Simmental), particularly those with heavy, well-muscled hip areas. Nearly all cases have been delivered in anterior presentation by means of forced extraction. Femoral nerve paresis/paralysis and fracture of the ribs and vertebrae have additionally been observed in some such cases.[11]

A second condition resulting in separation of the proximal femoral epiphysis is epiphysiolysis. It is commonly encountered in humans and swine but has rarely been documented in cattle.[11] Epiphysiolysis involves gradual widening of the growth plate associated with increasing lameness, then a total separation of the two components, displacement, and sudden development of severe lameness.

Traumatic fracture of the proximal femoral physis can also occur in older animals as a result of trauma. Hull and coworkers[12] report successful treatment of animals ranging from 3 months to 2.3 years. The proximal physis is reported to close in cattle at 40 months of age.

A calf afflicted unilaterally can stand and ambulate but prefers to remain recumbent. The affected limb supports limited weight in most animals, but occasional calves bear considerable weight. The limb is typically held with only the toe touching the ground; the hock and stifle are flexed, with medial rotation of the whole limb. When the calf is forced to walk, crepitus can usually be felt over the greater trochanter. The same sign may also be elicited in a recumbent animal with manipulation of the limb involving flexion, extension, and rotation of the hip. More chronic cases show a generalized muscle atrophy of the limb in general and gluteal regions in particular.

The condition is usually diagnosed on the basis of a history of forced extraction, as well as the clinical signs. Differential diagnosis includes coxofemoral luxation, proximal femoral fracture, and pelvic fractures. The condition must be confirmed radiographically, and if repair is being considered, the opposite hip, the lumbosacral area, and the chest should also be radiographed. The pelvic views should include the extended and frog-leg positions.

Conservative, non-surgical treatment is not recommended for any potential breeding stock because such calves tend to remain in pain, grow at a reduced rate, and soon develop coxofemoral osteoarthritis. Femoral head excision is an alternative surgical procedure and usually produces a relatively pain-free hip in the short term. It may provide an economical alternative for calves intended for early slaughter purposes. However, it is unsuitable for bull calves intended for breeding.

The surgical treatment of choice currently recommended is reduction and fixation of the fragments using interfragmentary compression when possible. Implants used to obtain compression include cannulated screws,[31] other forms of lag screws,[19] and Knowles pins.[6] Steinmann pins have also been successfully used without compression in older animals.[12] The use of additional, antirotational implants is suggested when forces acting at the physis need to be controlled. Approximate pin sizes and insertion depths may be determined from the pelvic radiographs. A lateral approach to the affected hip is made, and small Kirschner wires are placed from the lateral proximal femur along the axis of the neck and into the femoral head. After intraoperative radiographs to confirm reduction and placement of the guide wires, the appropriate implants are inserted parallel to the guide wires and into the femoral head. Proper depth is determined from pin measurements and intraoperative radiographs (Fig. 17–14). The fragments are then compressed, and the soft tissues are closed in a routine manner. An alternative approach is greater trochanteric osteotomy, which may allow a clearer view of the reduced fracture. However, it usually is not necessary for the fragments to be visualized to obtain excellent realignment of the fracture ends. A risk of disruption of the osteotomy site also exists postoperatively, particularly in neonatal calves. Preoperative antibiotic therapy is initiated, and postoperative radiographs are taken over an estimated 2-month healing period. With the advent and increased use of more specialized implants such as the dynamic hip screw, which has been successfully used in foals, the future for surgical repair of slipped capital femoral epiphysis looks even more promising.

A limited number of long-term follow-ups suggest that the overall success rate for neonatal animals

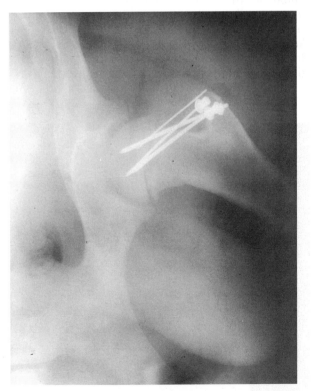

Figure 17–14. Radiograph of a slipped capital femoral epiphysis in a young calf. The fracture was successfully repaired by reduction and stabilization with Knowles pins.

intended for breeding may approach 40%. Complications include failure to heal, failure of the implants to function in the immediate postoperative period, conformational breakdown of the non-fractured limbs, and the development of osteoarthritis in the fractured hip, which may range from mild to debilitating. More detailed reports of procedures performed on animals ranging in age from 5 months to more than 2 years report success in 57% to greater than 90% of animals treated.[12, 31] These higher success rates may be related to improved surgical implants, improved bone consistency in older animals, minimal conformational changes developing in the healing phase, better case selection, or other factors not currently understood.

PREVENTION

Client education, anticipation of problems in high-risk dam/sire combinations, and increased use of cesarean section will reduce the number of proximal femoral physeal problems.

FRACTURES OF THE PELVIS

The bovine pelvis is a boxlike structure forming the junction between the hind limbs and the vertebral column. It is prone to fail when abnormally great forces are placed on it. Despite its crucial location, the pelvis is not a common site of fractures. The shape of this group of bones provides a basically strong, resilient structure, which requires failure of more than one element if a discontinuity is to occur. An exception to this rule is a broken or "knocked down" wing of the ilium, because this part of the girdle does not contribute to the boxlike structure.

Such fractures often have an association with trauma such as crowding through narrow doorways. A mild or moderate degree of lameness is possible, or the owner may recognize the problem only by observing asymmetry or absence of the normal contour of the pelvic region. Most such fractures need not be treated. The knocked down fragment occasionally results in a draining sequestrum and requires surgical removal. After excision, the recovery is usually uneventful. Replacement of displaced fragments for cosmetic or show purposes is problematic owing to the strong distracting forces of attached muscles.

When areas of the pelvis that are considered to compose the box are involved, radiographic evaluation is indicated for diagnostic and prognostic purposes. Affected animals are usually moderately to severely lame and exhibit crepitus on manipulation and ambulation. When fragments are displaced to a significant extent, rectal examination in a standing and moving animal is a valuable diagnostic aid, as is auscultation with a stethoscope. Radiographic examination, which may be demanded for valuable stock, requires heavy sedation or general anesthesia to obtain clear lateral, oblique, and ventrodorsal views (Fig. 17–15). Persistence and determination are then necessary to obtain excellent diagnostic radiographs, but even relatively low-power machines can produce adequate results with prolonged exposure times in all but the largest of animals (Fig. 17–16).

Fractures of the shaft of the ilium, ischium, or acetabulum are frequently related to breeding activity, such as when a female comes into heat in a pen with several other large females. In several recorded instances, pelvic fractures have occurred in more than one female during estrus synchronization and superovulation procedures. The repeated mounting activity, the possibility of slippery footing, and the size of the mounting cows are probably contributory factors. A similar etiology may well be responsible for occasional pelvic fractures in pens of young bull

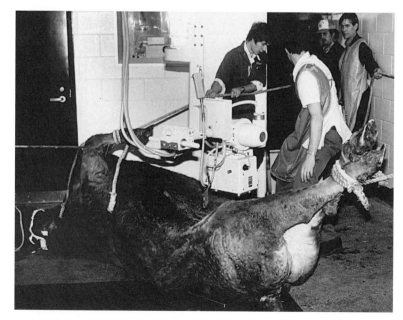

Figure 17–15. A young bull being positioned for radiographic diagnosis of a pelvic fracture. The animal is heavily sedated and held in position with ropes to allow the attendants to leave the room while radiographs are being taken. The x-ray beam is directed through the pelvis from its ventral aspect to a film that is contained in a protective box under the animal.

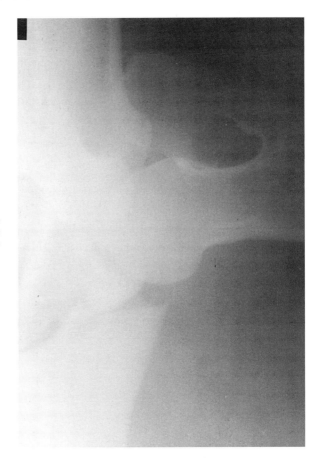

Figure 17–16. Radiograph of a non-articular pelvic fracture in a mature cow. The ischium is slightly displaced, and the articular surfaces of the hip are not involved. This radiograph was obtained using the methods described in Figure 17–15.

calves. These fractures less commonly occur in association with accidents involving motor vehicles or farm implements.

With the exception of the rare case of a draining tract associated with a knocked-down hip, surgery is not usually indicated in pelvic fractures. Shaft fractures heal reasonably well if the animal is confined for 1 or 2 months to a small pen or paddock with secure footing, despite the presence of more than one fracture of the pelvis. With displacement of the fractures into the pelvic cavity, the long-term effect may be severe interference with the birth canal, necessitating a cesarean section or culling from the breeding program. Acetabular fractures carry a very guarded prognosis, and slaughter is strongly advised.

Although long-term follow-up information is not available, personal observation suggests that young bulls suffering from multiple pelvic fractures neither grow nor ambulate well despite confinement, and their future as herd sires at pasture is usually bleak.

REFERENCES

1. Adams SB, Fessler JF: Treatment of radial ulnar and tibial fractures in cattle, using a modified Thomas splint cast combination. J Am Vet Med Assoc 183:430–433, 1983.
2. Ames KN: Comparison of methods for femoral fracture repair in young calves. J Am Vet Med Assoc 179:458–459, 1981.
3. Baird AN, Angel KL, Moll HD, et al: Upward fixation of the patella in cattle: 38 cases (1984–1990). J Am Vet Med Assoc 202:434–436, 1993.
4. Buchner H, Hönger D: Intrauterine Tibiafraktur bei einem Kalb. Wien Tierarztl Monatschr 76:221–223, 1989.
5. Crawford WH, Fretz PB: Long bone fractures in large animals: A retrospective study. Vet Surg 14:295–302, 1985.
6. Ferguson JG: Management and repair of bovine fractures. Comp Cont Ed Pract Vet 4:128–136, 1982.
7. Ferguson JG: Femoral fractures in the newborn calf: Biomechanics and etiological considerations for practitioners. Can Vet J 35:626–630, 1994.
8. Ferguson JG, Dehghani S, Petrali EH: Fractures of the femur in newborn calves. Can Vet J 31:289–291, 1990.
9. Gahlot TK, Chawla SK, Singh P, et al: Modified iron splint for tibial fracture repair in bovines. Indian Vet J 67:566–568, 1990.
10. Hamilton GF, Tulleners EP: Transfixation pinning of proximal tibial fractures in calves. J Am Vet Med Assoc 176:725–727, 1980.
11. Hamilton GF, Turner AS, Ferguson JG, Pharr JW: Slipped capital femoral epiphysis in calves. J Am Vet Med Assoc 172:1318–1322, 1978.
12. Hull BL, Koenig GJ, Monke DR: Treatment of slipped capital femoral epiphysis in cattle: 11 cases (1974–1988). J Am Vet Med Assoc 197:1509–1512, 1990.
13. Husa L, Bieger D, Fraser AF: Fluoroscopic study of the birth posture of the sheep fetus. Vet Rec 123:645–648, 1988.
14. Light TR, Ogden RN, Ogden JA: The anatomy of metaphyseal torus fractures. Clin Orthop Rel Res, 188:103–111, 1984.
15. Mickelsen WD: Correction of stifle lock in bovine dystocia. Vet Med Small Anim Pract 71:1047–1048, 1976.
16. Nelson DR, Huhn JC, Kneller SK: Surgical repair of peripheral detachment of the medial meniscus in 34 cattle. Vet Rec 127:571–573, 1990.
17. Nemeth F: Treatment of supracondylar fractures of the femur in large animals. Proc World Congr Dis Cattle 11:791–793, 1982.

18. Rakestraw PC, Nixon AJ, Kaderly RE, Ducharme NG: Cranial approach to the humerus for repair of fractures in horses and cattle. Vet Surg 20:1–8, 1991.
19. Smyth GB, Hatch P, Mason TA: Surgical repair of femoral neck fractures in two dogs and a calf. Vet Rec 105:248–251, 1979.
20. St.-Jean G, DeBowes RM: Transfixation pinning and casting of radial-ulnar fractures in calves: A review of three cases. Can Vet J 33:257–262, 1992.
21. St.-Jean G, Clem MF, DeBowes RM: Transfixation pinning and casting of tibial fractures in calves: Five cases (1985–1989). J Am Vet Med Assoc 198:139–143, 1991.
22. St.-Jean G, DeBowes RM, Hull BL, Constable PD: Intramedullary pinning of femoral diaphyseal fractures in neonatal calves: 12 cases (1980–1990). J Am Vet Med Assoc 200:1372–1376, 1992.
23. St.-Jean G, Hull BL: Conservative treatment of a humeral fracture in a heifer. Can Vet J 28:704–706, 1987.
24. Trostle SS, Wilson DG, Dueland RT, Markel MD: *In vitro* biomechanical comparison of solid and tubular interlocking nails in neonatal bovine femurs. Vet Surg 24:235–243, 1995.
25. Tryphonas L, Hamilton GF, Rhodes CS: Perinatal femoral nerve degeneration and neurogenic atrophy of quadriceps femoris muscle in calves. J Am Vet Med Assoc 164:801–807, 1974.
26. Tulleners EP: Management of bovine orthopedic problems. Part 1. Fractures. Comp Cont Ed Pract Vet 8:69–79, 1986.
27. Van Huffel X, Steenhaut M, Imschoot J, et al: Carpal joint arthrodesis as a treatment for chronic septic carpitis in calves and cattle. Vet Surg 18:304–311, 1989.
28. Verschooten F, DeMoor A, Steenhaut M, et al: Surgical and conservative treatment of infectious arthritis in cattle. J Am Vet Med Assoc 165:271–275, 1974.
29. Vijaykumar DS, Nigam JM, Singh AP, Chawla SK: Experimental studies on fracture repair of the tibia in the bovine. J Vet Orthop 3:6–12, 1984.
30. Welker FH, Modransky PD, Rings DM, Hull BL: Tarsal fractures in a heifer and bull. J Am Vet Med Assoc 195:240–241, 1989.
31. Wilson DG, Crawford WH, Stone WC, Frampton JW: Fixation of femoral capital physeal fractures with 7.0 mm cannulated screws in five bulls. Vet Surg 20:240–244, 1991.

Laminitis and Factors Predisposing to Lameness

Peter Ossent   *Switzerland*

Paul R. Greenough   *Canada*

Jos J. Vermunt   *New Zealand*

18

Laminitis

DEFINITIONS

LAMINITIS

Laminitis, a disease condition of the claw, has a complex etiology and uncertain pathogenesis. The condition is due to a disturbance in the microcirculation of the corium, with ensuing degenerative and possibly inflammatory changes at the dermal-epidermal junction. Sequelae include impaired horn production with diffuse softening and discoloration (subclinical laminitis); hemorrhages in the sole and heel; double soles, heels, and walls; ulcers in the sole and heel; white line lesions (separation); and, in chronic cases, deformation of the whole claw.

Subclinical laminitis, by definition, produces no immediate clinical signs. It is a chronic condition recognized only retrospectively by the delayed appearance of sequelae: deteriorated horn quality, hemorrhages in the sole, and an increase in the incidence of lesions such as sole ulcer, double soles, and white line disease.

Acute or subacute laminitis has a rapid onset. It evokes pain with various degrees and types of lameness and abnormal stance. Affected animals often stand "camped forward" (see p. 73) or may adopt bizarre positions (Fig. 18–1). Acute pain in a medial claw causes the animal to adopt a cross-legged stance (Fig. 18–2). The superficial veins of the hind limb may be engorged (Fig. 18–3). No alterations are visible in the foot other than initial hyperemia at the coronary band associated with warmth and increased pulsation.

Chronic laminitis is a condition developing over a prolonged period; successive bouts of laminitis eventually lead to a characteristic deformation of the claw, slipper foot (Fig. 18–4). The animal usually has difficulty in walking.

REVIEW OF THE LITERATURE

Laminitis was described in horses by Homer and Aristotle many centuries before Christ. Even etiological aspects were known to the ancient Greeks, who, among other things, wrote of "crithiasis" or barley disease.[21, 69] Although the etiology and pathogenesis have been extensively investigated in this species, many aspects, in particular pathogenesis, still remain unknown. The disease varies in severity from a very painful, life-threatening acute condition much feared by horse owners to one that produces only mild lameness, to chronic laminitis with deformation of the hoof.[26, 27, 38, 60]

Nilsson[58] produced an elegant monograph on bovine laminitis that served to initiate thought and research. He described the clinical picture and the histopathology and discussed the pathogenesis and etiology. He also introduced the concept that the etiology was multifactorial. Toussaint Raven[74] reported the important observation that many claw diseases, previously believed to be randomly occurring independent conditions, were more frequently encountered in animals affected with laminitis. Peterse[63, 65, 66, 67] substantiated aspects of the nutritional etiology of the disease in cattle, which he regarded predominantly to result in a "subclinical" form of laminitis.

Once the concept of subclinical laminitis became accepted, not only was the earlier literature reviewed but new histopathological studies were conducted[56]

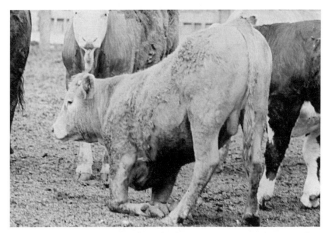

Figure 18–1. Acute pain in the foreclaws may cause an animal to crawl around on its knees. (Courtesy of E. D. Janzen, Western College of Veterinary Medicine, University of Saskatchewan, Saskatoon, Canada.)

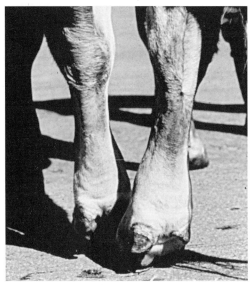

Figure 18–2. Acute laminitis can occasionally affect only the medial hind claws, in which case the animal may cross its limbs to relieve pain.

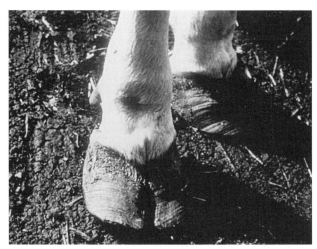

Figure 18–4. The foreclaws of a cow with chronic laminitis. The claw on the left is flat, and the toe is broken square. The coronary band has a fringe of frayed horn. Ripples are seen on the claw on the right.

and a significant number of publications dealing with the topic appeared.[8–10, 20, 76, 78–83] Of particular note were those suggesting that a high incidence of lameness can be correlated with the incidence of production diseases[71] or reproductive disorders.[17, 47] It was also suggested that the pathophysiological conditions that cause laminitis affect other important body organs, thereby causing heifers to fail to reach their expected productivity.[55]

Cumulative literature suggests that a combination

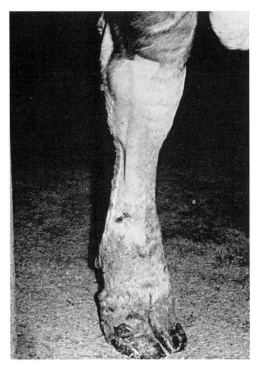

Figure 18–3. Engorgement of the subcutaneous veins in acute laminitis.

of factors influences the occurrence and severity of laminitis.[1–6, 11, 16, 45, 55, 56, 59, 63, 64, 72, 84] For this reason, an epidemiological approach to investigating and controlling lameness is justifiable.[30, 35, 54]

INCIDENCE

Subclinical Laminitis

It has been impossible to assess with accuracy the incidence of subclinical laminitis, let alone that of bovine lameness (see Chapter 1). In the past, criteria for recognizing the condition have been inconsistent, with the result that data in some instances may have been corrupted. Furthermore, effective surveys are handicapped by the fact that nutrition and management differ among countries, regions within a country, and even among farms. There is reason to believe that the incidence of subclinical laminitis has increased significantly during the past 15 years. In an analysis of clinical lameness cases during a period of 12 years—until 1993—a progressive increase of laminitis was observed; in the first 6-year period, the incidence was 6% but increased to 17% in the second half.[44] It is likely that improved knowledge and awareness may be the explanation for these increased numbers, but it is difficult to assess to what extent.

Subclinical laminitis is usually encountered in mature dairy cows, mostly in developed countries. The condition is of greatest concern in herds where intensive management is practiced.[57] Russell and colleagues[71] reported a herd incidence for all lesions of only 5%, of which 24.2% were either sole ulcers or white line disease. Assuming that subclinical laminitis was always the underlying condition, these results would suggest that in 1983 the overall average incidence of subclinical laminitis was only 1.3%. In contrast, a study also in the United Kingdom[15] revealed that 63% of the lesions, either sole ulcer or white line disease, were postulated with subclinical laminitis. The overall incidence of lameness in this survey was approximately 60%, which means that the incidence of subclinical laminitis was about 38%. These figures suggest a rising incidence of both lameness-producing lesions and laminitis.

Acute and Subacute Laminitis

Acute and subacute forms of laminitis are not common in cattle and usually occur in a single animal or a group that has accidentally gorged on large quantities of grain. The incidence of this form of laminitis in dairy cattle probably varies from 0.6%[70] to 1.2%.[13, 15] Subacute laminitis may occur in young beef bulls on feeding trials and in feeder calves that have been given high production rations rich in carbohydrates.[31, 36]

Chronic Laminitis

Chronic laminitis is encountered more commonly in older dairy cows and may be the third most common cause of culling, after reproductive failure and low production. Nevertheless, reliable figures for the incidence of chronic laminitis are not available, although it is suspected to be relatively high in dairy cows older than 5 years.

ETIOLOGY OF LAMINITIS AND PREDISPOSING FACTORS

Mainly observations in the field but also epidemiological surveys on bovine laminitis have revealed a wide spectrum of often interdependent etiological factors. Some factors such as those in carbohydrate overload or road founder were already known to the ancient Greeks; others have been discovered only recently. Many questions about cause still remain to be answered, and opinions on the significance of the various risk factors involved are controversial.

A complicating aspect is the difficulty of clearly separating purely etiological factors from merely predisposing factors. For example, animals fed identical rations under apparently comparable circumstances are not always affected in a similar manner. Although nutrition seems to be a key factor, this observation suggests that additional factors must be involved. Some of these are addressed next.

SYSTEMIC INSULT

Although many factors act systemically, it is only the claws that are obviously affected. Work by Danish researchers,[55] however, indicated that the media-

tors—in this case toxins—that evoked laminitis in the claws also affected internal organs such as the liver and kidneys. Furthermore, animals experiencing episodes of slight laminitis did not lactate as well as normal animals.

Acute laminitis frequently is coupled with the pathological conditions encountered in milk cows, such as acetonemia, lipomobilization (fat cow) syndrome, and abomasal displacement.[44, 58] Similarly, laminitic disorders are frequently associated with parturition.[22, 64, 70]

LACTIC ACIDOSIS

The classic hypothesis for the etiology of bovine laminitis closely follows that elaborated for horses. Research[36] has confirmed that a high level of carbohydrate in the diet is the most important cause of imbalance with laminitis. The frequency and quantity of feed consumed and the period of time over which the increased intake occurs are also important factors.[36, 50, 51, 57] Excessive levels of readily fermentable carbohydrate invoke an imbalance of rumenal homeostasis, with a selective increase of lactic acid (acidosis) caused by the activity of *Streptococcus bovis* and *Lactobacillus* species.[6, 45, 46, 67]

Lactic acid has been associated with the etiology of laminitis, but experimental attempts to produce laminitis in cattle failed,[1] although intraruminal injections of lactic acid did induce laminitis in sheep.[53]

ENDOTOXEMIA

These imbalances are frequently associated with rumenitis.[7, 29, 36] The low-pH environment is hostile to gram-negative organisms, and as they disintegrate, vasoactive endotoxins are released.

Endotoxins are assumed to be produced in severe inflammatory conditions such as mastitis or metritis (e.g., with retained placenta). Attempts at experimental induction of laminitis with endotoxins produced variable results.[9, 10, 56]

HISTAMINE

High levels of histamine in the blood have been recorded in the early stages of laminitis[49, 58, 73] and are thought to arise from disturbances in the gastrointestinal tract or the uterus.

FIBER QUALITY

Peterse considered the quantity and quality of fiber intake to be an important predisposing factor.[63] The fiber content of forage is measured in terms of neutral detergent fiber, part of which is soluble and contributes to the total digestible nutrients. The undigestible fiber or acid detergent fiber (ADF) has a very important buffering role in the rumen.

EXCESS PROTEIN

Cattle fed only grass also may have a high incidence of lameness with characteristics similar to laminitis.[20] The percentage of protein in rapidly growing grass can rise to greater than 30%, with a compensatory drop in the percentage of ADF. The excess protein (>16%) may be converted to amino acids and ammonia. Alternatively, protein may be degraded to toxic entities or may cause some allergic reaction. The mechanism causing grass founder is not known, but it causes very distinct problems for beef cattle in western Canada (see p. 289).

AVERAGE DAILY WEIGHT GAIN

The high incidence of subclinical laminitis in heifers has created an interest in the phenomenon of growth. Heifers that increase in weight at a rate in excess of 750 grams/day, between 3 and 15 months of age, have higher hemorrhage scores than animals that increase in weight at a slower rate.[34] With increased emphasis being placed on earlier first calving, it can be hypothesized that the younger the animal, the smaller will be the claw size and the greater will be the mechanical stress on the claw capsule.

A similar finding was recorded in studies with steers.[36] The fastest-growing beef bulls in feed trials commencing when the animals were 8 months of age showed clinical signs indistinguishable from subacute laminitis.[31]

Laminitis is not restricted to dairy cattle; accelerated weight gain in young beef bulls can bring about founderlike changes. It is highly probable that the feet of bulls can be ruined for life as a result of inappropriate management while they are still younger than 14 months.[36]

GENETIC PREDISPOSITION

Field observation would substantiate that animals react differently to the same insult. These differences may be attributed to genetic predisposition, although the precise nature of the susceptibility is not clear. Nilsson[58] observed a familial predisposition to laminitis, and others[3, 32, 48] mentioned a possible inherited susceptibility to laminitis. An inherited form of laminitis in Jersey cattle has been reported in South Africa,[19] the United States,[52] the United Kingdom,[23] and Zimbabwe.[39]

BREED SUSCEPTIBILITY

Friesian cattle are most susceptible to laminitis.[48, 58, 59] Swedish Friesians are more often affected by sole hemorrhages and sole ulcer than Swedish red-and-white cattle.[2] Grommers[37] detected a higher incidence of lameness in Dutch Friesians than in Dutch red-and-white cows, and Brochart[11] and Peterse[63] noticed a similar greater susceptibility to laminitis in Friesian cattle than in Holstein-Friesian cross cows. Similarly, Swiss Holstein Friesians (Schwarzfleck) were more affected than Simmentaler and Braunvieh.[44]

EXERCISE

Exercise is essential for normal blood flow through the claw, because a lack of movement with prolonged standing is conducive to pooling of blood in the claws. It has been suggested that management practice that interferes with exercise may be a factor that influences the occurrence of lameness.[85] Ward[83] reports that in one study, heifers at pasture lay for 9.35 hours/day, whereas animals confined in cubicles rested for only 6.25 hours/day. Heifers at pasture had free range, whereas heifers in relative confinement stood for long periods. Reduced exercise for animals that consume large quantities of carbohydrate may increase the risk of laminitis. Pregnant animals, particularly heifers that are allowed free range before suddenly being confined and introduced to a rich diet at calving, also may be particularly at risk.

MECHANICAL FACTORS

Locally acting factors influence the hoof directly. These are external trauma or trauma from within due to overburdening, resulting from abnormal claw or limb configuration. Furthermore, lack of movement (excessive standing) is regarded to be detrimental. Mechanical forces applied to the sole of the claw result from a permutation of claw size and shape, body weight, conformation of the limbs, claw hardness, and the quality of the surface over which the animal walks. Softer horn is conducive to bruising of the tissues that the horn capsule should protect. Bruising causes a local disturbance in the blood supply.

A clear indication that mechanical forces are involved in the development of lesions is that they occur far more frequently in the lateral hind and medial front claws—namely, those that bear most weight.[62, 75]

The consensus is that trauma may be a precipitating factor for laminitis or at least for lesions normally secondary to laminitis. Forced walking or walking on rough or stony roads may be a precipitating factor for such lesions,[12, 14] but it is not clear whether mechanisms similar to road founder, a form of laminitis in horses, are involved here.

BEHAVIOR

Behavior has been suggested as a predisposing factor in lameness[12, 18, 40, 41]; the effects of confrontation (between submissive heifers and dominant cows in the dry herd) could be considered a heritable character trait (see Chapter 19).

DEFICIENT KERATINIZATION

Deficiencies inherent in the keratinizing epidermis may be regarded as either local or systemic factors depending on the opinion of how they develop. Zinc and copper together with methionine (see Chapter 10) are known to be essential for keratinization; therefore, primary or secondary deficiencies of these nutrients can affect the quality of horn produced.

EPIDERMAL GROWTH FACTOR

An often overlooked hypothesis arises from Swedish work.[24, 25] Steers were used as a model for equine laminitis studies. It was discovered that receptors for epidermal growth factors (EGF) were present in the cell membranes of the horn matrix of the claws. EGF was found also in considerable amounts in the gastrointestinal tract and uterus, which are usually involved in the pathogenesis of laminitis. In addition to its mitogenic effect, this substance *(in vitro)* has the capacity to inhibit the differentiation of keratinocytes, a dominant morphological feature in the hoof matrix during the early stages of laminitis. This hypothesis might account for the irregularities in horn production that are noted in some cases of laminitis, and this mechanism readily fits into the sequence of events postulated to occur in the pathogenesis of laminitis.

Furthermore, the same researchers compiled a list of diverse substances in addition to EGF, ranging from cations, hormones, and vitamins, to bacterial toxins; all negatively influence keratinocyte differentiation. Yet another possibility, a deficiency of amino acids, is compatible with this theory of disturbances inherent in the keratinizing epidermis. A lack of cystine and methionine has been postulated to have a key role in equine laminitis.[43]

PATHOLOGY AND PATHOGENESIS OF LAMINITIS

Careful examination and interpretation of postmortem findings help to throw light on the pathogenesis of laminitis and of claw lesions, give insight into the order of events, and help to explain the nature of disorders in the horn capsule. The changes are best visualized in exungulated claws (Fig. 18–5).[61]

For most studies of the histopathological changes in laminitis, material taken from either induced hyperacute cases or chronic cases salvaged from the slaughterhouse has been used. Little information is available about the histopathological appearance of tissues affected with subclinical laminitis.

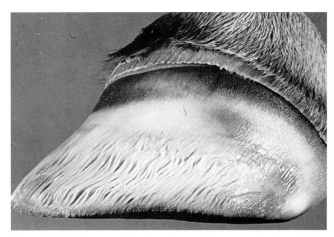

Figure 18–5. Exungulated claw showing the normal view of the corium in the wall region, with pink laminae and a pigmented parietal region. The sole and heel are also pink, and the inside surface of the horn capsule should be white. It is important to know that the corium of normal animals frequently has red patches due to passive congestion; thus, it is essential to correlate postmortem findings with the clinical signs before drawing conclusions about the significance of presumptive acute lesions.

Ultimately, all the theories brought forward to date on the pathogenesis of laminitis are best explained from the viewpoint focused on degenerative change in the epidermal-dermal junction of the claw. The sequence of events may be partitioned into three phases, discussed next.

PHASE 1

Physiopathology of the Dermis in Clinical and Subclinical Laminitis

MECHANICAL FACTORS

Localized pressure caused by disturbances in weight-bearing and prolonged standing lead to deficiencies in the blood supply through compression and injury of tissues.

SYSTEMIC FACTORS

The systemic etiological factors induce an initial response by releasing vasoactive substances or other mediators into the vascular system. The likelihood of a circulatory disturbance, although expressed somewhat simplistically, had been postulated for equine laminitis already in the 18th century.[42] Whether local or systemic, the primary reaction seems to be centered around the blood vessels of the corium. The reaction includes

- *Paralysis* (opening) *of the arteriovenous shunts* in the dermis of the wall beneath the coronary band[8, 68, 81, 82] (see Chapter 14) or

- *Inflammation in the dermis* (involving the laminae—hence the term *laminitis*) or

- *Both phenomena* occurring simultaneously or sequentially

INFLAMMATORY RESPONSE

In cattle, as opposed to horses, it is not clear to what extent and at which stage inflammatory cell components contribute to the disease process. There is no evidence that the primary insult episode of laminitis—despite the condition's designation—is more than a serious pathophysiological disturbance based on noninflammatory mechanisms. Certainly, their presence is not constant, and the term *laminitis* (i.e., an inflammation of the laminae) could be a misnomer when applied to cattle.

HEMOSTASIS

On the assumption that both shunting and inflammation do occur, it is nevertheless irrelevant which prevails, because both rapidly evoke similar reactions in the tissues. Open shunts cause the main flow of blood destined for the claw's corium (dermis) to bypass it and the blood within the claw to sludge, making the vessel walls prone to hypoxic damage. In addition, vessel wall paralysis due to toxins and the inflammatory reaction due to histamine, for example, in combination with influences of the nervous system induce vasodilation in the stratum vasculosum.[49] Vascular congestion with erythema of the corium (dermis) ensues for the duration of the acute process, particularly in the angle between the wall and sole. The circumferential arcade, a principal source of blood for the laminae, is located at this point (see p. 222).

HEMORRHAGE

Large hemorrhages occur around the apex of the distal phalanx as well as around its posterior border because both shunting and inflammation exert detrimental effects on the distended capillary walls and lead to diapedesis. Furthermore, after the vessel walls become permeable to fluid, exudation leads to generalized edema in the corium (Fig. 18–6).

THROMBOSIS

For anatomical reasons, the soft tissues in the hoof are in a unique predicament increasing their vulner-

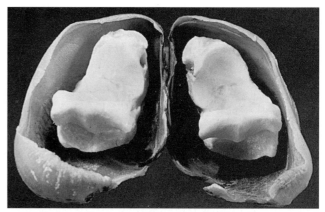

Figure 18–7. This caudal view of a macerated hoof demonstrates the limited space that the corium occupies between the hard horn capsule and the rigid skeletal components. It is not difficult to envisage the risk of lesions and pain developing from tissue compression after edema or displacement of the distal phalanx.

ability. The corium (dermis) is sandwiched in the rigid narrow space between the pedal bone and the horn capsule (Fig. 18–7). Any increase in the volume of the corium (i.e., swelling of the dermal tissues) amplifies the intraungular tissue pressure, which in turn reduces the blood flow and induces further pain. The formation of thrombi, which may be abundant in both large and small vessels, usually follows.[9, 49]

NECROSIS

A vicious circle with hypoxia and finally, analogous to the compartment syndrome in muscle, even tissue necrosis may develop.

Histopathology of the Dermal-Epidermal Junction During Acute Clinical Laminitis

A further special anatomical feature of the hoof is the interdigitating dermal-epidermal junction in the lamellar region of the wall. A greater part of the body weight bearing on the limb is suspended from the dorsal and side walls by this structure, whose integrity is imperative for normal weight-bearing.

During the normal horn growth of the claw wall, the lamellae glide past the laminae down toward the ground surface. Despite the presence of this seemingly vulnerable point, the laminar-lamellar interface fully supports a large proportion of the digital carrying forces by transferring them from the hoof wall to the corium's fibroelastic network, which inserts into the periosteum of the distal phalanx and finally the skeleton.

During the laminitic insult, the initial histopathological changes occur in the epidermis.[58] The germinal cells of the lamellae become reduced in number, take on a pyknotic appearance, and may become vacuolated (Fig. 18–8), enlarged, swollen, and disoriented (Fig. 18–9). Partial or complete disappearance of the onychogenic substance (the tonofibrils) (Figs. 18–10 to 18–12) from the stratum germinativum and

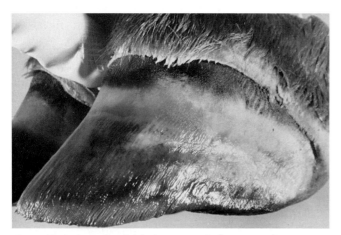

Figure 18–6. Acute laminitis in a severely lame cow. An exungulated claw with congestion, edema, and hemorrhage in the wall region, particularly in the laminae.

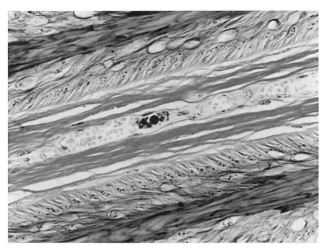

Figure 18–8. The dorsal border of the stratum lamellatum (×100, van Gieson stain). A fibrin-positive spot (shock globe) is seen in a capillary. To the right of the shock lobe is a spherical enlargement of the endothelium. This may be another shock globe covered by endothelium. Several cells in the stratum spinosum are vacuolated. (Courtesy of K. Mortensen, Royal Agriculture and Veterinary College, Copenhagen, Denmark.)

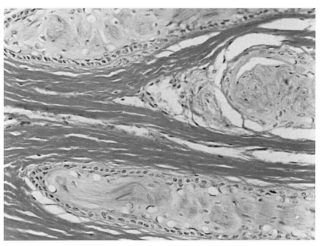

Figure 18–10. Induced endotoxemia in a 6-month-old calf, 24 hours after digital intra-arterial infusion of endotoxin. Marked edema, thickening of the endothelial cells, and several eosinophilic granulocytes are seen (×250, hematoxylin and eosin). (Courtesy of K. Mortensen, Royal Agriculture and Veterinary College, Copenhagen, Denmark.)

stratum spinosum occurs in the lamellar and solar regions, and the keratin pillar may contract away from the base of the laminae. In the matrices of the soft horn such as that of the periople and bulb, the keratohyalin granules decrease or disappear. In short, the cells of the lamellae and epidermis of the sole assume irregularities indicating degenerative change.

Inflammatory cells infiltrate the corium in the reactionary stages of an acute case or in chronically affected claws. Lymphocyte infiltration is seen around the base of the papillae, and histiocytes, granulocytes, plasma cells, and globular leukocytes

are also present. Mast cells, neutrophils, and eosinophils are not involved.

The multitude of changes described—such as vessel wall damage, edema, sludging of blood within the vessels, abnormal arteriovenous shunting, hypoxemia, tissue hypoxia, hemorrhage, and thrombosis—all implicate a reduced blood supply with fewer nutrients reaching the horn-producing tissues.

These basal epidermal cells, supplied from the underlying dermis, logically require more nutrients and oxygen than any other tissues in the vicinity because (1) these cells still multiply to a certain extent and (2) the phenomenon of claw wall growth, in which the horn "slides" past its underlying layers, is bound to stimulate considerable metabolic demands. Thus,

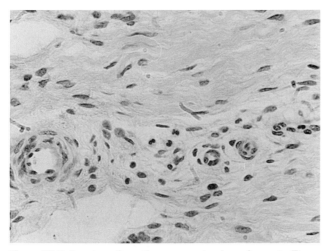

Figure 18–9. Laminae from the same animal as shown in Figure 18–4. Irregularities in shape are seen, with reduced or inactive horn production. Some of the cells in the stratum basale and spinosum are vacuolated and weakly stained. The keratogenic substance is reduced in amount and the keratin in the lamellae is distributed irregularly (×100, van Gieson stain). (Courtesy of K. Mortensen, Royal Agriculture and Veterinary College, Copenhagen, Denmark.)

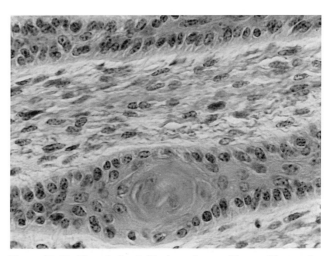

Figure 18–11. Chronic laminitis in a 4-year-old cow. Uneven lamella in an acidophilic body, loss of keratogenic substance, and local dislocation of the cells in the stratum basale. The number of fibroblasts in the corium is increased (×250, hematoxylin and eosin). (Courtesy of K. Mortensen, Royal Agriculture and Veterinary College, Copenhagen, Denmark.)

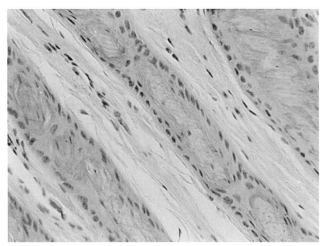

Figure 18–12. Subacute laminitis in a 13-month-old steer. The laminae are irregular in shape, islets or keratin is present, and the strata basale are reduced in number and are weakly stained (×100, hematoxylin and eosin). (Courtesy of K. Mortensen, Royal Agriculture and Veterinary College, Copenhagen, Denmark.)

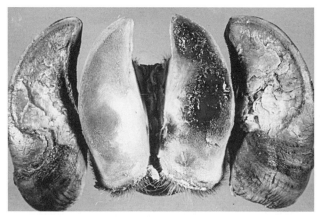

Figure 18–13. Subacute laminitis in a 2 1/2-year-old cow. The corium of one exungulated claw is practically unaffected. The other claw has a confluent dark red hemorrhagic area of necrosis in the corium immediately under a greater part of the distal phalanx. The most plausible explanation for these lesions is pressure necrosis due to sinkage of the skeletal components of the foot. Only one claw is affected because it was carrying more weight. Note that the horn of the sole and heel, at least the superficial layers, is friable, indicating that the animal was suffering from subclinical laminitis before the present severe bout of laminitis.

any deficiencies in the supply of nutrients and the exchange of essential substances affect the tissues of the dermal-epidermal junction in the laminar region.

Deficiency in keratinization, irrespective of causal mechanism, produces the same result: the keratin-producing cells synthesize structurally incompetent keratin, and the horn quality deteriorates. The claw's carrying mechanism no longer holds, and the lamellar-laminar link begins to separate by sliding apart like fingers being drawn from a glove. The claw, first for metabolic reasons and then for mechanical reasons, is no longer in a position to exert its carrying function; thus, the claw bone, and with it the whole animal, sinks within the horn capsule.

The laminitic state may persist in phase 1 without sinkage and without signs of lameness, resulting in the chronic state defined as subclinical laminitis. The horn is of inferior quality, diffusely softened, and discolored; escaped blood or blood fluids may be incorporated into the epidermal layers, staining them either pink or yellow. Hemorrhages in the horn tubules of the sole and heel give a brush-mark appearance.

PHASE 2

Compression of the Dermis (Corium) in the Sole and Heel

The already thin layer of soft tissues of the sole and heel under the distal phalanx is now at high risk of being compressed, even if no sinkage takes place and pressure due to edema and body weight increases. This causes a further episode of capillary damage, hemorrhage, ischemic necrosis, thrombosis, and cellular inflammatory reaction (Figs. 18–13 and 18–14). Further pain is induced, and severe lameness presents a threat to the animal's life. In a laminitic bout, part or all of the sole may be involved, depending on

the distribution of pressure, the magnitude of the insult, and the previous insult experience of the animal. The areas of necrosis are generally focal. The wall regions are reddened and edematous in the earlier stages of phase 2 but later revert to nearly normal color unless exudate has accumulated in the separated layers (Fig. 18–15).

Still no abnormality is visible to the clinician at this stage, although several weeks may have elapsed since the onset of laminitis.

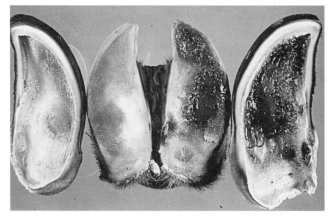

Figure 18–14. Subacute laminitis in a 2 1/2-year-old cow (same claws as shown in Fig. 18–13). The horn capsules have been turned over, and the walls have been sawn off to permit a view of the inner surfaces. It was evident that the lesions in the corium were no longer very fresh because the necrotic debris extended several millimeters into the sole horn. In the heel, a new horn layer is already being formed. It would have covered the lesion had the animal recovered. The extent of blood and debris incorporated into the sole horn is a useful index when estimating the duration of the process. This lesion was judged to be about 10 days old, but no relevant clinical details were available.

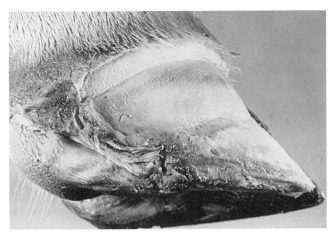

Figure 18–15. Side view of the corium of an exungulated claw. The original hemorrhage and necrosis were likely to have been at the angle between the wall and sole or heel in zone 3. With time, the necrotic material worked its way up the wall toward the coronary band. Nothing was visible in this claw before it was exungulated. Within weeks, however, the white line in zone 3 would have perforated.

Pathologically, the designation subacute laminitis has proved useful for this stage.

PHASE 3

Development of Lesions in the Capsule

Several weeks must pass before the changes in the corium and inner surfaces of the horn capsule become visible to the eye of the clinician. Sequelae of phase 2 are lesions in the horn capsule, which until relatively recently were regarded as independent claw diseases. However, each manifestation has a logical place in the sequence of events occurring after the laminitic episode or episodes.

CHANGES IN THE CORONARY BAND

The coronary band is a separate structure from the wall, although these structures are intimately connected (see Chapter 14). Under adverse circumstances, the band becomes irregular, rough, grooved, or thickened when the function of the periople, which is the dermis of the coronary band, is compromised. Although its etiology or pathogenesis is not known, the phenomenon is present in beef herds in which the incidence of grass founder is relatively high (Fig. 18–16).

CHANGES IN THE WALL

Horizontal ("Hardship") Grooves (see p. 111). When the function of the epidermal stratum germinativum in the papillary pegs that generate the structures of the wall is compromised for a short period (probably days), horn production may slow down, and a roughly horizontal groove—horn of reduced thickness—gradually emerges from beneath the coronary band. In some cattle, especially older,

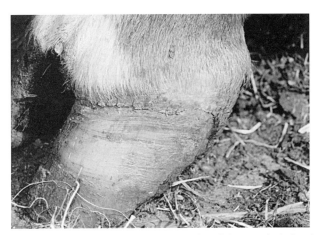

Figure 18–16. Rough coronary bands are found frequently in herds of beef cows with a high incidence of grass founder. The changes may be relatively mild, as in this case, or may appear as a swollen hard ridge, the border of which may be frayed. This phenomenon is also frequently present in claws affected by chronic laminitis.

chronically laminitic cows, a series of horizontal parallel grooves is present. Each groove is due to inhibited horn production, possibly as a result of successive bouts of laminitis.

Concave Dorsal Wall. From the kinked course of the wall horn tubules in such a groove, in sagittal section, it is evident that each groove marks a point at which the direction of growth alters by a few degrees, causing the dorsal surface of the claw eventually to become concave or buckled (Fig. 18–17).

Fissures. If the insult has been severe, the continuity of the wall is lost; this condition is referred to as a *fissure* (see p. 111). As a fissure grows distally,

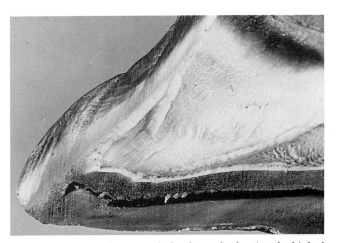

Figure 18–17. Sagittal section of a hoof capsule showing the kinked course of the white horn tubules against the dark horn of the dorsal wall in the region of a hardship groove. The kinks are in the shape of a wave that is exactly parallel to the parietal corium in the proximal wall where the horn was produced. The change of direction in growth occurred here and correlates with adverse events such as laminitic bouts. The lamellae are wider than normal. They become hyperplastic in chronic laminitis. Note the cross section of the innermost layer of normal white soft horn, which is 1 to 2 mm thick. A double sole is present.

it becomes mobile and forms a thimble. The animal experiences considerable pain until the loose fragment breaks away. The rough, ragged claws are termed *broken toes*.

Thus, the groove, fissure, thimble, and buckled and broken toe are different manifestations of the same phenomenon (see pp. 112–113). The importance of this phenomenon is that the measured progress of the groove or fissure can be used to calculate the date on which an insult may have occurred.

CHANGES IN THE LAMELLAR REGION

Extensive exudation in the acute phase or reactive hyperplasia in the chronic stage of laminitis leads to a widening of the laminar zone. Logically, any separation of the layers in the lamellar zone of the wall results in its becoming wider. Once the involved regions in the wall have grown down to the bearing surface of the claw, the changes eventually become visible as alterations in the white line, as a widening in zones 1, 2, and 3. Because the horn is softer than normal, it may erode and provide a port of entry for foreign matter and for infection, provided the corium is reached. In severe cases of separation combined with the accumulation of fluids, a double or hollow wall (seedy toe in horses) may result (Fig. 18–18).

CHANGES IN THE SOLE

The changes occurring in the sole may include hemorrhages in the horn (see p. 114), double soles, ulcers in the sole and toe (see pp. 101, 107), white line separation (see p. 104), and in chronic cases deformation of the whole claw.

A mechanical insult or episode of vascular disturbance leads to accumulations of transudate and hemorrhage or necrotic debris under the distal phalanx. Either the production of horn is hindered altogether, or the masses eventually grow out after they are incorporated within the sole by new horn produced by the basal cells of the epidermis to appear eventually at the ground surface. The tissues may recover, or the insult may be continuous and the animal may slowly adapt to the cause of the insult. In these cases,

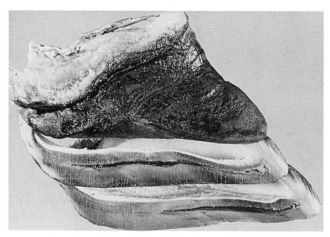

Figure 18–19. The horn capsule (axial view) has been sawn into three slices. In the sole and heel of the middle slice is a space that probably was originally filled with exudate and debris after a bout of laminitis. In the bottom slice, a second less serious double sole is present. This indicates that the first laminitic episode was not as serious as the second. Note the corresponding changes in the horn of the wall.

the most superficial horn is severely bloodstained, but the color shading reverts to normal in the horn most recently produced. These changes are best observed postmortem in claws that have been transected longitudinally (Fig. 18–19).

A single episode of laminitis with hemorrhage takes as long as 3 months to reach the bearing surface as a red-stained patch. Several layers of bloodstained horn may be seen in the same sole or heel when sectioned. In more severe cases, sufficient fluid or debris may accumulate to cause a separation at the dermal-epidermal junction, and the masses are incorporated into the horn, resulting in a double sole (see Fig. 18–18).

The tissues may recover. Alternatively, an ulcer develops when, in a focal area, tissue necrosis is severe and extensive enough to cause total cessation of horn production (Fig. 18–20 and 18–21).

Less severe and more diffuse, chronic changes lead to the production of inferior horn, which appears flaky, yellow, friable, and soft—as in subclinical laminitis.

The site of the lesions in the sole and heel depends on where the compression of the corium occurs. This in turn is dependent on the angle at which the distal phalanx sinks and on the bone's surface configuration. If the tuberositas flexoria—the most distal point of the sinking distal phalanx—causes the compression, the lesion is located in zone 4, adjacent to the "typical ulcer site." Correspondingly, toe lesions in zone 5 are caused by the tip of the distal phalanx, when the bone rotates. The inner edges of zone 2 and the abaxial parts of zone 1 are affected when the bone's sharp edge compresses the corium. Necrosis in the corium of the sole and heel is always focal, although the patches may coalesce. In an exungulated claw, bony protuberances or the sharp abaxial edges of bone are frequently palpable beneath the necrotic or hemorrhagic areas.

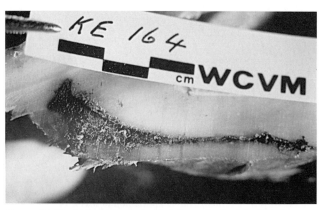

Figure 18–18. A double sole in the claw of a beef heifer that was culled because she was not pregnant. The space corresponds to the time she was turned out to grass in the spring.

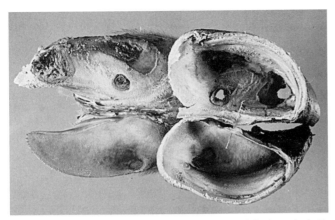

Figure 18–20. Chronic laminitis with ulceration of the horn in both the toe and at the typical site at the heel-sole junction. The corium was necrotic not only at these two sites but along the outer edge of the distal phalanx as well. The bone was easily palpable under the necrotic debris. Overall, the still viable corium of the sole and heel was far thinner than in a young animal. The corium of the other claw was slightly discolored in the heel, but the inner surface of the horn capsule was normal.

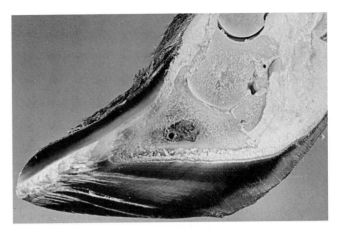

Figure 18–22. Chronic laminitic hoof (slipperfoot), sagittal section. The wall is concave, and it is plainly visible that it has progressively curved away from the normal direction of growth (i.e., parallel to the dorsal surface of the distal phalanx, in a dorsal direction). This has resulted in a wedge-shaped corium in the toe region and a severely widened, soft, and discolored white line (more than 1 cm thick). Note that the flexor surface is still parallel to the sole and heel horn (i.e., the distal phalanx has not rotated). The sole and heel horn is also far too thick owing to lack of wear and neglect.

DEFORMATION OF THE WHOLE CLAW IN CHRONIC LAMINITIS

A chronically laminitic claw is characteristically deformed and is referred to as a *slipper foot* (see p. 137). Multiple changes occur:

- Alternate grooves and ridges give the claw a washboard appearance.

- The hoof broadens and flattens.

- The horn wall, normally parallel to the dorsal surface of the distal phalanx, gradually changes its direction of growth to curve away, producing a con-

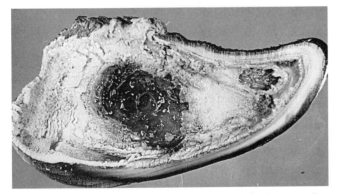

Figure 18–21. View of the horn capsule showing the inner surface of the sole and heel. (Hind right lateral claw of the same cow shown in Fig. 18–20). The wall horn has been removed. The lesions here are still in the subacute stage. The whole zone 4 (in the region of the flexor tubercle) is occupied by a deep hemorrhagic, necrotic mass. The apex of zone 5 (under the tip of the distal phalanx) is also focally affected, but here the necrosis is not (or no longer) hemorrhagic. This lesion is older than the other because the depression is several millimeters deeper. If sufficiently severe, such foci fully perforate the horn layer before the corium has a chance to recover, produce new horn, and enclose the necrotic masses.

cave dorsal wall as explained earlier. The corium becomes wedge shaped on section.

- The distal phalanx sinks away from the horn capsule in a distal direction. In chronic laminitis, successive episodes of laminitis may prevent the restitution of the wall structures because this would require enough time for the whole length of the wall to grow out.

- The lamellae widen in chronic laminitic claws as a result of hyperplasia, eventually producing a widened and vulnerable white line (Fig. 18–22).

Chronic displacement of the distal phalanx induces an increase of pressure in the corium. This pressure is constant and mild enough to cause sclerosis of the wall of blood vessels rather than tissue necrosis. Mantles are formed around nerve bundles. Thrombi may occlude blood vessels. Young animals appear to recover more readily from a laminitic incident, possibly because these individuals are still able to develop collateral circulation to take over the function of damaged vessels. Nevertheless, each time an animal suffers an episode of laminitis, more scar tissue is formed and the animal is less able to recover from the next insult (Figs. 18–23 and 18–24).

A diffuse proliferation of scar tissue in the corium is a consistent accompanying feature in chronic laminitis. Grossly, one may observe that the adipose tissue cushions in the heel are replaced by thick connective tissue layers. These reduce the elasticity and movement capacity of the weight-bearing corium.

Yet another sequel of the chronic compression and sclerosis of the corium under the distal phalanx in these chronically laminitic claws is that this layer becomes obviously thinner than normal. The cushioning function is reduced, and compression is transmitted to the sole and heel horn to produce two further morphological features:

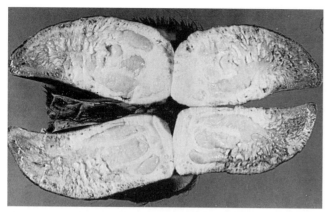

Figure 18–23. Normal exungulated claws showing the three normal yellow cushions of adipose tissue in the bulb. The corium has been removed by cutting along the flexor surface of the distal phalanx and parallel across the heel with a knife. The soft tissue was then turned over to allow a view of the inner surfaces. The caudal edge of the distal phalanx is just cranial to the cushions.

- The sole becomes convex and bulges (so-called dropped sole).

- A typical deep oblique furrow forms in the sole-heel junction, passing roughly along the border line between zones 4 and 6. Although it is not compressed directly, the bulb in these claws is still being drawn downward merely because it is connected to the actively sinking structures. Similar to the contents of a full bowl, the soft bulb overflows the upward curving edge of the heel horn, forming the inner wall of the furrow, and folding down again where the heel gets softer to form the outer wall of the furrow.

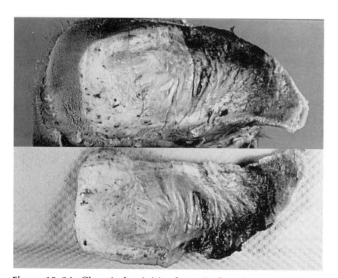

Figure 18–24. Chronic laminitic claw, similar view as in Figure 18–23. The whole corium on the flexor surface has been removed with a knife, turned over, and placed on a paper towel. It is only a few millimeters thick. Most of zone 5 is hemorrhagic. Zones 4 and 6 are totally sclerotic and have a reddish discoloration. This is a typical finding in claws with chronic inflammatory processes. The heel of the ulcerated claw in Figure 18–21 was similarly affected.

INVESTIGATING SUBCLINICAL LAMINITIS IN A DAIRY HERD

IDENTIFYING THE PROBLEM

At the time of the insult, there is usually no clinical evidence that the event is taking place. The investigator therefore has to depend on circumstantial evidence and historical indicators in order to assess the presence and severity of the condition.

Circumstantial evidence is provided by the presence of an increased incidence of diseases associated with laminitis—namely, sole ulceration, toe ulceration, white zone disease, and double sole. If these conditions account for 10% or more of the lameness in a herd, subclinical laminitis is likely. It is implicit that reliable records have been maintained in order for circumstantial evidence to prove of value. If the herd history suggests the probability of subclinical laminitis, a study of the historical indicators is appropriate.

Historical indicators are changes in the claw that have resulted from disturbance in claw growth patterns. In the first instance, they may be observed in a standing animal.

- Grooves, fissures, and thimbles suggest a short-term (up to 14 days) insult causing reduced (or absent) claw growth. The severity of the insult is reflected by the degree of the disruption of claw growth.

- Buckled claws suggest that an animal has been responding to a series of insults for a prolonged period. Broken toes indicate that fissures may have been present.

- An extensively rippled appearance of the wall indicates that disturbed horn growth has taken place. The rippling may be observed as a band of abnormal horn growth. In older cows, chronic laminitis (slipper foot) may be present.

At this time, no scientifically established guidelines are available to quantitate historical indicators. However, anecdotally it may be concluded that if more than 10% of cows older than 4 years have abnormal claw growth patterns, the probability of subclinical laminitis is quite high. Provided that losses from infectious diseases are excluded from the calculation, a culling rate for "feet and legs" of greater than 10% is suggestive of a laminitis problem. Low herd longevity and high culling rates accounted for by poor production or poor reproductive performance sometimes have an underlying correlation to lameness.

IDENTIFYING ASSOCIATIONS

Multiparous Cows

The growth of the claw provides a time scale for events in the life of the cow. The approximate date of an insult can be calculated by measuring the distance of the claw wall disturbance from the coronary band at the abaxial groove. Claw growth at this point takes place at a rate of 5 to 6 mm/month. Having calculated the date of the insult, possible associations to that date can be investigated:

- Peripartum nutritional changes
- Season of the year
- Changes in management
- The effect of temperature/rainfall on pasture
- Changes in forage quality

Primiparous Cows

Preparturient heifers and primiparous cows have not had time for insults to have caused demonstrable changes in the claw wall. Bergsten[5] has demonstrated that sole hemorrhages are twice as common in primiparous as in multiparous cows, and he also confirmed that sole hemorrhages are more commonly found in herds with a high incidence of laminitis than those with a low incidence. Therefore, accumulated sole hemorrhage scores can be used to evaluate the severity of an insult but with less certainty to

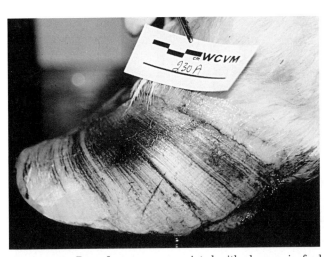

Figure 18–25. Deep fissures are associated with changes in feed such as from winter forage to spring grass. The fissure may be associated with vertical fissures. The black horizontal mark in the central part of the claw can be associated with mechanical stress on the weakened wall.

establish the date of that insult. Sole growth is relative to wear. Therefore, an animal maintained on concrete might replace the sole every 2 months. On softer surfaces, the replacement time would be considerably longer. Interpretation of sole hemorrhage scores therefore is somewhat subjective.

Grass Founder

Paul R. Greenough

Grass founder is a form of laminitis that has been reported in overconditioned ponies. Ongoing, unpublished studies of beef cows in western Canada indicate that grass founder also occurs in cattle.

Definition

Grass founder is characterized by anomalies of claw horn production that often appear similar to chronic laminitis in dairy cows.

Incidence

The condition affects many high-production herds of cows that are in excellent body condition and that calve early in the year. In two such herds, the incidence of claw abnormality was 35% and 67%, respectively.

Clinical Signs

The condition does not usually appear until the end of the first lactation. The first sign often is a rough or swollen coronary band (see Fig. 18–16). Horizontal fissures may be noticed during the second lactation (Fig. 18–25). Some animals show heavy rippling of the surface of the claw (Fig. 18–26), and vertical fissures are common (Fig. 18–27). Double sole and seedy toe (Fig. 18–28) have been encountered in maiden heifers. Thimbling is not uncommon (Fig. 18–29).

Etiology and Pathogenesis

Grass founder probably has a multifactorial etiology. Circumstantial evidence strongly suggests that, as in dairy cows, dramatic changes in nutrition and management are the most important factors. One scenario of change is from winter forage to fast-growing summer grass. During the grazing period, changes of pasture or alterations in pasture growth rate in response to climatic warmth and moisture may affect claw horn quality. The dramatic changes causing horizontal fissures are, however, most destructive to claw integrity.

Micronutrient imbalance may be implicated in the etiology of some herd problems, but practical infor-

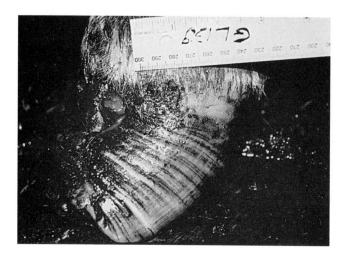

Figure 18–26. Rippled claw wall is very commonly encountered in the claws of beef cows. In this case, an associated vertical fissure has become infected. The animal was acutely lame.

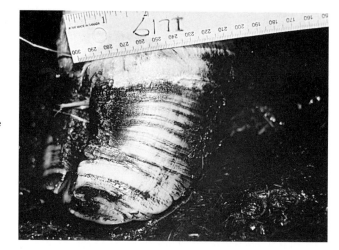

Figure 18–27. A vertical fissure extending from a horizontal fissure to the coronary band.

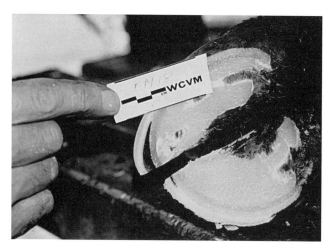

Figure 18–28. A maiden heifer with a seedy toe. The animal had never consumed any grain.

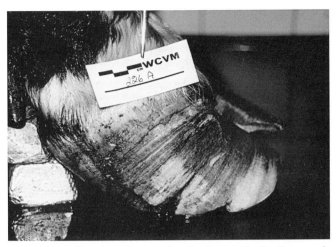

Figure 18–29. The claw of a cow shortly after producing its second calf. A horizontal fissure has grown distally to become a typical thimble. Note the general rough appearance of the claw.

mation to permit investigators to analyze this variable is insufficient.

Control

Control measures are discussed in Chapter 20.

REFERENCES

1. Andersson L: Frequency studies and clinical observations in bovine laminitis. Nord Vet Med 32:301–307, 1980.
2. Andersson L, Lundström K: The influence of breed, age, bodyweight and season on digital diseases and hoof size in dairy cows. Zentralbl Veterinarmed [A] 28:141–151, 1981.
3. Bazeley K, Pinsent PJN: Preliminary observations on a series of outbreaks of acute laminitis in dairy cattle. Vet Rec 115:619–622, 1984.
4. Bergsten C: Sole bruising as an indicator of laminitis in cattle. A field study. Proceedings of the 15th World Buiatrics Congress, Palma de Mallorca, Spain, 1988, pp 1072–1076.
5. Bergsten C: Digital disorders in dairy cattle with special reference to laminitis and heel horn erosion: The influence of housing, management and nutrition (dissertation). Skara, Sweden, Swedish University of Agricultural Sciences, Veterinary Institute, 1995.
6. Bergsten C, Andersson L, Wiktorson L: Effect of feeding intensity at calving on the prevalence of subclinical laminitis. Proceedings of the 5th International Symposium on Disorders of the Ruminant Digit. Dublin, Ireland, 1986, pp 33–38.
7. Blowey R: Diseases of the bovine digit. Part 1: Description of common lesions. In Practice 14:85–90, 1992.
8. Boosman R, Koeman J, Nap R: Histopathology of the bovine pododerma in relation to age and chronic laminitis. Zentralbl Veterinarmed [A] 36:438–446, 1989.
9. Boosman R: Bovine laminitis: Histopathologic and arteriographic aspects, and its relation to endotoxinaemia. Proefschrift, Utrecht, 1990.
10. Boosman R, Niewold TA, Mutsaers CW, Gruys E: Response of serum amyloid A concentration in cows given endotoxin as an acute-phase stimulant. Am J Vet Res 50:1690–1694, 1989.
11. Brochart M: Foot lameness of the cow, a multifactorial disease. In Wierenga HK, Peterse DJ (eds): Cattle Housing Systems, Lameness and Behaviour. Boston, Martinus Nijhoff, 1987, pp 159–165.
12. Chesterton RN: Examination and control of lameness in dairy herds. N Z Vet J 37:133–134, 1989.
13. Choquette-Lévy L, Baril J, Lévy M, St-Pierre H: A study of foot diseases of dairy cattle in Quebec. Can Vet J 26:278–281, 1985.
14. Clackson DA, Ward WR: Farm tracks, stockman's herding and lameness in dairy cattle. Vet Rec 129:511–512, 1991.
15. Clarkson MJ, Downham DT, Faull WB, et al: An epidemiological study to determine the risk factors of lameness in dairy cows. University of Liverpool, Veterinary Faculty, CSA 1370, Final report, 1993.
16. Colam-Ainsworth P, Lunn GA, Thomas RC, Eddy RG: Behaviour of cows in cubicles and its possible relationship with laminitis in replacement dairy heifers. Vet Rec 125:573–575, 1989.
17. Collick DW, Ward WR, Dobson H: Associations between types of lameness and fertility. Vet Rec 125:103–106, 1989.
18. David GP: Cattle behaviour and lameness. Proceedings of the 5th International Symposium on Disorders of the Ruminant Digit. Dublin, Ireland, 1986, pp 79–86.
19. De Boom HPA, Adelaar TF, Terblanche M: Hereditary laminitis of Jersey cattle, a preliminary report. Proceedings of the 3rd Congress of South African Genetic Society, 1968.
20. Dewes HF: Some aspects of lameness in dairy herds. N Z Vet J 26:147–148, 157–159, 1978.
21. Driesch von den A: Geschichte der Tiermedizin: 5000 Jahre Tierheilkunde. München, Callwey Verlag, 1989.
22. Eddy RG, Scott CP: Some observations on the incidence of lameness in dairy cattle in Somerset. Vet Rec 113:140–144, 1980.
23. Edwards GB: Hereditary laminitis in Jersey cattle. Proceedings of the 7th World Buiatrics Congress. London, UK, 1972, pp 663–668.
24. Ekfalck A: Studies on the morphology and biochemistry of the epidermal tissue of the equine and bovine hoof with special reference to laminitis (dissertation). Uppsala, Sweden, Swedish University of Agricultural Sciences, 1991.
25. Ekfalck A, Funkquist B, Jones B, Obel N: Presence of receptors for epidermal growth factor (EGF) in the matrix of the bovine hoof—a possible new approach to the laminitis problem. Zentralbl Veterinarmed [A] 35:321–330, 1988.
26. Garner HE: Pathophysiology of equine laminitis. Proceedings of American Association of Equine Practitioners 21:384–387, 1975.
27. Garner HE, Coffman JR, Hahn AW, et al: Equine laminitis of alimentary origin: An experimental model. Am J Vet Res 36:441–444, 1975.
28. Greenough PR: The subclinical laminitis syndrome. Bovine Pract 20:144–149, 1985.
29. Greenough PR: A review of factors predisposing to lameness in cattle. In Owen JB, Axford RFE (eds): Breeding for Disease Resistance in Farm Animals. London, CAB International, 1991, pp 371–393.
30. Greenough PR: Controlling lameness in dairy cows. In Phillips CJC (ed): Progress in Dairy Science. London, CAB International, 1996, pp 191–210.
31. Greenough PR, Gazek Z: A preliminary report on a laminitis-like condition occurring in bulls under feeding trials. Proceedings of the 5th International Symposium on Disorders of the Ruminant Digit. Dublin, Ireland, 1986, pp 63–68.
32. Greenough PR, MacCallum FJ, Weaver AD: Lameness in Cattle, 2nd ed. Philadelphia, JB Lippincott, 1981.
33. Greenough PR, Vermunt JJ: Evaluation of subclinical laminitis and associated lesions in dairy cattle. Proceedings of the 6th International Symposium on Disorders of the Ruminant Digit. Liverpool, UK, 1990.
34. Greenough PR, Vermunt JJ: Evaluation of subclinical laminitis in a dairy herd and observations on associated nutritional and management factors. Vet Rec 128:11–17, 1991.
35. Greenough PR, Vermunt JJ: In search of an epidemiologic approach to investigating bovine lameness problems. Proceedings of the 7th International Symposium on Disorders of the Ruminant Digit. Banff, Canada, 1994, p 186.

36. Greenough PR, Vermunt JJ, McKinnon JJ, et al: Laminitis-like changes in the claws of feedlot cattle. Can Vet J 31:202–208, 1990.

37. Grommers FJ: Veterinaire aspecten van de huisvesting van melkvee (PhD thesis). Utrecht, Rijksuniversiteit, 1967.

38. Hood DM, Stephens KA. Physiopathology of equine laminitis. Comp Cont Educ Pract Vet 3:S454–S459, 1981.

39. Hoyer MJ: Hereditary laminitis in Jersey calves in Zimbabwe. J S Afr Vet Med Assoc 62:62–64, 1991.

40. Irps H: The influence of the floor on the behaviour and lameness of beef bulls. *In* Wierenga HK, Peterse DJ (eds): Cattle Housing Systems, Lameness and Behaviour. Boston, Martinus Nijhoff, 1987, pp 73–86.

41. Kempens K, Boxberger J: Locomotion of cattle in loose housing systems. *In* Wierenga HK, Peterse DJ (eds). Cattle Housing Systems, Lameness and Behaviour. Boston, Martinus Nijhoff 1987, pp 107–118.

42. Kersting -. Unterricht, Pferde zu beschlagen. Göttingen, 1777. Cited by Racin, 1984 (see ref 69).

43. Larsson B, Obel N, Aberg B: On the biochemistry of keratinization in the matrix of the horse's hoof in normal conditions and in laminitis. Nord Vet Med 8:761–776, 1956.

44. Lischer CJ, Ossent P, Iselin U, Braun U: Diagnose der Klauenrehe beim Rind: 183 Fälle (1982–1993). Wien Tieraerztl Monatschr 81:108–116, 1994.

45. Livesey CT, Fleming FL: Nutritional influences on laminitis, sole ulcer and bruised sole in Friesian cows. Vet Rec 114:510–512, 1984.

46. Logue DN, Offer JE, Leach KA, et al: Lesions of the hoof in first-calving dairy heifers. Proceedings of the 8th International Symposium on Disorders of the Ruminant Digit. Banff, Canada, 1994, p 272.

47. Lucey S, Rowlands GJ, Russell AM: The association between lameness and fertility in dairy cows. Vet Rec 118:628–631, 1986.

48. Maclean CW: Observations on laminitis in intensive beef units. Vet Rec 78:223–231, 1966.

49. Maclean CW: The histopathology of laminitis in dairy cows. J Comp Pathol 81:563–569, 1971.

50. Manson FJ, Leaver JD: The influence of concentrate amount on locomotion and clinical lameness in dairy cattle. Anim Prod 47:185–190, 1988.

51. Manson FJ, Leaver JD: The effect of concentrate:silage ratio and hoof trimming on lameness in dairy cattle. Anim Prod 49:15–22, 1989.

52. Merrit AM, Riser WH: Laminitis of possible hereditary origin in Jersey cattle. J Am Vet Med Assoc 153:1074–1075, 1953.

53. Morrow LL, Tumbleson ME, Kintner LD, et al: Laminitis in lambs injected with lactic acid. Am J Vet Res 34:1305, 1973.

54. Mortensen K, Hesselholt M: Laminitis in Danish dairy cattle—an epidemiological approach. Proceedings of the 4th International Symposium on Disorders of the Ruminant Digit. Paris, France, 1982.

55. Mortensen K, Hesselholt M: The effects of high concentrate diet on the digital health of dairy cows. Proceedings of the International Production Congress. Belfast, N Ireland, 1986.

56. Mortensen K, Hesselholt M, Basse A: Pathogenesis of bovine laminitis (diffuse aseptic pododermatitis). Experimental models. Proceedings of the 14th World Congress on Diseases of Cattle. Dublin, Ireland, 1986, pp 1025–1030.

57. Moser EA, Divers TJ: Laminitis and decreased milk production in first-lactation cows improperly fed a dairy ration. J Am Vet Med Assoc 190:1575–1576, 1987.

58. Nilsson SA: Clinical, morphological and experimental studies of laminitis in cattle. Acta Vet Scand Suppl 4:9–304, 1963.

59. Nilsson SA: Recent opinions about cause of ulceration of the hoof in cattle. Nord Vet Med 18:241–252, 1966.

60. Obel N: Studies on the histopathology of acute laminitis (dissertation). Stockholm (Uppsala, Almquist & Wiksells Boktryckeri), 1948.

61. Ossent P: A simple procedure for the gross and histological examination of the bovine hoof. Schweiz Arch Tierheilkd 132:451, 1990.

62. Ossent P, Peterse DJ, Schamhardt HC: Distribution of load between the lateral and medial hoof of the bovine hind limb. Zentralbl Veterinarmed [A] 34:296–300, 1987.

63. Peterse DJ: Nutrition as a possible factor in the pathogenesis of ulcers of the sole in cattle. Tijdschr Diergeneeskd 104:966–970, 1979.

64. Peterse DJ: Prevention of laminitis in Dutch dairy herds. Proceedings of the 4th International Symposium on Disorders of the Ruminant Digit. Paris, France, 1982.

65. Peterse DJ, Korver S, Oldenbroek JK, Talmon FP: Relationship between levels of concentrate feeding and incidence of sole ulcers in dairy cattle. Vet Rec 115:629–630, 1884.

66. Peterse DJ, Van Vuuren AM: The influence of a slow or rapid concentrate increase on the incidence of foot lesions in freshly calved heifers. Proceedings of the EAAP Congress. The Hague, the Netherlands, 1984.

67. Peterse DJ, Van Vuuren AM, Ossent P: The effects of daily concentrate increase on the incidence of sole lesions in cattle. Proceedings of the 5th International Symposium on Disorders of the Ruminant Digit. Dublin, Ireland, 1986, pp 39–46.

68. Pollitt CC, Molyneux GS: A scanning electron microscopic study of the dermal circulation of the equine foot. Equine Vet J 22:79–87, 1990.

69. Racin Abdin-Bey M: Aetiologie und Pathogenese der Hufrehe beim Pferd; eine Literaturstudie (dissertation). Hannover, Tierärztliche Hochschule, 1984.

70. Rowlands GJ, Russell AM, Williams LA: Effects of season, herd size, management system and veterinary practice on the lameness incidence in dairy cattle. Vet Rec 113:441–445, 1983.

71. Russell AM, Rowlands GJ, Shaw SR, Weaver AD: Survey of lameness in British dairy cattle. Vet Rec 11:155–160, 1982.

72. Smart ME: Relationship of sub-clinical laminitis and nutrition in dairy cattle: A Canadian experience. Proceedings of the 5th International Symposium on Disorders of the Ruminant Digit. Dublin, Ireland, 1986, pp 51–62.

73. Takahashi K, Young BA: Effects of grain over-feeding and histamine injection on physiological responses related to acute bovine laminitis. Jpn J Vet Sci 43:375–385, 1981.

74. Toussaint Raven E: Lameness in cattle and foot care. Neth J Vet Sci 5:105–111, 1973.

75. Toussaint Raven E: Determination of weight-bearing by the bovine foot. Neth J Vet Sci 5:99–103, 1973.

76. Vermunt JJ: Predisposing causes of laminitis. Proceedings of the 8th International Symposium on Disorders of the Ruminant Digit. Banff, Canada, 1994, p 236.

77. Vermunt JJ: "Subclinical" laminitis in dairy cattle. N Z Vet J 40:133–138, 1992.

78. Vermunt JJ, Greenough PR: Observations on management and nutrition in a herd of Holstein dairy cows affected by subclinical laminitis. Proceedings of the 6th International Symposium on Disorders of the Ruminant Digit. Liverpool, UK, 1990.

79. Vermunt JJ, Greenough PR: Predisposing factors of laminitis in cattle. Br Vet J 150:151–164, 1994.

80. Vermunt JJ, Greenough PR: Lesions associated with subclinical laminitis of the claws of dairy calves in two management systems. Br Vet J 151:391–399, 1995.

81. Vermunt JJ, Leach DH: A macroscopic study of the vascular system of the bovine hind limb claw. N Z Vet J 40:139–145, 1992.

82. Vermunt JJ, Leach DH: A scanning electron-microscopic study of the vascular system of the bovine hind limb claw. N Z Vet J 40:146–154, 1992.

83. Ward WR: Recent studies on the epidemiology of lameness. Proceedings of the 8th International Symposium on Disorders of the Ruminant Digit. Banff, Canada, 1994, p 197.

84. Weaver AD: The prevention of laminitis in dairy cattle. Bovine Pract 14:70–72, 1979.

85. Zeeb K: The influence of the housing system on locomotory activities. *In* Wierenga HK, Peterse DJ (eds): Cattle Housing Systems, Lameness and Behaviour. Boston, Martinus Nijhoff, 1987, pp 101–106.

William G. Bickert   *United States*
Randy D. Shaver

Francisco A. Galindo   *Mexico*

Donald M. Broom   *United Kingdom*
Jan Cermak

19

Nutrition, Behavior, and Housing

NUTRITION

Randy D. Shaver

The total economic impact of lameness is considerable because of indirect adverse effects on intake, milk yield, and reproduction. Excessive grain or nonstructural carbohydrate (NSC) feeding, slug feeding of grain (feeding grain only twice daily), feeding sources of NSC that are rapidly fermented in the rumen, and feeding finely chopped silage are causative factors in the development of laminitis because of their propensity for inciting ruminal acidosis.[31]

Livesey and Fleming[23] reported an increase in clinical laminitis from 2 of 26 to 17 of 25 as concentrate-to-forage (C:F) ratio was increased from 50:50 to 60:40.[27] Wheat and barley, which are rapidly fermented in the rumen, were the sources of NSC in this trial. Other workers[26] observed an increase in lameness during weeks 3 to 22 of lactation as C:F ratio was increased from 44:56 to 58:42 with barley as the source of NSC. A similar trend was observed as C:F ratio was increased from 40:60 to 60:40 with barley as the source of NSC.[22]

This section of the chapter reviews the role of nutrition and feeding management in the development of lameness and discusses feeding guidelines for its prevention.

PREPARTUM ADAPTATION

The effects of social, environmental, and nutritional changes at calving on the incidence of laminitis in dairy cattle has been evaluated.[1, 33, 38] Herds with a high incidence of laminitis tended to put cows through more abrupt changes at calving than occurred in low-incidence herds. This underscores the need for specific feeding and management programs that allow prepartum and early postpartum cows to adapt gradually to social, environmental, and nutritional changes.

National Research Council[29] estimates dry matter intake (DMI) of dry cows at 1.8% to 2.0% of body weight (BW), or 12.5 to 13.5 kg for a 680-kg dry cow. However, intakes are not maintained at this level for the full dry period. Several trials reported a gradual decline (5% per week) in DMI starting 2 to 3 weeks before calving, followed by a rapid drop (30%) starting 3 to 5 days before calving.[36] Van Saun[40] reported a 15% decline in DMI between the close-up (last 2 to 4 weeks) and far-off (first 4 to 6 weeks) dry periods. DMI decline of 5% between weeks 3 and 2 prepartum, 5% between weeks 2 and 1 prepartum, and 30% during the last week prepartum approximates a 15% average reduction between the close-up and far-off dry periods.

This prepartum intake decline dictates that a separate ration with higher nutrient densities be fed to close-up dry cows to meet more closely their nutritional requirements. Assuming a far-off dry group DMI of 1.8% of BW and a 15% reduction in DMI between the far-off and close-up dry groups, DMI for the close-up dry group would average 10.0 to 10.5 kg per cow per day. This level of intake can be used to formulate nutrient densities of close-up dry group rations.

Lead feeding concentrates to close-up dry cows ("steaming up") is an important practice to improve energy intake in cows confronted with prepartum depression of intake and to adapt cows gradually to the higher starch content of lactation rations. This adaptation involves changes in the rumen microbial population. Dirksen and colleagues[12] reported that lead feeding of concentrates prepartum to increase starch intake and thereby increase ruminal volatile fatty acid (VFA) concentration increases the absorptive capacity of the ruminal papillae. These workers suggested that this was important for reducing ruminal acidosis and intake lag in early postpartum cows.

This knowledge of prepartum intake decline necessitates a reevaluation of lead feeding guidelines. A gradual addition of concentrates to dry cow rations starting 2 to 3 weeks before calving, at levels up to

1% of BW as concentrate dry matter, could result in feeding 80% concentrate and 20% forage during the last week prepartum. Limiting concentrate DMI to less than 0.75% of BW in the close-up dry period should provide a reasonable adaptation program, considering that prepartum intake decline limits total DMI of the close-up dry group to about 1.5% of BW. This would limit concentrate intake to about 50% of ration dry matter, or 5 kg per cow per day for a close-up dry group with a total DMI of 10.0 to 10.5 kg per cow per day. It should be noted that *concentrate* refers to all non-forage ingredients in the ration. One major advantage of feeding a total mixed ration (TMR) to close-up dry cows is that it provides the opportunity to maintain a constant C:F ratio as DMI fluctuates dramatically during the last prepartum week.

Close attention should be given to the environment in which close-up dry cows are housed and fed. Comfort, ventilation, and stall, lot, and feed bunk management are particularly important for such cows under the stress associated with prepartum intake decline and calving. Whenever practical, the close-up dry period can be used to adapt cows to their early postpartum environment. It appears that cows that undergo abrupt environmental and social changes at parturition are more prone to metabolic disorders.[1, 32] First-lactation heifers that are being introduced to new herd mates and the milking barn for the first time require especially careful management. Prepartum management is just as important as prepartum nutrition.

FEEDING LACTATING COWS

DRY MATTER INTAKE

Peak milk yield occurs before peak DMI in early lactation. It has been found[19] that intake data were best fit when separate equations were developed for each week postpartum up through week 5. Separate equations were also developed for the following periods: weeks 6 to 8, 9 to 13, and 14 to 20 postpartum. DMI did not peak until about 10 weeks postpartum for both multiparous and primiparous cows.

Estimated intakes and loss in BW are summarized below:

Multiparous Cows (41 kg 4% FCM)		Primiparous Cows (30 kg 4% FCM)
	kg DMI/day	
Week 1	16.6 (BW 636 kg)	14.1 (BW 545 kg)
Week 2	19.3	15.9
Week 3	21.2	17.3
Week 4	22.3	18.2
Week 5	23.9	18.9
Week 6–8	24.8 (BW 585 kg)	19.7 (BW 515 kg)
FCM, Fat-corrected milk		

DMI of an early postpartum group at these production levels and averaging 4 weeks postpartum with 65% multiparous and 35% primiparous cows aver-

ages about 20 kg per cow per day. This intake lag should be taken into account when formulating the TMR for early postpartum cows.

For component-fed herds, cows should be brought up gradually on concentrate intake during the first 6 weeks of lactation, with intake of forages relative to concentrates monitored closely to ensure that C:F ratio does not exceed 60:40. Cows should be consuming about 5 kg of concentrate dry matter at calving and be held at that level for 3 to 4 days. Intake of concentrate dry matter can then be increased at the rate of 0.25 kg/day for multiparous cows and 0.20 kg/day for primiparous cows until peak levels of concentrate feeding are achieved during the sixth week postpartum. This feeding schedule holds C:F ratios under 60:40, assuming normal forage intakes. Ruminal acidosis is often caused by having cows on full concentrates during the second week postpartum, resulting in C:F ratios of 70:30 or even 80:20.

Slug feeding of grain should be avoided. Feeding grain at least three to four times per day and offering some forage before grain can improve ruminal fiber digestion. Cows should always have access to roughage immediately after eating grain. Feeding the protein supplement simultaneously with the grain may improve rumen digestion by synchronizing ammonia and VFA in the rumen. Computer feeders advantageously deliver small amounts of concentrates (1 to 2 kg per meal) in frequent meals throughout the day, tending to stabilize rumen digestion by minimizing fluctuation of rumen pH and end-products of fermentation. However, improper management of computer feeders can result in an increased incidence of lameness. Increasing the feeding rate of concentrates too rapidly after calving, failing to calibrate the scales routinely, and the dispensing rate of concentrate from the feeders can cause ruminal acidosis. Overcrowding of feeders (more than 20 to 25 cows per stall) and placing the feeders in high-traffic areas (holding areas or parlor exits) force cows to wait in line for feeders and promote negative social interaction, which may increase lameness. Sudden changes in rations should be avoided whenever possible to help stabilize rumen digestion. It is recommended that major changes in dietary ingredients be made gradually during a 2-week period to permit ruminal flora adaptation.

CARBOHYDRATES

Carbohydrate nutrition is probably the most challenging aspect of feeding dairy cows and is the area most commonly associated with laminitis. Sufficient chemical fiber is needed to maintain rumen function, prevent ruminal acidosis, and keep cows on feed. Sufficient physical fiber is needed to promote rumination activity and saliva flow, maintain adequate rumen fill, and prevent displaced abomasum. Sufficient NSC is needed to provide adequate energy to support milk production and body condition requirements.

Fiber and NSC fractions must be balanced properly, particularly in early postpartum rations.

Carbohydrates account for about 70% of the dry matter in typical dairy rations. Total feedstuff carbohydrate can be separated into cell wall and non–cell wall components termed *fiber* and NSC, respectively. Neutral detergent fiber (NDF) contains lignin, cellulose, and hemicellulose, the indigestible or slowly digested components of feeds. Starch, sugars, and pectin make up the highly digestible carbohydrate or NSC fraction of feeds. By subtracting percent NDF, crude protein (CP), ether extract, and ash from 100, we can estimate percent NSC.

Dairy cows require a minimum amount of fiber and forage in their diet for proper chewing and rumination activity, to maintain rumen pH above 6.2 and acetate-to-propionate ratio above 2.5, and for proper rumen function. Fine chopping reduces the effective fiber content of forages. Maximum restrictions on dietary NSC help to prevent ruminal acidosis and hence the risk of laminitis.

Carbohydrate status of dairy cattle diets has traditionally been evaluated with regard to measures of structural carbohydrate content: NDF or acid detergent fiber (ADF). Evaluation of the carbohydrate status of milking cow rations should include

- Amounts of total ration and forage dry matter fed and consumed

- Concentrations of total ration NDF, ADF, and NDF from forage

- Proportion of forage in the ration and forage particle length

- Content of total ration NSC

- Ruminal fermentability of NSC for grains and byproduct feeds

- Frequency and sequence of feeding forage and grain in component-fed herds

One of the primary benefits of TMRs is an improved assessment of total ration and forage DMI. Because nutrients are contained in the dry matter portion of feedstuffs, regular accurate measurement of the moisture content of feeds is important so that the necessary ration adjustments can be made to maintain recommended nutrient intakes. This is particularly important for TMRs; moisture content of forages should be monitored on-farm at least weekly as well as each time a change in forage moisture content is apparent.

Many farms have three rations—namely, the one formulated by the nutritionist, the one fed by the feeder, and the one actually consumed by the cow. Carbohydrate feeding guidelines must be compared with the ration that the cow consumes. When the formulated ration "looks great on paper" relative to feeding standards but ruminal acidosis is apparent, the following steps are necessary:

- Determine how much wet total ration and forage is actually being consumed.

- Check the moisture content of wet forages, grains, and byproduct feeds to recalculate DMIs.

- Check NDF and ADF analyses on forages to ensure that estimates of fiber intakes are accurate.

- Check for proper feeding rates, scale calibration, and feed mixing.

MINIMUM FIBER AND FORAGE

The rations for high-producing, early-lactation cows must meet minimum fiber needs first, energy needs second. The first check should always be to ensure that minimum fiber and forage needs are being met. The following are the minimum fiber and forage guidelines (dry matter basis) for high-producing cows fed hay crop forage predominantly:

ADF 19% to 21%

NDF from forage 21%

Forage 40% to 45%

Total ration NDF 27% to 30%

The total ration NDF content generally is closer to 35% for rations containing barley or high-fiber byproduct-based concentrates, but minimum NDF from forage content and maximum NSC content must be closely monitored. The United Kingdom guidelines indicate that the total NDF ration should be 36% to 40%.

The Liverpool Survey[9] demonstrated that a high dry matter content in grass silage was closely associated with less lameness, as was a high-fiber content of silage. Both factors may have resulted in greater saliva production.

In formulating rations to contain at least 21% NDF from forage, the minimum percentage of forage in the ration dry matter should be calculated on hay crop forage-based rations. This results in a minimum percentage of forage in the ration dry matter ranging from 60% with low-fiber (35% NDF) forage to 40% with high-fiber (55% NDF) forage. Therefore, minimum amounts of forage DMI range from 13.6 to 9.1 kg per cow per day to meet minimum fiber needs in a range from low- to high-fiber forages for cows averaging 22.7 kg of total DMI. The first and most important calculation of the carbohydrate component is NDF from forage.

When byproduct fiber sources such as whole cottonseed are fed, hay crop forage-based rations with 18% NDF from forage should be adequate.[8] Rations with 50% or more well-eared corn silage in the forage dry matter should contain at least 23% NDF from forage. Here again, inclusion of whole cottonseed in the ration may allow a slightly lower level (21%) of ration NDF from forage.

Fineness of chop can alter the effectiveness of forage fiber for maintaining chewing activity. Forage in all hay crop silage (haylage, hay silage)–based rations should be chopped with the chopper set at a 0.95 cm theoretical length of cut (TLC) to provide

25% (weight basis) of the particles greater than 5 cm long. Forage particle length should be assessed in carbohydrate feed problems.

Hay crop silage chopped at a 0.64 cm TLC to provide only about 10% of the particles greater than 5 cm long needs to be fed with at least 2.5 kg of long hay to provide adequate effective fiber in the ration. Hay crop silage chopped at 0.48 cm TLC with less than 5% coarse particles should be fed with 4.5 kg of long hay. The lowest forage level may need to be set at 23% NDF from forage when finely chopped haylage is fed and no long hay is available. With TMRs, evaluate the particle size of the mix delivered to the feed bunk. Overmixing, resulting in a TMR that is too fine, should be corrected.

The effects of sodium bicarbonate buffers in hay crop silage–based rations have been small in research trials. However, adding buffers to rations containing finely chopped silage may help if saliva production is low owing to a low roughage value in the ration. Holsteins need to chew (masticate and ruminate) 11 to 12 hours/day to maintain normal rumen function. Addition of buffers at 0.75% of total ration dry matter is common with corn silage–based rations. Alfalfa is generally less hazardous for a potential ruminal acidosis than corn silage or other grasses because of its higher inherent buffering capacity. Also, the pH of alfalfa silage is generally higher than corn or grass silage (4.5 to 5.0 vs. 3.5 to 4.0). High dietary acidity is also a concern with high-moisture grains. Sodium bicarbonate buffer addition (e.g., 1%) to high-acidity rations is recommended.

NON-STRUCTURAL CARBOHYDRATE

NSC should not exceed 40% to 45% of ration dry matter. This upper limit should not be exceeded, because well-eared corn silage contains about 15 percentage units more NSC than alfalfa of a similar NDF content.

The optimum NSC ration is not well defined. New York workers suggest that 40% NSC is desired; West Virginia workers suggest 38% to 40%. Our work suggests that 35% to 38% NSC is acceptable. Byproduct feeds tend to be higher in fiber and lower in NSC than shelled corn. These feeds can help reduce the highly digestible carbohydrate load in a cow's rumen, particularly when incorporated into corn silage–based or high-grain rations. This may improve ruminal pH and fiber digestion.

When evaluating ration carbohydrates, it is important to consider inherent differences between feeds in the ruminal fermentability of carbohydrates. The NDF in soy hulls and beet pulp is highly fermentable in the rumen, and these feeds can be used to supply fermentable fiber in the ration as starch replacers. Inclusion of these ingredients in early postpartum TMRs allows the formulation of high-NDF, moderate-NSC diets of high energy density. However, they have limited value as forage replacers.

The NDF in whole cottonseed is effective in partially replacing forage NDF.[8]

Starch in barley and wheat is degraded more rapidly in the rumen than starch in corn. Steam flaking of grain increases starch digestion in the rumen. Starch in high-moisture grain is more rapidly degraded in the rumen than starch in dry grain. Starch in finely ground grain is degraded more rapidly in the rumen than starch in coarsely processed grain.

Acidosis can result when rates of starch degradation in the rumen are too fast. Caution is advised when feeding NSC sources with high ruminal degradability, such as barley or wet, finely ground high-moisture corn. The NSC content of rations with these highly fermentable grain sources should be limited to 35%. Adding sodium bicarbonate buffer to these rations is also recommended. However, it should not be fed at levels greater than 1% of ration; otherwise, the palatability of the ration may be affected. Avoid very wet (>35% moisture), finely ground, high-moisture corn. A medium to fine grind is preferred for dry corn and drier high-moisture (<25% moisture) corn, particularly when fed in a TMR.

PROTEIN

It has been suggested that feeding excess protein to dairy cattle may cause laminitis, but little research has investigated the level of dietary protein that may be of concern or established a mode of action.[31] Feeding excess protein may cause laminitis through conversion of the dietary amino acid histidine to histamine under high ruminal acidity, but no data have supported this theory.[30] One worker[6] suggested in a case study that toxins resulting from protein digestion and metabolism may cause laminitis through effects on claw keratin but provided no data to support this theory. It is possible that high ruminal and blood urea nitrogen levels may be related to the suggested increase in lameness when cows are fed excess protein. It has been reported[1] that four of five herds with a high incidence of laminitis were fed high-ammonia silage in a field study of five high- and five low-incidence herds. High-nitrate feeds or water may also have a role in the development of lameness, but experimental evidence is lacking.

An increase in lameness over weeks 3 to 26 of lactation occurred as dietary CP concentration was increased from 16% to 20%.[25] The rations were also high in degraded intake protein (DIP) because ration ingredients were grass silage, barley, and soybean meal. In another study,[24] 32 cows, during weeks 3 to 26 of lactation, were fed grass silage–based TMRs containing 21% CP formulated with either soybean meal or a supplement (meat and bone, blood, and fish meals) high in undegraded intake protein (UIP). No differences were found between low- and high-UIP rations for mean locomotion score, prevalence of lameness, or shape, growth, wear, or hardness of the claw. Lameness was a minor problem in this trial.

One theory[7] proposed that increasing the content

of dietary sulfur amino acids may improve claw growth and hardness through effects on claw keratin amino acid composition. During an 11-month study 50 Holstein cows were fed exclusively one of two sorghum silage–based TMRs containing 14.5%. Half of the animals were a control group, and the remainder were given a supplement of 30 grams of methionine hydroxy analogue (MHA) per day. MHA increased claw growth rate during the spring-summer period, had no effect on claw wear rate, and decreased claw hardness, cysteine, and disulfide bonding. Based on these results, the feeding of MHA to improve claw durability cannot be recommended. More research on the role of protein nutrition in the development of lameness in dairy cattle is needed. There is no evidence to suggest that formulating rations to meet National Research Council (NRC)[29] requirements for UIP and DIP is a problem.

Guidelines have previously been formulated to prevent laminitis in British dairy herds by controlling known predisposing factors.[43] These recommendations have been modified and expanded for North American conditions.

GUIDELINES FOR PREVENTING LAMENESS ASSOCIATED WITH LAMINITIS

1 Make all feed changes slowly!

2 Formulate rations to meet or exceed minimum NRC[29] guidelines for ADF and NDF. Rations should contain a minimum of 18% to 21% NDF from forage.

3 Silage should be chopped to contain 25% of the particles (weight basis) more than 5 cm long.

4 If silage is chopped too finely, consider feeding 2.5 to 4.5 kg of long or coarsely chopped hay per cow daily.

5 Do not exceed 35% to 40% NSC in the ration, depending on the grain source.

6 Control ruminal fermentability of supplemental NSC by partially substituting corn for barley or wheat and (or) including highly digestible fiber sources (i.e., beet pulp, soy hulls, or whole cottonseed) in the concentrate.

7 Supplement dietary buffers in early lactation. The recommended feeding rate of sodium bicarbonate is 0.75% to 1% of total ration dry matter.

8 Consider feeding a TMR to control C:F ratio. Closely monitor changes in forage moisture content and adjust rations accordingly.

9 For herds fed concentrates and forages separately, feed concentrates at least three to four times daily, monitor the intake of forages relative to concentrates to ensure that C:F ratio does not exceed 60:40, and gradually increase concentrate intake during the first 6 weeks of lactation. Never feed more than 4 kg of concentrate at one time.

10 Provide a steam-up ration 2 weeks before calving, with cows receiving concentrate up to 0.5% to 0.75% of BW or 3.5 to 5.0 kg per cow daily.

BEHAVIOR

Donald M. Broom

Francisco A. Galindo

A cow's susceptibility to lameness-producing disease depends to some extent on its environment. The environment of animals kept together in a building is not the same in all ways. For example, the way in which each cow interacts with its social and physical environment influences the duration and location of lying and standing. These individual behavioral responses determine the amount of time a cow's claws are exposed to damaging mechanical forces or to prolonged submersion in slurry. In this section, the effects of housing on the social behavior of dairy cows, its relationship with individual non-interactive behavior, and the relationship between individual time budgets and susceptibility to lameness are considered.

EFFECTS OF HOUSING ON SOCIAL BEHAVIOR OF DAIRY COWS

Modern housing systems for dairy cattle have been designed to make some management procedures more mechanized and easier to carry out. This is achieved by intensifying the use of space by the animals. These systems have important consequences for the social behavior of the animals. Several studies have compared the behavior of cattle, both when housed and at pasture.[15, 20, 21, 28, 32, 45] These have shown that the two aspects of behavior that are most disrupted when cows are housed at high density are

- Agonistic behavior
- Social facilitation (behavioral synchrony of the herd)

AGONISTIC BEHAVIOR

Reduced space usually results in resources being more clustered. Aggression thus increases, partly because cows have to compete more for eating and lying places and because a cow's individual space is more easily invaded.[37, 44] In a study of 40 cows observed during the winter and summer, the level of aggression in the herd, measured by the mean number of agonistic interactions during the day, was more than four times higher when the cows were housed than when they were at pasture.[16] This finding supports previous results in the literature.[28, 32, 45] In addition, some management procedures, such as constant altering of the group composition or not providing enough eating and lying places for all the cows, cause increased aggression.[46]

Although groups of cows can be classified as high, medium, and low ranking, according to success in agonistic interactions, the exact social status of each individual is not easy to calculate. Because dairy herds have a large number of individual animals and a low age distribution, they have a high frequency of non-linear dominance relationships—that is, where A dominates B, B dominates C, but C dominates A. The complexity of social relationships is one reason why some characteristics such as age or weight are not always reliable predictors of social status in dairy herds.[15] Individual differences in coping strategies of cattle in a social environment are important in relation to the incidence of lameness and other disease conditions.

SOCIAL FACILITATION

Social facilitation exists when behavior is initiated or increased in rate or frequency when an animal carries out that behavior.[14] It can be measured by the degree of synchronized behavior in a herd (number of cows performing the same behavior at the same time). Social facilitation is an important activity for cattle, which are a very social species. It can affect the rate of individual behaviors such as feeding and resting.[14] Several researchers report less synchrony of behavior when cows are housed than when they are at pasture.[20, 21, 28, 32, 45] Galindo and Broom[15] found that at pasture, between morning and afternoon milking, approximately 80% to 90% of the individuals showed behavioral synchrony. However, during the

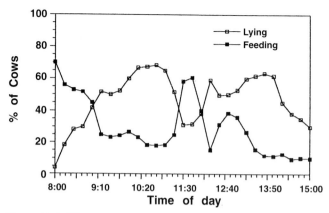

Figure 19–2. The percentage of dairy cows (n = 131) feeding and lying at the same time during the housing period.

same period when housed, only 50% to 60% of the cows showed synchronized behavior (Figs. 19–1 and 19–2).

A loss of synchrony is probably related to the increase in agonistic behavior.[28] It is important to know how relevant this is for the behavior of an individual cow.

SOCIAL BEHAVIOR AND INDIVIDUAL TIME BUDGETS

Social status affects individual behavior in cows. When sudden changes in the environment take place—for example, confining the cows, mixing of cows, or introduction of new members into the herd—stable dominance relationships are more difficult to maintain and agonistic interactions increase. Some animals try to adapt to these conditions by avoiding confrontations as much as possible, but not all cows do this. Some individuals are more successful than others and are able to choose feeding or lying places. Others have more difficulty in doing so and have to be active at less favored times, avoid activity when certain dominant animals are active, or tolerate less preferred places.

Galindo and Broom[15] found not only that the mean lying time for cows housed indoors was less than at pasture but also that the individual variation was higher (Table 19–1). A similar observation has also

TABLE 19–1. MEAN TOTAL LYING TIME AND COEFFICIENT OF VARIATION IN LYING TIME INDOORS AND OUTDOORS

Measure	Indoors	Outdoors	P Value
Total lying time (hours/day)	8.5 a	11.1 b	< 0.05
Coefficient of variation in lying time	20.91 a	12.52 b	< 0.01

Values for a and b in the same row are significantly different.
From Galindo F, Broom DM: The relationships between social behavior of dairy cows and the occurrence of lameness. Cattle Pract BCVA 1:360–365, 1993.

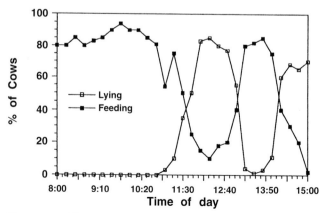

Figure 19–1. The percentage of dairy cows (n = 135) feeding and lying at the same time during the grazing period.

been reported by Singh and colleagues.[37] It is claimed that dairy cows should lie down for 9 to 14 hours, whether at pasture or in free stalls. Lying time is less at the beginning of lactation. Early in the housing period, first-lactation animals lie down for a significantly shorter period (6.25 hours) than adult cows (8.39 hours). This shorter lying time is significantly related to sole lesions. At pasture, on the other hand, first-lactation cows lie down for 9.35 hours and adult cows lie down for 10.20 hours.[38]

Lame cows at pasture graze for shorter periods and lie down longer than normal cows. Lame cows were found to have lower bite rates than normal cows. They enter the milking parlor later and are significantly more restless while being milked.[18]

When relating social rank with some non-interactive behaviors, a positive correlation ($r_s = 0.437$, P < 0.01) was found between the index of being displaced from a cubicle and the time spent in walking areas. Low-ranking cows spent significantly longer during the day in walking areas than high-ranking cows (58.8% and 40%, respectively) (Fig. 19–3). Also, low-ranking cows spent significantly longer (P < 0.01) standing in occupied or unoccupied cubicles with their hind feet in the passageway. This behavior probably indicates that low-ranking cows use cubicles not just to lie in but also as physical barriers to help avoid confrontations.[34]

INDIVIDUAL TIME BUDGETS AND LAMENESS

Several researchers have suggested that behavioral factors are of considerable importance in understanding the epidemiological pattern of lameness.[1, 5, 10, 11, 17, 39, 41] One study found a possible relationship between standing times and the incidence of laminitis in heifers.[10] In this study, the incidence of laminitis was

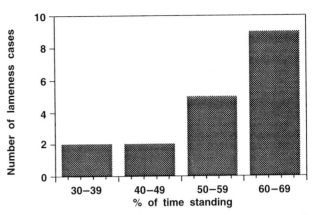

Figure 19–4. The number of cases of lameness according to the percentage of time walking and standing.

reduced considerably when the animals were encouraged to lie down by improving the bedding of cubicles. Singh and colleagues[37] found more hemorrhagic changes in the soles of the claws of individuals that spent longer standing, suggesting that these cows were potentially more likely to show lameness.

In one study,[16] the incidence of clinical lameness during 1 year in the group of cows was 42%. A total of 18 cases of infectious and non-infectious lesions was recorded. The animals that stood for longer times during the housing period had a higher incidence of sole and interdigital lesions. Of the 18 cases of lameness recorded, 14 cases (77.8%) developed in cows that spent more than 50% of the time standing (22 cows). In the group of cows that spent less than 50% of the time standing (18 cows), 4 cases of lameness were recorded (Fig. 19–4). The mean index of how much cows were displaced was higher in the group of cows that became lame (54) than in the rest of the herd (45.6). Other factors affecting individual lying times for a short period, such as estrus and stage of lactation, may also affect the likelihood of lameness.

CONCLUSIONS

- When housed, dairy cattle show more aggressive and asynchronous behavior than when at pasture.

- Housed cattle show more individual variation in the time spent lying, and low-ranking cows spent longer in walking areas and with their feet in slurry.

- Cows that have to stand for longer periods are more susceptible to digital lameness.

- In the design of housing systems for dairy cattle, systems that consider social behavior can reduce problems associated with individual adaptive responses and susceptibility to lameness (see p. 300).

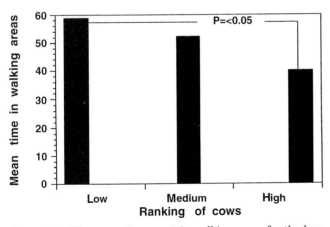

Figure 19–3. The mean time spent in walking areas for the low-, medium-, and high-ranking cows. These cows were ranked according to success in agonistic interactions.

HOUSING CONSIDERATIONS RELEVANT TO LAMENESS OF DAIRY COWS

William G. Bickert

Jan Cermak

Dairy farm profitability relies on sound management as well as quality animal environment. Both of these factors depend on the buildings and equipment on the dairy farm. Understanding the sometimes complex interactions involved, such as between cow comfort and barn design or between grouping strategies and the management plan, is essential when building new facilities as well as when remodeling existing ones.[2]

The buildings and equipment that a dairy farmer uses on a daily basis can serve the operation in the following ways:

- Enhance the farmer's ability to implement a management program

- Provide a quality environment for the animals

An up-to-date management program is a prerequisite before any change in facilities can be contemplated. This management program consists of a planned series of actions based on current recommendations as applied to a specific situation. The program must take into consideration the risk factors related to nutrition, health, and growth as well as other activities of the dairy farm operation. Because no single program suits everyone, decisions must be made about how current advances in technology and research can be incorporated into the program for the farm. Once the program has been developed, further decisions about implementation are needed.

Calves, heifers, and cows must be provided with an environment that permits them to grow, mature, reproduce, and maintain health. If the basic needs of the animals, which vary widely, are not being met, no amount of management can ensure success. A lack of understanding about the needs of the animals sometimes leads to an improper environment. For example, a warm barn for calves may have excessively high relative humidity owing to a lack of understanding of both the needs of the calves and the design and operation of the ventilation system. An environment detrimental to animals may result from an inappropriate ordering of the priorities being used for design—for example, a barn environment intended to keep people warm in winter rather than to meet the needs of the animals being housed.

The incidence of lameness in dairy cattle is related to a dairy farmer's management program and to the environment provided. The impact of deficiencies is sometimes obvious because of changes in the behavior or welfare of the animal. More often the interactions are more subtle. Stress is not always manifested as a pathological disorder, although several stressors collectively may have this effect. Thus, repercussions of unsuitable management practices or environmental conditions may be difficult to assess. Farmers can readily spot foot rot (phlegmon) or upper leg lameness. However, subtle changes in lying behavior of animals, frequency of visits to feeding sites, circulation patterns within the housing facility, bullying incidents, and so on, all relevant to cows' welfare, may go unnoticed.

Typical injuries occurring in cubicle houses of poor design and management include carpal hygroma, tarsal cellulitis, hematomas over the shoulder and the external angle of the ilium, adductor muscle damage, fractured ribs, extensive bruising, and teat injuries.

CHARACTERISTICS OF HOUSING DESIGN

The purpose of this chapter is to highlight some aspects of the design of housing that can contribute to enhanced animal welfare ("cow comfort") and that can lead to a reduction of economic loss to producers, especially those losses caused by lameness.

- Design of the space for circulation of animals, including spaces for lying down and for eating

- Texture and condition of floor surfaces from the standpoint of controlling skidding and avoiding excessively wet conditions underfoot

- Attributes of lying areas, especially free stalls, contributing to proper frequency and duration of resting periods

- Relationships between ventilation and condition of walking surfaces, free stall comfort and cleanliness, and feeding

- Possible interactions between certain management strategies and lameness

CIRCULATION AREAS

Potter and Broom[35] studied the behavior and welfare of cows in relation to free stall barn design and concluded that the space is used very competitively. They have established that the areas that are particularly intensively used are the spaces around clearways between rows of cubicles, around water drinkers, and at other prime sites within the building such as feeding areas, collecting yards, and entries and exits from the milking parlor. An underlying level of social aggression, promoted by social hierarchy of animals and the competitive use of space, can often result in sudden actions of avoidance, causing animals to slip and to fall on slurry-covered surfaces. This can lead to damage to legs, followed by upper leg lameness. The width of the passageways between the feed bunk and curb of the cubicles should be 3 to 3.5 meters when the feed fence is an integral part of the cubicle barn. This allows two cows to pass each other while others are feeding.

The layout of dairy units should reflect a compromise between the need for efficient movement of animals and materials and the provision of dry lying areas, mainly in free stalls or bedded pens. The relationship between feeding systems and spatial design for animal circulation and access to mangers has been documented in literature.[4]

Soft underfoot conditions allow a better weight distribution within the claw as well as between claws. Given free choice, cattle prefer yielding surfaces to hard floors. Locomotion is also greater on a soft surface than on a hard floor. Compression of the sole corium is directly related to the amount of time that cows spend standing, in particular where surface conditions are unyielding, as with concrete. The result of prolonged exposure to concrete is increased by mechanical trauma to the sensitive structures within the claw.

Cows confined to tie stalls or pens move less than cows in loose housing systems (cubicle), and locomotion of cows in a cubicle facility is reduced when the walking space (loafing area) is 3.0 square meters or less per cow. Low-ranking animals, such as first-lactation cows, whose movement is restricted by social factors, walk around less; they spend more time standing without moving rather than resting. Consequently, the increased pressure may cause injury to the corium of the sole.

PERSONAL SPACE

The crucial issue is to ensure that animals are free to move around in the feeding area and pass each other unhindered. The space is therefore defined in terms of a cow's body length and the width of the personal space of some 0.9 meter around a cow's head. Some typical examples of adequate solutions for the design of circulation space are shown in Figure 19–5.

MANURE REMOVAL

A reliable system of manure removal from circulation areas minimizes the exposure of claws to manure slurry and reduces the lubricating effects of slurry on concrete surfaces in order to provide a firm grip underfoot.

FLOOR SURFACES AND LAMENESS

Upper leg injuries and damage constitute some 12% of dairy cow lameness. Falls on slippery, slurry-covered floors are often the cause of trouble. From an engineering standpoint, grip on floors can be improved by removal of lubricating manure slurry and by provision of surface shapes and textures that tend to arrest claw skidding.

Dumelow and Albutt[13] examined the design of the optimum slip-resistant concrete floor surfaces for dairy cattle using a mechanical foot simulator rig that allowed precise measurement of the spatial dynamic movement of the mechanical foot on different surfaces. They concluded that for optimum slip resistance, floors for dairy cattle should be wood float finished and should have parallel grooves 10 mm wide running transverse to the direction of walking. The grooves should be spaced at 40-mm intervals. In the general circulation areas, a pattern of hexagons with 46-mm sides formed by 10-mm grooves improves the antislip properties of the concrete floor. A simple and equally effective grooving widespread in the United Kingdom is a rectangular pattern about 50 to 60 mm square and 10 mm deep.

On the other hand, concrete surfaces may have a texture that is too aggressive. Jagged edges, sharp points, and protruding aggregate due to improper finishing and texturing all may be injurious to the sole of the claw. Impressing a texture into the concrete surface is preferred over dragging rakes or other tools across the surface to create roughness. During the impressing process, wet concrete may cling to the tool and be pulled upward, creating a feathered edge that protrudes above the alley surface and becomes very sharp. This should be corrected by dragging a heavy concrete block or a weighted steel-blade scraper over the surface after the concrete is cured but before cows are introduced to the area. This procedure chips off sharp points, lessening their damaging effect. Equally injurious is broken or highly eroded concrete that has very rough and irregular surfaces. Such surfaces should be repaired by a qualified craftsman.

Frequent removal of slurry (e.g., twice daily) greatly helps to enhance foot/floor grip and reduces exposure of the claw horn to slurry and wetness. Prolonged contact between the claw horn and slurry leads to softening of the claw wall and increases the rate of abrasion. This could lead to other forms of claw lameness.

IDEAL CHARACTERISTICS OF A FREE STALL (CUBICLE)

Free stalls offer savings in both labor and bedding material over bedded manure pack housing. Much has been said and written about the free stall system, particularly the design of the free stall partition, the makeup of the stall bed, and relevant dimensions. Cleanliness and freedom from injury are two basic

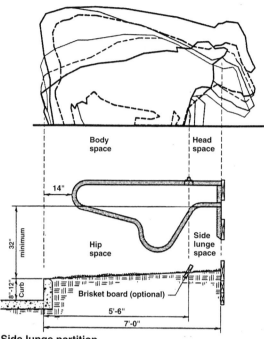

Side lunge partition
Cow thrusts her head under the lower rail of the partition into the adjacent freestall space

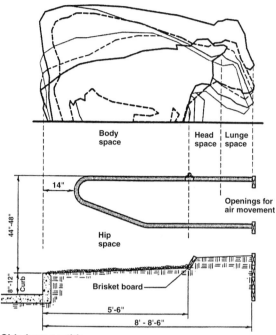

Side loop partition
A longer freestall platform allows the cow to thrust her head forward

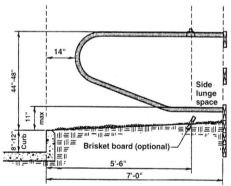

Wide loop partition
Cow thrusts her head over the lower rail of the partition into the adjacent freestall space

Side lunge freestall
Dimensions are for a 1400 lb (640 kg) cow

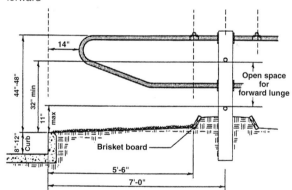

Head-to-head partition
Partitions mounted on posts and the cow thrusts her head forward using the space left open between facing freestalls

Forward lunge freestall
Dimensions are for a 1400 lb (640 kg) cow

Figure 19–5. Examples of adequate designs for providing personal circulation space for cows. Equivalents in cm are: 8″–12″ = 19–26 cm, 11″ = 24 cm, 14″ = 31 cm, 32″ = 70 cm, 44″–48″ = 97–106 cm, 5′6″ = 145 cm, 7′10″ = 185 cm, and 8′–8′6″ = 211–224 cm. (Redrawn from Bickert WG, Bodman GR, Brugger MF, et al: Dairy Freestall Housing and Equipment, 5th ed. Ames, IA, Midwest Plan Service, Iowa State University, 1995, p. 25.)

prerequisites that must be satisfied in order to promote cow welfare.

Spring-calving Friesian heifers randomly allocated either to Dutch Comfort cubicles bedded with rubber mats or to modified Newton Rigg cubicles without bedding were monitored until 2 months postpartum. Heifers in the Dutch Comfort system lay down significantly longer and spent less time standing half in the cubicles. Claw health deteriorated less in heifers in the Dutch Comfort system.[22]

REQUIREMENTS

- Provide cows with a lying surface that is both resilient and dry.

- Allow cows to enter stalls easily, lie down and rise naturally, and leave without interference.

- Reduce contact between the components of the stall and the body of the cow to minimize the potential for injury.

- Provide adequate numbers of cubicles to prevent competition for lying space, particularly between mature cows and heifers.

Cows prefer to lie down for 10 to 14 hours per day. When they are discouraged from doing so because of improperly designed stalls and uncomfortable lying surfaces, resting time is reduced. Prolonged standing compromises the perfusion of blood through the corium of the claw, and any stress caused by a nutritional insult is thus exacerbated. Additional stress is imposed on the joints of animals forced to stand for lengthy periods on concrete surfaces. Claw health is further compromised by extended exposure to manure slurry and possibly smooth surfaces. Thus, an effective free stall must be sufficiently attractive to a cow to cause it to choose to lie in the stall for 10 to 14 hours per day.

DIMENSIONS AND CONSTRUCTION OF A FREE STALL

The dimensions of a free stall (cubicle) should be related to the body weight and not just to the breed type of the animal. Small stalls and ill-designed partitions prevent cows from adopting natural body movement, and animals therefore struggle in a restricted space. Free stalls should allow cows to rise and lie down in a natural fashion. A cow rising from a lying position in the pasture lunges forward, transferring her weight forward to help raise her hindquarters, much like a springboard action (see Fig. 19–5). To achieve this natural movement, a cow must have sufficient space to thrust her head forward. If it cannot lunge forward, it must rise on its hind legs, which is more difficult. If restricted too much, it rises front legs first, like a horse.

Space allowances in a free stall represent a compromise. On the one hand, the free stall (cubicle) should be sufficiently spacious to accommodate a cow's movements and to allow it to be comfortable while lying. On the other hand, the stall space should be restrictive enough to limit defecating and urinating in the stall while the cow is either standing or lying. After all, the primary purpose of a free stall is to ensure that a cow's udder comes into contact with only a clean, dry surface when it lies down.

- Cubicle partitions must provide three areas of free space: for the head, the rib cage, and the loin-rump area.

- A 600-kg Friesian dairy cow has a forward space demand of 0.7 to 1.0 meter (measured from the carpus) to allow her to lunge forward when rising.

- To facilitate rising, provide a space for the cow to thrust its head during the lunge either forward or to the side.

- Sufficient opening between head-facing stalls allows cows to share space in the opposite stall during the lunge.

- If a cow's thrust of the head during the lunge is accommodated outside of the stall envelope (space sharing to the side or forward), provide a stall platform length of 215 cm.

- If the cow must lunge within the stall envelope, provide a stall platform length of 240 cm.

- Center-to-center spacing of cubicle partitions should be 110 cm for heifers, 115 cm for cows 550 to 650 kg, and 120 cm for cows weighing more than 650 kg.

- Position the top rail of the partition 115 to 120 cm above the top of the curb that is at the rear of the stall.

- A neck rail across the top rail of the stall partition, positioned 167 to 170 cm ahead of the alley side of the rear curb, reduces cows' manuring in the stall. The neck rail encourages cows to back up when rising and stops cows from moving too far forward when standing without being a nuisance to them. A neck rail that is too low hinders the rising movement.

- A brisket board is essential in a stall where the lunge space is forward. The brisket board prevents a cow from moving too far forward into the stall when in a lying position.

- Stall fronts and partitions should be open enough to allow ventilating air to move through the stall space to absorb moisture accumulating on the stall surface.

CURB HEIGHT

Ward[42] recommends using a curb that is 16 cm (6 inches) high to elevate the stall base above the alley. He found that curb height was closely related to lameness in a study of 37 farms in England and Wales. This relationship is not well understood. On the other hand, from a practical point of view, if water is used to flush manure from the alley, manure-laden water may flow into the stall bed if the curb is too low. Similarly, when slurry is removed by a straight-bladed scraper, the curb should be high enough to keep manure from overflowing into the stall bed when scraping a long alley. A curb that is too high, however, may cause a cow to stand half in and half out of a stall.

Slope the base of the free stall upward 4% from the rear to the front.

BEDDING

Free stalls must provide a clean, comfortable lying space for cows. The stall base and bedding act together to provide a resilient bed for a cow's comfort and a clean, dry surface to reduce the incidence of mastitis. Swollen hocks and knees usually result from a bed that does not provide sufficient cushion.

Bedding material added on top of the base absorbs moisture and manure introduced into the stall, adds resilience, makes the stall more comfortable, and reduces the potential for injuries. Possible materials are straw, sawdust, wood chips, sand, ground limestone, shredded newspaper, rice hulls, corn stalks, and peanut hulls. Choice of bedding material may influence selection of a manure-handling and storage system. Excessive straw or other organic material builds up a substantial crust in storage, creating problems with agitation at time of emptying. The use of short, fine bedding material reduces the amount of debris dragged into the manure alley.

Sand

A bed of sand (15 cm minimum) maintained in the stall area can act as both a base and bedding in a free stall. Sand contributes to a cow's comfort, is beneficial to udder health, and keeps cows clean. In addition, sand kicked into the alleys improves footing. Every 1 to 4 weeks, sand is added to the front of the stall bed, leaving it to the cow to work it toward the rear of the stall. Sand is replenished before the front of the stall bed becomes lower than the rear, a condition that makes it difficult for cows to rise and causes them to lie diagonally in the stall. Such behavior increases the likelihood that cows will deposit manure in the stall and thus be dirtier.

Unfortunately, design criteria for long-term storage of sand-laden dairy manure are ill defined. Large quantities of sand (as much as 16 to 34 kg per stall per day) are incorporated into the manure. Sand-laden manure, especially with added rainwater or milking center effluent, is too soupy to be handled conveniently as a semi-solid. When the system is designed for a liquid, sand causes excessive wear on pumping equipment, besides settling out in storage.

Most dairy farmers using sand in free stalls must spread manure daily.

Mattresses

Mattresses 3 to 4 inches thick, over hard stall bases such as concrete or well-compacted earth, can provide a satisfactory cushion. A bedding mattress consists of bedding material sandwiched between fabric, heavyweight polypropylene, or other material. Various materials are used as a filler, such as long or chopped straw, poor-quality hay, sawdust, shavings, and shredded or ground rubber. A small amount of bedding (chopped straw) maintained on top of the mattress helps keep the surface dry.

MANAGEMENT OF FREE STALLS

Proper free stall management includes daily inspection and removal of wet bedding and manure, as well as periodical additions of dry bedding. Neglected free stalls with excessive moisture or accumulations of manure may cause bacterial populations to exceed critical values, markedly increasing the rate of udder infections. Also, for stalls with bases that must be replenished, such as sand, always maintain an upward slope of the base toward the front. This upward slope helps position cows more squarely in the stall when lying down, contributing to stall cleanliness.

If a cow can lie and rise easily and its bed is comfortable, it will more likely use the free stalls.

After it was recognized that deficiencies of poor-quality cubicles (incorrect dimensions, poor bedding) could lead to a high incidence of lameness, which was not restricted to first-lactation cows, farms in some areas began a trend back to straw yards. The lying time is likely to be longer and may almost reach that period spent at pasture. A straw yard must have about one third of the area separated off by wood sleepers. It must have a concrete surface capable of being scraped and must give access to a feed area extending the length of the yard. To maintain clear and dry conditions, optimal for claw health, a considerable quantity of straw is needed through the winter season. Straw must be added daily, and during the winter period, the straw must be removed one or more times. Provide at least 4.5 square meters (50 square feet) of bedded area per cow.

VENTILATION AND THE AERIAL ENVIRONMENT

Good ventilation is defined as optimal flow of air that is distributed evenly and equally throughout a facility in a manner that provides a healthy environment for the occupants. High humidity in winter and heat buildup in summer should be avoided. Concentrations of disease organisms, noxious gases, and dust are minimized. Good air quality, which is conducive to good health and animal welfare, is a result of proper ventilation.

While contributing directly to good health, good ventilation has indirect benefits as well:

- Good ventilation dries moisture from alley surfaces, reducing the potential for slipping by the animals. Dry alley surfaces minimize wetting as well.

- Good ventilation in the free stall area increases total lying time of confined animals, especially during hot weather.

- Good ventilation in the feed manger area increases the amount of time that cows spend eating, especially when in confinement during hot weather.

- Well-ventilated cattle buildings have less condensation on the underside of roof surfaces. Dripping condensation, which in extreme cases could soak bedding in free stalls and bedded pens, is thus reduced.

Barns with natural ventilation have proved to be effective as well as low cost. Bickert and Stowell[3] described the design and operation of natural ventilation systems for dairy free stall barns in temperate climates. In general, a cold free stall barn designed for natural ventilation has these minimum characteristics: (1) no insulation, (2) open ridge and eaves, and (3) sidewalls that open. Basically, the barn is to provide a sunshade in the summer and a windbreak in the winter.

MANAGEMENT GROUPING

Viewing a dairy or livestock herd as a series of management groups is an integral aspect of a farmer's management program. A group is simply a collection of animals that have sufficiently similar needs in such areas as nutrition and environment that we can view these animals collectively. That is, in terms of day-to-day management, we can think of them as the same. As herd sizes grow, it becomes simply too much to think about each and every animal each and every day.

In general, animals are housed in groups in order to implement certain management practices. Some examples of how particular management practices may influence the incidence of lameness on a dairy farm follow:

- Groups of older heifers housed in free stalls during the year before parturition, having already experienced use of stalls, will likely demonstrate a higher rate of free stall use as primiparous animals (see p. 313).

- Primiparous cows segregated in a group separate from multiparous cows are subject to less bullying by the older animals.

- From a nutrition standpoint, high-producing cows have a lower incidence of laminitis when fed a separate ration during the 2 to 3 weeks prepartum. Maintaining DMI during this critical time helps avoid numerous other health-related problems as well.

- High-producing cows receiving a TMR are likely to experience fewer health-related problems, including lameness, as a result of feeding concentrates and forages mixed together in known proportions. Associated with this practice is the ability to separate cows into different groups, generally according to milk production level but also according to size or age.

A sound management program is essential for a successful livestock operation and for effective barn design. The management plan defines the particular groups of animals and their needs according to nutritional requirements, medical treatments and other procedures, and breeding. The resultant strategy specifies the total number of groups as well as the number per group. In order for a farmer to implement provisions of the management program, the barn and related facilities must allow cows to be grouped according to the predetermined strategy. In some cases, more than one group can be housed in the same facility. An important point is that each group can be viewed separately for management purposes. In large dairy and livestock operations, separate facilities may be provided for each group; however, a predetermined management program that describes the grouping strategy is a fundamental feature of the barn design process.

A dairy or livestock facility is a complex assembly of interrelated subsystems. Sound structural design and farmstead layout are essential but not sufficient. Recommendations of experts from all subject matter areas must be integrated into designs. Moreover, a long-range plan is an essential aspect of facility planning. In fact, major construction or remodeling must not proceed unless the farmer has formulated a vision 10 to 15 years into the future. The stakes are just too high.

The message is that a plan on the back of an old envelope is not enough. Farmers must use consultants and other sources of assistance, providing adequate lead time for formulating a plan that meets all criteria that have been discussed. In the ideal situation, a farmer engages a facilities designer who has a responsibility to produce designs that

- Enhance the ability to implement current management recommendations as defined in the farmer's individualized management program

- Provide a quality environment for the animals

- Are reliable, durable, low cost, environmentally acceptable, and based on sound engineering design

SORTING, HANDLING, AND RESTRAINT

Provide means of restraining calves, heifers, and cows for medical examination, treatments such as vaccinations and dehorning, weighing, artificial insemination, estrus synchronization, pregnancy checking, and other procedures as needed.

- Include provisions for observing animals for signs of heat, injury, and so on and a means of separating an animal from the rest of the group.

- As a general rule, one person should be able to separate and restrain an animal.

- Do not examine or treat dairy animals in the milking parlor.

Each management group must be provided with a method of restraint. The choice of method varies with age or size and the particular housing facility. Options include rope and halter (for smaller animals), individual stanchions, head gates, and gang-lock stanchions. Use these in combination with corrals, chutes, and pens. Provide the capability of lifting individual feet of animals to allow for inspection and treatment of the claws and associated areas (see pp. 127–129).

Provide a loading chute with solid sides for receiving and shipping animals. Provide a holding pen to contain animals before loading.

Give primary consideration to safety in all cases: the safety of the persons handling, examining, and treating the animals and the safety of the animals themselves.

REFERENCES

1. Bazeley K, Pinsent PJN: Preliminary observations on a series of outbreaks of acute laminitis in dairy cattle. Vet Rec 115:619–622, 1984.
2. Bickert WG: Designing Dairy Facilities to Assist in Management and to Enhance Animal Environment. Proceedings of the 3rd International Dairy Housing Conference. Orlando, FL, 1994.
3. Bickert WG, Stowell RR: Design and Operation of Natural Ventilation Systems in Dairy Free Stall Barns. Proceedings of the 4th International Livestock Environment Symposium. Coventry, UK, 1993.
4. Cermak J: Forage Feeding Systems for Cattle—A Review. Farm Buildings and Engineering 1:1984.
5. Chesterton RN, Pfeiffer DU, Morris RS, Tanner CM: Environmental and behavioural factors affecting the prevalence of foot lameness in New Zealand dairy herds—a case control study. N Z Vet J 37:135–142, 1989.
6. Chew KH: Subacute/chronic laminitis and sole ulceration in a dairy herd. Can Vet J 13:90–93, 1972.
7. Clark AK, Rakes AH: Effect of methionine hydroxy analog supplementation on dairy cattle hoof growth and composition. J Dairy Sci 65:1493–1502, 1982.
8. Clark PW, Armentano LE: Effectiveness of NDF in cottonseed and dried distiller's grains (abstract). J Dairy Sci 75(Suppl 1):233, 1992.
9. Clarkson MJ, Downham DY, Faull WB, et al: An Epidemiological Study to Determine the Risk Factors of Lameness in Dairy Cattle. Report CSA 1379, Liverpool University Leahurst, Neston, S. Wirral, L64 7TE, 1993.
10. Colam-Ainsworth P, Lunn GA, Thomas RC, Eddy RG: Behaviour of cows in cubicles and its possible relationship with laminitis in replacement heifers. Vet Rec 125:573–575, 1989.
11. David GP: Terminology and pathogenesis associated with laminitis in cattle. Proceedings of the 6th International Symposium on Disorders of Ruminant Digit. Liverpool, UK, 1990, pp 1–5.
12. Dirksen GU, Liebich HG, Mayer E: Adaptive changes of the ruminal mucosa and their functional and clinical significance. Bovine Pract 20:116–120, 1985.
13. Dumelow JR, Albutt R: The effect of floor design on skid resistance in dairy cattle buildings. Update in cattle lameness. Proceedings of the 6th International Symposium Diseases of the Ruminant Digit. Liverpool, UK, 1990, pp 130–134.
14. Fraser AF, Broom DM: In Farm Animal Behaviour and Welfare, 3rd ed. London, Ballière Tindall, 1990.
15. Galindo F, Broom DM: The relationships between social behaviour of dairy cows and the occurrence of lameness. Cattle Pract BCVA 1:360–365, 1993.
16. Galindo F, Broom DM: How does social behaviour of dairy cows affect the occurrence of lameness (abstract)? Appl Anim Behav Sci 41:272–273, 1994.
17. Greenough PR, Vermunt JJ: Evaluation of subclinical laminitis in a dairy herd and observations on associated nutritional and management factors. Vet Rec 128:11–17, 1991.
18. Hassall SA, Ward WR, Murray RD: Effects of lameness on behaviour of cows during the summer. Vet Rec 132:578–580, 1993.
19. Kertz AF, Reutzel LF, Thomson GM: Dry matter intake from parturition to midlactation. J Dairy Sci 74:2290, 1991.
20. Krohn CC, Munksgaard L: Behaviour of dairy cows kept in extensive (loose housing/pasture) or intensive (tie stall) environments. Appl Anim Behav Sci 37:1–16, 1993.
21. Krohn CC, Munksgaard L, Jonasen B: Behaviour of dairy cows kept in extensive (loose housing/pasture) or intensive (tie stall) environments. Appl Anim Behav Sci 34:37–47, 1992.
22. Leonard FC, O'Connell J, O'Farrell K: Effect of different housing conditions on behaviour and foot lesions in Friesian heifers. Vet Rec 134:490–494, 1994.
23. Livesey CT, Fleming FL: Nutritional influences on laminitis, sole ulcer, and bruised sole in Friesian cows. Vet Rec 114:510–512, 1983.
24. Logue DN, Lawson A, Roberts DJ, Hunter EA: The effect of two different protein sources in the diet upon incidence and prevalence of lameness in dairy cattle (abstract). Anim Prod 48:636, 1989.
25. Manson FJ, Leaver JD: The influence of concentrate amount on locomotion and clinical lameness in dairy cattle. Anim Prod 47:185–190, 1988.
26. Manson FJ, Leaver JD: The influence of dietary protein intake and of hoof trimming on lameness in dairy cattle. Anim Prod 47:191–199, 1988.
27. Manson FJ, Leaver JD: The effect of concentrate: silage ratio and of hoof trimming on lameness in dairy cattle. Anim Prod 49:15–22, 1989.
28. Miller K, Wood-Gush DGM: Some effects of housing on the social behaviour of dairy cows. Anim Prod 53:271–178, 1991.
29. National Research Council: Nutrient requirements of dairy cattle, 6th rev ed. Washington, DC, 1988. National Academy Press, 1988.
30. Nocek JE: Laminitis: A mysterious cause of lameness. Hoard's Dairyman, Sept 1982, p 1185.
31. Nocek JE: Management of foot and leg problems in dairy cattle. Prof Anim Sci 1:1–7, 1985.
32. O'Connell, Giller PS, Meaney W: A comparison of dairy cattle behavioural patterns at pasture and during confinement. Ir J Agric Res 28:65–72, 1989.
33. Pehrson BG, Shaver RD: Displaced abomasum: Clinical data and effects of peripartal feeding and management on incidence. Proceedings of the AABP World Buiatrics Congress, St Paul, MN, 1992.
34. Potter MJ, Broom DM: The behaviour and welfare of cows in relation to cubicle house design. Curr Top Vet Med Anim Sci 40:129–147, 1987.
35. Potter MJ, Broom DM: Behavior and welfare aspects of cattle lameness in relation to building design. Update in cattle lameness. Proceedings of the 6th International Symposium on Diseases of the Ruminant Digit. Liverpool, UK, 1990, pp 80–84.
36. Shaver RD: TMR strategies for transition feeding of dairy cows. Proceedings of the Minnesota Nutrition Conference. Bloomington, MN, 1993.

37. Singh SS, Ward WR, Lautenbach K, et al: Behaviour of first lactation cows during housing and at pasture and its relationship with sole lesions. Vet Rec 133:469–474, 1993.
38. Singh SS, Ward WR, Murray RD: Aetiology and pathogenesis of sole lesions causing lameness in cattle: A review. Vet Bull 63:303–315, 1993.
39. Tranter WP, Morris RS: A case study of lameness in three dairy herds. N Z Vet J 39:88–96, 1991.
40. Van Saun RJ: Nutritional management of the dry cow. Proceedings of the Michigan Dairy Management Conference. Grand Rapids, MI, 1992.
41. Ward, WR: Cattle behaviour, stockmanship and bovine lameness. Cattle Pract, BCVA 1:332–337, 1993.
42. Ward WR: Recent Studies on the Epidemiology of Lameness.

Proc VIII Internat Symp Disorders Ruminant Digit. Banff, Canada, 1994, pp 197–203.
43. Weaver AD: The prevention of laminitis in dairy cattle. Bovine Pract 14:70–72, 1979.
44. Wierenga HK: The influence of space for walking and lying in a cubicle system on the behaviour of dairy cattle. Curr Top Vet Med Anim Sci 24:171–180, 1983.
45. Wierenga HK: The social behaviour of dairy cows: Some differences between pasture and cubicle system. Proceedings of the International Congress of Applied Ethol Farm Animals. Dordrecht, Netherlands, 1986, pp 135–138.
46. Wierenga HK: Behaviour of dairy cows under modern housing and management (PhD thesis). Wageningen, Netherlands, Agricultural University, 1991.

Jos J. Vermunt *New Zealand*

Paul R. Greenough *Canada*

20

Management and Control of Claw Lameness—An Overview

This chapter presents an overview of the concept of preventing or controlling lameness in a group of cattle. Although the repetition of some information in previous chapters is inevitable, readers are asked to refer to the appropriate chapters for specific data, details, and references. This chapter is, consequently, not referenced.

Changes in the etiology and incidence of lameness have occurred during the past two decades. Progress in identifying and understanding the risk factors involved has been slow and incomplete. These factors are associated with management, genetic makeup, housing, animal behavior, nutrition, and feeding systems. Significant changes have taken place to accommodate the increasing herd size and the production potential of modern dairy cows. Cubicles (free stalls) are favored over tie stalls and straw yards, and concrete has taken the place of pasture. These changes have been accompanied by an increase in the incidence of lameness.

MOTIVATION FOR THE CONTROL OF LAMENESS

Adoption of control measures by farmers depends to a large extent on a veterinarian's ability to convince them that the control of herd lameness is cost effective. Useful arguments and data on the economic importance of lameness were well documented in Chapter 1.

Most lameness is a direct result of pain; therefore, lameness has serious implications in respect to animal welfare. In some countries such as the United Kingdom, animal welfare issues have become a major motivating factor in the drive to reduce the incidence of lameness.

THE MULTIFACTORIAL CONCEPT

Awareness of the importance of methods for investigating and controlling herd lameness is growing. As

is the case with many production diseases, the cause of herd lameness is multifactorial and often difficult to identify with certainty.

Risk factors, either alone or in conjunction with one another, influence the severity and prevalence of lameness. Surveys have quantified the amount of the lameness (see Chapter 1) and recorded the incidence and prevalence of lameness-causing conditions. Evaluating which risk factor(s) may be causing problems in an individual herd requires a systematic investigation. It is a prerequisite that adequate, relevant herd data be collected regularly and expertly analyzed.

EPIDEMIOLOGICAL INVESTIGATION

Epidemiological methods provide practitioners with a tool that can be used as an aid in a systematical analysis of a herd lameness problem. An analysis identifies and prioritizes risk factors and acts as the basis for designing a control or prevention program for a herd.

CONFIRM THAT A PROBLEM EXISTS

Lameness problems can be fickle in their prevalence, varying according to season and factors that are not immediately identifiable. It is not surprising that farmers tend to wait until they have an obvious and well-established problem before they are willing to act. Unfortunately, delays can lead to an irreversible disease process in some animals.

Both veterinarians and stockpersons must learn to be sensitive to the quantity of lameness that exists. One disease may be more prevalent during one season than it was during the previous comparable period (e.g., interdigital dermatitis and interdigital phlegmon). An overall incidence may increase almost imperceptibly year after year (e.g., laminitis). In some cases (e.g., digital dermatitis), the increased prevalence may be so rapid that the institution of expensive and labor-intensive control measures cannot be delayed.

Guidelines that must trigger an investigative process are uncertain, but it is preferable to err on the side of caution. An annual incidence of 10% of animals in a herd showing signs of lameness, due to any cause, is the maximum level economically acceptable today. In a few years, this figure will become unacceptable as stockpersons become increasingly aware of the true economic cost of lameness and the serious animal welfare concerns involved. Many would consider 7% a more acceptable figure for a thorough investigation. Using the annual incidence alone to trigger the investigative process is unwise. If the prevalence of a condition rises by 5% in any given month, an immediate herd investigation should be implemented.

DEFINE THE PROBLEM

A common error is to reach a false conclusion as a result of insufficient "expert" study of the lesions identified. In a dairy unit, an aggressive outbreak of digital dermatitis may mask concurrent subclinical laminitis. In a beef operation, the significance of an unusual incidence of vertical fissures can be masked by an outbreak of interdigital phlegmon (foot rot, foul). When the incidence of lameness is based only on the attending veterinarian's reports, the data may be skewed. If treatment by the farmer is omitted from the records, the incidence is underestimated and a full investigation delayed.

To complicate the matter still further, a possibility is that diseases of the digit are still evolving. The appearance of super foul and the uncertainty about possible new synergisms that may be occurring between digital pathogens (digital dermatitis) are causes for concern. Accurate and long-term recording of findings is becoming imperative for larger, intensively managed dairy herds.

To enable a veterinarian to confirm the existence of a herd lameness problem, it is essential that a detailed record be made for each incident of lameness (case). Farmers must take an active role in data recording. They should be provided with lameness data capture forms (such as Fig. 1–2, or any other system that uses internationally recommended terminology, severity scores, and claw zones). The data must be regularly transferred to an appropriate analytical computer database.

An initial inspection of the claw characteristics of all mature cows in a herd can provide an extremely valuable insight into the status of the claw health of the herd. Regular claw trimming (e.g., twice yearly) is an excellent means of monitoring claw health. The trimmer must be well informed and willing to keep detailed records on the forms provided. The attending practitioner thus has a convenient means of monitoring the occurrence of lesions and the incidence of lameness.

Each lameness incident (case) must be correctly and completely described. Criteria for a case may be simple, such as one lesion in the interdigital space, or more complex, such as lameness in which more than one lesion is present in one or more claws. When the number of defined cases exceeds those acceptable for a specific period for that group of cattle, then the problem (outbreak) is real and an epidemiological study should be implemented to investigate possible risk factors or causes. A new case in the same animal is defined as one that occurs after more than 28 days in the same claw or in any claw other than the one first affected.

For example, the criteria for confirming a subclinical laminitis problem are as follows:

- More than 5% of all cattle have been lame within 1 year as a result of disorders generally recognized as being associated with subclinical laminitis.

- More than 50% of all cases of lameness occur within 60 days after calving.

- More than 25% of any particular lactation group have sole hemorrhages.

WHICH INDIVIDUALS ARE INVOLVED?

Determine if the problem is present in individuals or a group of animals. Factors that define cattle are age, breed, lactation number, days in milk or dry, level of production, and body weight or condition score. Information should be collected from affected and non-affected animals. Lameness incidence can be compared between groups.

In the absence of accurate observation and data, erroneous conclusions may be reached. For example, a superficial study may identify the majority of cases of lameness to be present in mature animals, but close investigation may reveal that the lesions causing the lameness are first seen in heifers. Controlling a problem in chronically affected mature animals may prove to be impossible, but the long-term solution may lead to improving the management of young animals.

WHEN DID THE PROBLEM START?

Defining the problem within a time frame (temporal pattern of occurrence) can often identify the factors that caused it. The chronological progress of problems with obvious clinical signs (such as lameness) can be easily monitored. The temporal pattern of subclinical problems (e.g., sole hemorrhages associated with laminitis) may be more difficult to establish if the problem was not noticed until it was well established within the dairy herd. Repeated sampling or examination (claw trimming) may be necessary to determine how the problem is progressing. Findings may be illustrated by plotting the incidence against time. For example, lameness might be high at midlactation in first-calf dairy heifers.

However, the appearance of sole hemorrhages might be highest when the heifers joined the mature dry cows. Social confrontation, reduced exercise, changed nutrition, exposure to concrete, and cubicle training are some of the risk factors that would then be reviewed.

The most valuable key in defining a calendar of events is the claw itself. The rate of displacement (position) of a hardship groove or reaction ridge (see p. 111) can establish the approximate period during which an insult occurred. Similar information can be gleaned from a study of the pattern of sole hemorrhages. Changes in horn quality can indicate the ability of an animal to adjust to changes in management. An alteration of the texture of the coronary band can signal stress that occurred 4 to 8 weeks previously, and erythema of the skin around the coronary band or accessory digits may suggest an ongoing insult.

If a serious problem exists in a herd, the claws of all animals older than 18 months should be evaluated by a veterinarian. For dairy cows, this can usually be conducted during milking and can be initially based on the findings taken from one fore and one hind extremity. The hind limb balance (stability, see p. 123), claw shape, and quality would be noted; however, an in-parlor visual, non-tactile approach has limitations. Several cows with abnormal claw characteristics should have each leg elevated for a thorough inspection in conditions of secure restraint.

WHERE AND UNDER WHAT CONDITIONS IS THE AFFECTED GROUP LOCATED?

Finding a cluster of morbidity in one location often provides a clue to the source of the problem. In dairy operations, animals may be located in different production groups, housed in different facilities, or grazed on different pasture. Replacements may be moved among several housing facilities before entering the milking herd. Each location or the management associated with it may have characteristic risk factors (concrete, slats, ventilation, hygiene, and so on). Risk factors such as ration and days postpartum are often related to location.

Animal behavior and human stewardship are other factors to be considered. For example, poor management of heifers entering the milking herd or crowding cattle along trackways needs to be evaluated.

Similar factors apply to the management of beef cattle. Winter supplementary feed or grassland management may be significant in a cow-calf operation. Certain regions or pastures may have distinct trace element characteristics. The captive environment of the feedlot may also have special features such as space, bedding, and health care monitoring.

WHY IS THE PROBLEM PRESENT?

After completion of a study to determine the animal groups affected, the characteristics of the environment, and time factors, a hypothesis can often be developed. One or more risk factors may appear to be related to the problem under investigation. A herd investigation occasionally results in rapid identification of an easily correctable causal factor (e.g., lameness due to interdigital dermatitis). More than one risk factor is likely to be implicated. In such cases, control measures (such as the use of a medicated footbath) can be put in place and the herd problem (or outbreak) rapidly resolved.

More commonly, however, several risk factors for the problem are identified but a single causal factor is not apparent. This occurs when the problem is truly multifactorial (e.g., laminitis) or because further, more detailed investigation is required to determine the cause. In a multifactorial scenario, it may be necessary to use advanced epidemiological analysis techniques to identify the most important factors.

Inability to pinpoint the exact underlying cause of a herd problem does not mean that intervention cannot be successful. Correction of management deficiencies that are known to be risk factors often resolves the problem. For example, an analysis of herd lameness data may reveal that lactating cows confined indoors on concrete have a greater incidence of lameness due to sole ulcers than dry cows in a paddock. Ensuring that the cows are getting plenty of exercise and access to softer underfoot surfaces (e.g., straw yard) may correct the problem.

Any investigation of a herd problem should generate an action list so that the farm manager achieves a clear understanding of the steps that need to be taken to control the problem and prevent a recurrence. Subsequent monitoring is necessary to determine whether the problem has been resolved and to remain informed of new developments.

ECOPATHOLOGY

The term *ecopathology* is being used to describe the science of studying the relationship between disease and various risk factors that may predispose an animal to a disease. Ecopathological study defines the characteristics of each risk factor. The significance of each risk factor varies in relation to other risk factors with which it may have synergistic and cumulative effects. Ecopathology provides the basis for understanding, prioritizing, and monitoring risk factors.

Although the etiology of an infectious disease may differ from that of a disease such as laminitis, multiple risk factors can still influence the outcome of an incident to a greater or lesser extent.

RISK FACTORS

COW COMFORT

Numerous investigators have emphasized the importance of housing in relation to claw lesions. However, little experimental research has been conducted on the influence of housing on claw health. Clinical studies of lame herds have identified several predisposing factors, which include sudden introduction to cubicles and concrete walking surfaces, lack of bedding and exercise, and poor cubicle and housing design (see Chapter 19).

Concrete. The concrete surface on which cows walk has received a great deal of attention. When smooth, it is slippery, making footing tenuous, and when rough enough to give reasonable grip, it is very abrasive and causes damage to the horn. In general, indoor surfaces are too smooth and outdoor surfaces too rough (claw stability, see Chapter 9). Lameness is reduced where walking surfaces are satisfactory (see p. 301). Severe problems may arise on new concrete, which is often extremely abrasive.

Cubicle Design. The use of cubicles is related to their comfort. A negative correlation exists between the use of cubicles and the incidence of lameness. Resting time is adversely affected in situations with poorly designed cubicle partitions and when cubicle dimensions do not meet the space requirements of the animal (see p. 303). The number of cubicles should exceed the maximum number of cows.

Selective breeding for larger animals may cause previously adequate housing to become restrictive. Many cubicles are too small for the modern Holstein dairy cow. Cattle refuse to use uncomfortable cubicles in which they have difficulties in rising. Poor cubicle use may require modification of cubicle partitions and dimensions (see p. 303).

From another perspective, if cows lie longer in cubicles, their exposure to slurry in the passageways is reduced. The environmental challenge to the claws is thus lowered, and the likelihood of falls on slippery concrete is less.

Bedding. The importance of a soft resting area in relation to lameness has been recognized. Soft bedding results in longer resting times and less lameness, thus supporting the importance of the burden factor (compressive stress or loading). Cows lie down for longer periods in straw yards and on pasture than in cubicles, particularly if the cubicles have inadequate bedding. Cows that lie down for shorter periods are more likely to become lame. A combination of straw yard and concrete area (70:30) adjacent to the feeding area has many advantages for cows' comfort but is expensive in bedding and labor costs associated with the removal of old bedding (see p. 304).

Passageway Design. Space between rows of cubicles, around drinking troughs, in collecting yards, and at entries and exits is used very competitively. The available space in these strategic sites must be generous to ease movement and avoid aggressive confrontation. Very narrow passageways may create a problem for subordinate cows (see p. 301).

Computer feeding stalls positioned at the dead end of single passageways can lead to crowding and insufficient opportunity to escape competitive social interactions. Having sufficient computer stalls for the number of cows in the herd is also important. Standing in line while waiting for a turn reduces feeding as well as resting time.

Most investigators believe that adverse housing conditions and changed patterns of behavior result in an increased incidence of lameness (see p. 300). Certainly, some of this lameness is a direct result of injury. However, it is also thought that animals that are stressed are more prone to claw diseases. Careful observation of the animals for aggressive behavior and the amount of time spent resting or standing may provide a useful indicator of the importance of this environmental factor.

EXERCISE

Locomotion maintains adequate blood circulation in the claws, supplying nutrients and oxygen to the keratin-producing tissues. In intensive dairy systems, cows are maintained in relative physical confinement (overcrowded) and have limited opportunity for exercise. A significant reduction in the amount of exercise decreases the rate of blood perfusion of the corium. This state reduces the rate of toxin removal, causes anoxia, and increases intraungular pressure.

Recommendations

- Keep concrete surfaces clean and in a fit state of repair; make sure they are non-abrasive but not slippery.

- Provide comfortable resting areas; straw yards are better than cubicles. Cubicles must have plenty of bedding and the correct dimensions.

- Ensure that a cubicle and feeding place are available for each cow.

- Ensure correct cubicle dimensions, height of curb, and position of divisions and neck rail.

- Separate dry cows from the milking herd and keep them on dirt or grassed areas.

- Allow lactating cows as much exercise as practicable, preferably outdoors on pasture, as well as a loafing area or a dirt lot.

- Design cubicle rows and passageways and locate computer feeders in such a manner that cows can move and walk freely and avoid aggressive confrontation.

- Make sure that slurry does not accumulate in the passageways.

NUTRITION
(see Chapter 19)

Concentrates. Large amounts of concentrate in the diet and high concentrate-to-silage ratios result in a greater prevalence of lameness. Cows fed concentrate according to yield appeared to be more affected than those fed a flat-rate or complete diet. More lameness occurs in cows fed higher amounts of concentrate and less forage (see p. 293). These effects are additive, because they are more noticeable during the second lactation.

Protein. Protein fed at high percentages, particularly rumen-degradable protein, has also been implicated as a factor in increased lameness.

Sulfur-containing amino acids contribute to the sulfur bonds that give horn tissue the strength and resilience needed to minimize lameness. It has been suggested that a diet supplemented with protein high in sulfur-containing amino acids (proteins from animal origin) may either be less harmful or possibly have a preventive quality when compared with a plant protein–based diet.

Zinc Deficiency. Zinc deficiency has been implicated in lameness in dairy cattle. Zinc is important in claw horn formation and is present in reduced quantities in the horn of cattle with claw lesions. A zinc derivative, zinc methionate, is now commercially available.

Biotin supplementation is of value for improving the quality of claw horn in pigs and hoof horn in horses. In due course, it may also prove beneficial in cattle.

Recommendations

STOCKMANSHIP

A study of lameness in dairy cows conducted by the University of Liverpool has found that the prevalence of lameness was correlated highly significantly and inversely with the knowledge, level of training, and awareness of the farmers. Other factors related to stockmanship that have been associated with lameness are a stockperson's impatience and the use of a biting dog while herding the cows.

VETERINARY TRAINING AND SKILL

In some countries, a veterinarian's knowledge of lameness may be limited to the treatment of interdigital phlegmon and some simple surgical procedures. In other countries, such as Italy and Spain, veterinary practices may specialize in claw trimming and care. Undergraduate veterinary training rarely reflects the economic and welfare implications of lameness in cattle. The anatomy and pathology of the digit are often absent from the curriculum, as is detailed instruction on topics such as claw trimming and bovine laminitis. Such deficiencies may be remedied by appropriate extramural study (practice student experience), as well as postgraduate seminars and short courses.

Recommendations

- Encourage farmers and stockpersons to acquire extra training to increase their awareness and to enable them to recognize and deal with lameness problems.
- Use patience while assembling and herding cows, and drive cows gently over tracks and through gateways; the herd should be allowed to drift to and from the milking shed or parlor.
- Do not use a biting dog, motorbike, or tractor to herd cows.
- Dairy cattle veterinarians should attend short courses or workshops to learn proper claw care.

FARM TRACKS

Recommendations

- Physically walk all the farm tracks as part of a herd lameness investigation.
- Ensure that the width of the main track is at least 5 meters for herds of 200 cows or more.
- Use fine, non-abrasive or easily crushable material (e.g., sand, pumice, or sandstone) rather than coarse gravel on the surface of the track.
- Ensure that the track is firm, correctly crowned to promote drainage from the center of the track, and well drained along the sides.
- Fill holes and repair any broken section by either grading, rolling, or both.
- Avoid steep slopes and eliminate any areas of potential bunching.
- Ensure that excellent underfoot conditions are maintained year-round at gateways and drinking troughs.
- Remove adjacent hedges or keep them well trimmed to enable the sun and wind to dry out the track.
- Direct track expenditure toward those parts nearest to the milking shed when improvements are necessary.
- Avoid use of farm machinery on the cattle track.
- Eliminate factors that make cows reluctant to enter the holding yard and milking shed (e.g., shadows, slippery concrete, electrified backing gates, and stray voltage).
- After every milking, clean the yard and the concrete apron linking the main track with the yard; ensure that water does not accumulate at the yard entrance.
- Separate herds for heifers and older cows, especially on farms with large herds (more than 200 cows).

FUNCTIONAL CLAW TRIMMING
(see p. 129)

Horn wear is decreased and horn growth is increased by claw trimming. Therefore, corrective claw trimming to stimulate the growth of healthy horn may help in the control of lameness.

Claw trimming can be beneficial, but only if carried out correctly. Training in the correct technique seems essential; otherwise, trimming may increase the incidence of lameness (see Chapter 9).

Recommendations

- Provide regular claw care (i.e., inspection and trimming).

- Do not trim just before turnout or calving; one recommended time is at drying off.

- People who trim claws should be trained to use the correct technique.

- Heifers should have their claws trimmed only lightly before entry into a loose housing system or confinement on concrete.

FOOTBATHS
(see p. 133)

Footbaths are used to remove dirt and abrasive material and to bring claws and interdigital skin in contact with a disinfecting, astringent chemical. The use of permanent (concrete) footbaths has declined in favor of portable equipment. Formalin and copper sulfate are the most widely used agents (see p. 134). The human health hazard associated with the use of formalin is likely to restrict its legal use in some countries. Other chemical agents such as iodides and cresols rapidly fail owing to the organic matter in the washing fluid.

Footbaths containing antibiotic solutions have been used in the control and treatment of digital dermatitis. The antimicrobial activity and concentration of these products decrease significantly after a herd has used the bath, possibly because of absorption by feces and soil particles (see p. 134).

Recommendations

- Footbath use as part of a regular claw care program is essential because it reduces a number of conditions affecting the area between the claws.

- Make sure that cows do not drink from a medicated footbath, which could cause antibiotic residues in the milk or disturbances of the ruminal microflora.

GENETIC CONSIDERATIONS
(see pp. 77–78)

Claw measurements are significantly correlated to the prevalence of claw disease, longevity, and lifetime performance. Clinical lameness and digital disease are associated with long, very low-angled toes (less than 45°) and deep heels (high ratio of toe height to heel height). Claw measurements of young Holstein cows are associated with their future economic value (see p. 77).

Excessively straight legs (post legs) are positively correlated with a high incidence of joint, tendon, and claw diseases (see p. 78). The mean value of the hock angle of Holstein heifers is 167.3° (range 154.3° to 177.4°), and the angle decreases with age.

When making correlations between conformation traits and lameness, avoid confusing cause and effect. In animals older than 2 years, the combined effects of age and management can change both hock angulation and claw shape and size. Claw shape traits should be measured on young bulls during performance testing. Selection of bulls based on claw measurements is a suitable method to increase longevity of their daughters and to reduce the prevalence of claw disorders (see pp. 76–77).

Recommendations

- Select bulls that sire offspring with shorter, steeper claws in addition to high milk yield.

- Select bulls with a hock angle of 170° or less in breeding programs for herd replacements.

- Consider the use of crossbred cows.

REARING REPLACEMENT STOCK

Recommendations

- Monitor the growth rate of heifers, particularly during their second year.

- Start at breeding age to train heifers to the system that they will join after parturition.

- In systems requiring housing, allow heifers to adapt (for about 8 weeks) to reduced exercise and to walking on a concrete surface before introducing them to the main herd.

- Alternatively, keep heifers and cows in a straw yard during early lactation (up to 8 weeks) and only then transfer to cubicles, thus avoiding major postpartum stress.

- Avoid introducing single heifers to the main herd; transferring heifers in groups of four or five may reduce the amount of bullying.

- Ensure at least one cubicle per cow and, if passage fed, one feed space per cow. This minimizes confrontation between dominant cows and those lower in the social hierarchy (mainly heifers).

- Group together similar classes of cattle such as first-calving cows, particularly in large herds on grass.

- Handle first-calf cows carefully during the first 60 days of lactation.

CONTROLLING SPECIFIC DISEASE PROBLEMS

CONTROL OF DISEASES OF THE DIGITAL SKIN
(see Chapter 7)

Digital Dermatitis

Digital dermatitis can be successfully controlled by passage through a footbath containing oxytetracycline, 5 to 6 grams/liter, or 150 grams of a mixture of lincomycin and spectinomycin (Lincospectin 100, Upjohn) in 200 liters of water. Bathing should take place daily for 3 days and then be repeated in 10 to 14 days. For optimal effect, the heels of the cows should be washed before they enter the footbath. Equally important is the need for improved hygienic measures to reduce the environmental challenge. Periodical topical treatment may be beneficial in animals or herds that fail to respond to routine antibiotic footbaths. The heels of every animal should be sprayed once daily for 5 days using an antibiotic solution containing oxytetracycline, 25 mg/mL of 20% glycerin and deionized water. None of these products is licensed for use in a footbath, and antibiotic contamination of the milk is a potential risk. This is particularly the case in herds in which teats are not routinely washed and wiped before milking.

Interdigital Dermatitis

Control measures must include improved sanitation (i.e., improving the environment, thereby reducing the amount of slurry) and corrective claw trimming. Additionally, animals may be provided with a drier environment (e.g., turned out onto pasture or a dry lot). In the Northern Hemisphere, routine use of a formalin (5%) or copper sulfate (10%) footbath should commence on a weekly basis in October. More frequent footbaths may be necessary later in the winter, when lameness tends to increase.

Interdigital Phlegmon (Foot Rot; Interdigital Necrobacillosis)

Control of interdigital necrobacillosis is difficult. A reduced incidence can be expected if regular foot bathing using formalin or copper sulfate is practiced. Also, adequate drainage around drinking and feeding areas and reduction in the amount of slurry on passageways (increase of scraper use), on tracks, and near gateways are important control steps. Once a case has become open, environmental spread of the causal organisms leads to severe contamination where cattle traffic is heaviest. It is advisable to isolate affected cows or to use a protective boot.

Organic iodides such as ethylenediamine dihydroiodide have been commonly used as a feed additive to prevent interdigital necrobacillosis in cattle. In several countries, its use for dairy cattle is now prohibited.

Interdigital Skin Hyperplasia (Corn; Fibroma; Interdigital Wart; Limax)

Control of interdigital skin hyperplasia should be directed toward the control of all interdigital diseases. Because the condition in some cases may be inherited, dairy cattle that are affected symmetrically during their first lactation should be culled.

CONTROL OF DEFECTS OF THE CLAW CAPSULE

Vertical Fissures
(see p. 109)

Control of vertical fissures is difficult, but regular claw trimming may help. Supplementation with zinc or copper or both may also prove useful if a deficiency can be demonstrated.

Horizontal Fissures
(see p. 111)

Horizontal fissures are rarely a herd problem. If numerous cases are encountered, the investigator should assume that certain factors predisposing to laminitis exist at the herd level.

Normal Overgrowth
(see pp. 124, 135)

Claw overgrowth may have a heritable component, but most overgrown claws are acquired as a result of insufficient wear or increased growth of the horn capsule. Regular claw trimming is recommended but only if performed by a skilled operator. Regular removal of old horn probably accelerates the growth of new, sound horn.

Corkscrew Claw
(see p. 135)

Most workers consider corkscrew claw to be heritable, and animals with this defect should not be used for breeding replacement animals. Unfortunately, cows may not show this condition until they are older than 4 years. Bulls rarely develop this deformity in an advanced form. However, some bulls have lateral hind claws that are more concave than the opposing medial claws. It is wise not to use such animals for breeding purposes, unless their ancestry has been carefully scrutinized for the defect.

Slipper Foot
(see p. 137)

Slipper foot is synonymous with chronic laminitis. Reducing laminitis in a herd reduces the incidence of this condition.

Laminitis and Associated Claw Lesions

Lesions such as sole ulcer, white line disease, double sole, and possibly heel erosion are directly related to subclinical laminitis. The control of this problem is dealt with in more detail in Chapter 18.

DISCUSSION

The causes of lameness in dairy cattle are numerous. Environment—particularly housing and walking surfaces, nutrition, and feeding strategies—poses potential risk factors. Consequently, interest in controlling herd lameness is likely to increase in the future, accelerated by the present trend toward ever more intensive management practices. Fortunately, excellent research models have been developed, and ample evidence has pointed out the direction for future research.

Identification of faults in the total management of a herd is often extremely difficult. A thorough investigation of any herd problem inevitably takes time. However, a single herd examination often produces leads that require a multidisciplinary approach such as involvement of a nutritionist or farm building engineer.

A very important and specific problem that requires urgent further study is digital dermatitis. The incidence is increasing rapidly, and significant economic losses are being reported.

Another profitable topic for future study is development of recommendations for genetic selection of dairy cattle to increase resistance to digital disease and improve longevity. The dairy industry is only slowly becoming aware of the important long-term role of claw shape, size, and quality.

Heifer management is emerging as one of the most important and urgent matters that require attention. Pressure from the industry to bring animals into milk production at an earlier age has to be considered in relation to a possible reduction in longevity. Increasing evidence shows that permanent damage to the claws of young dairy cattle can occur before maturity. Abnormal behavior as a reaction to the inadequacy of modern livestock facilities also requires further study.

Finally, the most important factor is that veterinary education and subsequent transfer of knowledge to dairy farmers have failed to keep up with the helpful information that has become available through research during the past few years. Several pocketbooks, directed toward farmers, have been devoted exclusively to lameness, and videos that demonstrate claw trimming are available. A good example for the future is the work of the Centre d'Ecopathologie, Villeurbanne, France, which has directed significant resources toward helping farmers and veterinarians alike develop a better understanding of lameness problems.

Index

Note: Page numbers in *italics* refer to illustrations; numbers followed by t refer to tables.